POLYMERS *for* DENTAL *and* ORTHOPEDIC APPLICATIONS

POLYMERS *for* DENTAL *and* ORTHOPEDIC APPLICATIONS

Edited by
Shalaby W. Shalaby
Ulrich Salz

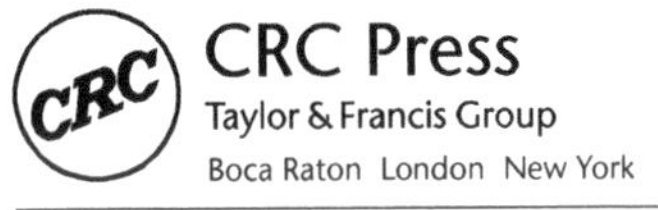

CRC Press is an imprint of the
Taylor & Francis Group, an **informa** business

CRC Press
Taylor & Francis Group
6000 Broken Sound Parkway NW, Suite 300
Boca Raton, FL 33487-2742

First issued in paperback 2019

ISBN-13: 978-0-8493-1530-5 (hbk)
ISBN-13: 978-0-367-38985-7 (pbk)

Library of Congress Cataloging-in-Publication Data

Shalaby, Shalaby W.
Polymers for dental and orthopedic applications / Shalaby W. Shalaby, Ulrich Salz.
p. cm.
Includes bibliographical references and index.
ISBN 0-8493-1530-1
1. Polymers in dentistry. 2. Polymers in medicine. I. Salz, Ulrich. II. Title.

RK655.5S53 2006
617.9--dc22 2006048288

Visit the Taylor & Francis Web site at
http://www.taylorandfrancis.com

and the CRC Press Web site at
http://www.crcpress.com

Preface

This is the second volume in the series covering advances in polymeric biomaterials. The first volume was dedicated to the general area of absorbable and biodegradable polymers and discussed, in a unique, evolutionary format, the technological and clinical significance of this family of polymers of fast-growing significance. As a second volume in the series, the present book is prepared using a similarly unique evolutionary format in 13 of its 14 chapters, with the first chapter introducing the main events propelling the use of polymers for dental and orthopedic applications.

This volume was prepared because over the past two decades there have been phenomenal achievements in the science and technology of polymers relative to their use as biomaterials. These were paralleled by major milestones in the clinical applications of polymers. And this book is designed to address and bridge advances made in both areas, with a focus on their use of polymers in dental and orthopedic applications. The book is designed to cover most recent topics in a unique manner with technology evolution and clinical impacts being the principal themes. It provides a unique illustration of the conceptual development of contemporary biomaterials and processes for meeting targeted clinical needs and offers a concise perspective for future development. Following the introductory chapter (covering the developing synergism between polymer technology and contemporary clinical needs) the book's 13 main chapters follow the noted discovery format.

The volume's 14 chapters are prepared by fewer authors than commonly found in edited books. These authors have comprehensive knowledge and experience in industrial product development, bioengineering, education, and/or clinical applications. The contents of Chapters 2 through 14 are designed to provide in-depth technical material of interest to industrial, academic, and clinical readers as well as food for thought for technical managers and strategic planners. Each of these chapters provides a concise conclusion and perspective for the future.

Chapters 6, 8, 10, 12, and 13 provide extensive coverage of the most critical areas in orthopedics of interest to biomaterial scientists and engineers as well as clinicians. The areas of articulating joint repair and replacement, polymeric composites, and tissue engineering received special attention in these chapters. Meanwhile, Chapters 2, 3, 4, 5, and 7 are dedicated to the discussion of polymeric materials for dental and maxillofacial applications. Contents of these chapters are designed to provide the reader with extensive coverage, in one volume, of key scientific and clinical aspects. In a carefully tailored approach, Chapters 9, 11, and 14 provide integrated coverage of topics of common interest to dental and orthopedic scientists, engineers, and clinicians. This is intended to strengthen a long-ignored bridge between the dental and orthopedic communities, including tissue engineering and management of infection.

The editors express their sincere gratitude to all contributors for their highly informative chapters on cutting-edge technologies and their enthusiastic response to making contributions to the book. The comprehensive nature of the chapters and their extensive biographies will make this volume a valuable source, well-suited for use by graduate students, industrialists, clinicians, and educators with interest in development or investigation of polymeric biomaterials for dental and orthopedic applications.

Acknowledgment

The editors express their gratitude to Dr. Joanne E. Shalaby of Poly-Med, Inc., for her guidance and valuable contributions during the compilation and integration of the diverse segments of the book.

Editors

Shalaby W. Shalaby is currently president and director of R&D at Poly-Med, Inc., Anderson, South Carolina. After completing his undergraduate training in chemistry and botany as well as pharmacy in Egypt at Ain Shams and Cairo Universities, he enrolled at the University of Massachusetts at Lowell to complete his graduate studies toward an M.S. degree in textiles, a Ph.D. degree in chemistry, and a second Ph.D. degree in polymer science. Following the completion of his graduate training and 2 years of teaching and a postdoctoral assignment, Dr. Shalaby spent 4 years as a senior research chemist at Allied Signal, Polymer Research Group. Subsequently, he joined Ethicon/Johnson & Johnson to start an exploratory group on polymers for biomedical applications, with some focus on new absorbable and radiation-sterilizable polymers. Before joining Clemson University in the summer of 1990, Dr. Shalaby headed the Johnson & Johnson Polymer Technology Center. His previous research activities pertained to the molecular design of polymeric systems with a major focus on biomedical and pharmaceutical applications. At Clemson University, his research activities addressed primarily the molecular and engineering design of bioabsorbable systems, high performance composites, radiostabilization of polymers, and new aspects of radiation processing. He has supervised or co-supervised 35 M.S. and Ph.D. thesis projects. After joining United States Surgical Corporation in 1993 as a corporate research scientist/senior director, Dr. Shalaby directed his efforts toward the establishment of new R&D programs pertinent to surgical and allied products and assessment of new product opportunities through technology acquisition. In late 1994, as president of Poly-Med, Inc., Dr. Shalaby directed his industrial efforts toward focused R&D of polymeric materials for biomedical and pharmaceutical applications. Since 1994, he has been appointed an adjunct or visiting professor at four universities. He has more than 110 patents and 300 publications, including nine books. Dr. Shalaby's awards include the Johnson & Johnson's Phillip Hoffman Award for Outstanding Scientist, 1979; Small Business Administration's Tibbetts Award for outstanding contributions to the SBIR program, 1988; and Society for Biomaterials' Technology Innovation and Development Award, 2006.

Ulrich Salz studied chemistry at the Albert-Ludwigs University of Freiburg (Germany) and completed his Ph.D. in 1984 in organic chemistry. He entered the dental field in 1985 by joining the Kulzer Company (Germany) and becoming involved in the development of composites, denture base materials, and materials for nondental technical applications. In 1988 he joined Ivoclar-Vivadent, A.G. (Liechtenstein), where he was responsible for the development of a broad range of products. At the moment, he is very much involved in the development of dental adhesive systems. He has more than 35 patents and 20 peer-reviewed publications.

Contributors

Bruce L. Anneaux, M.S.
Poly-Med, Inc.
Anderson, South Carolina

J.M. Antonucci, Ph.D.
National Institute of Standards & Testing
Washington, D.C.

Mark Borden, Ph.D.
Globus Medical, Inc.
Phoenixville, Pennsylvania

Rebecca A. Caldwell, Ph.D.
Greenville Memorial Hospital
Greenville, South Carolina

Meng Deng, Ph.D.
Ethicon, Inc.
Somerville, New Jersey

Sunita P. Ho, Ph.D.
University of California
San Francisco, California

Martine LaBerge, Ph.D.
Department of Bioengineering
Clemson University
Clemson, South Carolina

Norbert Mozner, Ph.D.
Ivoclar-Vivdent, A.G.
Schaan, Liechtenstein

Jiro Nagatomi, Ph.D.
Department of Bioengineering
Clemson University
Clemson, South Carolina

Sheila D. Nagatomi, M.S.
Poly-Med, Inc.
Anderson, South Carolina

Shawn J. Peniston, M.S.
Poly-Med, Inc.
Anderson, South Carolina

Ulrich Salz, Ph.D.
Ivoclar-Vivadent, A.G.
Schaan, Liechtenstein

Marc Shalaby, M.D.
Department of Medicine
Lehigh Valley Hospital
Allentown, Pennsylvania

Shalaby W. Shalaby, Ph.D.
Poly-Med, Inc.
Anderson, South Carolina

Waleed S.W. Shalaby, M.D., Ph.D.
Gynecologic Oncology Specialists
Lehigh Valley Hospital
Allentown, Pennsylvania

Mei-Shu Shih, Ph.D.
SkeleTech, Inc.
Bothell, Washington

D. Skrtic, Ph.D.
National Institute of Standards & Testing
Washington, D.C.

Guigen Zhang, Ph.D.
Department of Engineering
University of Georgia
Athens, Georgia

Jörg Zimmermann, Ph.D.
Ivoclar-Vivadent, A.G.
Schaan, Liechtenstein

Table of Contents

SECTION A Introductory Notes

SECTION B Development and Application of New Systems

SECTION C Development in Preparative, Processing, and Evaluation Methods

SECTION D Advanced Biomaterials, Technologies, and Sought Applications

Section A

Introductory Notes

1 Events Propelling the Use of Polymers in Dental and Orthopedic Applications

Waleed S.W. Shalaby and Shalaby W. Shalaby

CONTENTS

1.1 INTRODUCTION

Since the beginning of civilization, events leading to our current technologically advanced society occurred in parallel or in series. The respective outcomes were often parallel and independent, but continuously cumulative. Pertinent to the contents of this book are events that have propelled the clinical application of polymers in the dental and orthopedic fields. Specifically, this pertains to (1) technological achievements in polymer science and technology, (2) unmet clinical needs based on and advances in dental and orthopedic procedures, (3) improved understanding of the pathophysiology of disease processes with interventions targeted at both treatment and prevention, and (4) the need to optimize patient function based on changes in the aging population demographics, overall healthcare needs, and cost of medical care. Most of these events are noted in different chapters of this book. However, a few less obvious events, which directly affect advances in the clinical applications of polymers, are noted in this chapter.

1.2 TECHNOLOGICAL EVENTS

These events pertain to (1) development of new absorbable or biodegradable, synthetic, biosynthetic, and modified natural polymers with upgraded or unique properties, (2) development of novel injectable polymeric, bioactive formulations, (3) development of new processes to modulate the properties of biomedical polymers and implants therefrom, (4) advancement in the development of new absorbable and nonabsorbable composites with exceptional properties, (5) innovative approaches to electrostatic spinning of absorbable polymers, (6) development of new techniques for producing absorbable scaffolds for tissue ingrowth, and (7) genesis of tissue engineering and fast-growing advances thereof.

1.2.1 Development of New Synthetic, Biosynthetic, and Modified Natural Polymers

Among the new, absorbable, synthetic copolymers are (1) the segmented copolyesters with prolonged strength retention profiles suitable for producing long-term, load-bearing implants for use in orthopedic applications, (2) cyanoacrylate-based systems, such as absorbable and nonabsorbable tissue adhesives for use in adjoining small bone fractures, as bone sealants in attachment of support structures to articulating joint components, and as dental sealants and adhesives, and (3) amphiphilic, high impact-resistant polymers for use in cartilage tissue engineering.[1,2] For biosynthetic polymers, there have been consistent improvements in the properties of the polyhydroxyalkanoate family of polymers through controlled changes in molecular weight and composition.[1] Another class of polyesters produced by bacterial fermentation are polythioesters, which were first discussed in *Advanced Materials and Processes* September 2001, p. 27. They were described as being biocompatible and less likely to become infected by microbes because of the presence of sulfur in their backbones. Modified forms of chitosan and hyaluronic acid continued to be the subject of many investigators interested in producing bioactive injectable formulations of joint intracapsular administration.[3,4]

1.2.2 Development of New Processes to Modulate Properties of Biomedical Polymers and Implants

The first of these processes entailed the development of the orthogonal solid-state orientation process to upgrade the modulus of both absorbable and nonabsorbable implant materials toward matching the modulus of typical bone.[5] The second type of processes dealt with surface functionalization of orthopedic and dental implants to permit their osseointegration with surrounding bone tissues.[6,7] Such surface functionalizations were associated with introducing covalently bonded phosphonic, sulfonic, and dicarboxylic acid moieties, which could be used to immobilize calcium ions among other positively charged bioactive agents.[6–9] Orthopedic and dental implants having phosphonic acid–bearing surfaces, with or without calcium ion immobilization, have been shown to encourage osseointegration with surrounding bone tissues.[10–13] Phosphonic, sulfonic, and succinic acid–bearing polymer surfaces have been shown *in vitro* to immobilize calcium ions and support the proliferation of osteoblasts, which are vital to the success of existing and future dental and orthopedic implants.[14,15] Polymeric biomaterials with acid-bearing surfaces have also shown promise in reducing infectious complications by retarding or inhibiting bacterial attachment. In the area of bone-growth promotion through electrostimulation, acid-bearing polymeric surfaces can be rendered electroconductive by direct polymerization of monomers, such as pyrrole. It is expected that this technology will find application in a variety of orthopedic devices. However, the area with the greatest versatility is the surface immobilization of bioactive agents through ionic linkages. This allows for the effective tailoring of novel implants with new and targeted drugs to overcome specific clinical shortcomings.[15–18] The polymer phosphonylation technologies were further extended to prepare phosphonylated polymers for use in bone-compatible binders or bone cement in dental applications.[19] These included phosphonylated polymethyl methacrylate and polyethers.[19,20]

1.2.3 Advanced Fiber and Microfiber Processing

Over the past decade there have been substantial developments in the areas of fiber and microfiber processing. This is expected to play a key role in future use of biomedical polymers for orthopedic applications. First and foremost in these processes is the production of microfibers by electrostatic spinning of absorbable polymers for use in tissue and bone tissue engineering as described in Chapter 13. Self-reinforced composites of nonabsorbable polymers, such as ultrahigh molecular weight polyethylene, as discussed in Chapter 8, represent the second area of advanced processing that is most relevant to the development of high load-bearing polymeric implants as preferred alternatives to the current metallic counterparts. The third area of advanced processing is the growing field of bone and cartilage tissue engineering. Many of these processes incorporate so-called crystallization-induced microphase separation to prepare microporous, absorbable, and nonabsorbable foams to simulate a continuous cellular structure.[21–23]

1.3 MEDICALLY RELATED EVENTS

Medically related events that have attracted the interest of clinicians to using polymers in dental and orthopedic applications fall into three categories: (1) clinical, (2) biomedical engineering, and (3) damage-controlled associated events.

1.3.1 Clinically Related Events

Among the fastest growing clinical needs are those associated with rupture and degeneration of intervertebral discs from primary degenerative or deformative disorders, spondylolisthesis, traumatic bone fractures, and tumor metastasis. In an effort to meet these needs, special forms of an engineering thermoplastic, polyether–ether ketone, has been developed and reported to show promise as an alternative to metal implants presently used for vertebral fusion.[24] Vertebral fractures from trauma and/or comorbid conditions, such as osteoporosis, can produce severe and chronic ambulatory, occupational, and neurological deficits. Complications of vertebral compression fractures include deep venous thrombosis, acceleration of osteoporosis, loss of height, respiratory or gastrointestinal disturbances, as well as emotional and social problems secondary to unremitting pain and loss of independence. Osteoporotic vertebral compressions usually remain subclinical and progress gradually; however, some patients develop an acute severe pain syndrome with limited mobility and functional deterioration. One approach toward corrective treatment has been the use of injectable bone cement for anterior spinal column augmentation.[25] Percutaneous vertebroplasty is a newer technique in which the cement is injected though a needle into a painful fractured vertebral body. This stabilizes the fracture, allowing most patients to discontinue or significantly decrease analgesics and resume normal activity. It is expected that these interventional, yet minimally invasive, procedures may shorten recovery time and eliminate the need for extended nursing and rehabilitation care.

In the dental area there has been a significant growth in the use of esthetically appealing tooth-colored restorations as discussed in Chapter 2. More specifically, this has been the case for the restoration of anterior lesions, as well as for treatment of smaller and medium-sized defects in the posterior region. Direct composite fill materials have been the subject of significant research and development with impressive clinical results. Commercially available restorative composites contain a mixture of various cross-linkable dimethacrylate, glass and/or silicon dioxide fillers, and a photoinitiator. They are cured *in situ* by irradiation with visible light. New and continuing efforts on the development of polymeric composites focus on the reduction of polymerization-induced shrinkage, improved biocompatibility and osteoconductive behavior, and increased longevity through increased wear resistance. This has prompted the development and implementation of novel monomer–polymer systems to optimize filler particles to provide unique surface properties while maximizing the filler–matrix interaction. The new monomers include those that are cyclic, liquid crystalline, branched, and radiopaque as well as organic-inorganic hybrid polymers (ormocers) and composite materials composed of an ion-leachable glass embedded in a polymeric matrix (compomers). The growing interest in nanotechnology has led to a new focus on nanoparticulate fillers. Recently, there has been a renewed awareness for the role of dental restoratives as depots for the local release of bioactive agents to prevent tooth decay and minimize dental caries. As a result, a number of contemporary investigators are developing bioactive restorative composites to provide sustained fluoride release for caries inhibition.

1.3.2 Biomedical Engineering Driven Events

The genesis of these events is attributed to a multidisciplinary approach by clinicians and bioengineers. As discussed in Chapters 5 and 6, this has led to advances in maxillofacial bone augmentation and replacement, and total joint replacement techniques. However, one of the most challenging clinical problems is discogenic back pain. The etiology relates to chronic intervertebral disc degeneration, which is the predominate cause of disability in patients over the 50, a fast-growing fraction of the aging population.[26] Current treatment modalities are rapidly evolving into a multidisciplinary effort that follows a logical, orderly algorithm. Various nonoperative and operative treatment strategies have been tried with varying degrees of success. Treatment often involves patient education, physical therapy, alternative medicine options, and pharmacotherapy. If these fail, surgical intervention is usually recommended. Minimally invasive techniques such as intradiscal electrothermal therapy, radiofrequency ablation, percutaneous endoscopic laser discectomy, and cryoablation are challenging more conventional surgical approaches. Early results are promising in terms of symptomatic relief and early return of function. Discectomy is a common surgical approach in which the degenerated disc is removed followed by either fusion with the adjoining vertebrae or replacement with an intervertebral disc (allograft or prosthetic implant). Intervertebral fusion has the advantage of maintaining spinal stability and decreasing mobility; however, it becomes more challenging when multiple disc levels are involved or in the cervical region where maintaining motion is optimal. Challenges associated with the use of allografts include long-term viability and mechanical stability. Meanwhile, the use of prosthetic devices is limited by the loss of performance due to mechanical factors such as wear or fatigue.[27–29] The challenges and limitations of the aforementioned treatments led to recent studies on the generation of new, intervertebral discs by tissue engineering methods. The emphasis has been to develop composites to better simulate the biomechanical and biochemical behavior of the native disc. A recent example of this technology has been described using a composite tissue-engineered disc composed of an outer shell of polyglycolic acid mesh, seeded with an annulus of fibrous cells with an inner core of nucleus pulposus cells seeded into an alginate gel.[30] Composite implants retained both gross shape and regional arrangements of tissues for 16 weeks in an athymic mouse model. Tissue-engineered discs showed progressive tissue formation with time, as indicated by deposition of extracellular matrix and changes in mechanical properties. By 16 weeks, the biochemical composition and mechanical properties of tissue-engineered intervertebral discs were similar to that of native tissue. The results of this study demonstrate the feasibility of creating composite, tissue-engineered intervertebral implants with composition and properties similar to native tissue.[30]

1.3.3 Damage-Control Associated Events

Most of these events are associated with the so-called damage control surgeries, which represent an outgrowth of clinical experience from trauma surgery encountered by military personnel and civilians. Advances have been most evident in the delivery of surgical and intensive care unit (ICU) care on the battlefields of Iraq with improved survival as compared with prior conflicts. This has led to better approaches to areas of urban violence and civilian traumas. The latter not only pertains to motor vehicle accidents and work-related injuries, but also to injuries from natural disasters, such as hurricanes, floods, and earthquakes. The principles for damage control were first described for the management of patients with devastating, penetrating injuries to the abdomen. As discussed in a number of reviews edited by Hirshberg and Mattax, the same principles can be applied to injuries to the pelvis, head and neck, and extremeties.[31] Damage control is the initial control of hemorrhage and contamination followed by intraperitoneal packing and rapid closure. This is followed by resuscitation to normal physiology in the ICU and subsequent definitive reexploration. Resuscitation efforts from shock may include rewarming, large-volume intravenous fluid hydration, blood products, vasoactive drugs, and mechanical ventilation. The next level of care is to provide necessary available monitoring of physiology, with periodic assessment of pain control, level of consciousness, intake and output, and appropriate endpoints for shock resuscitation. Thereafter, care is focused on organ-specific support for central nervous system (CNS) injury, pulmonary failure, cardiovascular collapse, and renal dysfunction. For illustration, discussion in this chapter is limited to damage control for devastating pelvic and extremity injuries, which have been addressed earlier by Henry et al.[32] These authors discussed (1) the general principles of care involving immediate airway control, circulation, pelvic fracture and concomitant blood loss, as well as pelvic fractures and concomitant urethral injuries, (2) damage control of blunt pelvic fractures, (3) damage control of penetrating pelvic injuries, and (4) damage control of extremity injury and mangled extremities.

1.4 SOCIOECONOMIC EVENTS

Increase in the average lifespan in United States and worldwide may be attributed to improved standards of living and access to health care. However, osteoporosis is becoming particularly prevalent and a major health problem. Osteoporosis is a skeletal disorder characterized by compromised bone strength, which predisposes the individual to an increased risk of fractures of the hip, spine, and other skeletal sites. The clinical consequences and economic burden of this disease call for measures to assess individuals who are at high risk to allow for appropriate intervention. Many risk factors are associated with osteoporotic fracture, including low peak bone mass, hormonal factors, the use of certain drugs (e.g., glucocorticoids), cigarette smoking, low physical activity, low intake of calcium and vitamin D, race, small body size, and a personal or a family history of fracture. The seriousness of osteoporotic fractures may be more complicated by other comorbid states such as diabetes, peripheral vascular diseases, and obesity. Accordingly, osteoporosis and associated complications evoke the need for creative corrective measures not only from therapeutic perspective, but also from the orthopedic surgical one. Conversely, young people who are 20 to 40 years in age, who are quite active in sport and related exercise regimens, are likely to be subjects with a high incidence of bone fracture. These patients, by the nature of their active lifestyle, require a fast recovery and resumption of activities. This, again, presents a challenge to the orthopedic community to develop means for fast recovery and shortened immobilization periods.

Limited ability to manage infections is another medical problem associated with aging. Increasing numbers of aging patients with articulating joint diseases aggressively pursue artificial joint replacement. A good fraction of these patients have to deal with device-related infections, which are difficult to cure without a second surgery. This creates a new demand for improved procedures, more effective infection therapies, and longer-lasting implants. All the medical problems discussed earlier can be aggravated in overweight patients, who represent an increasing fraction of the population in modern societies.

1.5 CONCLUSION AND PERSPECTIVE ON THE FUTURE

Impressive advances in the use of polymeric biomaterials in dental and orthopedic applications are convincingly related to equally impressive advances made in biomaterials science and engineering over the past decade. Wide acceptance of their use has inspired a new breed of technologically oriented and highly skilled clinicians. The extraordinary collaborative efforts of the clinicians with their colleagues in science and engineering are evident and timely to meet the challenges of present-day complex clinical problems outlined in this chapter. Of the growth areas noted in the chapter, the authors foresee the following to be of paramount significance in the next 10 years or so: self-reinforced composites with bonelike properties, electrospun microfibers and bioactive forms thereof, absorbable scaffolds for *in situ* cartilage and bone tissue engineering, and surface activated implants for augmentation and/or replacement of bone and cartilage.

REFERENCES

1. Shalaby, S.W. and Burg, K.J.L., Absorbable/biodegradable polymers: Technology evolution, in *Absorbable/Biodegradable Polymers,* Shalaby, S.W. and Burg, K.J.L., Eds., CRC Press, Boca Raton, FL, 2004, Chap. 1.
2. Shalaby, S.W. and Shalaby, W.S.W., Cyanoacrylate-based systems as tissue adhesives, in *Absorbable/Biodegradable Polymers,* Shalaby, S.W. and Burg, K.J.L., Eds., CRC Press, Boca Raton, FL, 2004, Chap. 5.
3. Shalaby, S.W., DuBose, J.A., and Shalaby, M., Chitosan-based systems, in *Absorbable/ Biodegradable Polymers* Shalaby, S.W. and Burg, K.J.L., Eds., CRC Press, Boca Raton, FL, 2004, Chap. 6.
4. Shalaby, S.W. and Shalaby, W.S.W., Hyaluronic acid-based systems, *Absorbable Biodegradable Polymers* Shalaby, S.W. and Burg, K.J.L., Eds., CRC Press, Boca Raton, FL, 2004, Chap. 7.
5. Shalaby, S.W., Johnson, R.A., and Deng, M., Process of Making a Bone Healing Device, U.S. Patent No. 5,529,736, 1996.
6. Shalaby, S.W. and Rogers, K.R., Polymeric Prosthesis Having a Phosphonylated Surface, U.S. Patent No. 5,558,517, 1996.
7. Allan, J.M. and Shalaby, S.W., Surface phosphonylation of low-density polyethylene, *J. Appl. Polym. Sci.*, 76(13), 1870, 2000.
8. Hylton, D.M., Latour, R.A. Jr., and Shalaby, S.W., Effect of surface sulfonation of low-density polyethylene (LDPE) on platelet adhesion, *Trans. Soc. Biomater.*, 26, 465, 2003.
9. Shalaby, S.W. and Vaughn, M.A., Surface Functionalized Absorbable Medical Devices, U.S. Patent Application Serial No. 60/662,852, 2005.
10. Allan, J.M., Wrana, J.S., Kline, J.D., Gerdes, G.A., Anneaux, B.L., Budsberg, S.E., Farris, H.E., and Shalaby, S.W., Bone ingrowth into phosphonylated PEEK rabbit tibial implants, *Sixth World Biomaterials Congress, Trans. Soc. Biomater.* II, 631, 2000.
11. Anneaux, B.L., Hollinger, J.O., Budsburg, S.C., Fulton, L.K., and Shalaby, S.W., Surface activated PEEK-based endosteal implants, *7th World Biomaterials Congress, Trans. Soc. Biomater.*, 27, 967, 2004.
12. Anneaux, B.L., Taylor, M.S., Johnston, S.A., and Shalaby, S.W., Biomechanical properties of osseointegrated PEEK-based and metallic endosteal implants, *Trans. Soc. Biomater.,* 28, 129, 2005.

13. Anneaux, B.L., Taylor, M.S., Shih, M., Fulton, L.K., and Shalaby, S.W., Histomorphometric evaluation of osseointegration of metallic and PEEK-based endosteal dental implants, *Trans. Soc. Biomater.*, 28, 431, 2005.
14. Shalaby, S.W., Surface Functionalized Absorbable Medical Devices, U.S. Patent Application Serial No. 60/662,852, 2005.
15. Shalaby, S.W., Surface Electroconductive Biostable Polymeric Articles, U.S. Patent Application Serial No. 60/662,908, 2005.
16. Atkins, G.G., Barefoot, S., LaBerge, M., Dooley, R.L., and Shalaby, S.W., Effect of surface-modified LDPE on bacterial cell attachment, *Trans. Soc. Biomater.*, 24, 507, 2001.
17. Shalaby, S.W., Gregory, R., and Allan, J.M., Molecularly Bonded Inherently Conductive Polymers on Substrates and Shaped Articles Thereof, U.S. Patent No. 5,849,415, 1998.
18. Shalaby, S.W. and Allan, J.M., Modulated Molecularly Bonded Inherently Conductive Polymers on Substrates with Conjugated Multiple Lamellae and Shaped Articles Thereof, U.S. Patent No. 6,117,554, 2000.
19. Shalaby, S.W., High Strength Fibers of *l*-Lactide Copolymers, ε-Caprolactone, and Trimethylene Carbonate and Absorbable Medical Constructs Thereof, U.S. Patent No. 6,342,065, 2002; European Patent No. 1057844, 2004.
20. Shalaby, S.W., Phosphonylated Derivatives of Aliphatic Heterochain and Acrylate Polymers and Applications Thereof, U.S. Patent No. 6,551,580, 2003.
21. Shalaby, S.W. and Roweton, S.L., Continuous Open Cell Polymeric Foam Containing Living Cells, U.S. Patent 5,677,355, 1997.
22. Shalaby, S.W. and Roweton, S.L., Microporous Polymeric Foams and Microtextured Surfaces, U.S. Patent No. 5,847,012, 1998.
23. Shalaby, S.W., and Roweton, S.L., Microporous Polymeric Foams and Microtextured Surfaces, U.S. Patent No. 5,898,040, 1999.
24. Toth, J.W., Wang, M., Estes, B.T., Scifert, J.L., Seim, H.B., III, and Turner, A.S., Polyether-ether ketone as a biomaterial for spinal application, *Biomaterials*, 27, 324, 2006.
25. Verlaan, J-J., Oner, F.C., and Dhert, W.J.A., Anterior augmentation with injectable bone cement, *Biomaterials*, 27, 290, 2006.
26. Hasset, G., Hart, D.J., Manek, N.J., Doyle, D.V., and Spector, T.D., Risk factors for progression of lumbar spine disc degeneration: the Chingford study, *Arthritis Rheum* 48, 3112, 2003.
27. Thomas, J., Lowman, A., and Marcolongo, M., Novel associated hydrogels for nucleus pulposus replacement, *J. Biomed. Mater. Res.*, 67A(4), 1329, 2003.
28. van Ooij, A., Oner, F.C., and Verbout, A.J., Complications of artificial disc replacement: a report of 27 patients with the SB Charite disc, *J. Spinal Disord. Tech.*, 16, 369, 2003.
29. Kostuik, J.P., Intervertebral disc replacement. Experimental study, *Clin. Orthop.*, 337, 27, 1997.
30. Mizuno, H., Roy, A.K., Zaporojan, V., Vacanti, C.A., Ueda, M., and Bonassar, L.J., Biomechanical and biochemical characterization of composite tissue-engineered intervertebral discs, *Biomaterials*, 27, 362, 2006.
31. Hirshberg, A. and Mattox, K.L., Eds., *The Surgical Clinics of North America: Damage Control Surgery*, Surgical Clinics, Saunders, Philadelphia, 1997, 77(4).
32. Henry, S.M., Tornetta, P., III, and Scalea, T. M, Damage control of devastating pelvic and extremity injuries, in *The Surgical Clinics of North America: Damage Control Surgery*, Hirshberg, A. and Mattox, K.L., Eds., Saunders, Philadelphia, 1997, 77(4), p. 879.

Section B

Development and Application of New Systems

2 Composites for Dental Restoratives

Norbert Moszner and Ulrich Salz

CONTENTS

2.1 INTRODUCTION

2.1.1 General Description of Dental Restoratives

Aesthetic, tooth-colored dental restorations are becoming increasingly popular all over the world. For the restoration of anterior lesions, as well as for the treatment of smaller and medium-sized defects in the posterior region, direct composite filling materials are state of the art. For larger defects, prefabricated ceramic restorations such as inlays, onlays, veneers, and crowns are attached to the tooth structure with composite-based luting cements in combination with the adhesive technology. Because of the complexity of this topic, the present review concentrates only on polymer-based restorative composites rather than on the adhesive technology to facilitate comprehensibility.

By definition, a composite is a mixture of several components; in the case of dental filling composites, the mixture consists of an organic matrix and inorganic fillers. Usually, the organic matrix is based on methacrylate chemistry, especially cross-linking dimethacrylates like 2,2-*bis*[4-(2-hydroxy-3-methacryloyloxypropyl) phenyl]propane (Bis-GMA), ethoxylated Bis-GMA (EBPDMA), 1,6-*bis*-[2-methacryloyloxyethoxycarbonylamino]-2,4,4-trimethylhexane (UDMA), dodecanediol dimethacrylate (D_3MA), triethyleneglycol dimethacrylate (TEGDMA), or *bis*-methacryloyloxymethyltricyclo[5.2.1.02,6] decane (TCDMA) are used (Figure 2.1). The free-radical polymerization of the matrix monomers leads to a three-dimensional

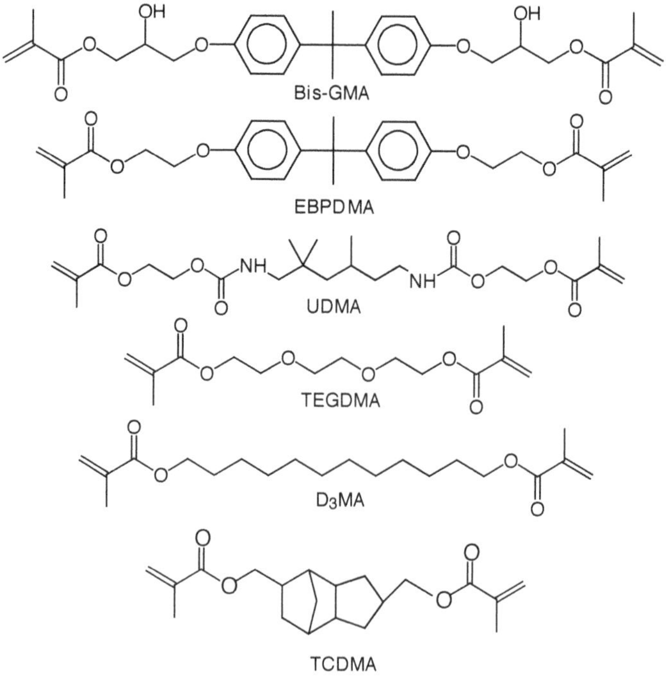

FIGURE 2.1 Dimethacrylates mostly used in dental composite filling materials.

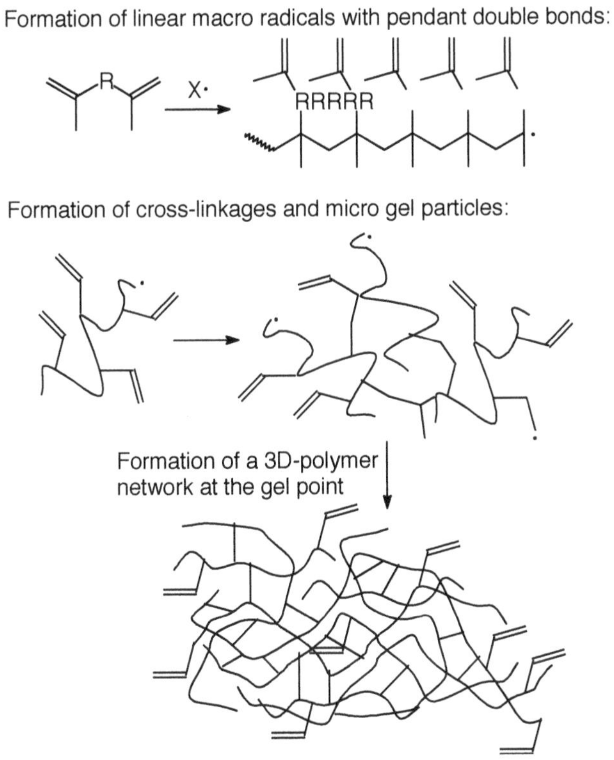

Formation of linear macro radicals with pendant double bonds:

Formation of cross-linkages and micro gel particles:

Formation of a 3D-polymer network at the gel point

FIGURE 2.2 Mechanism of the cross-linking radical polymerization.

network, which is formed by the mechanism shown in Figure 2.2.[4,5] After the initiation of the polymerization by an initiator radical, linear propagating macro radicals are formed because only one double bond per monomer molecule is involved at the time in the polymerization process. During the subsequent chain propagation, the macro radicals form microgel particles. At what is known as the gel point, a three-dimensional (3D) polymer network is built up. The time between the initiation and the gel point is called gel time (Figure 2.3). The gel time for the polymerization of dimethacrylates is in the range of a few seconds (Figure 2.3). However, to get a nearly complete monomer conversion and a high double-bond conversion, a longer polymerization time is needed (20–60 s).

Most of the direct filling materials are light curing composites, which harden by irradiation with visible light in the wavelength range 400–500 nm. Nearly all composite manufacturers are using camphor quinone as the photoinitiator.[6] The absorption maximum of camphor quinone is at 468 nm (Figure 2.4). Amines, such as ethyl *p*-dimethylaminobenzoate, are used as accelerators, and thereby the initiation radicals are formed via proton and electron transfer. In some cases, conventional photoinitiators, which absorb light of the UV-A region in particular, are added to increase the concentration of primary radicals (Figure 2.5).

100 % rel. Conversion
Monom.
Convers.
80
(%)
60
40
20
Exposure
Period
Gel Point
TEGDMA
Dark Reaction
MMA
10
20
30
40
s
50
Time
Induction + Inhibition Period

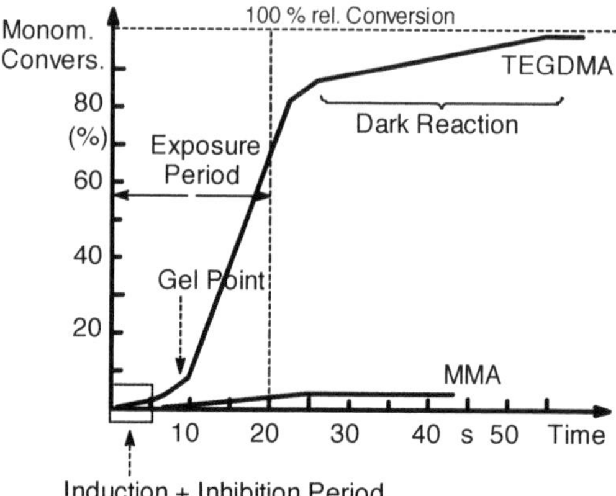

FIGURE 2.3 Course of cross-linking photopolymerization.

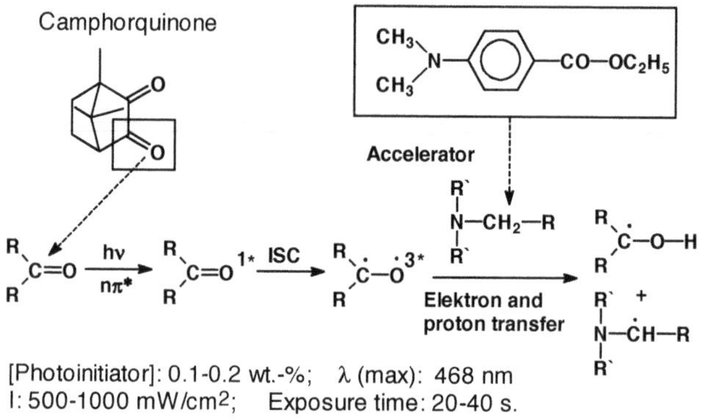

Camphorquinone
Accelerator
hv
nπ*
ISC
Elektron and
proton transfer
[Photoinitiator]: 0.1-0.2 wt.-%; λ (max): 468 nm
I: 500-1000 mW/cm2; Exposure time: 20-40 s.

FIGURE 2.4 Initiator system for the photopolymerization of dental composites.

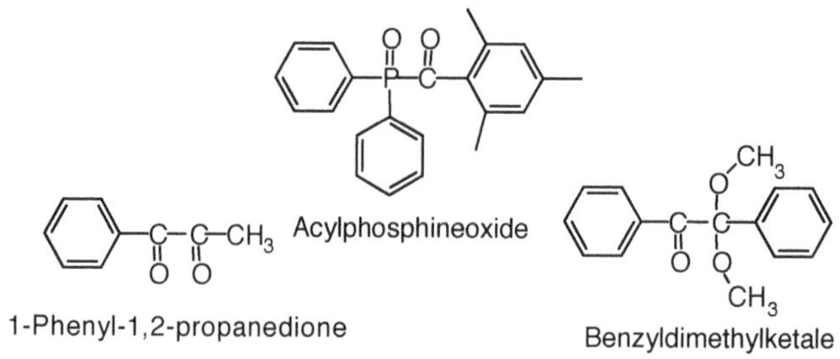

Acylphosphineoxide
1-Phenyl-1,2-propanedione
Benzyldimethylketale

FIGURE 2.5 Photoinitiators absorbing light in the wavelength range of 400 nm.

The photopolymerization is induced by irradiation with halogen lamps, emitting light in the wavelength range of 380–500 nm.[8] Recently, new light units have been brought onto the market, such as plasma-arc lights and blue-light light-emitting diodes (LED).[8–10] In this respect, confusion has arisen because of the mismatch of the emission spectra of these new lamps with the absorption spectra of the initiator systems, insufficient light output, and too short irradiation times. Composite luting cements are often dual curing, i.e., they incorporate a combination of photoinitiator and a chemically initiating redox system (for example amine and peroxide).

Cross-linking polymerization results in the composite being hardened because of the build-up of a 3D polymer network. In general, even at a high monomer conversion, not all double bonds are consumed and radical centers are also present. The reason for this is the low flexibility of the formed polymer network at room temperature. Not all double bond radicals are available because with increasing network density, the flexibility of the polymer chains is reduced. Therefore, the residual double bond content of the formed polymer network is increasing with the functionality of the corresponding monomer (see Table 2.1).[11,12] The degree of double bond conversion of a Bis-GMA/TEGDMA composite largely correlates with the values of the pure monomers (Table 2.1), which means that the addition of, for example, a quartz filler to the monomer matrix does not significantly influence the double bond conversion.[13]

The selection of appropriate monomers for the formulation of a composite strongly influences the reactivity, viscosity, and polymerization shrinkage of the composite paste, as well as the mechanical properties, water uptake, and swelling by water uptake of the cured composite. The polymerization shrinkage of low molecular monomers is higher than that of high molecular monomers (Table 2.2). However, high molecular monomers are very viscous (Table 2.3).

There is a correlation between the filler load of the composite, its polymerization shrinkage, and the viscosity of the composite. Therefore, favorable special mixtures of high molecular monomers and reactive diluents in combination with different fillers are used in dental composites.

TABLE 2.1
Double Bond Conversion of the Radical Polymerization of Methacrylates with Different Functionality at Room Temperature

Monomer	Functionality	% Reacted C:C Bonds
Methyl methacrylate (MMA)	1	99.5
Decanediol dimethacrylate	2	78.0
TEGDMA	2	68.2
Bis-GMA	2	56.0
Trimethylolpropane trimethacrylate	3	41.7

TABLE 2.2
Polymerization Shrinkage (ΔV_p) of Dental Monomers

Monomer	ρ_{mon} (g/cm³)	ρ_{poly} (g/cm³)	ΔV_p (%)
TEGDMA	1.072	1.250	14.3
TCDMA	—	—	7.1
UDMA	1.110	1.190	6.7
Bis-GMA	1.151	1.226	6.1

ρ_{mon} = density of monomer; ρ_{poly} = density of polymer

2.1.2 State of the Art of Dental Restoratives

Because of the major influence of the fillers on the physical properties, the classification of dental filling composites is based on the type and the particle size of fillers used in them (Figure 2.6).[14] In general, two types of composites are available on the market: microfill and hybrid composite filling materials. Microfill composites are based on nanofillers with a particle size in the range of 10–250 nm. Furthermore, a differentiation between homogenous and heterogeneous microfills is made. To enhance their handling properties and achieve a higher load, heterogeneous microfill composites contain prepolymer particles that are based on a homogeneous microfill material. The inorganic part of hybrid composites consists of about 70–80% glass fillers and 20–30% nanofillers. A scanning electron microscope (SEM) investigation published by Hosoda et al. confirmed that this characterization is still valid for modern type composite filling materials.[15] The following subdivision has been made: traditional, microfill, microfill-type, hybrid, hybrid-type, and semihybrid or highly filled composite. In the literature, a hybrid material is described.[16] Analogous to the microfills, this hybrid material may be called a heterogeneous hybrid composite because prepolymerized splinter polymerizates, based on a glass-filled polymer matrix, are used in them (see Figure 2.7).

The fillers used in dental composites directly influence the radiopacity, abrasion resistance, flexural modulus, and thermal coefficient of expansion. Polymerization shrinkage largely correlates with the volumetric amount of the filler in the composite.

TABLE 2.3
Correlation between the Molecular Weight and the Viscosity of Monomers

Monomer	Molecular Weight (g/mol)	Viscosity (mPas)
TEGDMA	286	100
TCDMA	332	110
UDMA	470	5,000–10,000
Bis-GMA	512	500,000–800,000

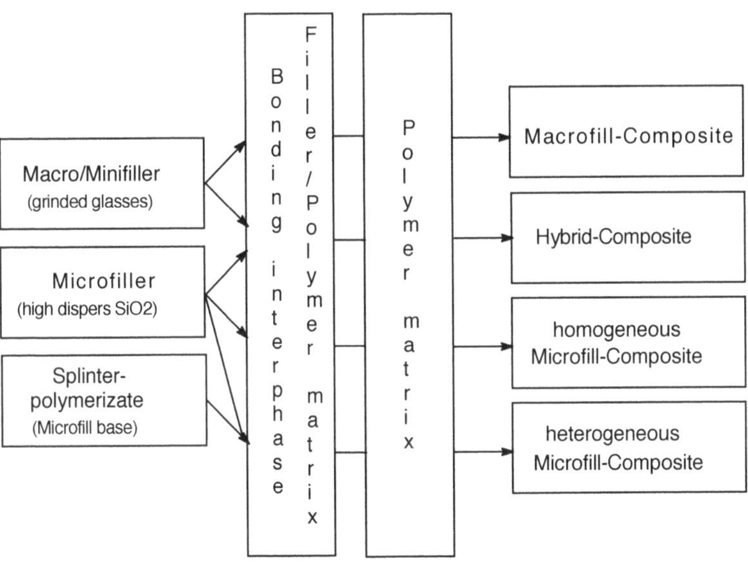

FIGURE 2.6 Classification of composite filing materials.

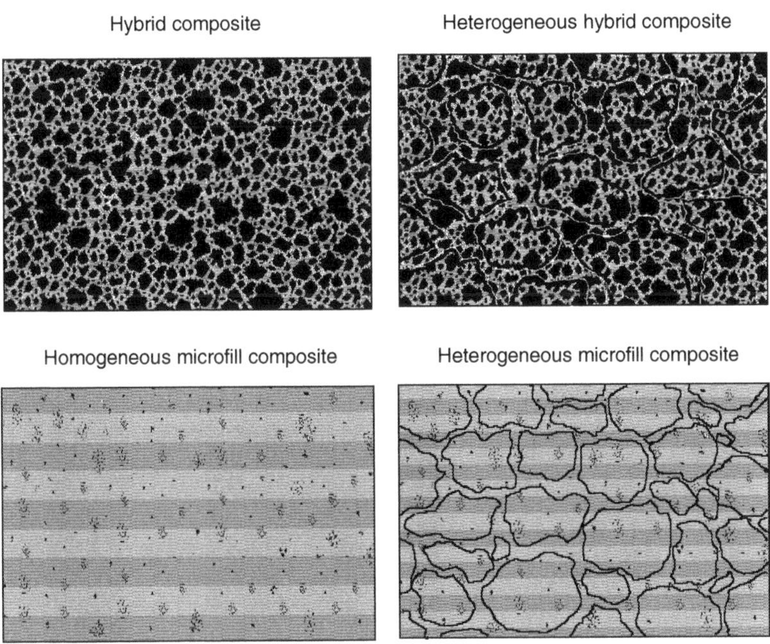

FIGURE 2.7 Schematic of the various dental filling composite types.

TABLE 2.4
Type of Fillers and Filler Size used in Dental Composites

Filler composition	Particle size
Highly dispersed silicon dioxide	10–40 nm
Radiopaque, finely ground barium or strontium silicate glasses	0.7, 1.0,1.5 μm, or larger
Radiopaque, finely grinded Ba-/Sr-fluoro silicate glasses	1.0, 1.5 μm or larger
Ground quartz glass	1.0–1.5 μm
Ytterbiumtrifluoride, yttriumtrifluoride	100–3000 nm
Si-/Zr-mixed oxide	250–500 nm (3.5 μm)
Titanium-, zirconium-, and aluminum oxides used as opacifier	250–500 nm
Splinter polymerizate mainly based on silicon dioxide	10–100 μm

Many modern dental composites use the fillers listed in Table 2.4. In general, dental filling composites contain a mixture of at least two different fillers. Ytterbiumtrifluoride serves mainly as radiopacifier, yttrium fluoride, fluorosilicate glasses, or sparingly soluble fluoride salts are added to composites for fluoride release.

The particle size distribution of nanoparticle filler systems is nearly monodisperse, but in many cases agglomerates are present. Because of the milling process, the ground glasses have a relatively broad particle size distribution (Figure 2.8 and

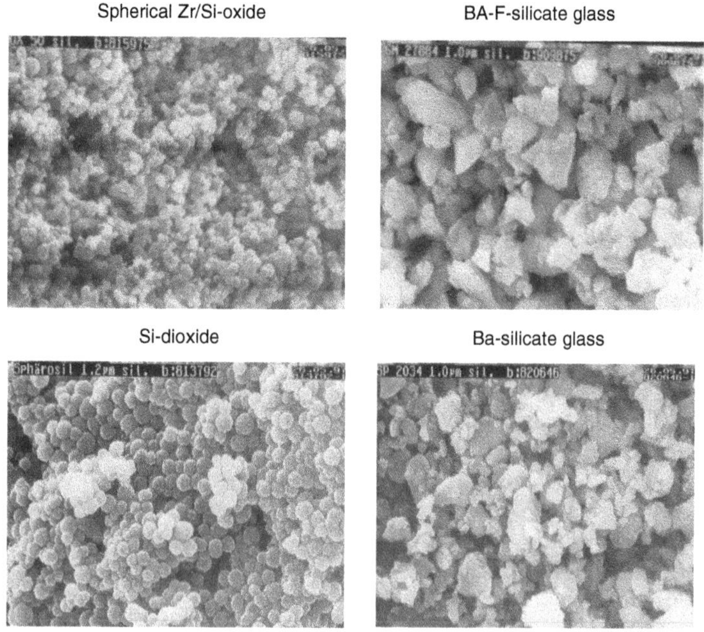

FIGURE 2.8 SEM pictures of different fillers used in dental composites.

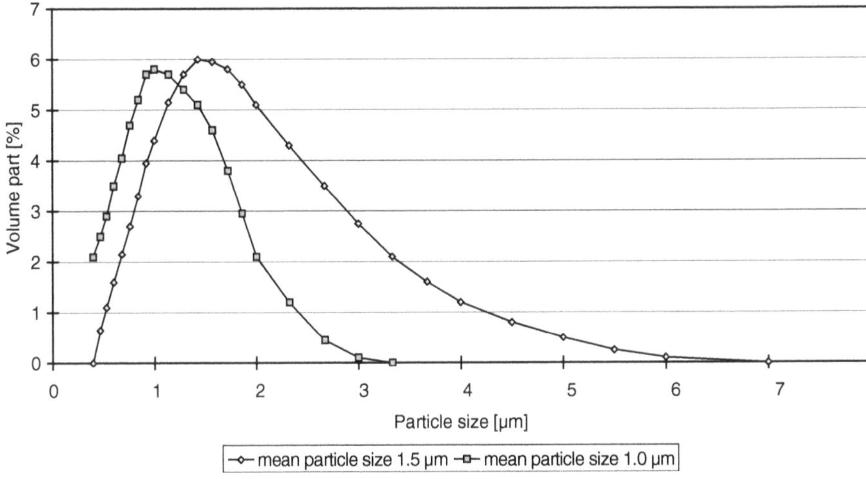

FIGURE 2.9 Particle size distribution of a barium glass filler with mean particle size of 1.5 or 1.0 µm, respectively.

Figure 2.9). The abrasion resistance of the cured composite is strongly influenced by the particle size of the fillers. In the case of ground glasses, the mean particle size is less crucial than the maximum particle size. Ground glass fillers with a relatively small difference in the mean particle size of about 1 µm show a relatively significant difference in the maximum particle size of about 4 µm (Figure 2.9). This difference has significant effects on the surface smoothness and the abrasion behavior of a composite. In the case of microfill-based splinter polymerizates, the particle size has no influence on abrasion behavior. Abrasion resistance is comparable with the polymer matrix admixed with pure silicon dioxide.

In Table 2.5 some physical properties of composite filling materials are listed in correlation with the type of filler, particle size of the filler, and filler load. In the case of hybrid composites, the filler load has an effect on the flexural strength and the flexural modulus (see Table 2.5: fine particle hybrid, mean particle size (mp) 1.0 µm compared with flowable fine particle hybrid, mp 1.0 µm). Heterogeneous microfill composites show only a correlation between filler load and flexural modulus. More coarsely ground mean particle size fillers as well as higher loads influence the flexural modulus of hybrid composites (fine particle hybrid, mp 1.0 µm compared with a fine particle hybrid, mp 1.5 µm).

Table 2.6 shows the composition of a fine particle hybrid composite (Tetric Ceram/Ivoclar Vivadent) and a heterogeneous microfill composite (Heliomolar/Ivoclar Vivadent).

2.1.3 Improvements of Dental Composites

The clinical performance of a filling material largely depends on the indication for which it is used. The stress effect on restorations in the posterior region is much more pronounced than the stress effect on restorations in the anterior region. According to the literature, the average life cycle of hybrid composite posterior MOD

TABLE 2.5
Correlation between Type of Filler, Filler Load, and the Physical Properties of a Composite

Type of Composite	Filler Type	Filler Load (wt%)	ΔV_p[a] (vol%)	Flexural Strength (MPa)	Flexural Modulus (MPa)
Fine particle hybrid (mp[b]: 1.0 μm)	Ba-glass, Ba-F-glass, YbF_3, Zr/Si-oxide	78	3.2	135	9,000
Fine particle hybrid (mp: 1.5 μm)	Ba-glass, Si-oxide, YbF_3, Zr/Si-oxide	81	2.7	135	11,000
Flowable fine particle hybrid (mp: 1.0 μm)	Ba-glass, Ba-F-glass, YbF_3, Zr/Si-oxide	69	3.6	95	5,100
Heterogeneous microfill-composite	Si-oxide, YbF_3, splinter-polymer	78	2.4	110	6,500
Flowable, heterogeneous microfill composite	Si-oxide, YbF_3, splinter-polymer	59	ne	110	4,100

[a] Polymerization shrinkage, 24-h value.
[b] Mean particle size.

restorations placed in general practices is 4 years, compared with 8 years for amalgam restorations. To improve the clinical performance of composite filling materials, a large number of investigations are currently being conducted.[17] The main topics are as follows:

- Reduction of the polymerization shrinkage to improve marginal adaptation and avoid recurrent caries
- Release of fluoride or other substances to reduce recurrent caries
- Improvement of mechanical properties
- Improvement of biocompatibility by reducing the elution of components.

TABLE 2.6
Composition of a Fine Particle Hybrid and a Heterogeneous Microfill Composite

	Tetric Ceram (Ivoclar-Vivadent)	Heliomolar (Ivoclar-Vivadent)
Monomer mixture	Bis-GMA, UDMA, TEGDMA	Bis-GMA, UDMA, D_3MA
Fillers	Ba-silicate glass, Ba-fluoro-silicate glass, ytterbiumtrifluoride, Zr/Si-mixed oxide	Pyrogenic silicon dioxide, prepolymer, ytterbiumtrifluoride
Filler particle size	40 nm–3.5 μm	40-250 nm (SiO_2, YbF_3)
Classification	Fine particle hybrid composite	Heterogeneous microfill composite

2.2 FILLER-COMPONENT-BASED IMPROVEMENTS OF DENTAL RESTORATIVES

2.2.1 Reduction of Shrinkage Stress

During polymerization, of TEGDMA for example, only a slow change of density is observed in the pregel phase (see Figure 2.10). After the viscous flow of the liquid material, which is not cross-linked at that stage, no shrinkage stress builds up. After the gel point, the polymerization system behaves like a viscoelastic solid. Because of the gel effect, the change in density is accelerated, resulting in an increase in internal contraction stress. About 80% of the polymerization shrinkage of cross-linking dimethacrylates results in internal stress buildup (Figure 2.10). Polymerization contraction stress can be partly compensated for by flow after the gelation of the composite.[18] On the other hand, each prolongation of the pregel phase leads to a reduction of internal stress at the same volume shrinkage. This means that the parameters that influence the polymerization shrinkage in general have an effect on the buildup of compressive stresses in the material. Figure 2.11 lists the parameters that have the strongest influence on shrinkage stress. In the case of light curing composites (LC), a much higher stress is built up compared with composites initiated by a redox initiator system (CC).[19] Because hardening occurs faster with the light curing system than with the redox initiated system, there is less time to reduce internal stress by relaxation of the polymer chains. A slight stress reduction can be achieved by a step-by-step modulation of the light energy, starting the irradiation process with low light intensity and then increasing the light intensity (soft-start polymerization).[20,21] The clinical relevance of soft-start polymerization remains questionable; some investigators found an advantage with regard to *in vitro* marginal adaptation of the light curing filling material to the tooth structure, and some did not find such an advantage.[22,23] Analogous to the polymerization kinetics, the chance

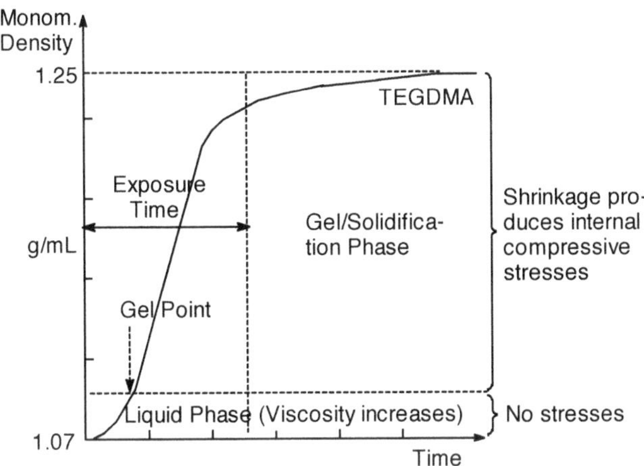

FIGURE 2.10 Correlation between polymerization shrinkage and shrinkage stress.

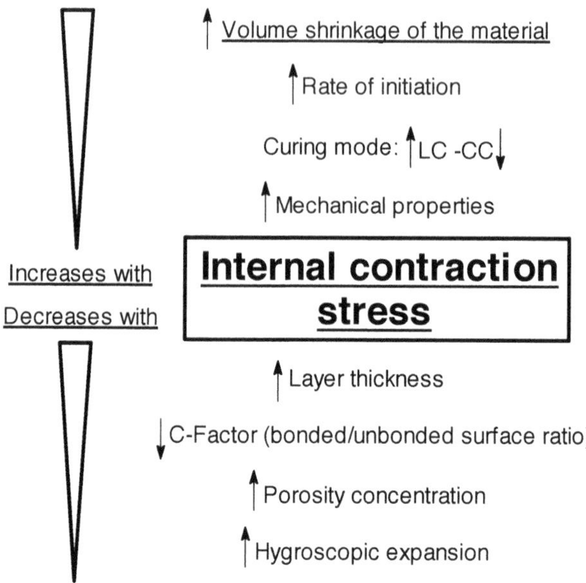

FIGURE 2.11 Parameters influencing internal stress build-up by polymerization shrinkage.

for stress reduction is less possible in materials with a high flexural modulus compared with more flexible materials.

The polymerization shrinkage of composite filling materials and internal stress buildup are not a problem in restorative dentistry because marginal gaps are the result of the shrinkage stress that builds up at the interface of the filling material and the cavity walls. Besides the monomer composition of the composite and the polymerization kinetics, the amount of stress that builds up at the interface largely depends on the geometry of the tooth cavity, which can be expressed with the C-factor. The C-factor is the ratio of bonded to unbonded surfaces.[24] Figure 2.12 illustrates the C-factor for a mesial–occlusal (MO) filling.

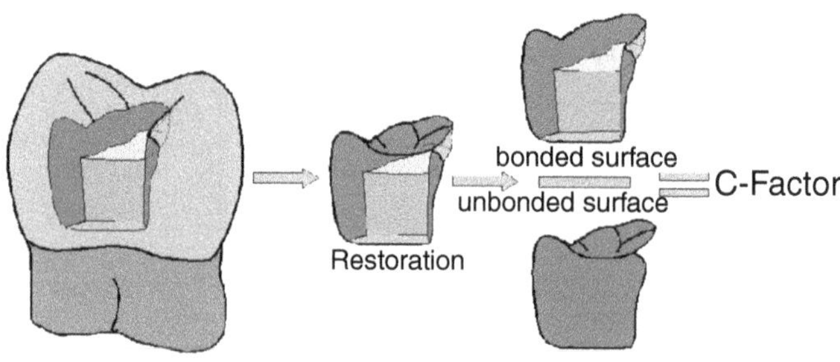

FIGURE 2.12 Illustration of the C-factor in the case of an MO-filling.

The porosities incorporated into a two-component material reduce the shrinkage stress due to the enlargement of the unbonded surfaces.[25] However, the porosities in a restorative weaken the material and cause discoloration at the surface. The addition of nonbonded nanoparticles to a composite, as described in the literature, has the same effect on polymerization contraction stress reduction as porosities.[26,27]

Usually, the surfaces of silicate fillers are conditioned with a methacrylate functionalized silane, such as the frequently used γ-methacryloxypropyl trimethoxy silane, to create covalent links between the filler particles and the organic matrix by copolymerization. Condon and Ferracane silanized aerosol-type silicon dioxide with a non–methacrylate-functionalized silane to include nonbonded surfaces in the composite (see Figure 2.13).[26] Additional reduction of shrinkage stress could be achieved by incorporating methacrylated styrene–allyl alcohol copolymer.[27] Only a slight deterioration of the mechanical properties compared with the silanization with methacrylate-functionalized silane was observed.[26,27] Other attempts to reduce polymerization shrinkage, or shrinkage stress, through the inorganic parts of the composite include the addition of ammonia-modified montmorillonite (NH_3/MMT) or porous fillers.[28,29] Composites containing ammonia-modified montmorillonite raise their temperature during curing, which causes the NH_3/MMT-particles to expand and counteract polymerization shrinkage. The addition of porous silicon dioxide filler particles with a mean particle size of 0.5–50 μm and a size of porosities in the range of 20–120 nm increases the abrasion resistance and reduces the polymerization shrinkage of composite filling materials.[29] Use of this method results in the linear polymerization shrinkage being reduced by 50% and the abrasion resistance being increased by 100%. The effect of porous fillers on the abrasion resistance was confirmed by others, while the reduction of polymerization shrinkage couldn't

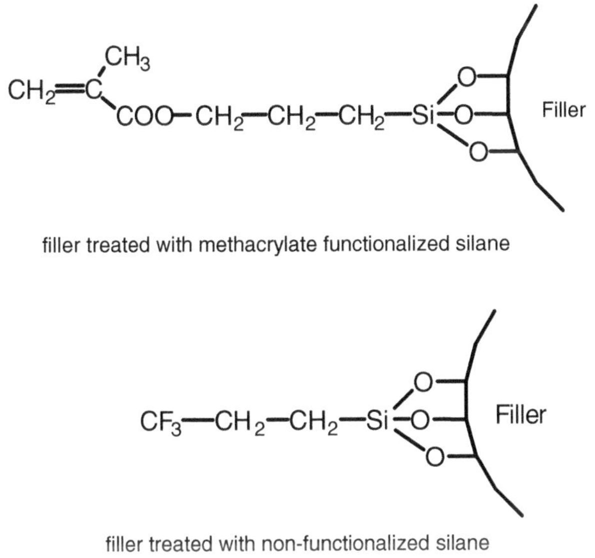

FIGURE 2.13 Filler treated with methacrylate-functionalized and nonfunctionalized silane.

be reproduced.[30,31] There is a potential of reducing the polymerization contraction stress through the inorganic parts of a composite filling material. Further *in vitro* and *in vivo* studies have to confirm this potential.

2.2.2 Nanoparticles and Composite Reinforcement

At present many investigations are being carried out to improve the properties of composite materials, such as abrasion resistance, rheology, or mechanical properties. For instance, *in situ* formed layered silicate nanofillers increase the strength and toughness of acrylic nanocomposites.[32] The literature describes organopolysiloxane particles of 5–200 nm of diameter, among others, as compact modifiers for dental materials.[33] Because of the low interaction between these particles, the load of the corresponding composite could be increased, resulting in reduced polymerization shrinkage.

Most dental composites contain particulate fillers. Composites are reinforced by incorporating fibers or whiskers, in particular. However, fiber reinforced dental filling composites are seldom described in the literature. The gradual addition of silanized short-cut glass fibers to a Bis-GMA/TEGDMA based composite resulted in an increase in the elastic modulus and a decrease in the tensile strength.[34] Xu et al. and Xu[36]used ceramic single-crystalline whiskers as fillers to reinforce composites. The filler mass fraction ranged from 0 to 70%. Compared with microfill and hybrid composites, the whisker reinforced material showed significantly higher flexural strength values. Whiskers exhibit some potential for being used to reinforce composite filling materials; however, at least the whiskers described in Xu et al.[35] and Xu[36] are not that easy accessible. Recently, nanoparticles, such as tantalum oxide [37,38] or zirconium oxide,[35] have been incorporated into dental composites to reinforce them, to improve their radiopacity, or to produce transparent materials.[37,39] In the case of nonsilicate filler, surface modification with methacrylate silanes is less efficient.[38] Tantalum oxide or zirconium oxide nanoparticles were therefore surface functionalized with phosphate methacrylates (Figure 2.14), zirconates, or aluminozirconates (Figure 2.15).[37,39]

Nanoparticles have the tendency to agglomerate. In this case, the refractive index of the particles has to be adjusted to the refractive index of the polymer matrix to obtain translucent materials. By means of the sol–gel process, mixed oxide particles can be prepared that have a refractive index that depends on the ratio of the different metal ions used.[40]

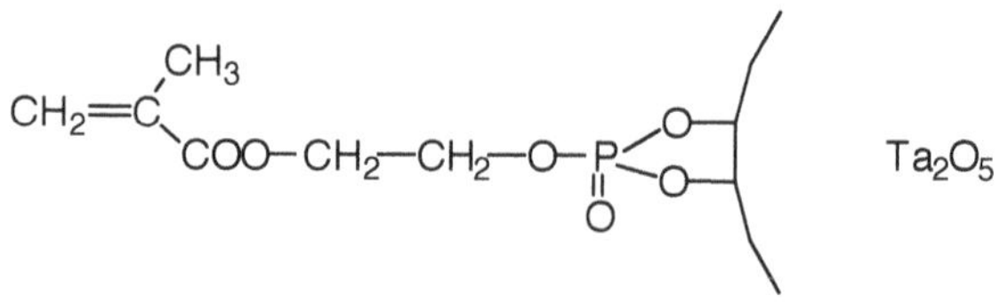

$$CH_2{=}C(CH_3){-}COO{-}CH_2{-}CH_2{-}O{-}P({=}O)(O{-})_2 \quad Ta_2O_5$$

FIGURE 2.14 Tantalum oxide nanoparticle functionalized with a phosphate methacrylate.

$CH_2{=}C(CH_3){-}COO{-}CH_2{-}CH_2{-}O{-}Zr(O{-})_3$ ZrO_2

FIGURE 2.15 Zirconium oxide nanoparticle functionalized with a methacryl zirconate.

2.2.3 Condensable and Flowable Composites

Composites with different consistencies have been available on the market for a few years. In addition to conventional composites with a pasty consistency, so-called condensable and flowable composite filling materials are available. The buzz word "condensable" is somewhat marketing driven and is supposed to imply that the handling properties are similar to those of amalgam. Composites are neither condensable nor do they have working or curing characteristics similar to those of amalgam. Against such a background, the catch phrase "condensable" is increasingly replaced by the term "packable."[41,42] Packable composites are characterized by less stickiness and a stiffer viscosity than conventional composites. As a result, they can be placed using a technique that somewhat resembles the technique employed to place amalgam restorations. They are therefore preferred for fabrication of posterior restorations.[43] Packable composites have a composition similar to conventional composites. However, they feature a higher filler load or higher concentration of thickening fine particle fillers than conventional restorative filling composites. In some cases these features are realized by adding a certain amount of coarse fillers or even fiber fragments to the composite (see SEM Figure 2.16). Flexural strength and modulus are due to the higher filler load in most packables, which are somewhat higher than those of conventional composites.[44] The packable composites tested in the literature, however, showed a wide range of mean values for the physical properties.

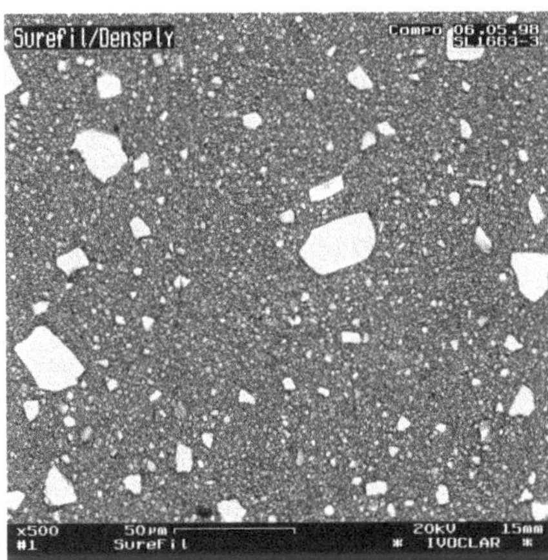

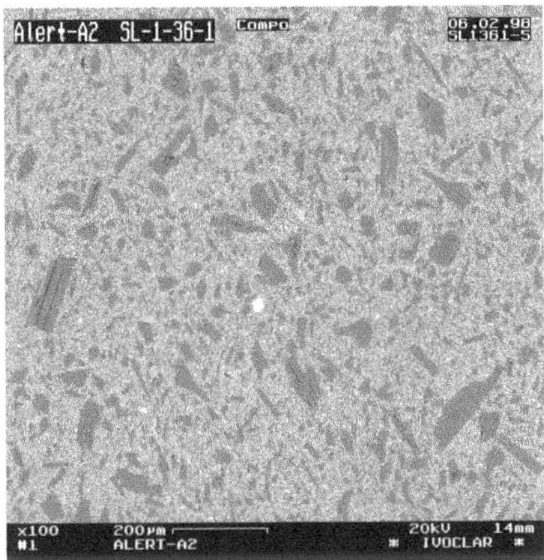

FIGURE 2.16 SEM pictures of two commercially available packable composites.

Compared with conventional filling composites, the polymerization contraction stress of packable composites is significantly higher.[46]

Given their high stiffness, packable composite pastes require the preapplication of a flowable composite to enhance marginal adaptation.[47] Flowable composites have a filler load in the range of 52–68 wt% and most of them are fine particle hybrids. Flowable composites, which were initially introduced for the restoration of cervical defects, are in general predestined for small cavities. Because of their favorable wetting properties, they are conveniently used as an initial layer in big cavities.[48,49] Because of their low filler load, the volumetric polymerization shrinkage of flowable composites is higher than that of conventional or packable composites.[50]

2.2.4 Bioactive Restoratives

The most frequent reason for replacing dental fillings is recurrent caries, regardless of the type of filling material used.[51,52] Plaque accumulates in the gaps that form around the filling after a certain service time. In some cases, plaque accumulation causes the formation of secondary caries. A method to decrease the incidence of recurrent caries is to incorporate additional preventive substances into the filling material to prevent demineralization and support remineralization of the tooth structure adjacent to the restoration.

Fluoride ions are known to alter the tooth structure (fluorohydroxyapatite formation) and render it less soluble to acids produced by cariogenic bacteria. Fluoride release can be achieved from the organic as well as from the inorganic part of the composite restorative. The patent literature mainly describes examples of fluoride ion containing monomeres or polymers (Figure 2.17).[54,55] Glasspoole et al. recently described a filling composite in which tetrabutylammonium tetrafluoroborate was incorporated as the fluoride source.[56] The cumulative fluoride release from this experimental composite was comparable with that of glass ionomer materials.

In most materials, fluoride release is achieved from the inorganic part of the composite. Barium or strontium fluorosilicate glasses are often used for this purpose. In some cases, the fluoride released from added fluoride salts, such as strontium or sodium fluoride, or potassium hexafluorotitanate.[57,58] Glass ionomers are the most widely investigated fluoride releasing restorative materials.

Fluoride release is largely determined by the solvent in which the test specimens are stored and changes depending on the pH value. The amount of fluoride released in deionized water is about twice as high as in artificial saliva.[59] At a low pH value, more fluoride is released than at neutral conditions.[60] This means that fluoride is released on demand, for instance in response to the acids produced by the cariogenic

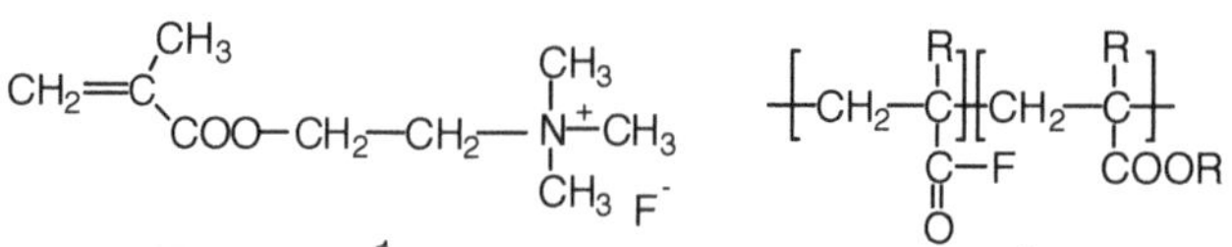

FIGURE 2.17 Example of a fluoride-containing monomer 1 and a fluoride-releasing polymer 2.

bacteria. In many cases, fluoride-releasing restoratives can be recharged by fluoridating agents that are applied within the scope of oral hygiene.[61] Besides measuring the level of fluoride release, a number of studies are investigating the effect of fluoride release on the adjacent tooth structure, either by examining the fluoride uptake of enamel and dentin or by assessing the prevention of demineralization or the acceleration of remineralization.[62–64]

In contrast to the *in vitro* investigations, which confirmed that particular glass ionomers have a preventive effect against demineralization of tooth structure, a comparative study, which used the same test setup *in vitro* and *in vivo*, did not show any preventive effect for glass ionomers *in vivo*.[65] To some degree, these results have been confirmed by investigations on the clinical behavior of dental restoratives placed in general dental practices.[51,52] In response to this situation, dental restoratives with additional beneficial effects have been developed to prevent the formation of secondary caries. There are several mechanisms that help achieve this aim, such as release of substances that have an antimicrobial effect to combat cariogenic bacteria and that support the remineralization of the tooth structure by buffering the acids produced by the cariogenic bacteria.

Some glass ionomers show antibacterial properties against *Streptococcus mutans* and Lactobacilli.[66] However, it is unclear if these properties are attributable to released fluoride, a low pH-value, or the effect of eluated metal ions, such as zinc, silver, or aluminum ions. Silver ions have also been incorporated into silica glass filler, prepared by means of the sol–gel method, to supply antibacterial properties to composite filling materials.[67]

Antimicrobial substances like chlorhexidine or triclosan have been added to restorative materials too.[68,69] The problem with physically bonded antimicrobials is that the drugs are released in high amounts in an initial burst rather than "on demand." Imazato et al. synthesized an antibacterial monomer 3 (Figure 2.18), which can be incorporated into a composite by copolymerization.[70] Here the disadvantage is that such a composite shows only an antimicrobial effect by direct surface contact of the bacteria.

Human saliva has a highly preventive effect against caries.[71] Because of the high content of calcium and phosphate ions, the chemical equilibrium between demineralization and remineralization is shifted in the direction of remineralization. This natural mechanism of prevention has been copied by adding amorphous calcium phosphate (ACP) as filler to restorative composite materials. The mechanical properties of such composite materials are lower than those of ACP-free controls.[72] When coated with ACP-filled composites, artificial caries lesions recovered 71% of their lost mineral.

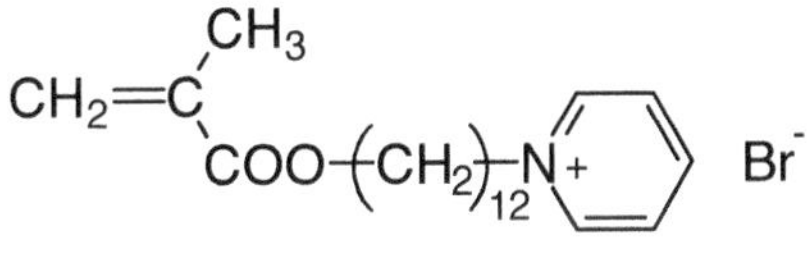

$$CH_2{=}C(CH_3)COO{-}(CH_2)_{12}{-}N^{+}C_5H_5\ \ Br^{-}$$

3

FIGURE 2.18 Antibacterial monomer 12-methacryloyloxydodecylpyridinium bromide 3.

Besides having a high concentration of calcium and phosphate ions, human saliva shows an enormous buffering capacity to neutralize acids produced by cariogenic germs. A restorative material introduced in the literature tries to combine the remineralizing and buffering effect of natural saliva with the preventive effect of fluoride.[74,75]

In conclusion, there is a clinical demand for materials inhibiting the formation of secondary caries. Bioactive materials have a high potential to fulfill these requirements, but there must be a balance between release of active ingredients (effectiveness) and the longevity of the corresponding filling. Release on demand is a mechanism that helps prevent the formation of secondary caries. However, the disadvantage of this new concept is that besides the fluoride release, only very few, if any, long-term clinical results are currently available.

2.2.5 Special Additives

Fluorescent dyes make composites look like natural tooth substance even when exposed to ultraviolet (UV) light. As a consequence, it is generally fairly difficult to distinguish between the tooth-colored composites and the natural tooth structure. For esthetic reasons, the close similarity between tooth structure and composite is very important. However, if there is a need to remove a composite filling or to remove the excess of a composite luting cement, dentists may find it very hard to differentiate between the tooth-shaded restorative material and the natural tooth structure. A method to facilitate optical differentiation is to add to the composite a fluorescent dye that absorbs light within the wavelength range of 360–480 nm and shows a fluorescent maximum in the range of 480–600 nm.[76] To render the composite visible, the light within the wavelength range of 360–480 nm has to be filtered out. Another approach to render restoratives visible is to use photochromic dyes. Photochromic dyes change their appearance by irradiation with light; they may for example change from colorless to red (see Figure 2.19). Two systems are known, reversible and nonreversible color change. In general, photochromic dyes should be reversible. In the special case of photochromic dental composites, some dyes lose their photochromic properties by radical polymerization.[77] If an all-ceramic crown is cemented with a photochromic composite cement, the red shaded cement can be easily detected and therefore removed during cementation. After polymerization the red shade completely disappears.[77]

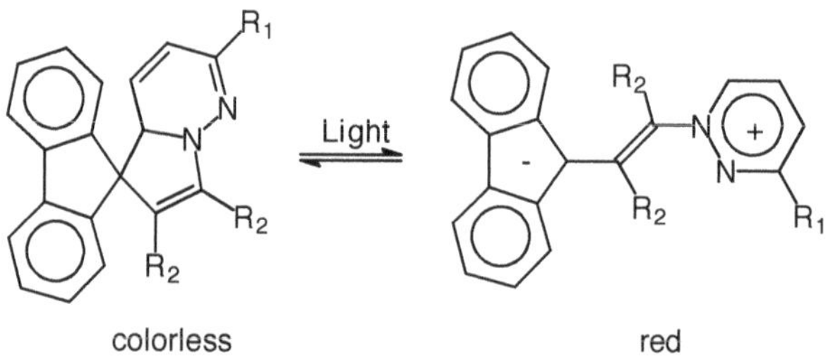

FIGURE 2.19 Photochromic dye system added to dental composites.

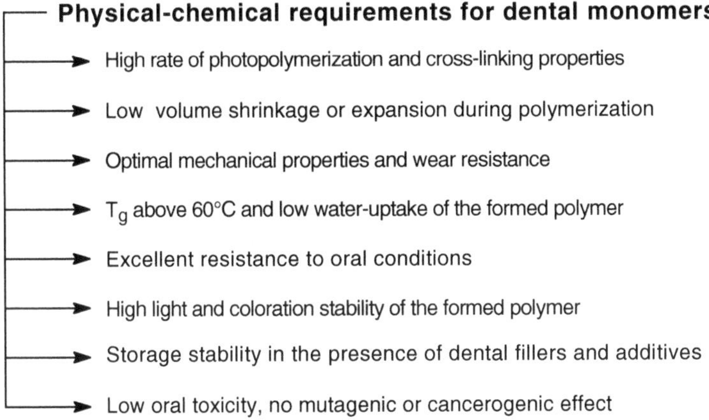

Physical-chemical requirements for dental monomers
High rate of photopolymerization and cross-linking properties
Low volume shrinkage or expansion during polymerization
Optimal mechanical properties and wear resistance
Tg above 60°C and low water-uptake of the formed polymer
Excellent resistance to oral conditions
High light and coloration stability of the formed polymer
Storage stability in the presence of dental fillers and additives
Low oral toxicity, no mutagenic or cancerogenic effect

FIGURE 2.20 Basic requirements for monomers in dental composites.

2.3 NEW MONOMERS FOR DENTAL RESTORATIVES

At present, the monomer matrix systems of dental filling composites are mainly based on a mixture of dimethacrylates and have to fulfill a number of basic requirements with regard to the reactivity, stability, or toxicity of the monomers used and the properties (strength, stiffness, stability) of the formed polymer network (Figure 2.20). In this context, the development of new monomers for restorative filling materials is predominantly motivated by the will to overcome the main shortcomings of resin composites, i.e., marginal leakage due to polymerization shrinkage and insufficient abrasion resistance. The objective is to create composites that can fulfill new functions, such as releasing fluoride ions or exhibiting anticariogenic effects or antiplaque action.

Furthermore, cross-linking monomers that improve the mechanical and processing properties of the composite are synthesized. These composites demonstrate reduced water uptake, radiopacity, or self-adhesion to dentin or enamel.

A review of the dental monomer systems used is presented by Peutzfeldt.[2] the following sections, the development of recent dental monomers is described, focusing on the polymer-chemical aspects of the following systems in particular: ring-opening monomers with the potential of low shrinkage, cross-linking monomers with a new architecture (mesogenic units, hyperbranched structures or nanoparticles), and acidic monomers used in compomers.

2.3.1 Ring-Opening Monomers

2.3.1.1 Causes of Polymerization Shrinkage

Polymerization shrinkage is produced during the chain propagation process, in which the monomer units are more closely connected to one another in the polymer chain than they are in the starting monomer phase. This is demonstrated in Figure 2.21 for the polymerization of MMA. In the liquid bulk monomer, which shows a density of 0.940 g/cm^3, the distance between the MMA molecules is characterized by the van der

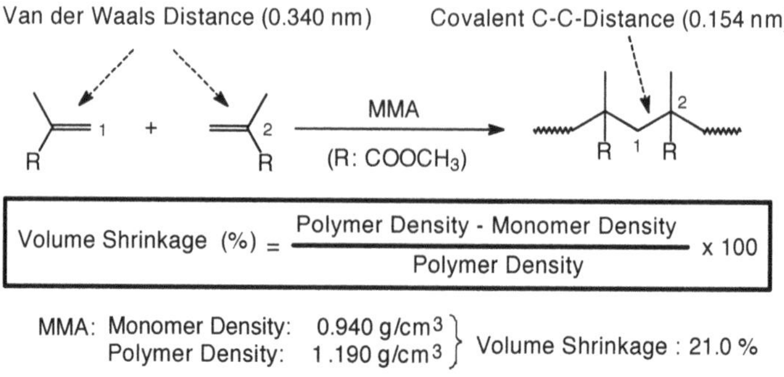

Van der Waals Distance (0.340 nm) Covalent C-C-Distance (0.154 nm)

MMA (R: $COOCH_3$)

$$\text{Volume Shrinkage (\%)} = \frac{\text{Polymer Density - Monomer Density}}{\text{Polymer Density}} \times 100$$

MMA: Monomer Density: 0.940 g/cm^3; Polymer Density: 1.190 g/cm^3 } Volume Shrinkage : 21.0 %

FIGURE 2.21 Volume shrinkage as a result of bond changes during the polymerization of MMA.

Waals distance (VWD) of about 0.340 nm. In the polymer the distance between the monomer units is about 0.154 nm, which corresponds with the distance of covalent carbon–carbon (C–C) bonds (CD). This results in an increased density of poly(MMA) (1.190 g/cm^3) and subsequently a volume shrinkage of about 21.0%. In composites, polymerization shrinkage causes a number of problems (Figure 2.22). For example, polymerization shrinkage produces internal stress. Internal stress, in turn, produces microvoids or microcracks, which impair the mechanical properties of a composite. In composites used for dental restoratives, the most serious problem is that polymerization shrinkage impairs the adhesion to the tooth surface, which leads to the formation of marginal gaps. Therefore, a considerable number of studies have been carried out to find new ways of reducing the volume shrinkage during the polymerization of the monomer matrix.

2.3.1.2 Shrinkage Reduction by Ring-Opening Polymerization of Cyclic Monomers

With regard to the reduction of polymerization shrinkage, the application of cyclic monomers has received the most attention. It is well known that cyclic compounds

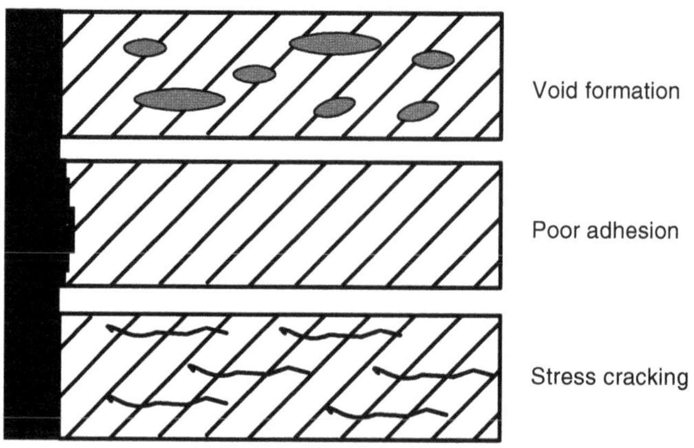

FIGURE 2.22 Typical problems associated with the polymerization shrinkage.

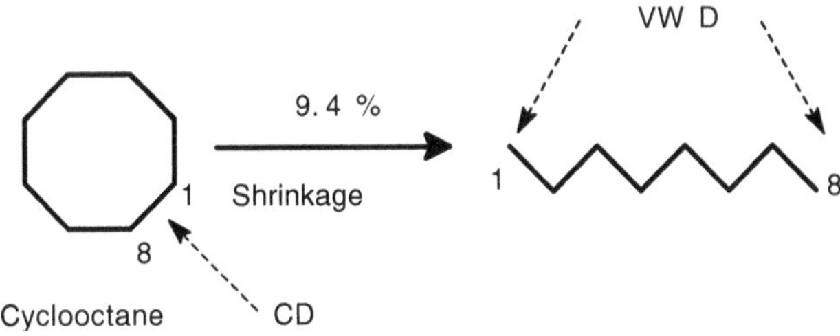

FIGURE 2.23 Volume shrinkage during the ring-opening of cyclo-octane.

possess higher densities than their linear counterparts because they are able to arrange themselves in an orderly and close fit manner in the liquid state.[78] principle, therefore, the ring-opening polymerization of cyclic monomers produces less shrinkage than the polymerization of linear monomers. For example, in the case of the ring-opening polymerization of cyclooctane (density: 0.834 g/cm^3), which has a similar molecular weight as MMA, the polymerization shrinkage, which is calculated on the basis of the density of medium density polyethylene (0.92 g/cm^3) is only 9.4% (Figure 2.23). The degree of volume changes during the ring-opening polymerization is influenced by the ring size, number of rings per volume unit, and the ring-opening effect. For example, this means, that the larger the rings, the smaller the shrinkage. Moreover, the shrinkage can be further reduced by increasing the number of reactive rings per monomer molecule. Based on this fact, Bailey first reported the expanding monomer concept of the double ring-opening polymerization of bicyclic monomers in 1972, which is schematically demonstrated in Figure 2.24.

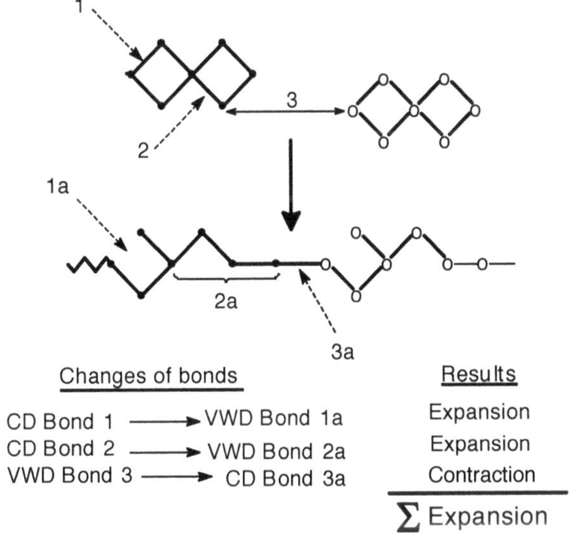

FIGURE 2.24 Bond changes according to Bailey's concept of expanding monomers.

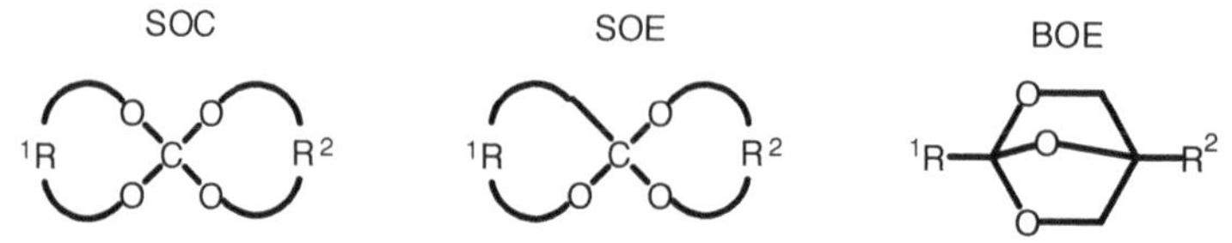

FIGURE 2.25 Examples of Bailey's basic structures for expanding monomers.

According to this concept, at least two bonds would have to shift from a CD to near VWD for every bond that undergoes a change from VWD to a CD during the ring opening of bicyclic monomers.

2.3.1.3 Spiro Orthocarbonates

About 20 years ago, Bailey patented the polymerization of polycyclic ring-opening monomers, such as spiro orthocarbonates (SOC), spiro orthoesters (SOE), or bicyclic orthoesters (BOE) (Figure 2.25), which show a near-zero shrinkage or expansion during their polymerization. Bailey's concept initiated many important fundamental studies and some applied investigations on the synthesis and ring-opening polymerization of expanding monomers.[80–82] The first example of an SOC investigated in a dental resin formulation was the crystalline SOC 4 (3,9-dimethylene-1,5,7,11-tetraoxaspiro[5.5]undecane) (Figure 26).[83] The monomer was used as a slurry in a free-radical polymerizable resin composition based on conventional dimethacrylates (Bis-GMA and ethyleneglycol dimethacrylate).

However, the crystalline SOC 4 was partially left undissolved and unreacted in the resin cured at ambient temperature. Therefore, a number of free-radical polymerizable SOC 5–9 were synthesized for dental applications (Figure 2.27).[84–86]

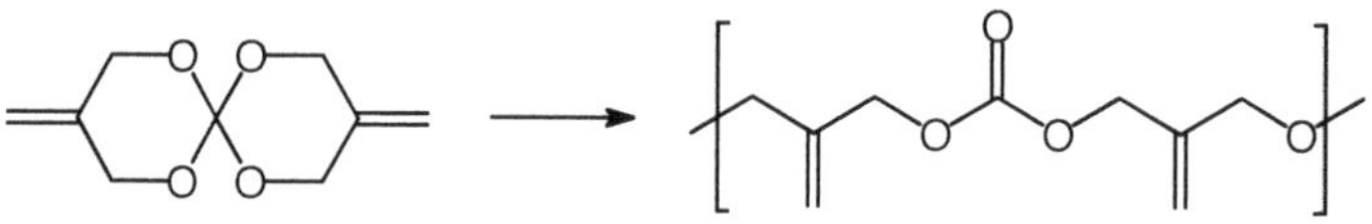

FIGURE 2.26 Double ring-opening polymerization of 4.

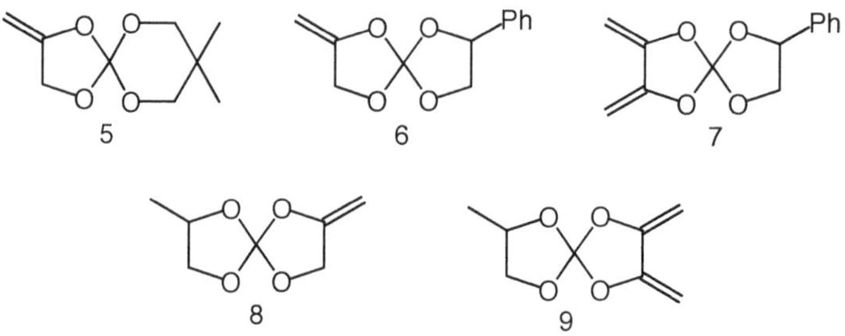

FIGURE 2.27 Liquid SOC 5–9 investigated in dental composites.

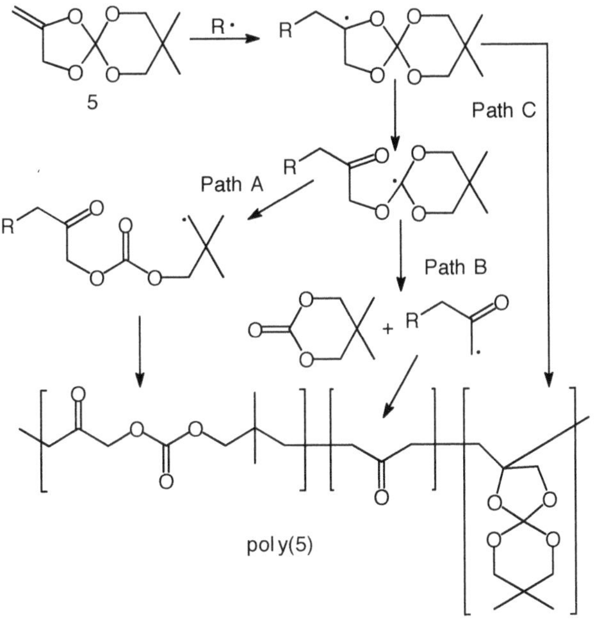

FIGURE 2.28 Proposed mechanism for the free-radical polymerization of SOC 5.

These monomers demonstrated melting points below room temperature, depending on the substituents of the SOCs. The polymerization behavior of SOCs 5–7 were investigated using pure monomers and combinations with Bis-GMA, EBPDMA, or TEGDMA. For the free-radical homopolymerization of SOC 5 in the presence of di-*tert*-butylperoxide (DTBP) at 130°C, it was found that the polymerization took place by means of several competing pathways. In addition to the desired double ring-opening (path A), a single ring-opening with a concomitant elimination of a cyclic carbonate molecule (path B), and a non–ring-opening vinyl polymerization (path C) occurred (Figure 2.28). The degree of ring-opening varied between 45 and 85%. In comparison with the monofunctional SOCs 5 and 6, the 2,3-(bismethylene)–substituted SOC 7 was more reactive. However, in a mixture with the dimethacrylate EBPDMA, it did not demonstrate any storage stability. The free-radical polymerization of the low viscosity SOCs 8 and 9 was investigated in bulk in the presence of DTBP at 130°C and in solution in the presence of azobisisobutyronitrile (AIBN) at 65 in comparison to MMA.[87] The difunctional SOC 9 was more reactive than the SOC 8 monomer. However, the spectroscopic investigation of the formed poly(8) and poly(9) showed that primarily vinyl polymerization with only a low degree of ring-opening occurred. This finding was also confirmed by the polymerization shrinkage of SOC 9 of about 12.5%, which was similar to that of TEGDMA ($\Delta V = 12.0\%$), a frequently used dental diluent dimethacrylate. To improve the free-radical ring-opening tendency of SOCs, researchers synthesized various designed SOCs, for example, based on seven-membered rings and using radical stabilizing benzyl groups.[88] The most promising monomers 10 and 11 (Figure 2.29) showed a degree

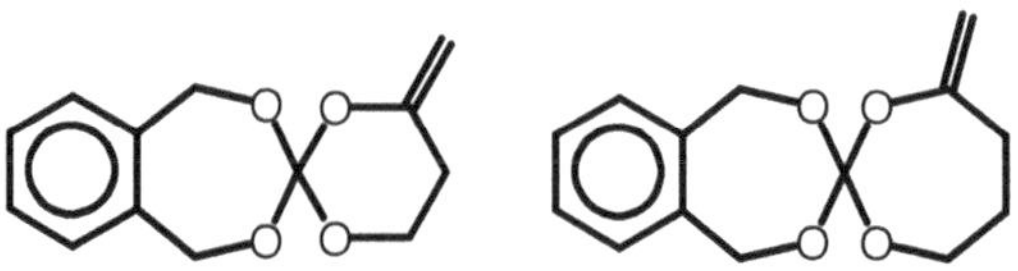

10 (mp 73-74 °C) 11 (mp 88-90 °C)

FIGURE 2.29 Designed SOC 10 and 11 for free-radical-ring-opening polymerization.

of ring-opening of 89 and 42%, respectively. Unfortunately, SOCs 10 and 11 were crystalline compounds. Generally, the evaluation of SOCs in dental composite formulations showed the following serious disadvantages in the application of methylene-substituted SOC-monomers for free radically cured composites:

- The crystalline SOCs showed only a limited solubility in methacrylate based compositions. Therefore, the incorporation of a high SOC content in a composite formulation is almost impossible.
- The SOCs are less reactive than methacrylates, which significantly prolonged the necessary irradiation time.
- The low degree of ring-opening at room temperature results in a significant reduction of the shrinkage potential.
- The sensitivity of the SOCs to water, acidic compounds, and fillers decrease the storage stability of the uncured composites pastes.
- The polymers formed by the free-radical ring-opening polymerization of the SOCs show only a low UV-light stability and therefore the cured composites tend to be vulnerable to discoloration.

2.3.1.4 Cationic Ring-Opening Polymerization of SOCs and Cyclic Ethers

Nevertheless, the usefulness of SOCs as expanding monomers was first demonstrated for high-strength industrial composites based on the cationic ring-opening polymerization.[89,90] In this context, the most promising expanding SOC candidates were six-membered SOCs because the five- and seven-membered SOCs were reported to polymerize with elimination of small molecules in the presence of a cationic initiator.[14] Given these findings, cationic polymerizable, non–methylene-substituted, six-membered SOCs 12–15 (Figure 2.30) were evaluated as a component of photo-curable epoxy resins.[91–95] The crystalline SOC 12 (*trans*/*trans*-2,3,8,9-di(tetramethylene)-1,5,7,11-tetraoxaspiro[5.5]undecane, mp: 77°C) was polymerized in the presence of a cationic photoinitiator (4-octyloxyphenyl)-phenyliodonium hexafluoroantimonate by irradiation with UV light under ring-opening with an expansion of about 3.5 vol%.[91,92] In contrast, the influence of 30 wt% SOC 16 on the shrinkage of a UV-light cured three-component epoxy mixture based on diglycidyl ether of bisphenol A, 3,4-epoxycyclohexanemethyl-3,4-epoxycyclohexane carboxylate (DECHC), and vinylcyclohexene dioxide (weight ratio: 5:4:1) was negligibly small.[93] In this context, it is interesting to mention that the pure epoxy mixture

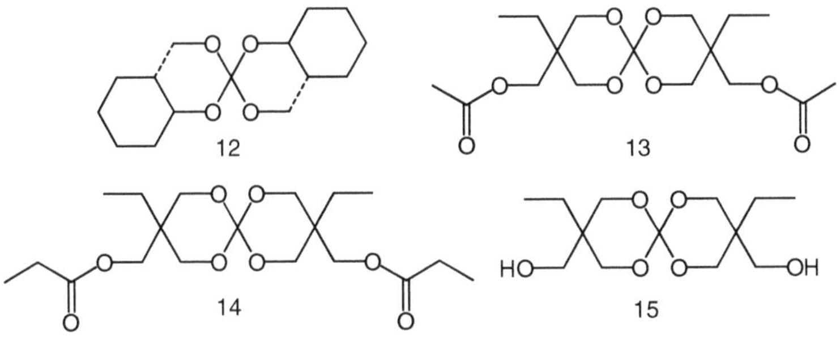

FIGURE 2.30 Cationic polymerizable SOC 13–15 evaluated for dental composites.

showed a polymerization shrinkage of only 0.3 vol%. The SOCs 13–15 were more reactive in a mixture of, for example, DECHC and poly(THF) (80/20), compared with SOC 13. However, the addition of SOC to the initial epoxy–polyol mixture resulted in a significant decrease in the reactivity of the UV-light–cured mixture.

In recent years, the application of cationic photopolymerizable epoxy-monomer based compositions for dental fillings have found increasing attention in patent applications.[96–98] Particularly, cross-linking cycloaliphatic epoxy compounds were of interest because they demonstrate significantly lower shrinkage than dental methacrylate resins. Moreover, these epoxy resins should be reactive enough to be cured by cationic photopolymerization in an acceptable time frame and to an adequate depth using a dental visible light (VL) source. Figure 2.31 shows one example of the composition of a proposed VL-cured composite that contained a mixture of two cationic polymerizable diepoxides: cycloaliphatic epoxide 16 (3,4-epoxycyclohexyl-methyl-3,4-epoxycyclohexane-carboxylate), which was more reactive than glycidyl compounds, and the diglycidyl ether of bisphenol A, which improved the mechanical properties of the cured composite. The poly(THF) as polyol influenced the physical properties in the permanently cured composition and the speed of photocure. Camphorquinone (CQ), which is currently the most frequently used photoinitiator in VL-curing dental filling materials, acted as the VL-sensitizer, while diphenyliodonium

Monomer:	9.43% Diglycidyl ether of bisphenol A
	9.14% Cycloaliphatic diepoxide 16
	4.66% Poly(THF) (molecular weight: 250)
Filler:	76.55% Quartz
Initiator:	0.11% CQ (visible light sensitizer)
	0.11% Iodonium salt 17

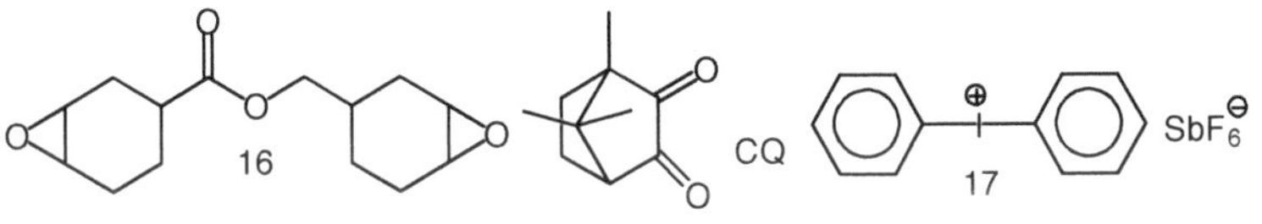

FIGURE 2.31 Composition (wt%) of a composite based on VL-curable epoxy resins.

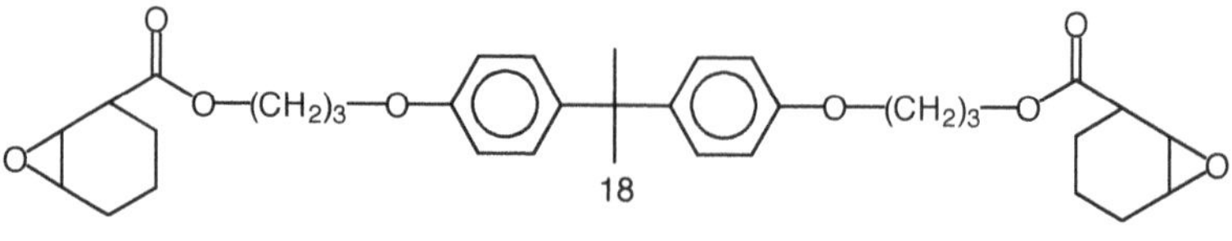

FIGURE 2.32 Bis-GMA-like cycloaliphatic epoxide 18.

hexafluoroantimonate 15 was used as the photoinitiator. Patented variations of these basic epoxy resin compositions mainly concern cycloaliphatic diepoxides, for example, the epoxides 16 and 18 (Figure 2.32); the application of other cationic photoinitiators, such as aromatic sulfonium or ferrocenium salts; and the addition of accelerating low basic amines, such as ethyl 4-dimethylaminobenzoate (EDMAB).[98] In addition to epoxy resins, oxetanes were evaluated for dental application.[99,100] The reactivity of oxetanes is mainly controlled by the ring stress and the basicity of the ring oxygen. The ring stress of oxetanes is similar to that of oxiranes. However, oxetanes demonstrate a higher basicity. Therefore, photoinitiators, such as sulfonium and iodonium salts, can be used for the cationic polymerization of oxetanes. The ring-opening polymerization of oxetanes was also characterized by a significantly lower shrinkage compared with methacrylates (Figure 2.33). From the investigated oxetanes, monomer 19, which contained a hydroxy group, showed the highest polymerization rate, while esters and urethanes were either nonpolymerizable or reacted with very low rates only. In addition, it was found that the polymerization reactivity of oxetanes was substantially affected by the type of atmosphere used. In an air atmosphere, oxetane photopolymerization showed an induction period, while the polymerization of oxetanes was greatly accelerated in nitrogen.[101] Generally, composites based on cyclic ethers showed some advantages in comparison with dimethacrylate materials, such as the lower polymerization shrinkage, no (epoxides) or low oxygen sensitivity, excellent adhesion properties, and chemical durability of the formed polymers. Furthermore, hybrid systems with methacrylates can be prepared, using the cyclic ethers as a basis. In spite of these advantages, the use of cationic ring-opening polymerization of cyclic ether currently also creates a number of problems, such as the lower cure speed at room temperature, sensitivity to bases (amines, urethanes or fillers), restricted storage stability in the presence of acidic impurities, and the toxicological risk of the epoxides and cationic photoinitiators. These problems have not been completely solved to date.

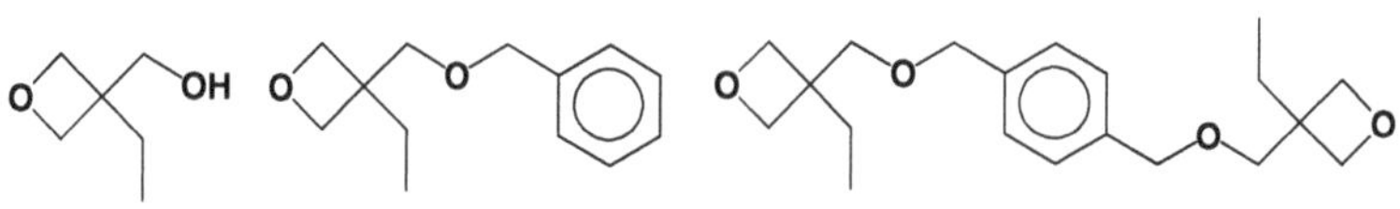

FIGURE 2.33 Volume shrinkage during the cationic photopolymerization of oxetanes 19–21 in the presence of *bis*-[4-(diphenylsulfonio)-phenyl]-sulfide-*bis*-hexafluorophosphate.

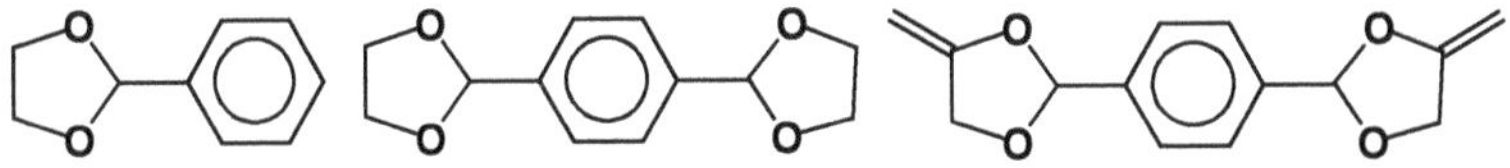

FIGURE 2.34 Non-inyl 22/23 and vinyl 1,3-dioxolanes 24 evaluated for dental composites.

2.3.1.5 Cyclic Acetales, Allyl Sulfides, and Vinylcyclopropanes

Among the heterocyclic monomers that show little or no volume changes upon polymerization, cyclic ketene acetals have found great interest because these monomers can undergo both free-radical and cationic ring-opening polymerization.[102] Thus, various 1,3-dioxolanes (Figure 2.34) were evaluated by Reed as a monomer component of VL-cured dental composites based on EBPDMA and the photoinitiator system CQ/EDMAB.[103] In contrast to the nonvinyl cyclic acetals 22 and 23, the composite based on a mixture of EBPDMA with the difunctional cyclic vinyl acetal 24 showed a tensile strength similar to that of the control example with only EBPDMA. In this context, a free-radical ring-opening mechanism under the formation of poly(alkylene-ether-ketone) was proposed for monomer 25 (2-phenyl-4-methylene-1,3-dioxolane, Figure 2.35). In the presence of DTBP at a temperature of about 125°C, monomer 25 underwent a mixed polymerization mechanism involving the elimination of benzaldehyde (Figure 2.36).[104] Monomer 25 also underwent an exclusive cationic ring-opening polymerization in the presence of photoinitiators, for example, such

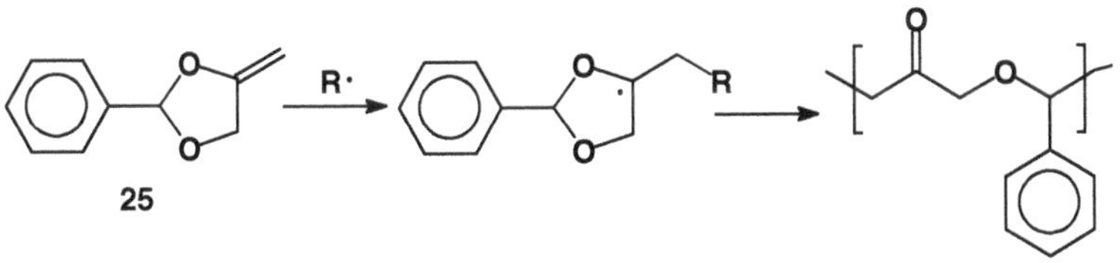

FIGURE 2.35 Proposed mechanism of free-radical ring-opening polymerization of monomer 25.

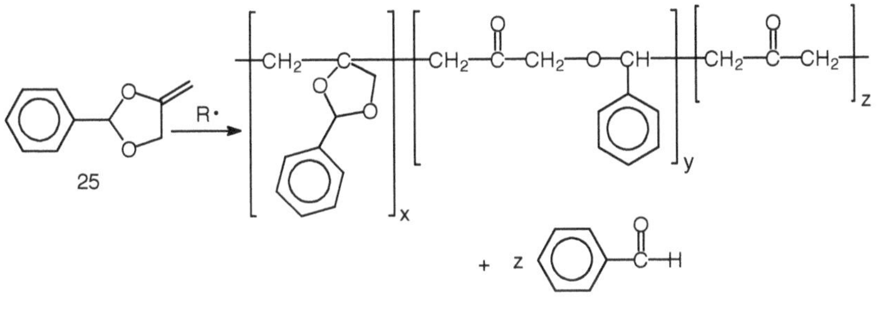

FIGURE 2.36 Formation of benzaldehyde in the polymerization of 25 in the presence of DTBP at 120°C.

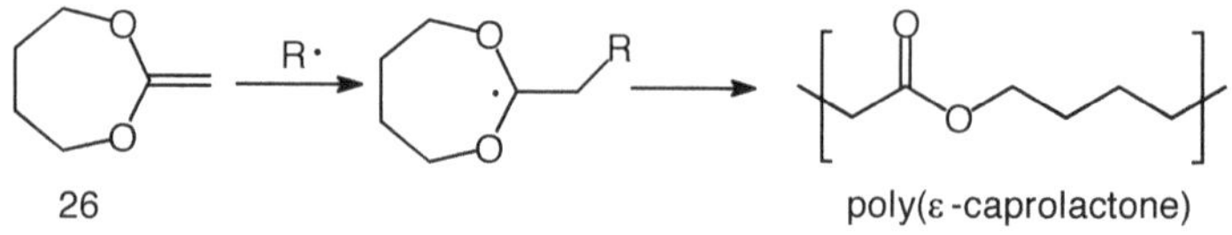

FIGURE 2.37 Mechanism of free-radical ring-opening polymerization of monomer 26.

as tris(methylphenyl)sulfonium hexafluoroantimonate or 4-(decyloxyphenyl) phenyliodonium hexafluoro-antimonate.[105] The glass transition temperatures (T_g) of the formed poly(alkylene-ether-ketone)s were in the range of 26–35°C, which was too low for dental applications. More promising polymers with a T_g between 52 and 67°C were synthesized by the copolymerization of 24 with 25.[106] Analogous to cyclic vinyl monomer 25, the seven-membered cyclic ketene acetal 2-methylene-1,3-dioxepane 26 underwent nearly complete ring-opening polymerization and resulted in essentially pure poly(ε-caprolactone) if polymerized with the free-radical initiator AIBN or with the photoinitiator benzoin isopropyl ether (Figure 2.37).[107] Furthermore, it was found that the free-radical ring-opening polymerization of 26 was accompanied by intramolecular hydrogen transfer during propagation under the formation of a flexible, branched polyester.[108] The 2-methylene-1,3-dioxepanes as electron-rich olifins were very sensitive to water and nucleophilic compounds, such as amines or alcohols. Furthermore, composite pastes based on conventional dental glass fillers and 2-methylene-1,3-dioxepanes were not storage stable and demonstrated a tendency to spontaneous hardening after some days, which is probably caused by the acidic silanol surface groups of the glass filler particles.[109] Finally, 2-methylene-1,3-dioxepanes were significantly less reactive than methacrylates, which resulted in an unacceptable increase in the curing times. In contrast to the cyclic ketene acetals, cyclic allyl sulfides are stable in the presence of water, and these monomers, for example, 6-methylene-1,4-dithiepane 27 or 3-methylene-1,5-dithiacyclooctane 28 (Figure 2.38), readily survived the exposure to aqueous bases and acids.[110] The cyclic allyl sulfides underwent a free-radical ring-opening polymerization in the presence of AIBN under formation of high molecular crystalline homopolymers. Therefore, they showed a shrinkage of about 8.6 (27) and 6.7% (28), respectively. In this context, various liquid difunctional 6-methylene-1,4-dithiepanes, for example, monomers 29–31 (Figure 2.39), were synthesized.[111] They formed cross-linked polymers and were, therefore, interesting for composites. For the application of cyclic allyl sulfides in the dental field, the main problems were the significantly lower reactivity of these monomers in comparison with methacrylates and the high flexibility of the amorphous structure of the formed polymers.

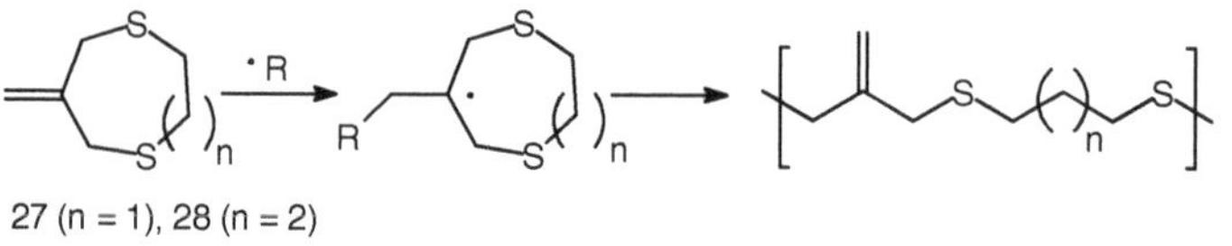

FIGURE 2.38 Free-radical ring-opening polymerization of cyclic allyl sulfides 27 and 28.

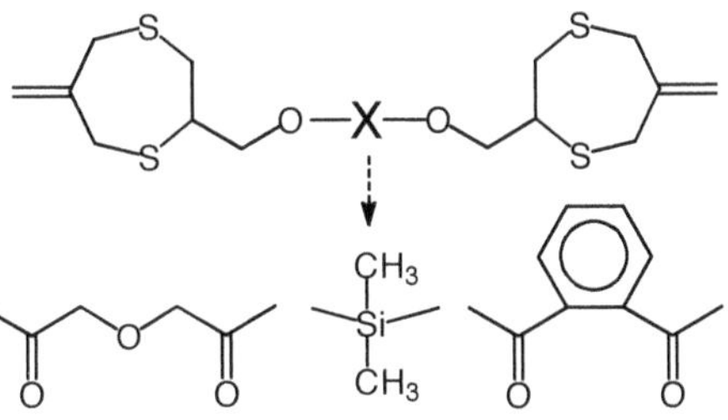

FIGURE 2.39 Structure of liquid difunctional 6-methylene-1,4-dithiepanes 29–31.

2-Vinylcyclopropanes (VCP) are also well-known as low-shrinking free-radical polymerizable monomers.[112] The free-radical ring-opening tendency of the relatively easily accessible 1,1-disubstituted VCP is increased by both radical-stabilizing and electron-withdrawing groups. Therefore, the free-radical bulk polymerization of 1,1-diethoxycarbonyl-2-vinylcyclopropane 32 in the presence of AIBN at 60°C yielded a polymer with almost exclusively 1,5–ring-opened repeating units A, whereas at higher temperature, for example, at 80°C (DBPO), polymers with additional units, probably cyclobutane rings B, were formed (Figure 2.40).[113] Based on these results, the synthesis of cross-linking 1,1-disubstituted VCPs 33–35 (Figure 2.41) was developed.[114,115]

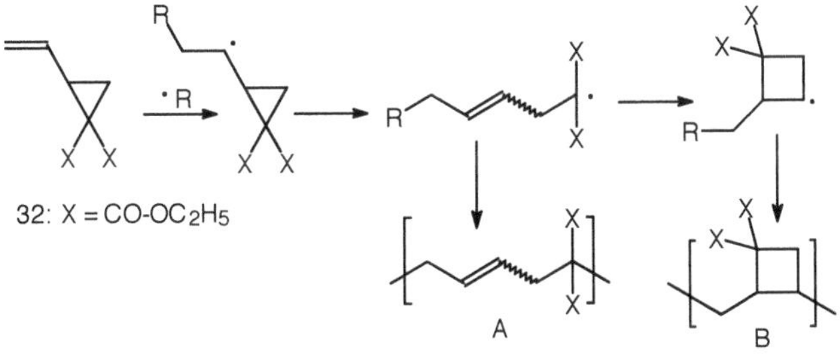

FIGURE 2.40 Free-radical ring-opening polymerization of VCP 32.

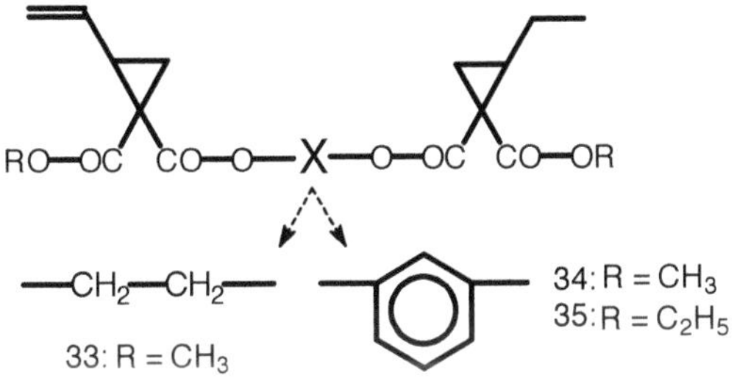

FIGURE 2.41 Cross-linking 1,1-disubstituted 2-vinylcyclopropanes 33–35.

Monomers 33 and 35 were viscous liquids, while monomer 34 was a crystalline compound. The monomers 34 and 35 were polymerized in bulk in the presence of AIBN at 65°C and resulted in hard transparent polymers, which were completely insoluble in organic solvents. In this respect, bulk polymerization was accompanied by a change in volume of +1.0% (34) and 3.9% (35), respectively. The expansion in volume was explained with the transition of the denser structure of the crystalline monomer to the less compressed structure of the amorphous polymer formed. The cross-linking VCPs 35 showed a low oral toxicity (LD_{50} > 2000 mg/kg), no mutagenicity, and a lower cytotoxicity than the commonly used cross-linking methacrylates. Moreover, the cross-linking VCP were stable in the presence of humidity, acid or basic impurities, as well as inorganic fillers, such as silica or glass powder. These properties and the low volume shrinkage during the polymerization of the cross-linking VCPs make them attractive as a monomer component in dental filling materials. Thus, monomer 35 was able to modify the shrinking kinetics of dental composites, yielding a reduced amount of marginal failure and microleakage in *in vitro* experiments.[116]

In general, it can be summarized that although the polymerization shrinkage has been one of the main shortcomings of resin-based composites since their introduction, the ring-opening polymerization of cyclic monomers has not been successfully achieved for commercial dental filling materials to date. This is mainly caused by the excessive basic requirements, which have to be fulfilled (Figure 2.20) by the monomers used for composite restoratives.

2.3.2 Liquid-crystalline Monomers

2.3.2.1 Liquid-Crystalline State and Liquid-Crystalline Polymers

Liquid crystalline (LC) compounds show a LC state in their phase diagram, which on the one hand has the viscosity of liquids, and on the other hand shows the physical anisotropic characteristic of crystalline solids. An LC phase is found only in those substances whose molecules have a pronounced shape anisotropy. These so-called mesogenic molecules, have, for example, a rod- or disk-shaped structure. In the case of thermotropic LC compounds, the LC phase is formed by the melting of the LC compound. The structure of the LC phase, which is determined by the chemical composition of the mesogenic group, is classified into three types: nematic, cholesteric, and smectic phase.[117] For example, in the nematic phase, the molecules tend to be parallel to the common axis, and the preferred axis of orientation varies from point to point in the medium, whereas in a smectic A phase the molecules are parallel to one another and are arranged in layers (Figure 2.42). In the case of LC polymers, the macromolecules have a rigid rod- or disklike structure or contain mesogenic groups as monomer units. In LC main chain polymers, the mesogenic group is located in the polymer main chain.[118] In LC side chain polymers, the mesogenic group is attached to the polymer main chain in a side-chain–like manner (Figure 2.43). In the context with LC thermosets, a number of papers and patents have been issued on LC cross-linking monomers.[119] The polymerization of these monomers resulted in isotropic or anisotropic LC networks, depending on the monomer structure (mesogenic, spacer, and polymerizable group) and the conditions of the cross-linking polymerization. The favorable properties of LC monomers with a designed molecular

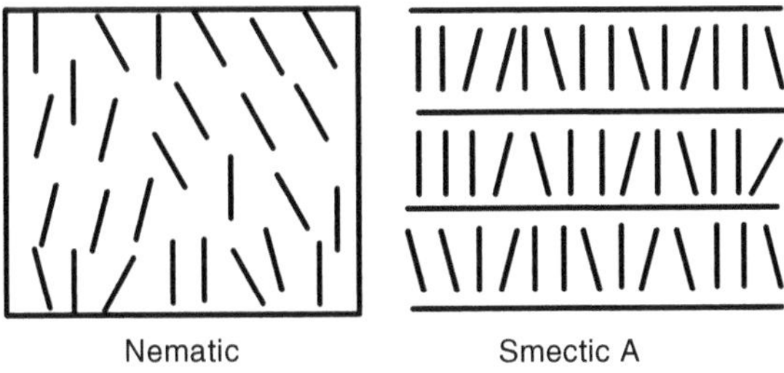

FIGURE 2.42 Schematic representation of molecular arrangements in LC nematic and smectic A phases.

structure are as follows: relatively low viscosity and lower polymerization shrinkage of the preordered monomers than that of the corresponding ordinary linear monomers. Accordingly, it was shown that the photoinitiated polymerization of LC diacrylates, for example, 1,4-phenylene *bis*[4-(6-acryloyloxy)alkyloxybenzoate]s (Figure 2.44), proceeded at a significantly higher rate in the LC state than in the crystalline state, led to a high degree of conversion of the acrylate groups, and was accompanied by a lower polymerization shrinkage than that commonly observed for conventional diacrylates.[120,121] Maximal reduction of shrinkage was achieved if the polymerization of the LC cross-linking monomer resulted in an amorphous polymer network rather than in a polymer network with a LC structure.

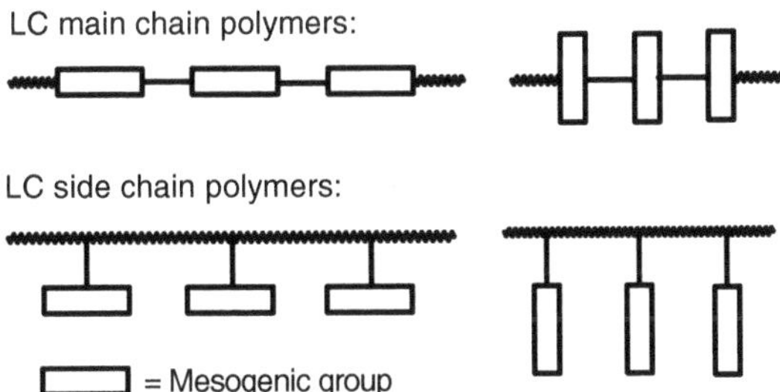

FIGURE 2.43 Structure of LC main and side chain polymers with rodlike mesogenic groups.

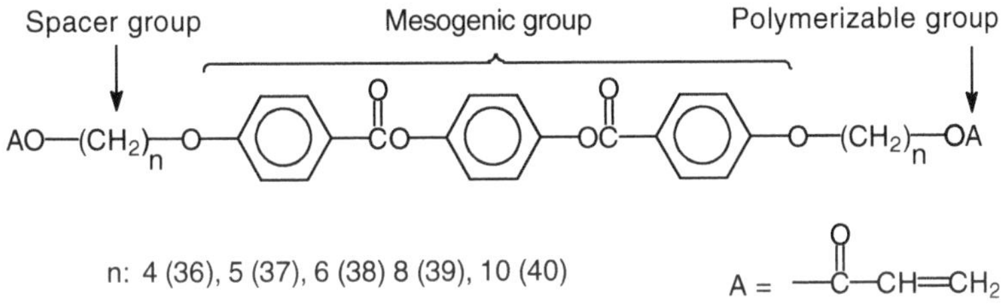

Spacer group Mesogenic group Polymerizable group

AO—(CH2)n—O—C6H4—CO—O—C6H4—O—OC—C6H4—O—(CH2)n—OA

n: 4 (36), 5 (37), 6 (38) 8 (39), 10 (40)

A = —C(=O)—CH=CH2

FIGURE 2.44 Examples of LC diacrylates.

2.3.2.2 Liquid-Crystalline Cross-linkers

In addition to the ring-opening polymerization of cyclic monomers, use of preordered, i.e., LC, cross-linkers is the second basic concept used to achieve a low-shrinkge photopolymerization system. Unfortunately, almost all of the described di(meth)acrylates melted at temperatures higher than 80°C, resulting in complicated curing conditions, as well as restricted practical relevance. To circumvent these problems, researchers had to synthesize new LC di(meth)acrylates that exhibited a melting temperature near or below room temperature. This was achieved by modifying the spacer length, introducing suitable substituents in the mesogenic group, and varying the mesogenic group, respectively.[122–124] It was very delicate to achieve a balance between introducing pendant groups on the LC molecules to reduce the temperature range of the crystalline phase stability and avoiding too much structural perturbation of the monomer structure, which may result in the loss of the LC character. Some successful examples are diacrylate 41 (Figure 2.45), which is a nematic LC monomer that demonstrated a polymerization shrinkage of approximately 2.1 vol%, and monomer 42, for which a volume contraction of about 1.3 vol% was measured during photopolymerization.[122,123] A decrease of the transformation temperature of LC monomers was also achieved by the preparation of a mixture of two LC monomers or of a solution of a low-melting crystalline monomer and a comonomer as the solvent. Finally, branched LC bismethacrylates were proposed as an additional group of ambient-temperature LC cross-linking methacrylates.[125,126] The general structure of these branched monomers consisted of a rigid linear bismethacrylate central unit, linked with mesogenic groups via flexible alkyl spacers, as shown by bismethacrylates 43 and 44 (Figure 2.46). The branched structure was expected to impede crystallization yet not disable the mesophase formation. The branched monomer 43 exhibited a nematic phase between 18 and 67°C, while monomer 44 showed both a stable smectic C* phase (15–34°C) and a cholesteric phase (34–58°C). The photopolymerization of the branched bismethacrylates at ambient temperature resulted in cross-linked anisotropic polymer networks without remarkable changes in the

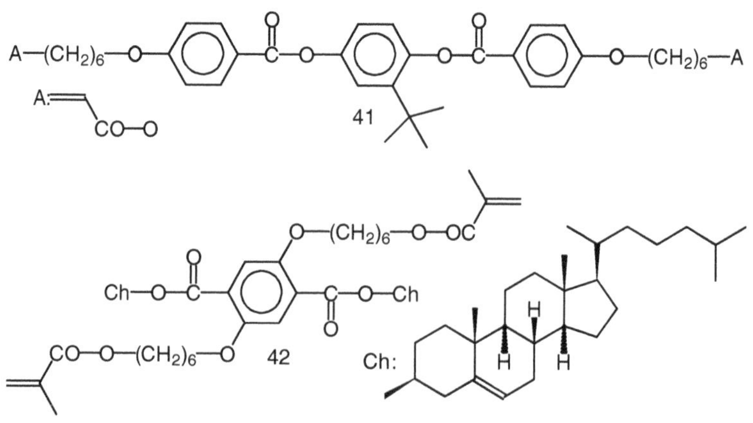

FIGURE 2.45 Cross-linking LC di(meth)acrylates 41 and 42.

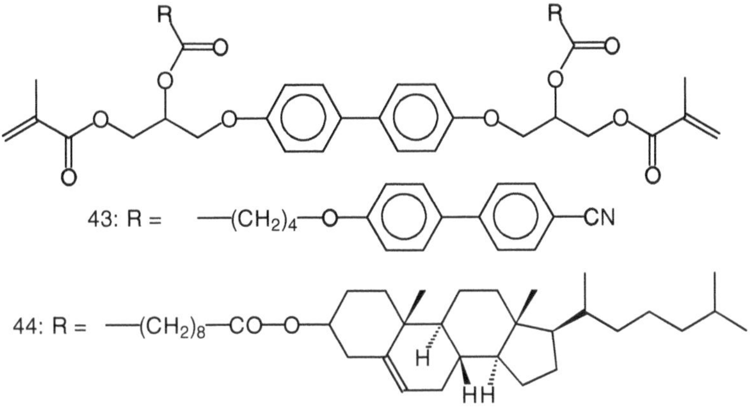

43: R = —(CH2)4—O—⟨◯⟩—⟨◯⟩—CN

44: R = —(CH2)8—CO—O—

FIGURE 2.46 Branched ambient-temperature LC bismethacrylates 43 and 44.

structure of the mesophase. In other words, the LC structure of the monomers was "frozen in" by the photoinduced cross-linking. In the case of monomer 43, the volume shrinkage during photopolymerization was approximately 2.5%. In summary, ambient-temperature LC cross-linking monomers are very promising as matrix monomers for photopolymerizable composites because of their low polymerization shrinkage, relatively low viscosity, and high monomer conversion. However, additional components of a composite, such as isotropic liquid comonomers or fillers may influence the LC formation. Furthermore, the synthesis of a LC monomer is more expensive. In addition, the resulting polymer network tends to be more flexible, which may impair the mechanical properties.

2.3.3 Branched and Dendritic Monomers

2.3.3.1 Branched and Dendritic Polymers

In the past decade dendrimers and hyperbranched polymers have received enormous attention as new polymer materials because their properties differ significantly from those of linear polymers.[127–131] These cascade polymers are globular macromolecules with a great number of reactive end groups that are characterized by a highly branched structure in which all bonds converge to a focal point or core (Figure 2.47). In contrast to hyperbranched polymers, dendrimers are perfect monodisperse macromolecules with a regular three-dimensional architecture. Dendrimers are built of AB_x-monomers coupled in several layers around a central core molecule where each layer is called a generation (Figure 2.47: first, second, third generation). Therefore, the degree of branching (DB), which defines the ratio of branched, terminal, and linear units in the polymer structure, is 100% in dendrimers. Hyperbranched polymers show a DB less than 100%, and exhibit a broad molar mass distribution and a statistical distribution of the functional groups throughout the structure. The physicochemical properties of dendrimers and hyperbranched polymers are sometimes in contrast to the behavior of linear polymers. For example, they show

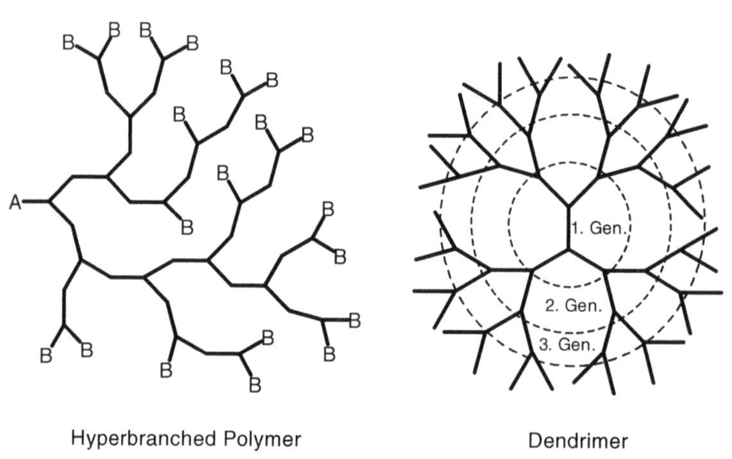

Hyperbranched Polymer

Dendrimer

FIGURE 2.47 Schematic representation of a hyperbranched polymer and dendrimer.

a higher solubility and a lower solution viscosity compared with the linear analogs, which is important for their application in composites. The synthesis of a regular dendrimer is in general a multistage reaction, which includes an extension and deprotection stage for every generation. For example, in case of the first commercialized poly(propylene imine) dendrimers, the extension stage is an exhaustive Michael-type addition of acrylonitrile to an amine (core), followed by the reduction of the nitrile groups to primary amines (Figure 2.48).[132] In contrast to this, hyperbranched polymers can be rapidly prepared, often in a one-stage process, and are a more economical replacement for perfect dendrimers in special applications.

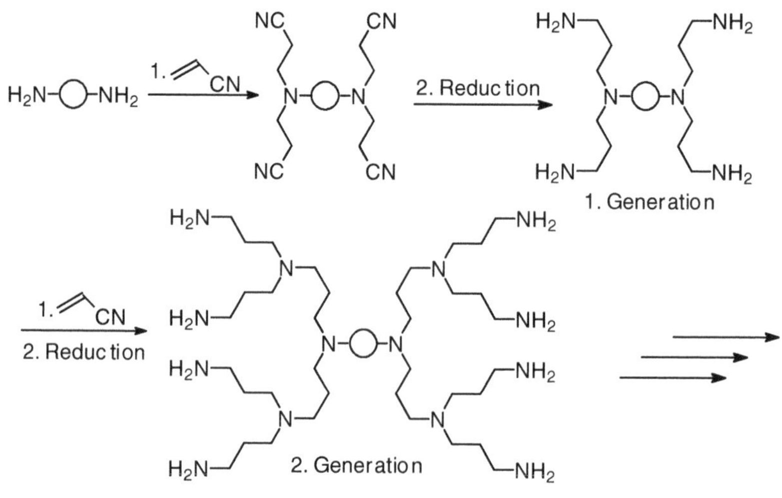

FIGURE 2.48 Synthetic scheme of poly(propylene imine) dendrimers.

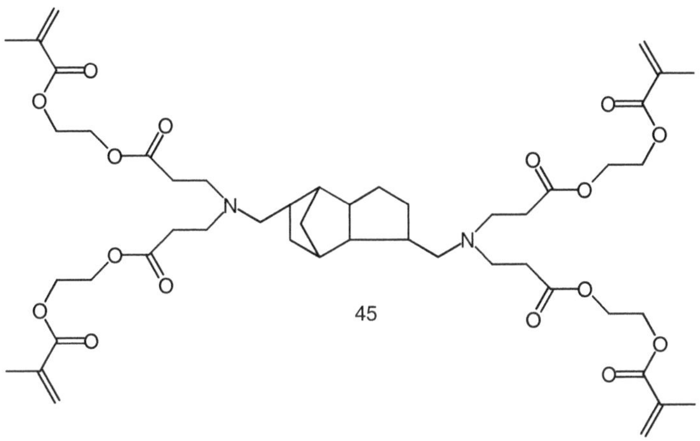

45

FIGURE 2.49 Branched low viscous tetramethacrylate 45.

2.3.3.2 Branched and Dendritic Methacrylates

The volume shrinkage should be lower when the number of polymerizable moieties is reduced by using larger molecules. In this context, dendrimers or hyperbranched polymers may represent an interesting alternative. Therefore, these polymers were synthesized and evaluated for dental composites, which demonstrated both low viscosity and low polymerization shrinkage at the same time.[133,134] The branched methacrylate 45 (Figure 2.49), for example, was synthesized by simple Michael addition of technical 3,(4),8,(9)-*bis*(aminomethyltricyclodecane and 2-(acryloyloxy) ethyl methacrylate. Monomer 45 (molecular weight: 931) showed both a lower viscosity η of about 150 mPa·s in comparison to Bis-GMA (molecular weight: 512; η: approximately 1000 Pa·s) and a lower polymerization shrinkage of approximately 2.9% (Bis-GMA: 6.0%). According to these results, the polymerization shrinkage of a corresponding VL-cured composite based on a monomer mixture of 45 and Bis-GMA (3.5:1.5) with a filler content of approximately 72% was as low as 1.1%. Unfortunately, the flexural strength (52 MPa) and the modulus of elasticity (5960 MPa) of this composite were also lower. This finding was true for branched methacrylates with more flexible aliphatic spacers in particular.[133] Branched macromonomers and hyperbranched polyester methacrylates showed a similar behavior. In other words, they demonstrated low monomer viscosity and low polymerization shrinkage, as well as high flexibility of the formed polymer networks and poor mechanical properties of the corresponding composites. More promising results were obtained by starting from dendritic Boltron® polyols (Perstorp, Sweden), which were modified by the reaction with methacrylic anhydride or methacryloyl chloride.[135,136] The addition of the obtained hyperbranched multimethacrylates to a mixture of Bis-GMA/TEGDMA (1:1) resulted in both improved mechanical properties and reduced free monomer leaching. Recently, a series of aliphatic and aromatic hyperbranched polyesters were synthesized and functionalized with methacrylic acid and carboxylic acids.[137] The synthesis of the aliphatic polyester using trimethylolpropane (TMP)

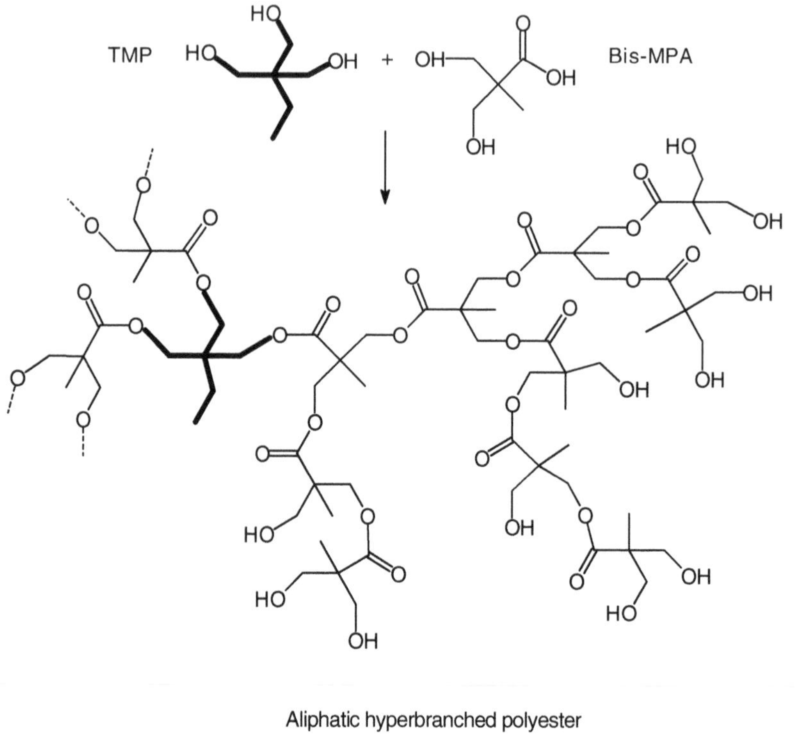

Aliphatic hyperbranched polyester

FIGURE 2.50 Synthesis of a hyperbranched polyester starting from TMP and Bis-MPA.

and 2,3-bishydroxymethylpropionic acid (Bis-MPA) (Figure 2.50) resulted in viscous polymers with a DB of 0.47 and a degree of polymerization (P_n) of 16.5. The solid aromatic hyperbranched polyesters, which were synthesized using TMP and 2,2-bis (4-hydroxypheny)pivalonic acid, showed a similar DB (0.48) and a higher P_n (30.5). The methacryloyl terminated aliphatic hyperbranched polyesters showed a relatively low viscosity ranging from 200–364 Pa·s and exhibited a low volume shrinkage (1.9 to 3.6%) during their photopolymerization. The corresponding dental composites, which were prepared using these methacryloyl terminated aliphatic hyperbranched polyesters in combination with a Ba-alumosilicate glass filler, showed a volume shrinkage of only 0.5 to 1.5%. Finally, it was found that flexible dendritic methacrylates can be used to modify the rheological behavior of composites.[138] The dendritic cross-linking plurifunctional methacrylates were synthesized by the Michael addition of 2-(acryloyloxy)ethyl methacrylate with the aminofunctional poly(propyleneimine) dendrimers from DSM (Netherlands). Depending on the generation of the starting dendrimer, plurifunctional methacrylates with 32 (dendrimers of the second generation) to 128 methacrylic groups per molecule (dendrimers of the fifth generation) were obtained. It was surprising that all synthesized dendritic methacrylates were liquids. The methacrylated dendrimer of the fifth generation, for example, demonstrated a viscosity of approximately 7 Pa·s, although the calculated molecular weight of this plurifunctional monomer was about 30,700. This occurrence can be explained by both the high flexibility of the poly(propyleneimine) dendrimer structure and the well-known fact that the intrinsic viscosity of dendrimers did not increase linearly with molecular weight.[129] According to the flexibility of the obtained dendritic monomers, almost every methacrylic double bond took part in the free-radical polymerization in the presence of AIBN. Starting from a mixture of these dendritic methacrylates (20%) with Bis-GMA (approximately 40%), UDMA (20%), and TEGDMA (20%), a composite paste with a filler content of approximately 80% was prepared. After the kneading procedure, the paste obtained was a fine-grained, dry-looking material. However, it turns into a paste with a flowable consistency under compressive or shear stress and, therefore, can be processed like amalgam. The explanation of this rheological behavior is that the dendritic methacrylates acted as a molecular sponge for the diluent monomer. When exposed to compressive or shear stress, the dendrimers release the monomer.

Basically, hyperbranched or dendritic methacrylates are very promising monomers for the preparation of low-shrinking composites because of their relatively low viscosity and efficient incorporation into the formed polymer network. However, for a successful application in dentistry, those monomers that will produce polymer networks with improved mechanical properties have to be synthesized.

2.3.4 Monomers for Compomers

One type of photocurable dental filling material is represented by composites known as compomers, also referred to as polyacid-modified composite resins.[139,140] The term "compomer" is a combination of the terms *compo*site and glass iono*mer* and is used to describe water-free, single-component, light-cured composites consisting of acid-modified dimethacrylate reinforced with silanized calcium-, strontium- or barium-aluminium-fluorosilicate glass particles (Figure 2.51), which were well-known from glass ionomers.[141] Compomers were developed to improve the physical properties and the clinical handling of glass-ionomer cements, which were formed by the acid–base reaction of an aqueous polymeric acid and an ion-leachable glass. The structure of proposed compomer monomers is characterized by the presence of at least two polymerizable methacrylic residues and acid groups, such as the bis(2-hydroxyethyl methacrylate) esters of an aliphatic butane 1,2,3,4-tetracarboxylic

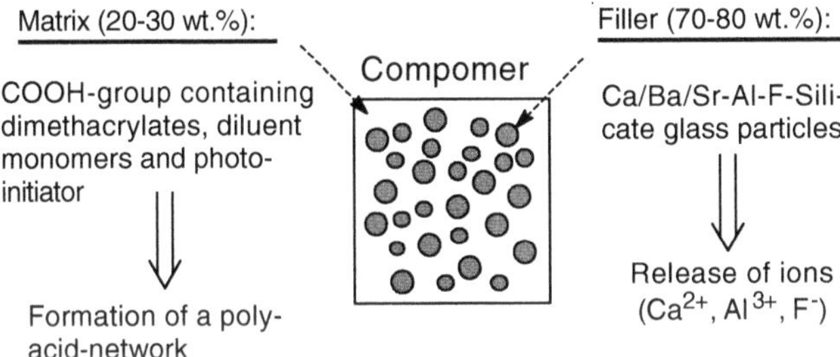

FIGURE 2.51 Composition of a compomer.

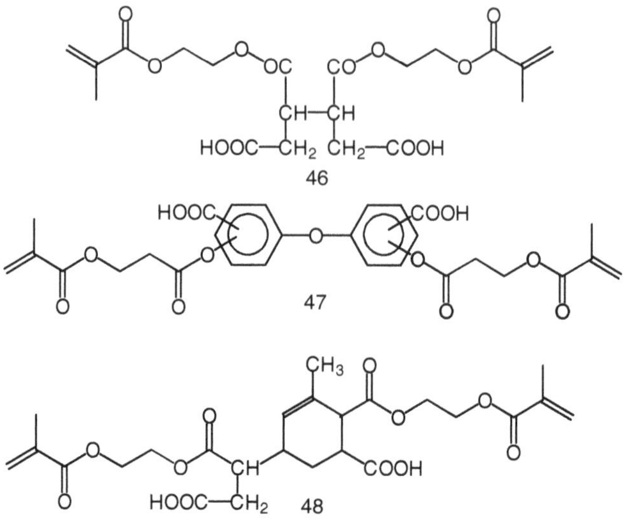

FIGURE 2.52 COOH-containing dimethacrylates 46–48 for copomers.

acid 46, of an aromatic tetracarboxylic acid 47, or a cycloaliphatic or tetracarboxylic acids 48 (Figure 2.52).[143–146] Finally, compomers based on oligomeric polyacids, for example, the reaction product of oligomeric poly(acrylic acid) (P_n of about 10) with glycidyl methacrylate (GMA) were prepared (49, Figure 2.53).[147] Basically, these compomer monomers were able to react simultaneously with the methacrylate groups by free-radical polymerization and by an acid–base neutralization reaction, with the cations released from the glass particles by the action of water. However, in the absence of water, the neutralization reaction did not occur and, therefore, the setting of compomers can only be achieved by VL-initiated polymerization of the monomers under the formation of a polymeric covalent network. In the presence of water from the environment, a limited acid–base reaction was observed.[148] This acid–base reaction of irradiated materials stored in water took place on the surface and reached a saturation point after approximately 4 weeks. Moreover, it was discovered by means of electron spin resonance spectroscopy that the storage of

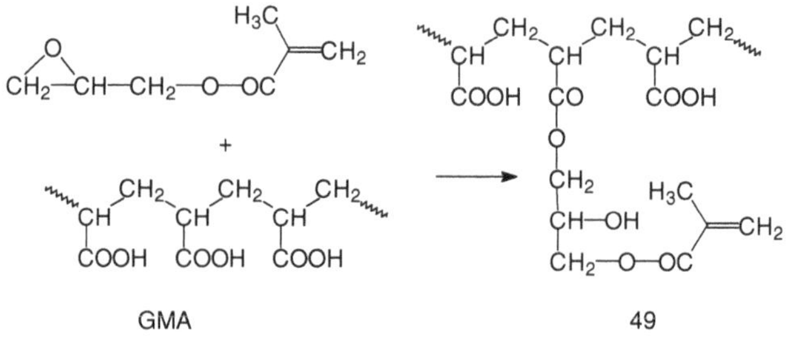

FIGURE 2.53 Synthesis of GMA-modified poly(acrylic acid).

TABLE 2.7
Properties of Composites, Compomers, and Glass-Ionomer Cements (GIC)

	Composite	Compomer	GIC
Flexural strength (MPa)	100–145	90–125	30–60
Compressive strength (MPa)	280–480	200–260	100–200
Modulus of elasticity (GPa)	10–25	5–8	5–20
Release of fluoride ions (μg/cm^2)	0–10	30–60	50–600

VL-cured compomers in water or ethanol also influenced the life cycle of the free radicals that were trapped.[149] All compomers showed a decrease in both compressive and flexural strength, which is caused by water-induced degradation of the matrix–filler interface in the compomers. Although compomers were developed to combine the favorable properties of composite resins (high values of mechanical properties, good clinical handling, and low effect of water on the material's stiffness) and glass–ionomer cements (no polymerization shrinkage, adhesion to the tooth structure, and fluoride release), their behavior (Table 2.7) is more similar to that of composite resins than to that of glass ionomers.[150,151]

2.3.5 Ormocers

In addition to the classical composite filling materials, which are based on cross-linking dimethacrylates and inorganic fillers, a new type of inorganic–organic hybrid dental materials, known as ormocers have been developed.[152,153] Ormocer stands for *or*ganically *mo*dified *cer*amic. The aim was to improve the composites by improving marginal adaptation, abrasion resistance, and biocompatibility. *In vitro* studies confirmed that ormocers demonstrate favorable abrasion resistance.[154] Their marginal adaptation is comparable with that of conventional composites in conjunction with the adhesive technology.[155,156] Improvement in biocompatibility can only be achieved if no diluting monomer, such as TEGDMA, is used to reduce the viscosity of the corresponding condensate. Ormocers can be prepared by sol–gel processing of organofunctional metal alkoxides such as chloro or alkoxy silanes, which contain polymerizable groups P or functional groups R (Figure 2.54). The hydrolysis of these silanes resulted in oligomeric polysiloxanes (Figure 2.55).[157]

These oligomers may replace the conventional monomers in the dental composites. The composite in a second stage is hardened by linking the the polymerizable groups and forming a three-dimensional network (Figure 2.56). The hybrids formed are composites in which the organic and inorganic components are combined on a nanoscopic or molecular scale. Therefore, these materials not only show the properties of both pure organic and inorganic components, but they also have the potential of providing properties that have been unknown to date and that make these materials very attractive for use in dental materials. In addition to alkoxy silanes, other metal alkoxides, such as Ti, Zr or Al alkoxides, can be condensated or cocondensated with

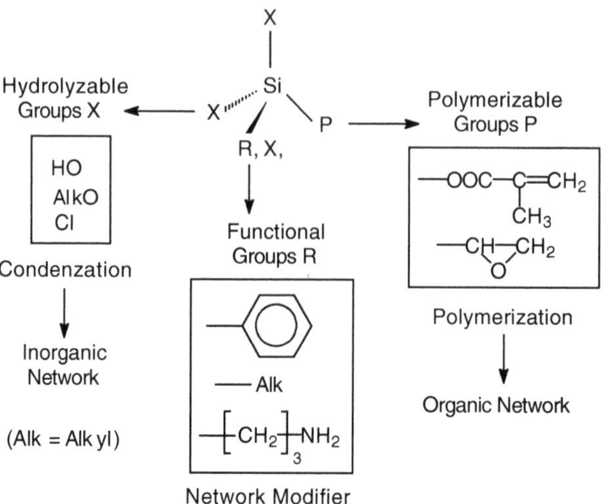

FIGURE 2.54 Chemical structure variations of ormocer silanes.

alkoxy silanes (Figure 2.56).[158,159] An example of a methacrylate functionalized alkoxy silane used in dentistry is reaction product 50 of (3-isocyanatopropyl)-triethoxysilane (IPTES) with glycerol dimethacrylate (GDMA) (Figure 2.57).[153,157] The main problem is that the condensates of silane 50 show a very high viscosity, comparable with that of Bis-GMA. A high filler load and good handling properties of the composite are obtained by diluting the condensate with a low viscous monomer such as TEGDMA. In this case, the biocompatibility requirements are no longer fulfilled. Recently, the cross-linking silanes 51 were synthesized, the condensates of which demonstrate a viscosity in the range of 1–15 Pa·s.[160] By Michael addition of 2-acryloyloxyethylmethacrylate (AEMA) with (3-aminopropyl)triethoxysilane (APTES) the methacrylate-functionalized amino silane 51 was obtained in a yield

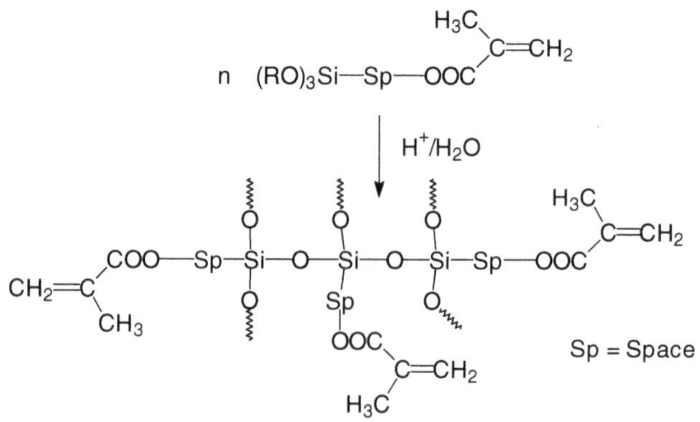

FIGURE 2.55 Hydrolytic condensation of a trialkoxysilanemethacrylate under formation of Si-O-Si nanostructures.

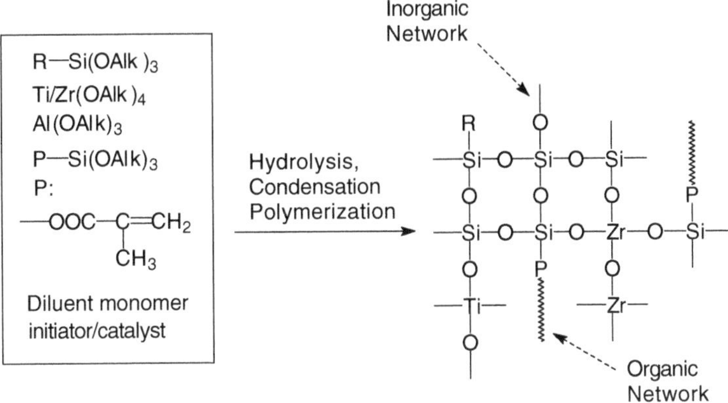

FIGURE 2.56 Formation of an organic-inorganic hybrid material by hydrolytic condensation and polymerization of functionalized alkoxy silanes.

of 99% (Figure 2.58). The hydrolytic condensation of alkoxy silanes in the presence of ammonium fluoride (NH_4F), for example, results in linear and branched oligomeric amorphous Si-O-Si structures.

The problem of methacrylate-functionalized silanes is that the polymerization shrinkage of their condensates is still too high, which has been confirmed by *in vitro* investigations. The marginal adaptation of ormocer composites is comparable with that of conventional composites.[155,156] This was the reason for combining non- or low-shrinking polyreaction systems with the sol–gel process. It is well known that the thiolene polyaddition proceeds with a low volume contraction. Suitable norbornene silanes have already been synthesized (Figure 2.59).[161,162] The reaction of the corresponding condensates with pentaerythritol tetra(3-mercaptopropionate) (PETMP) showed a volume contraction of only 0.5%.[163] The resulting polymers are relatively flexible, which means that the corresponding composites show low mechanical properties.

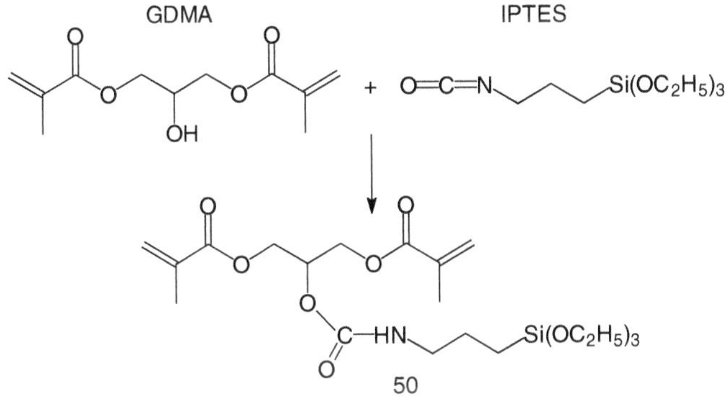

GDMA + IPTES → 50

FIGURE 2.57 Synthesis of silane 50 by the reaction of IPTES with GDMA.

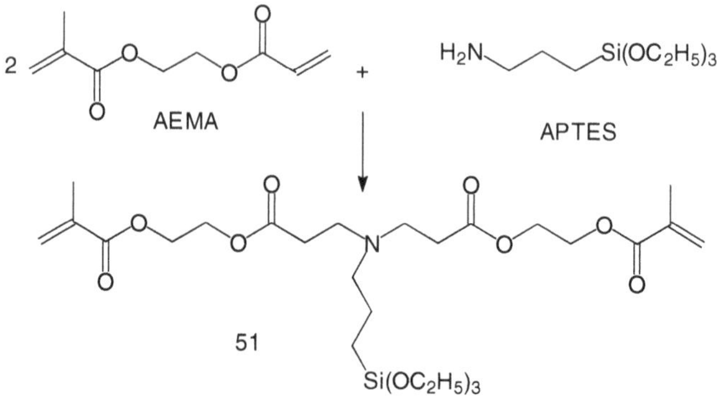

FIGURE 2.58 Synthesis of silane 51 by Michael addition of AEMA with APTES.

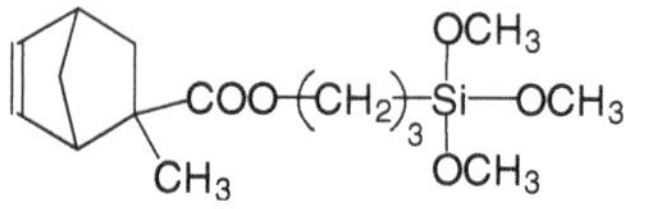

FIGURE 2.59 Example of a norbornene-functionalized silane 52.

Composite filling materials based on the ormocer technology that are currently available on the market are not pure ormocer systems. Diluent monomers are used to adjust the viscosity of the condensate. To avoid elusion of unreacted substances, a biocompatible formulation should at least be free of monomer. Furthermore, a substantial improvement of the abrasion resistance, compared with the conventional dental composites, has to be achieved.

2.3.6 Fluorinated Bis-GMA Analogs and Substitutes

At present, most of the commercially available VL-curing restorative materials contain Bis-GMA, which was synthesized by Bowen from bisphenol A and GDMA.[164] The reason for the dominance of Bis-GMA is that this bulky, difunctional monomer has relatively low polymerization shrinkage (≈6.0%), rapid hardening by free-radical photopolymerization, and low volatility. Furthermore, it results in cured materials that exhibit favorable mechanical properties. However, the deficiencies of Bis-GMA, i.e., the high viscosity (1.0–1.2 kPa·s at 23°C), the water susceptibility, and the relatively low degree of double-bond conversion of light-cured Bis-GMA-based materials and their proneness to brittle fracture and wear, have stimulated the development of fluorinated Bis-GMA analogs and monomers, which may substitute for Bis-GMA.

2.3.6.1 Fluorinated Bis-GMA Analogs

Fluorocarbon-containing polymers have low surface energies, are highly hydrophobic, and display excellent resistance to softening in conjunction with a wide range of

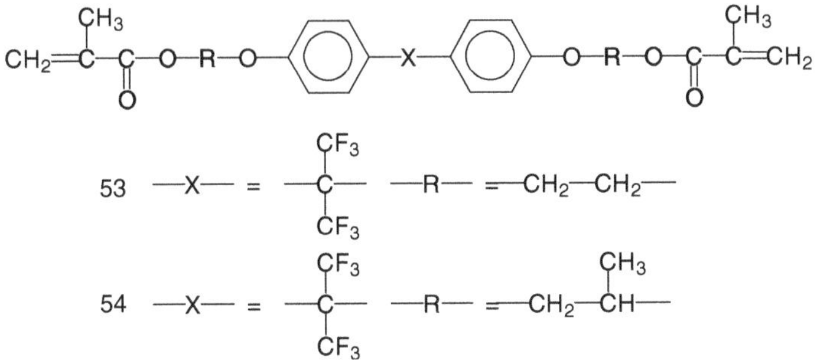

FIGURE 2.60 Structure of semifluorinated Bis-GMA analogs 53 and 54.

chemicals. Furthermore, the potential resistance to staining and microbial attachment, as well as the generally good biocompatibility, make fluorinated polymers very attractive for dental application. For example, the new semifluorinated aromatic dimethacrylate monomers 53 and 54 (Figure 2.60) demonstrated a significantly lower viscosity (0.8–1.3 Pa·s) and exhibited a higher conversion of methacrylate double bonds for isothermal polymerization at 80°C.[165] Moreover, materials based on 53 and 54 showed a lower water uptake and thus higher Vickers hardness values of water-saturated samples compared with Bis-GMA-based materials.[166] The influence of the monomer structure and fluorine content on resin and composite properties was systematically studied using dimethacrylate monomers 55–58 (Figure 2.61) with varying fluorine content and distribution as a basis.[167–170] Resin formulations based on dimethacrylates 55–58 were prepared with equimolar proportions of

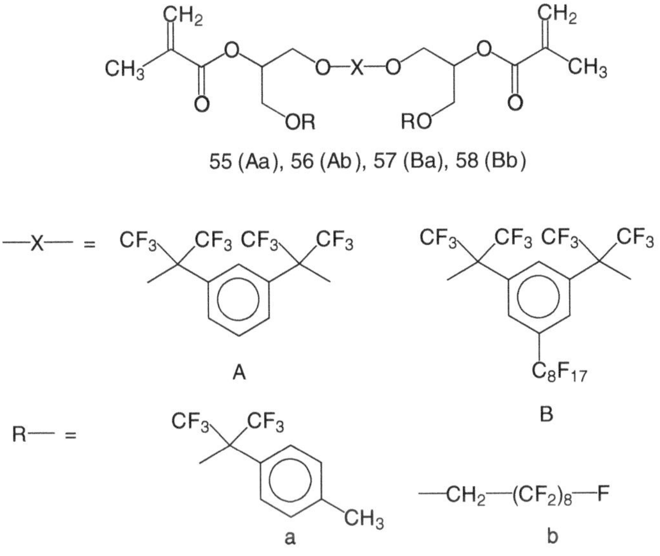

FIGURE 2.61 Structure of fluorinated monomers 55–58.

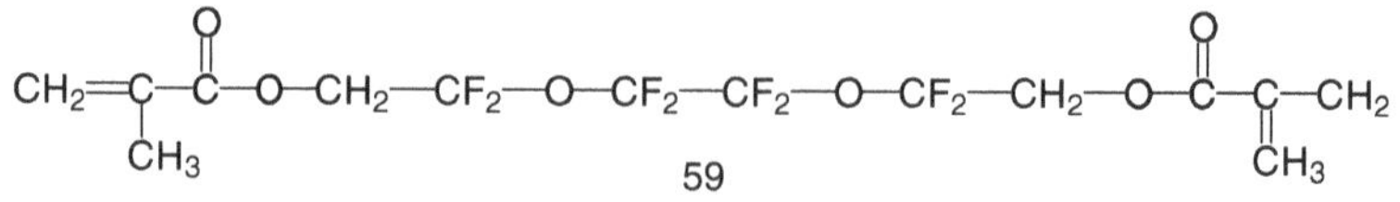

FIGURE 2.62 Fluorinated triethyleneglycol dimethacrylate 59.

1,10-decamethylene dimethacrylate, as well as of 0.2 wt% of CQ and 0.8 wt% of EDMAB as the photoinitiators. Fused quartz (60 wt%) was mixed with the resins to provide photopolymerizable composite pastes. The results of the investigation of the VL-cured materials showed that, on the one hand, the use of bisphenol A, or its fluorinated analog, as a core structure in the monomers provided composites with the highest mechanical strength, while, on the other hand, the placement of fluorine in the extended perfluoroalkyl chains did not decrease water absorption and resulted in lower mechanical strength compared with the use of alternate fluorinated aromatic terminal groups.[169] Furthermore, an alternative approach to fluorinated Bis-GMA analogs is the use of fluorinated dimethacrylate-reactive diluents, for example, fluorinated triethyleneglycol dimethacrylate 59 (Figure 2.62), which resulted in a decrease in both water absorption and polymerization shrinkage.[171–173]

2.3.6.2 Bis-GMA substitutes

In the context of the discussion about the estrogenicity of bisphenol A, Bis-GMA impurities, or degradation products, the new urethane dimethacrylates 60–63 (Figure 2.63) were synthesized by the reaction of the commercially available α,α,α',α'-tetramethyl-*m*-xylylene diisocyanate (TMXDI) with OH-group-containing monomers, like 2-hydroxyethyl or hydroxypropyl methacrylate, which can be used to substitute Bis-GMA in dental composites.[174,175] TMXDI combines the advantageous properties of aliphatic (low tendency to discoloration) and aromatic (stiffness) diisocyanates. Therefore, the photopolymerization of the urethane dimethacrylates 60–63 resulted in UV-light stable polymer networks with properties similar to those of Bis-GMA. Moreover, the mechanical properties of photocured materials based on these monomers were less affected by storage or boiling in water. Based on another approach of urethane chemistry, new methacrylate carbamoyl isocyanurate resins were evaluated for the use in dental restoratives.[176] These crosslinkers were

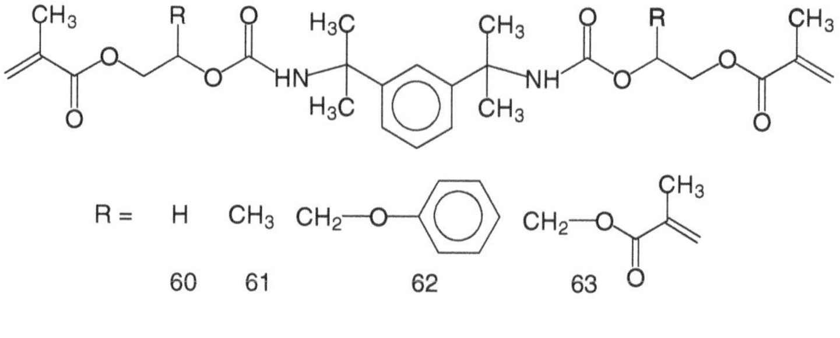

FIGURE 2.63 Bis-GMA substitutes on the bases of urethane dimethacrylates 60–63.

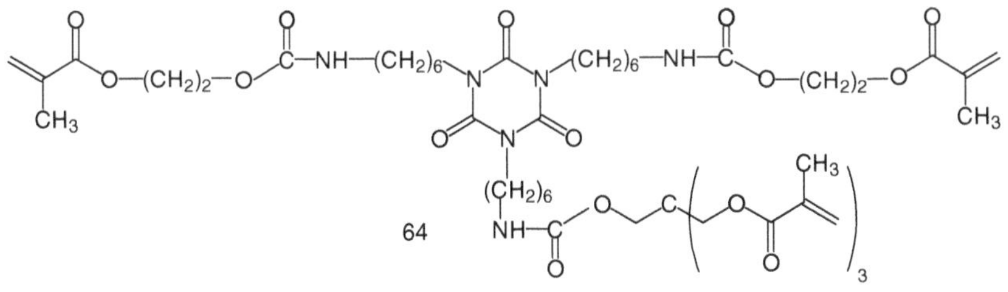

64

FIGURE 2.64 Ethylenically unsaturated carbamoyl isocyanurate 64.

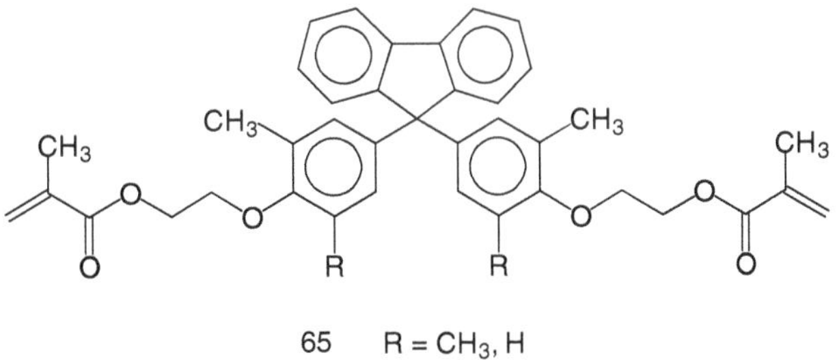

65 R = CH_3, H

FIGURE 2.65 Fluorene-based dimethacrylates 65.

synthesized by the stage-by-stage reaction of a triisocyanato-isocyanurate with one or more OH-group–containing monomers. For example, the reaction of the isocyanurate derived from hexamethylene diisocyanate with 2-hydroxyethyl methacrylate and pentaerythritol trimethacrylate resulted in monomer 64 (Figure 2.64). The physical properties of cured highly filled composites based on monomer 64, for example, were superior to those of comparable conventional Bis-GMA based restoratives. New fluorene based dimethacrylates 65 (Figure 2.65) were synthesized, which resulted in VL-cured matrix resins exhibiting higher, water saturated T_g (59–63° compared with Bis-GMA (53°C).[177] Furthermore, the resins based on 65 showed a greater resistance to creep and fracture. In general, the substitution of Bis-GMA in restorative composites may contribute to substantial improvements of dental filling materials as far as the increase of the degree of double-bond conversion, the reduction of the water absorption, and the improvement of staining, creep, and wear resistance are concerned.

2.4 CONCLUSION AND PERSPECTIVE ON THE FUTURE

The efforts to improve the clinical performance and the handling of restorative composite filling materials is mainly focused on the reduction of polymerization shrinkage as well as on the improvement of biocompatibility, wear resistance, and processing properties. Polymerization shrinkage, which impairs marginal adaptation, can be reduced by using cyclic monomers polymerizing by means of a ring-opening mechanism. Unfortunately, the presently described free-radical polymerizable cyclic monomers show a lower reactivity than methacrylates, are not stable in the presence of typical dental fillers, or result in polymers with disadvantageous properties such as high flexibility, low hydrolytical stability, or high water uptake. In the case of cationic polymerizable cyclic monomers, it is nescessary to increase the reactivity of the monomers and solve the problems concerning toxicology, and the sensitivity to bases and water. The contribution of liquid-crystalline, hyperbranched, or dendritic monomers to the reduction of polymerization shrinkage is more limited than that of the cyclic monomers. Therefore, the combination of these monomer structures with ring-opening groups seems to be promising. Biocompatibility and wear resistance can be improved by means of ormocers and fluorine-containing monomers. The incorporation of polymerizable cyclic groups is also very attractive in conjunction with theses matrix monomers.

REFERENCES

1. Ruyter, I.E. and Oeysaed, H., Composites for use in posterior teeth: composition and conversion, *J. Biomed. Mater. Res.*, 21, 11–23, 1987.
2. Peutzfeldt, A., Resin composites in dentistry: the monomer systems, *Eur. J. Oral. Sci.*, 105, 97–116, 1997.
3. Schmitt, W., 1978. Dentalmassen, DE Patent No. 2,816,823, 1978.
4. Zhu, S. and Hamielec, A., Kinetics of polymeric networks synthesis via free-radical mechanisms — polymerization and polymer modification, *Makromol. Chem. Macromol Symp*, 63, 135–182, 1992.
5. Anseth, K.S., Wang, C.M., and Bowman, C.N., Reaction behaviour and kinetic constants for photopolymerizations of multi(meth)acrylate monomers, *Polymer* 35(15), 3243–3250, 1994.
6. Stansburry, J.W., Curing dental resins and composites by photopolymerization, *J. Esthet. Dent.*, 12, 300–308, 2000.
7. Park, Y-J., Chae, K-H., and Rawls, H.R., Development of a new polymerization system for dental light-cure composite resins, *Dent. Mater.*, 15, 120–127, 1999.
8. Davidson, C.L. and de Gee, A.J., Light-curing units, polymerization, and clinical implications, *J. Adhes. Dent.*, 2(3), 167–173, 2000.
9. Peutzfeldt, A., Sahafi, A., and Asmussen, E., Characterization of resin composites polymerized with plasma arc curing units, *Dent. Mater.*, 6(5), 330–336, 2000.
10. Knezevic, A., Tarle, Z., Meniga, A., Sutalo, J., Pichler, G., and Ristic, M., Degree of conversion and temperature rise during polymerization of composite resin samples with blue diodes, *J. Oral. Rehabil.*, 28(6), 586–591, 2001.
11. Cowperthwaite, G.F., Foy, J.J., and Malloy, M.A., The nature of the crosslinking matrix found in dental composite filling materials and sealants, in *Biomedical and Dental Applications of Polymers*, Koblitz, F.F., Ed., Plenum Press, New York, 1981, pp. 379–385.
12. Moore, J.E., Photopolymerization of multifunctional acrylates and methacrylates, *Coat. Plast. Prep.*, 36, 747–753, 1976.
13. Imazato, S., McCabe, J.F., Tarumi, H., Ehara, A., and Ebisu, S., Degree of conversion of composites measured by DTA and FTIR, *Dent. Mater.*, 17, 178–183, 2001.
14. Lutz, F., Phillips, R.W., Roulet, J.-F., and Imfeld, Th., Komposits — Klassifikation und Wertung, *Schweiz. Mschr. Zahnheilk.*, 93, 914–929, 1983.
15. Hosoda, H., Yamada, T., and Inokoshi, S., SEM and elemental analysis of composite resins, *J. Prosthet. Dent.*, 64, 669–676, 1990.

16. Yearn, J.A. and Sakuma, T., Composition for Dental Restorative Material, GB Patent No. 2,263,115, GC, 1993.
17. Hickel, R., Dasch, W., Janda, R., Tyas, M., and Anusavice, K., New direct restorative materials — FDI commission project, *Int. Dent. J.*, 48, 3–16, 1998.
18. Davidson, C.L. and De Gee, A.J., Relaxation of polymerization contraction stresses by flow in dental composites, *J. Dent. Res.,* 63, 146–148, 1984.
19. Kinomoto, Y., Torii, M., Takeshige, F., and Ebisu, S., Comparison of polymerization contraction stresses between self- and light-curing composites, *J. Dent.*, 27, 383–389, 1999.
20. Silikas, N., Eliades, G., and Watts, D.C., Light intensity effects on resin-composite degree of conversion and shrinkage strain, *Dent. Mater.*, 16, 292–296, 2000.
21. Yap, A.U., Ng, S.C., and Siow, K.S., Soft-start polymerization: influence on effectiveness of cure and post-gel shrinkage, *Oper. Dent.*, 26(3), 260–266, 2001.
22. Yoshikawa, T., Burrow, M.F., and Tagami, J., A light curing method for improving marginal sealing and cavity wall adaptation of resin composite restorations, *Dent. Mater.*, 17(4), 359–366, 2001.
23. Friedl, K.H., Schmalz, G., Hiller, K.A., and Markl, A., Marginal adaption of Class V restorations with and without "softstart-polymerization," *Oper. Dent.*, 25(1), 26–32, 2000.
24. Feilzer, A.J., De Gee, A.J., and Davidson, C.L., Setting stress in composite resin in relation to configuration of the restoration, *J. Dent. Res.*, 66, 1636–1639, 1987.
25. Alster, D., Feilzer, A.J., De Gee, A.J., Mol, A., and Davidson, C.L., The dependence of shrinkage stress reduction on porosity concentration in thin resin layers, *J. Dent. Res.*, 71, 1619–1622, 1992.
26. Condon, J.R. and Ferracane, J.L., Reduction of composite contraction stress through non-bonded microfiller particles, *Dent. Mater.*, 14, 256–260, 1998.
27. Condon, J.R. and Ferracane, J.L., Assessing the effect of composite formulation on polymerization stress, *J. Am. Dent. Assoc.*, 131, 497–503, 2000.
28, Liu, C.-F., Collard, S.M., and Armeniades, C.D., Constant-volume polymerization of composites by addition of ammonia-modified montmorillonite, *Am. J. Dent.*, 3, 44–50, 1990.
29. Heindl, D. and Erdrich, A., 1997. Füllstoff auf Siliciumdioxid Basis, Verfahren zu seiner Herstellung und seine Verwendung, DE Patent No. 19615763 (to Hereaus Kulzer GmbH), 1997.
30. Luo, J., Lannutti, J.J., and Seghi, R.R., Effect of filler porosity on the abrasion resistance of nanoporous silica gel/polymer composites, *Dent. Mater.*, 14, 29–36, 1998.
31. Soltesz, U., Polymerisationsschrumpfung einiger neuer Komposit-Füllungswerkstoffe, *Zahnärztl. Mitteil.*, 88(11), 52–54. 1998.
32. Muelhaupt, R., Dietsche, F., Doell, W., and Thomann, R., Acrylic nanocomposites containing organoclay nanofillers: Morphology development, properties, and fracture behaviour, 219th American Chemical Society National Meeting, 26–30, 2000.
33. Ebenhoch, J., Kreis, G., Hierstetter, T., and Geck, M., Organopolysiloxanpartikel enthaltende acrylathaltige Zusammensetzung, DE Patent Application 19816148 (to Wacker-Chemie GmbH), 1999.
34. Krause, W.R., Park, S.H., and Straup, R.A., Mechanical properties of BIS-GMA resin short glass fiber composites, *J. Biomed. Mater. Res.*, 23, 1195–1211, 1989.
35. Xu, H.H., Smith, D.T., Schumacher, G.E., Eichmiller, F.C., and Antonucci, J.M., Indentation modulus and hardness of whisker-reinforced heat-cured dental resin composites, *Dent. Mater.*, 16, 248–254, 2000.

36. Xu, H.H., Dental composite resins containing silica-fused ceramic single-crystalline whiskers with various filler levels, *J. Dent. Res.*, 78, 1304–1311, 1999.
37. Chan, D.C., Titus, H.W., Chun, K.H., Wellinghoff, S.T., and Rawls, H.R., Radiopacity of tantalum oxide nanoparticle filled resins, *Dent. Mater.*, 15, 219–222, 1999.
38. Furman, B.R., Rawls, H.R., Wellinghoff, S.T., Dixon, H., Lankford, J., and Nicolella, D., Metal-oxide nanoparticles for the reinforcement of dental restorative resins, *Crit. Rev. Biomed. Eng.*, 28, 439–443, 2000.
39. Furman, B.R., Rawls, H.R., Norling, B.K., and Wellinghoff, S.T., Mechanically Strong and Transparent or Translucent Composites Made Using Zirconium Oxide Nanopatricles, Intl. Patent Application No. PCT WO 00/69392 (to Southwest Research Institute), 2000.
40. Taira, M., Toyooka, H., and Miyawaki, H., Studies on radiopaque composites containing ZrO2-SiO2 fillers prepared by the sol-gel process. *Dent. Mater.*, 9, 167–171, 1993.
41. Tyas, M.J., Jones, D.W., and Rizkalla, A.S., The evaluation of resin composite consistency, *Dent. Mater.*, 14, 424–428, 1998.
42. Leinfelder, K.F., Bayne, S.C., and Swift, E.J., Packable composites: overview and technical considerations, *J. Esthet. Dent.*, 11, 234–249, 1999.
43. Jackson, R.D. and Morgan, M., The new posterior resins and a simplified placement technique, *J. Am. Dent. Assoc.*, 131, 375–383, 2000.
44. Manhart, J., Kunzelmann, K.-H., Chen, H.Y., and Hickel, R., Mechanical properties and wear behavior of light-cured packable composite resin, *Dent. Mater.*, 16, 33–40, 2000.
45. Kelsey, W.P., Latta, M.A., Shaddy, R.S., and Stanislav, C.M., Physical properties of three packable resin-composite restorative materials, *Oper. Dent*, 25(4), 331–335, 2000.
46. Chen, H.Y., Manhart, J., Hickel, R., and Kunzelmann, K-H., Polymerization contraction stress in light-cured packable composite resins, *Dent. Mater.*, 17(3), 253–259, 2001.
47. Leevailoj, C., Cochran, M.A., Matis, B.A., Moore, B.K., and Platt, J.A., Microleakage of posterior packable resin composites with and without flowable liners, *Oper. Dent* 26(3), 302–307, 2001.
48. Bayne, S.C., Thompson, J.Y., Swift, E.J., Stamatiades, P., and Wilkerson, M., A characterization of first-generation flowable composites, *J. Am. Dent. Assoc.*, 129, 567–577, 1998.
49. Unterbrink, G.L. and Liebenberg, W.H., Flowable resin composites as "filled adhesives": literature review and clinical recommendations, *Quintessence Int.*, 30, 249–257, 1999.
50. Labella, R., Lambrechts, P., Van Meerbeek, B., and Vanherle, G., Polymerization shrinkage and elasticity of flowable composites and filled adhesives, *Dent. Mater* 15, 128–137, 1999.
51. Wilson, N., Burke, F., and Mjör, I.A., Reasons for placement and replacement of restorations of direct restorative materials by a selected group of practitioners in the United Kingdom, *Quintessence Int.*, 28, 245–248, 1997.
52. Burke, F., Cheung, S.W., Mjör, I.A., and Wilson, N.H., Restoration longevity and analysis of reasons for the replacement of restorations provided by vocational dental practitioners and their trainers in the United Kingdom, *Quintessence Int.*, 30, 234–242, 1999.
53. Ten Cate, J.M., Current concepts on the theories of the mechanism of action of fluoride, *Acta Odontol. Scand.*, 57, 325–329, 1999.
54. Fife, W.K., Zeldin, M., and Rubinsztajn, S., Fluoride Ion Releasing Dental Materials, Int'l Patent Application No. PCT WO 96/22761 (to Indiana University), 1996.

55 Masuhara, E., (Meth)acryloyl Fluoride-Containing Polymer and Dental Material Containing the Same, Int'l Patent Application No. PCT WO 82/01708, 1982.
56. Glasspoole, E.A., Erickson, R.L., and Davidson, C.L., A fluoride-releasing composite for dental applications, *Dent. Mater.*, 17(2), 127–133, 2001.
57. Geurtsen, W., Leyhausen, G., and Garcia-Godoy, F., Effect of storage media on the fluoride release and surface microhardness of four polyacid-modified composite resins ("compomers"), *Dent. Mater.*, 15, 196–201, 1999.
58. Nowak, R., Wanek, E., and Gangnus, B., Fluoride Releasing Dental Composite Material, EP Patent Application No. 0717977 (to Thera Patent GmbH), 1996.
59. Carvalho, A.S. and Cury, J.A., Fluoride release from some dental materials in different solutions, *Oper. Dent.*, 24, 14–19, 1999.
60. Karantakis, P., Helvatjoglou-Antoniades, M., Theodoridou-Pahini, S., and Papadogiannis, Y., Fluoride release from three glass ionomers, a compomer, and a composite resin in water, artificial saliva, and lactic acid, *Oper. Dent.*, 25, 20–25, 2000.
61. Vieira, A.R., de Souza, I.P., and Modesto, A., Fluoride uptake and release by composites and glass ionomers in a high caries challenge situation, *Am. J. Dent.*, 12, 14–18, 1999.
62. Yamamoto, H., Iwami, Y., Unezaki, T., Tomii, Y., and Tuchitani, Y., Fluoride uptake around cavity walls; two-dimensional mapping by electron probe microanalysis, *Oper. Dent.Operative Dent.*, 25, 104–112, 2000.
63. Donly, K.J., Segura, A., Wefel, J.S., and Hogan, M.M., Evaluating the effects of fluoride-releasing dental materials on adjacent interproximal caries, *J. Am. Dent. Assoc.*, 130, 817–825, 1999.
64. Francci, C., Deaton, T.G., Arnold, R.R., Swift, E.J., Perdigao, J., and Bawden, J.W., Fluoride release from restorative materials and its effects on dentin demineralization, *J. Dent. Res.*, 78, 1647–1654, 1999.
65. Kakaboura, A., Papagiannoulis, L., and Eliades, G., In vivo vs in vitro anticariogenic potential of aesthetic restorative materials, *J. Dent. Res.*, 77, 658 Abstr. 209, 1998.
66. Herrera, M., Castillo, A., Baca, P., and Carrion, P., Antibacterial activity of glass-ionomer restorative cements exposed to cavity-producing microorganisms, *Oper. Dent.*, 24: 286–291, 1999.
67. Kawashita, M., Tsuneyama, S., Miyaji, F., Kokubo, T., Kozuka, H., and Yamamoto, K., Antibacterial silver-containing silica glass prepared by sol-gel method, *Biomaterials* 21, 393–398, 2000.
68. Ericson, D., Antibacterial Dental Materials. Intl. Patent Application No. PCT WO 89/10736, 1990.
69. Imazato, S., Torii, M., and Tsuchitani, Y., Antibacterial effect of composite incorporating Triclosan against Streptococcus mutans, *J. Osaka Univ. Dent. Sch.*, 35, 5–11, 1995.
70. Imazato, S., Ebi, N., Tarumi, H., Russell, R.R., Kaneko, T., and Ebisu, S., Bactericidal activity and cytotoxicity of antibacterial monomer MDPB, *Biomaterials*, 20, 899–903, 1999.
71. Hall, H.D., Protective and maintenance functions of human saliva, *Quintessence Int* 24, 813–816, 1993.
72. Park, M.S., Eanes, E.D., Antonucci, J.M., and Skrtic, D., Mechanical properties of bioactive amorphous calcium phosphate/methacrylate composites, *Dent. Mater.*, 14, 137–141, 1998.
73. Skrtic, D., Hailer, A.W., Takagi, S., Antonucci, J.M., and Eanes, E.D., Quantitative assessment of the efficacy of amorphous calcium phosphate/methacrylate composites in remineralizing caries-like lesions artificially produced in bovine enamel, *J. Dent. Res.*, 75, 1679–1686, 1996.

74. Salz, U., Aktive Substanzen in Dentalmaterialien, *Phillip J.*, 14, 296–297, 1997.
75. Fontana, M., Gonzalez-Cabezas, C., Wilson, M.E., and Appert, C., In vitro evaluation of a "smart" dental material for its efficacy in preventing secondary caries using a microbial artificial mouth model, *Am. J. Dent.*, 12, Spec. No. 8–9, 1990.
76. Rheinberger, V., Salz, U., and Ott, G., Verfahren zur optischen Unterscheidung eines Dentalwerkstoffes sowie Dentalwerkstoff dafür, DE Patent No. 3939998 (to Ivoclar AG), 1991.
77. Salz, U., Burtscher, P., Rheinberger, V., and Dürr, H., Photochrome Dentalmaterialien, DE Patent No. 19520016 (to Ivoclar AG), 1996.
78. Sadhir, R.K. and Luck, R.M., Monomers that expand during polymerization, in *Expanding Monomers*, Sadhir, R.K. and Luck, R.M., Eds., CRS Press, Boca Raton, FL, 1992, pp.21–61.
79. Bailey, W.J. and Sun, R.L., The polymerization of a spiro ortho ester, *Polym. Prepr* 13(1), 281–286, 1972.
80. Bailey, W.J., Polycyclic Ring-Opened Polymers, U.S. Patent No. 4,387,215, 1983.
81. Brady, R.F., Recent advances in the development of expanding monomers: synthesis, polymerization and volume change, *J. Macromol. Sci.-Rev. Macromol. Chem. Phys* C32, 135–181, 1992.
82. Takata, T. and Endo, T., Recent advances in the developments of expanding monomers: synthesis, polymerization and volume change, *Prog. Polym. Sci.*, 18, 839–870, 1993.
83. Thomson, V.P., Williams, E.F., and Bailey, W.J., Dental resins with reduced shrinkage during hardening, *J. Dent. Res.*, 58, 1522–1532, 1979.
84. Stansbury, J.W. and Bailey, W.J., Evaluation of spiro orthocarbonate monomers capable of polymerization with expansion as ingredients in dental composite materials, in *Progress in Biomedical Polymers*, Gebelein, C.G. and Dunn, R.L., Eds., Plenum Press, New York, 1990, pp. 133–139.
85. Stansbury, J.W., Synthesis and evaluation of new oxaspiro monomers for double ring-opening polymerization, *J. Dent. Res.*, 71, 1408–1412, 1992.
86. Stansbury, J.W., Ring-opening polymerization of methacrylate-substituted spiro orthocarbonates, *Polym. Prepr.*, 33(2), 518–519, 1992.
87. Moszner, N., Zeuner, F., and Rheinberger, V., Polymerization of cyclic monomers. 1. Radical polymerization of unsaturated spiro orthocarbonates, *Macromol. Rapid Commun.*, 16, 667–672, 1995.
88. Sanda, S., Takata, T., and Endo, T., Synthesis and radical polymerization of spiro orthocarbonates bearing exomethylene groups, *J. Polym. Sci.: Part A: Polym. Chem* 32, 323–332, 1994.
89. Bailey, W.J., Matrices that expand on curing for high strength composites and adhesives, *Mater. Sci. Eng.*, A126, 271–279, 1990.
90. Takata, T. and Endo, T., Ionic polymerization of oxygen-containing bicyclic, spiro-cyclic and related expandable monomers, in *Expanding Monomers*, Sadhir, R.K. and Luck, R.M., Eds., CRC Press, Boca Raton, FL, 1992, pp. 63–152.
91. Byerley, T.J., Eick, J.D., Chen, G.P., Chappelow, C.C., and Millich, F., Synthesis and polymerization of new expanding dental monomers, *Dent. Mater.*, 8, 345–350, 1992.
92. Millich, F., Eick, J.D., Chen, G.P., Byerley, T.J., and Hellmuth, E.W., Determination of density changes with expansion polymerization, *J. Polym. Sci.: Part B, Polym. Phys.*, 31, 729–33, 1993.
93. Eick, J.D., Byerley, T.J., Chappel, R.P., Byerley, T.J., Bowles, C.Q., and Chappelow, C.C., Properties of expanding SOC/epoxy copolymers for dental use in dental composites, *Dent. Mater.*, 9, 123–127, 1993.

94. Chappelow, C.C., Pinzino, C.S., Power, M.D., and Eick, J.D., Photopolymerization of epoxy/polyol mixtures containing spiro orthocarbonates, *J. Dent. Res.*, 76, 40. 1997.
95. Chappelow, C.C., Eick, J.D., and Pinzino, C.S., Polymeric Compositions and Composites Prepared from Spiro Orthocarbonates and Epoxy Monomers, U.S. Patent No. 5,808,215, 1998.
96. Wictorin, L. and Larsson, A., Photopolymerizable Composition, Intl. Patent Application No. PCT WO 95/30402 (to ORALEG AB), 1995.
97. Kaisaki, D., Mitra, S.B., Schultz, W., and Devoe, R., Visible-Light Curable Epoxy System with Inhanced Depth of Cure, Int'l Patent Application No. PCT WO 96/13538 (to 3M Company), 1996.
98. Oxman, J. and Jacobs, D.W., Ternary Photoinitiator System for Curing of Epoxy Resins, Intl. Patent Application No. PCT WO. 98/47046 (to 3M Company), 1998.
99. Nuyken, O., Böhner, R., and Erdmann, C., Oxetane photopolymerization — a system with low volume shrinkage, *Macromol. Symp.*, 107,125–138, 1996.
100. Schaefer, R., Heindl, D., Schödel, D., Nuyken, O., Böhner, R., and Erdmann, C., Polymerizable Materials, U.S. Patent No. 5,750,590 (to Heraeus Kulzer), 1998.
101. Sasaki, H. and Kuriyma, A., Photoinitiated cationic polymerization of 3-ethyl-3-(phenoxymethyl)-oxetane in nitrogen atmosphere, *Polym. Mat. Sci. Eng.*, 72, 475–476, 1995.
102. Bailey, W.J., Ring-opening polymerization, in *Comprehensive Polymer Science* Allen, G. and Bevington, J.C., Eds., Pergamon, Oxford, Vol. 3, 1989. pp. 283–320.
103. Reed, B., Stansbury, J., and Antonucci, J., Ring-opening dental resins systems based on cyclic acetals, *Polym. Prepr.*, 33(2), 520–521, 1972.
104 Cho, I., Kim, B.-G., Park, Y.-C., Kim, C.-B., and Gong, M.-S., Photoinitiated free-radical ring-opening polymerization of 2-phenyl-4-methylene1,3-dioxolane, *Macromol. Chem., Rapid Commun.*, 12, 141–146, 1991.
105. Belfield, K.D. and Abdelrazzaq, F.B., Novel photoinitiated cationic copolymerizations of 4-methylene-2-phenyl-1,3-dioxolane, *J. Polym. Sci. Part A: Polym. Chem.*, 35, 2207–2219, 1997.
106. Belfield, K.D. and Abdelrazzaq, F.B., Photoinitiated cationic cross-linking of 4-methylene-2-phenyl-1,3-dioxolane with 2,2-(1,4-phenylene)bis(4-methylene-1,3-diox-olane), *Macromolecules*, 30, 6985–6988, 1997.
107. Endo, T., Okawara, M., and Bailey, W.J., Photoinitiated ring-opening polymerization of 2-methylene-1,3-dioxepane, *J. Polym. Sci.: Polym. Lett. Ed.*, 21, 373–380, 1983.
108. Jin, S. and Gonsalves, K.E., A study of the mechanism of free-radical ring-opening polymerization of 2-methylene-1,3-dioxepane, *Macromolecules*, 30, 3104–3106, 1997.
109. Moszner, N., Völkel, T., Rheinberger, V., and Klemm, E., Polymerization of cyclic monomers. 3. Synthesis, radical and cationic polymerization of bicyclic 2-methylene-1,3-dioxepanes, *Macromol. Chem. Phys.*, 198, 749–762, 1997.
110. Evans, R.A. and Rizzardo, E., Polymerizable Monomers and Polymers, Intl. Patent Application No. PCT WO 96/19471 (to CSIRO), 1996.
111. Evans, R.A. and Rizzardo, E., Free-radical ring-opening polymerization of cyclic allylic sulfides, *Macromolecules*, 29, 6983–6989, 1996.
112. Moszner, N., Zeuner, F., Völkel, T., and Rheinberger, V., Synthesis and polymerization of vinylcyclopropanes, *Macromol. Chem. Phys.*, 200, 2173–2187, 1999.
113. Sanda, F., Takata, T., and Endo, T., Radical polymerization behavior of 1,1-disubstituted 2-vinylcyclopropanes, *Macromolecules*, 26, 1818–1824, 1993.
114. Moszner, N., Zeuner, F., and Rheinberger, V., Polymerization of cyclic monomers. 4. Synthesis and radical polymerization of bi- and trifunctional 2-vinylcyclopropanes, *Macromol. Rapid Commun.*, 18, 775–780, 1997.

115. Moszner, N., Zeuner, F., Völkel, T., and Rheinberger, V., Polymerization of cyclic monomers. VII. Synthesis and radical polymerization of 1,3-bis[(1-alkoxycarbonyl-2-vinylcyclopropane-1-yl)carboxy]benzenes, *J. Appl. Polym. Sci.*, 72, 1775–1782, 1999.
116. Moszner, N., Völkel, T., Zeuner, F., and Rheinberger, V., Radical ring-opening monomers for dental composites, *Polym. Prepr.*, 38(2), 86–87, 1997.
117 Noel, C. and Navard, P., Liquid crystal polymers, *Progr. Polym. Sci.*, 16, 55–110, 1991.
118. Finkelmann, H., Liquid crystalline polymers, *Angew. Chem. Int. Ed. Engl.*, 26, 816–824, 1987.
119. Mormann, W., Liquid crystalline thermosets, *Trends Polym. Sci.*, 3, 255–261, 1995.
120. Hikmet, R.A., Zwerver, B.H., and Broer, D.J., Anisotropic polymerization shrinkage behaviour of liquid-crystalline diacrylates, *Polymer*, 33, 89–95, 1992.
121. Doornkamp, A.T., Albertda, G.O., and Tan, Y.Y., Kinetic study of the photoinitiated polymerization of a liquid crystalline diacrylate monomer by DSC in the isothermal mode, *Polymer*, 33, 2863–2867, 1992.
122. Ritter, H., Draheim, G., Moszner, N., and Salz, U., Dentalmaterialien auf der Basis von flüssig-kristallinen Monomeren, DE Patent Application No. 195,25,941 A1 (to Ivoclar AG), 1997.
123. Rawls, H.R., Wellinghoff, V.T., Norling, B.K., Leamo, S.H., Swynnerton, N.F., and Wellinghoff, S.T., Low shrinkage resins from liquid crystal diacrylate monomers, *Polym. Prepr.*, 38(2), 167–168, 1997.
124 Wellinghoff, V.T., Wellinghoff, S.T., Norling, B.K., and Rawls, H.R., Reduced shrinkage dimethacrylate liquid crystal resins, *J. Dent. Res.*, 76, 279, 1997.
125. Hölter, D., Frey, H., Mülhaupt, R., and Klee, J.E., Liquid crystalline thermosets based on branched bismethacrylates, *Macromolecules,* 29, 7003–7011, 1996.
126. Hölter, D., Frey, H., Mülhaupt, R., and Klee, J.E., Ambient temperature liquid-crystalline bismethacrylates based on cholesterol: cholesteric and smectic thermosets, *Adv. Mat.*, 10, 864–868, 1998.
127. Matthews, O.A., Shipway, A.N., and Stoddart, J.F., Dendrimers — branching out from curiosities into new technologies, *Prog. Polym. Sci.*, 23, 1–56, 1998.
128. Fischer, M. and Vögte, F., Dendrimers: from design to application — a progress report, *Angew. Chem. Int. Ed. Engl.*, 38, 884–905, 1999.
129. Bosman, A.W., Jansen, H.M., and Meier, E.W., About dendrimers: structure, physical properties and applications, *Chem. Rev.*, 99, 1665–1688, 1999.
130. Malmström, E. and Hult, A., Hyperbranched polymers: a review, *J. Macromol. Sci.-Rev. Macromol. Chem. Phys.*, C37, 555–579, 1997.
131. Voit, B., New developments in hyperbranched polymers, *J. Polym. Sci.: Part A: Polym. Chem.*, 38, 2505–2525, 2000.
132. De Brabander-van den Berg, E.M., and Meijer, E.W., Poly(propylenimin)-Dendrimere: Synthese in grösserem Massstab durch heterogen katalysierte Hydrierungen, *Angew. Chem.*, 32, 1370–1372, 1993.
133. Klee, J.E., Neidhart, F., Flammersheim, H.-J., and Mühlhaupt, R., Monomers for low shrinking composites. 2. Synthesis of branched methacrylates and their application in dental composites, *Macromol. Chem. Phys.*, 200, 517–523, 1999.
134. Klee, J.E., Walz, U., Hölter, D., Frey, H., and Mühlhaupt, R., Branched macromonomers and their application in dental composites. 3. Monomers for low-shrinking composites, *Angew. Makromol. Chem.*, 269, 71–75, 1998.
135. Wan, Q., Schricker, S.R., and Culbertson, B.M., Studies on synthesis and characterization of hyperbranched multi-methacrylates and their potential applications, *Polym. Prepr.*, 41(1), 101–102, 2000.

136. Wan, Q., Schricker, S.R., and Culbertson, B.M., Hyperbranched multi-methacrylates: their applications in dental resin systems, *Polym. Prepr.*, 41(1), 155–156, 2000.
137 Klee, J.E., Schneider, C., Hölter, D., Burgath, A., Frey, H., and Mühlhaupt, R., Hyperbranched polyesters and their application in dental composites: monomers for low shrinking composites, *Polym. Adv. Techn.*, 12, 1–9, 2001.
138. Moszner, N., Völkel, T., and Rheinberger, V., Synthesis, characterization and polymerization of dendrimers with methacrylic end groups, *Macromol. Chem. Phys.*, 197, 621–631, 1996.
139. Krejci, I., Standortbestimmung in der konservierenden Zahnmedizin, *Schweiz. Monatsschr. Zahnmed.*, 103, 614–619. 1993.
140. McLean, J.W., Nicholson, J.W., and Wilson, A.D., Proposed nomenclature for glass-ionomer dental cements and related materials, *Quintessence Intern.*, 25, 587–589, 1994.
141. Nicholson, J. and Anstice, M., The development of modified glass-ionomer cements for dentistry, *Trends Polym. Sci.*, 2, 272–276, 1994.
142. Wilson, A.D. and McLean, J.W., *Glass Ionomer Cements*, Quintessence Publishing, Chicago, 1988.
143. Blackwell, G.B., Dental/Medical Composition and Use, U.S. Patent No. 5,218,070 (to Dentsply Corp), 1993.
144. Hammersfahr, P.D., Compomers and hydromers for use in restorative dental procedures, *Polym. Prepr.*, 38(2), 131–132, 1997.
145 Lu, K., Huang, C.-T., and Hammersfahr, P.D., Dental Composition and Method, U.S. Patent No. 5,338,773 (to Dentsply Corp), 1994.
146. Fischer, U., Untersuchung des radikalischen Polymerisationsverhaltens von monomeren Carbonsäuremethacrylaten, dissertation submitted for diploma, Hohere Technische Lehranstalt Chur, Switzerland 1995.
147. Rumphorst, A., Salz, U., Gianasmidis, A., Völkel, T., Moszner, N., and Rheinberger, V., Radikalisch polymerisierbarer Dentalwerkstoff, DE Patent Application 198,18,210 A1, (to Ivoclar AG) 1999.
148. Eliades, G., Kakaboura, A., and Palaghias, G., Acid-base reaction and fluoride release profiles in visible light-cure polyacid-modified composite restoratives (compomers), *Dent. Mat.*, 14, 57–63. 1998.
149. Tiba, A., Culbertson, B.M., and Berliner, L.J., Electron spin resonance (ESR) spectroscopy studies of compomer type dental restoratives, *J. Macromol. Sci.-Pure Appl. Chem.*, A39, 1445–1457, 1998.
150. Meyer, J.M., Cattani-Lorente, M.A., and Dupuis, V., Compomers: between glass-ionomer cements and composites, *Biomaterials*, 19, 529–539, 1998.
151. Attin, T. and Buchalla, W., Werkstoffkundliche und klinische Bewertung von Kompomeren, *Dtsch. Zahnärtzl. Z.*, 53, 766–774, 1998.
152. Hickel, R., Moderne Füllungswerkstoffe, *Dtsch. Zahnärztl. Z.*, 52, 572–585, 1997.
153. Wolter, H., Storch, W., and Ott, H., New inorganic/organic copolymers (ormocer for dental applications, *Mat. Res. Soc. Symp. Proc.*, 346, 143–149, 1994.
154. Bauer, C.M., Kunzelmann, K-H., and Hickel, R., Simulierter Nahrungsabrieb von Kompositen und Ormoceren®, *Dtsch. Zahnärztl. Z.*, 50, 635–338, 1995.
155. Manhart, J., Hollwich, B., Mehl, A., Kunzelmann, K-H., and Hickel, R., Randqualität von Ormocer- und Kompositfüllungen in Klasse-II-Kavitäten nach künstlicher Alterung, *Dtsch. Zahnärztl. Z.,* 54, 89–95, 1999.
156. Haller, B. and Schuster, P., Randqualität eines Ormocers (Admira) und eines Feinhybridkomposites (Arabesk Top) in Klasse-II-Kavitäten, *Dtsch. Zahnärztl.* 55, 331–335, 2000.

157. Wolter, H., Glaubitt, W., and Rose, K., Multifunctional (meth)acrylate alkoxysilanes a new type of reactive compounds, *Mat. Res. Soc. Symp. Proc.*, 271, 719–724, 1992.
158. Wolter, H. and Storch, W., Dentalharzmasse, Verfahren zu deren Herstellung und deren Verwendung, DE Patent No. 4,133,494 C2 (to Fraunhofer-Gesellschaft), 1996.
159. Paul, P. P, Organic-Inorganic Hybrid Composites for Dental Restorative Material, U.S. Patent No. 6,005,028 (to Southwest Research Institute), 1999.
160. Moszner, N., Völkel, Th., Cramer von Clausbruch, S., Geiter, E., and Batliner, N., Synthesis and new cross-linking trialkoxysilane methacrylates and upon it based light curing composites, *Macromol. Mater. Eng.*, 287, 339–347, 2002.
161. Jacobine, A.F., Glaser, D.M., and Nakos, S.T., Photoinitiated cross-linking of norbornene resins with multifunctional thiols, *ACS Symp. Ser.*, 417, 160–175, 1990.
162. Moszner, N., Schöb, W., and Rheinberger, V., Synthesis, characterization and thiol-ene polymerization of hydrolyzed/condensed norbornenyl silic acid ester, *Polym. Bull* 73, 289–295, 1996.
163. Rheinberger, V., Moszner, N., Salz, U., Wolter, H., Storch, W., and Baeuerlein, H., Dental Material, U.S. Patent No. 5,889,132 (to Ivoclar AG), 1999.
164. Bowen, R.L., Dental Filling Material Comprising Vinyl Silane Treated Fused Silica and a Binder Consisting of the Reaction Product of Bis-Phenol and Glycidyl Acrylate, U.S. Patent No. 3,066,112, 1962.
165. Sankarapandian, M., Shobba, H.K., Kalachandra, S., Taylor, D.F., Shultz, A.R., and McGrath, J.E., Synthesis of new dental composite matrix dimethacrylates, *Polym. Prepr.*, 38(2), 92–93 1997.
166. Sankarapandian, M., Shobba, H.K., Kalachandra, S., and McGrath, J.E., Characterization of some aromatic dimethacrylates for dental composite applications, *J. Mater. Sci.: Mater. Med.*, 8, 465–468, 1997.
167. Stansbury, J.W., Antonucci, J.M., and Scott, G.L., Photocured composites based on dimethacrylate monomers of varied fluorine content, *Polym. Prepr.*, 36(1), 831–832, 1995.
168. Stansbury, J.W., Choi, K.M., and Antonucci, J.M., Considerations in the development of semi-fluorinated methacrylate dental resins and composites, *Polym. Prepr.*, 38(2), 96–97, 1997.
169. Stansbury, J.W. and Antonucci, J.M., Dimethacrylate monomers with varied fluorine content and distributions, *Dent. Mater.*, 15, 166–173, 1999.
170. Choi, K.M. and Stansbury, J.W., New families of photocurable oligomeric fluoromonomers for use in dental composites, *Chem. Mater.*, 12, 2704–2707, 1996.
171. Wang, G., Culbertson, B.M., Xie, D., and Seghi, R.R., Physical property evaluations of perfluorotriethylene glycol dimethacrylate as a potential reactive diluent in dental composite resins, *J. Macromol. Sci.-Pure Appl. Chem.*, A36, 225–236, 1999.
172. Wang, G., Culbertson, B.M., Xie, D., and Seghi, R.R., Effect of fluorinated triethylene glycol dimethacrylate on the properties of unfilled, light-cured dental resins, *J. Macromol. Sci.-Pure Appl. Chem.*, A36, 237–252, 1999.
173. Wang, G., Culbertson, B.M., and Seghi, R.R. Strength, abrasive wear, and durability properties of dental composites containing a fluorinated dimethacrylate reactive diluent *J. Macromol. Sci.-Pure Appl. Chem.*, A36, 373–388, 1999.
174. Mariotti, A., Söderholm, K.-J., and Johnson, S., The in vivo effect of bisGMA on murine uterine weight nucleic acids and collagen, *Eur. J. Oral. Sci.*, 106, 1022–1027, 1998.

175. Moszner, N., Völkel, T., Fischer, U.K., Klester, A., and Rheinberger, V., Synthesis and polymerisation of new multifunctional urethane methacrylates, *Angew. Makromol. Chem.,* 265, 31–35, 1999.
176. Mitra, S.B., Dental composites prepared from resin matrices containing ethylenically unsaturated carbamoyl isocyanurates, *Polym. Prepr.*, 38(2), 103–104, 1997.
177. Culbertson, B.M., Tiba, A., Sang, J., and Liu, Y.N., Synthesis, characterization and evaluation of new fluorene-based dimethacrylates for formulating dental composites, *Polym. Adv. Technol.*, 10, 275–281, 1999.

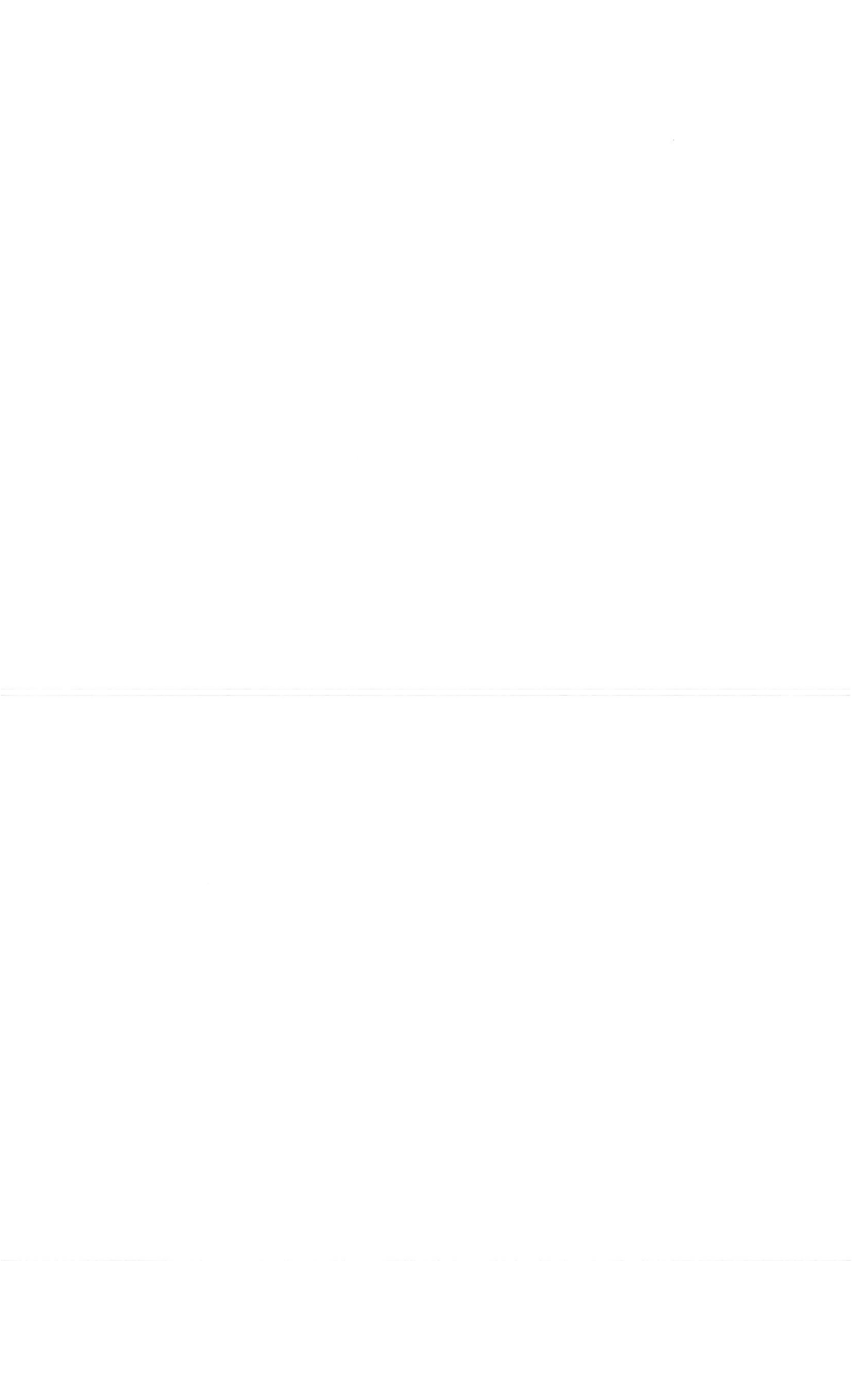

3 Enamel and Dentin Adhesion

Ulrich Salz, Norbert Moszner, and Jörg Zimmermann

CONTENTS

3.1 INTRODUCTION

3.1.1 Clinical Requirements

The main goals of restorative dentistry are to restore a tooth's health, function, and esthetic appearance, and to prevent recurrent caries.[1] In contrast to the mainly function-focused reparative dentistry of the twentieth century, restorative dental therapy is more concerned with a minimally invasive approach, which starts with caries diagnosis and risk assessment as a basis for a proper treatment decision. Based on the result of the assessment, different scenarios for the management of initial caries lesions are established: noninvasive management by arresting the caries process and remineralization or surgical intervention.[4,5] In the case of operative treatment, a minimally invasive preparation technique is demanded. The principles of cavity design for amalgam restorations established by Black and his concept of "extension for prevention" are no longer valid.[6,7] The current concept is "prevention of extension": retentions no longer have to be prepared.[8,9] However, it was not until the breakthrough of effective enamel–dentin adhesives in the 1980s and 1990s that the dental community was able to establish the concept of minimally invasive restorative therapy.[1]

In the last couple of years, the desire of patients for esthetic restorations has significantly increased. Therefore, tooth shaded, invisible fillings with invisible margins are demanded as well as esthetic crowns, inlays, and veneers that are bonded with an invisible composite luting cement according to the adhesive technique.

In the field of caries prevention, the sealing of fissures with a low-viscosity composite-based fissure sealant has been established for many years. In this technique, the fissure sealant is fixed to the tooth structure by the acid etch technique.[10] The success of this measure is very much dependent on the long-term marginal adaptation.

A further application of the adhesive technique in dentistry is the bonding of brackets to enamel for orthodontic treatment.

3.1.2 Postoperative Sensitivity

One of the first clinical signs of marginal disintegration and insufficient seal of open dentinal tubules, respectively, is postoperative sensitivity.[11–14] Sensitivity is primarily related to the pulpal nerve response to fluid pressure changes caused by fluid shifts in the tubules (hydrodynamic theory, Figure 3.1).[12,14] Changes in the local ionic concentration produce fluid flows by osmotic pressure: Thermal and mechanical pressure changes may induce flow. In any case, proper sealing of the tubules is the key factor to inhibiting fluid movements and thereby preventing sensitivity.[15–17]

In general practice, the dentist is mainly confronted with the following types of sensitive dentin: hypersensitive exposed tooth necks or as already described postoperative sensitivity following restorative treatment. For the treatment of hypersensitive teeth, two strategies are available. First, the pain threshold of pulp sensory nerves subjacent to the exposed dentin can be lowered by reducing nerve activity. Potassium salts, especially KNO_3 and KCl, are recommended for this purpose.[18,19] The statements regarding the efficiency of this treatment, however, are controversial.[20,21]

Second, certain physicochemical mechanisms can lead to a reduction of the permeability and sensitivity of exposed dentin:

- Topical application of agents forming precipitates, for example, potassium oxalate[18]
- Topical application of spherical polymer particles of the dimensions of dentinal tubules (diameter 2 to 5 μm) with an affinity to dentin to block the tubules mechanically[22,23]
- Closing the tubules by coagulation of proteins in the dentin liquor by the application of, for example, glutaraldehyde[24]
- Blocking the tubules by applying a topcoat in the form of a dentin adhesive: for example, a similar effect as that created by glutaraldehyde is caused by the acid monomers used in dentin adhesives.[25–28]

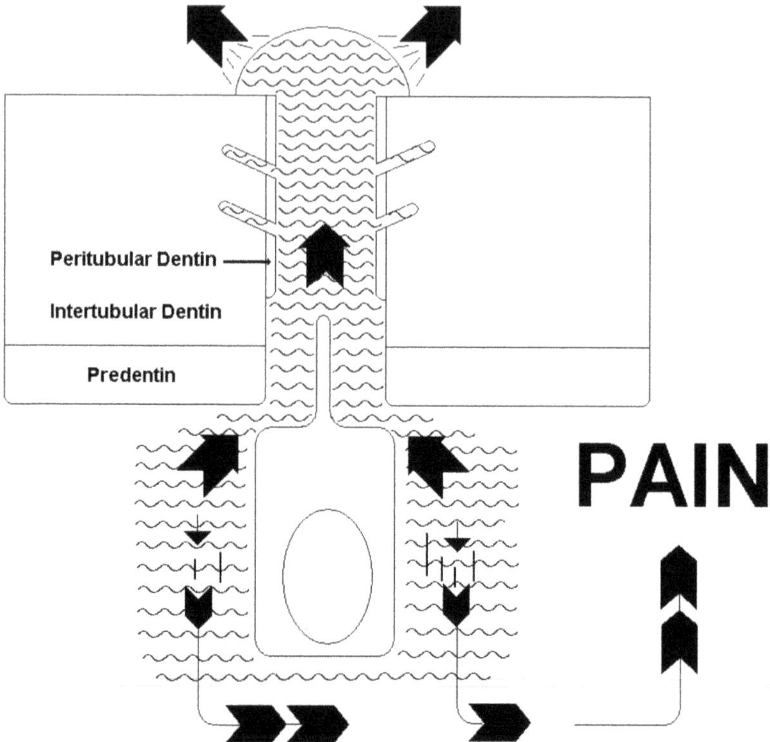

FIGURE 3.1 Schematic of the hydrodynamic mechanism of dentin sensitivity in which fluid shifts across dentinal tubules, indirectly stimulating pulpal nerves.

To avoid postoperative sensitivity in adhesive filling therapy, perfect margins or a sufficient sealing of the dentin surface are required. This leads to a perfect hybridization of the intertubular and the peritubular dentin and the occlusion of the dentinal tubules. Cervical preparations with margins in the cementum are prone to higher levels of postoperative sensitivity because small amounts of cementum are inadvertently removed during finishing and polishing and dentinal tubules are opened.[11]

3.1.3 Reasons for the Replacement of Fillings

In the long term, marginal disintegration can contribute to marginal discoloration, secondary (recurrent) caries, as well as pulpal complications.[29] If cariogenic bacteria are incompletely removed by excavation from the cavity floor, they will reinvade the cavity. From investigations with fissure sealants, it is known that the activity of residual bacteria in the fissure can be stopped by establishing a proper and long lasting seal.[30]

Selected surveys of Mjör et al. in general dental practices in Scandinavia, the United Kingdom, and the United States during the 1980s and 1990s indicate that more replacements than initial restorations have been done.[31–34] The principal reason

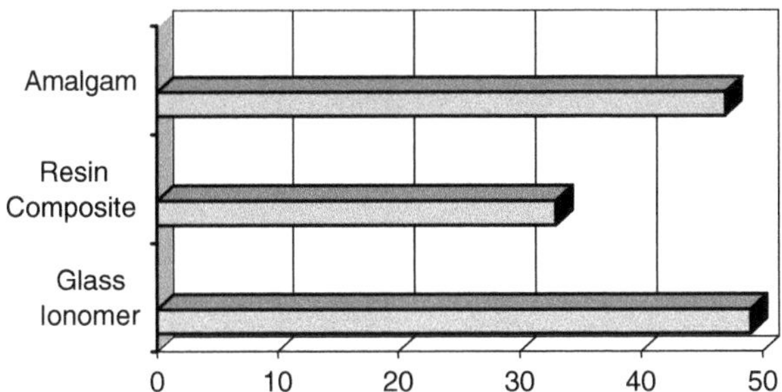

FIGURE 3.2 Percentage of restorations with the diagnosis of secondary caries. (Source: Mjör, I. A, *Quintessence Int.*, 27, 171–174, 1996.)

for the replacement of restorations is secondary caries, independent of the type of restorative material used (amalgam, composite, or glass ionomer; see Figure 3.2).[31,34] The clinical difficulty of secondary caries diagnosis lies in the differentiation between stained restoration margins, real secondary caries, and residual caries. Further investigations showed that the diagnosis of secondary caries in many cases could not be confirmed after removing the filling material.[35] Many discolored marginal areas showed no caries activity. In some cases a new primary caries was found adjacent to the existing filling.[35]

3.1.4 Evolution of the Adhesive Technique

In Table 3.1, the main adhesion systems in restorative dentistry are listed: the adhesion between the composite and the tooth substances, enamel and dentin, as well the composite–metal and composite–ceramic adhesion. Good adhesion between the tooth substances dentin and enamel and the composite filling or luting materials is very important for the direct as well for the indirect restorative technique. In the case of indirect restorations, sound adhesion to lab or chairside fabricated ceramic restorations is also necessary. Usually, after chemical or mechanical surface roughening, a coupling agent such as a methacrylate-functionalized silane is applied to establish a covalent chemical link between the ceramic restoration and the composite luting material.[36]

TABLE 3.1
Composite-Adhesive Systems in the Restorative Dentistry

Interface	Surface Conditioning	Adhesive System
Metal–composite	Sandblasting	Silicatization, silanization, metal primer
Ceramic–composite	HF-etch, sandblasting	Silanization
Dentin–composite	Phosphoric acid etch, self-etching primer	Adhesive monomer systems
Enamel–composite	Phosphoric acid etch, self-etching primer	Methacrylate bonding agents, adhesive monomer systems

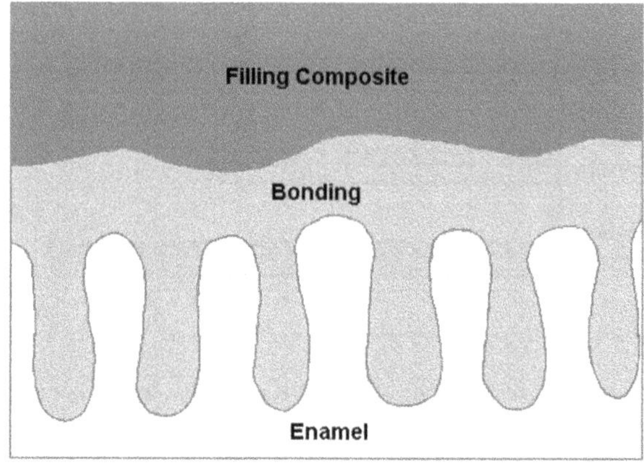

FIGURE 3.3 Schematic of the mechanical interlocking of a composite on etched enamel.

As early as in 1955, Buonocore suggested creating micromechanical retentions on enamel by etching with phosphoric acid (Figure 3.3) to obtain clinically durable adhesion between the tooth structure and the methacrylate polymerized on top.[37] time, this procedure became established in restorative therapy as the acid etch technique. At the time, Buonocore used 85% phosphoric acid, others have also tried hydrochloric, nitric, lactic, citric, pyruvic, poly(acrylic acid), or EDTA for conditioning the tooth surface.[38–43] Phosphoric acid is still the material of choice. A lot of further *in vitro* investigations have shown that a concentration of 35 to 40% phosphoric acid is optimal for enamel etching.[44,45] In contrast, Shinchi et al. did not observe any dependence between the tensile bond strength and the concentration of the phosphoric acid.[46] The conditioning time should be in the range of 20–40 s. Because of its low acid solubility, fluoridated enamel has to be etched for 120 s.[47] Before acid etching deciduous teeth, a thin layer of aprismatic enamel should be removed using a burr. Afterward the teeth should be conditioned again with phosphoric acid for 120 s. Newer investigations are questioning such long etching times.[49] After etching, the acid is thoroughly rinsed off with water and the etched enamel surface dried with oil-free air.

Three types of etch patterns are known.[50] Type 1 shows a honeycomb-like appearance. In the Type 2 etch pattern, the peripheral regions of the prisms are dissolved leaving the prism cores relatively intact (Figure 3.4). Type 3 is a more unstructured etch pattern.

Micromechanical interlocking is then obtained by *in situ* polymerization of a methacrylate-based resin in the acid-induced porosity. Scanning electron microscope (SEM) and transmission electron microscope (TEM) investigations showed that beside the micromechanical retention, as shown in Figure 3.3, a resin infiltration zone was formed.[51]

For the adhesion to dentin, the smear layer produced during cavity preparation has to be removed by acid-etch treatment, which, in the case of the total-etch technique, results in the creation of a 3 to 5 μm deep demineralized zone in the dentin surface.[52] In 1956, Buonocore et al. tried to improve dentin adhesion by etching dentin with hydrochloric acid, though with minor success.[53] Fusayama et al.

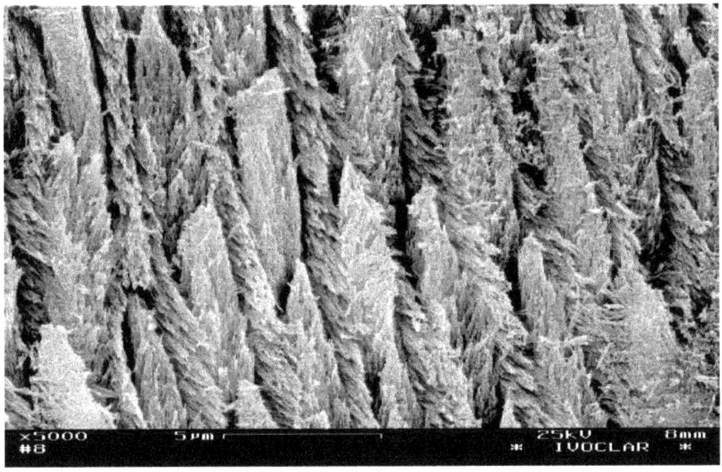

FIGURE 3.4 SEM image of a type 2 etch pattern.

achieved an increase in the tensile bond strength from 16.8 kg/cm^2 to 62.3 kg/m by etching the dentin surface with 40% phosphoric acid.[54] The adhesive they used was Clearfil Bond System-F (Kuraray).

Collagen fibrils are almost completely denuded of hydroxyapatite by acid etching (Figure 3.5), forming a microretentive interpenetrated polymer network with the applied dimethacrylate-based resins. This interlock was first described by Nakabayashi et al. and is commonly referred to as the "hybrid layer."[55] Furthermore, Bowen and coworkers developed a number of monomers, tailormade for the wet dentin surface.[56–73]

"Total etch" adhesives require the simultaneous application of acid to enamel and dentin, after which the acid needs to be rinsed off. This step is very technique sensitive

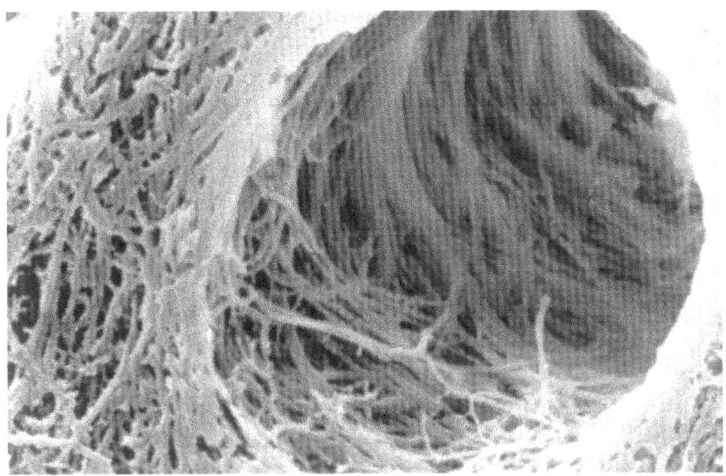

FIGURE 3.5 SEM of a dentin surface etched with phosphoric acid.

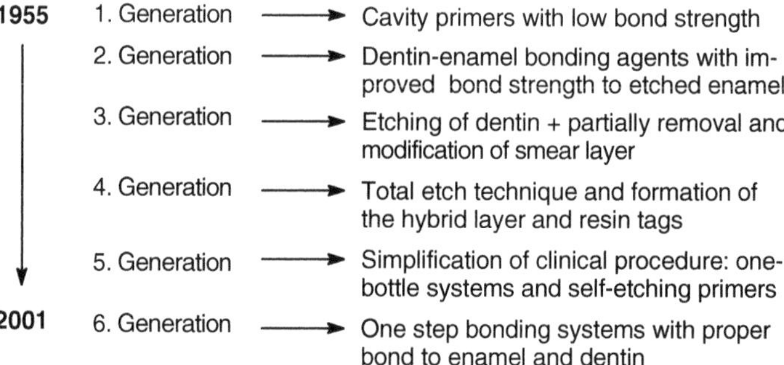

FIGURE 3.6 Evolution of bonding systems from the first generation to current bonding materials of the sixth generation.

and has a major influence on the function of the adhesive. Many systems are extremely sensitive to the application technique, the application time, and the remaining moisture on the dentin, which is very difficult to control by the general practitioner.[74]

The concept of "self-etching" adhesives is based on the use of polymerizable acidic monomers that simultaneously condition and prime dentin and enamel. Therefore, the self-etching primers eliminate the technique-sensitive rinsing step. The most common systems involve two application steps: the dentin and enamel conditioning step with the self-etching primer followed by the application of an adhesive resin. One of the first acid monomers to be developed was 4-META (4-methacryloyloxyethyl trimellitate anhydride), which still is very often used in self-etching primer systems.[75,76] Clinically, it has been shown that self-etching systems are low in technique sensitivity with regard to the dentin surface conditions (dry, wet, moist, etc.) resulting in a very low level of postoperative sensitivity. The low risk of postoperative sensitivity is the consequence of the obvious fact that dentin decalcification and the penetration of dentin by the acid monomers occurs to the same depth. There is no nanoleakage in the hybrid layer, or in the words of Nakabayshi, nonhybridized, decalcified dentin does not exist.[77]

Because of the great number of bonding materials and the different types that have been developed and the considerable evolution of bonding systems, a review of bonding materials from the first to the current sixth generation (Figure 3.6) has been conducted.[78]

3.2 CHARACTERIZATION AND PRETREATMENT OF ENAMEL AND DENTIN

3.2.1 Histology of Enamel and Dentin

3.2.1.1 Enamel

Enamel is the hardest tissue in the human body. Its composition and properties are quite different from those of dentin, cement, or bone tissues. Enamel consists of 97 wt% mineral, about 1 wt% organic material, and 2 wt% water.[79] The organic component of mineralized enamel contains soluble and nonsoluble proteins, enameline, and small amounts of carbon hydrates and lipids. The crystalline enamel rods build the structure of the enamel. The crystallites are hexagonal rods with a thickness of about 20–60 nm and a length of some micrometers. Between the rods, the organic component forms a thin gel-like network.

3.2.1.2 Dentin

The main part of the human tooth consists of dentin. Dentin encloses the pulp and generates a functional unit with it. Compared with enamel, dentin is a less mineralized tissue. It consists of 70% hydroxyapatite, 20% organic material, and 10% water.[79] The hydroxyapatite crystals are integrated into the organic matrix in a disordered way. The main part of this matrix consists of Type I collagen and collagen-like compounds. From a morphological point of view, we can differentiate between the odontoblasts, the dentin tubules with the periodontoblastic area, and the peritubular and intertubular dentin as shown in Figure 3.7.

Dentin can be divided into primary, secondary, and tertiary dentin. Primary dentin is the major component of the crown and root dentin and is formed before the tooth has reached occlusion. The outer layer of the primary dentin is called the mantle dentin. This layer is about 150 mm thick and differs from the rest of the primary dentin. Mantle dentin is the first dentin formed by the newly differentiated odontoblasts and has larger collagen fibers and is slightly less mineralized than the rest of the primary dentin. Secondary dentin is formed after the tooth has come into occlusion. Compared with primary dentin, the formation of secondary dentin is a much slower process continuing over the life span of the tooth, narrowing the pulp camber. Tertiary dentin is produced in response to trauma or disease and has an irregular appearance. During dentin formation, the odontoblasts produce a dentin matrix with collagen fibers that are perpendicular to the odontoblast process. As the odontoblasts move toward the center of the pulp, mineral is deposited in the matrix, starting in foci called calcospherites.

During dentin formation, dentinal tubules are formed around the odontoblastic processes as they move away from the dentin–enamel junction. The tubules are small circular canals with a diameter of about 0.9 μm at the dentin–enamel junction, gradually increasing to about 2.5 μm near the pulp. As a result of growth during dentinogenesis, the tubules show a slight S-curve from the dentin–enamel junction

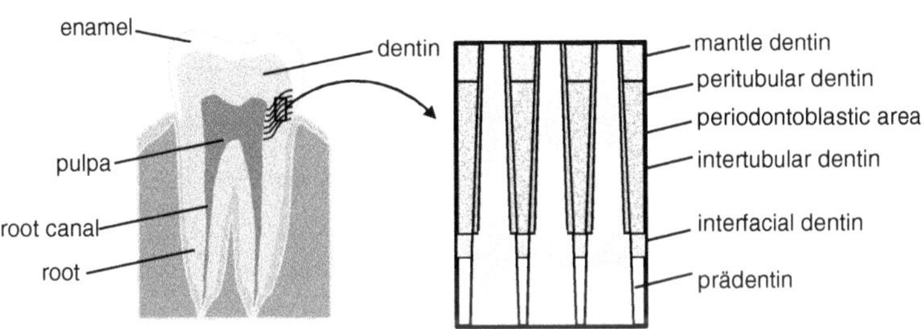

FIGURE 3.7 Schematic description of tooth and dentin tubuli composition.

to the pulp. The tubules number about 10,000 per mm^2 close to the dentin–enamel junction and about 45,000 per mm^2 near the pulp. Perpendicular to the tubules, small branches called microtubules or canalicules can be seen. The canalicules are less than 0.1 μm in diameter, and some of the branches may enter the adjacent main tubule. Dentin tubules are surrounded by peritubular dentin that is about 40% more mineralized than the rest of the dentin, which is called intertubular dentin. Like enamel, dentin exhibits dark deposit lines. These are called the lines of von Ebner. If mineralization of the dentin is disturbed, for example, by vitamin D deficiency, a less mineralized cloudlike dentin, called interglobular dentin, is formed.

The junction between enamel and dentin is uneven and made up of a series of ridges, which increase the surface area between the enamel and dentin. This increases the contact surface area, enhancing the attachment between enamel and dentin.

3.2.1.3 Chemical and Histological Buildup of Sclerotic Modified Dentin

The theory of caries formation was introduced by Miller in 1883.[80] He assumed that microorganisms or plaque at the tooth surface with adequate substrate supply produce organic acids, which are able to demineralize the tooth surface. Dentinal caries occurs normally as a result of enamel or cement caries. Initially the enamel surface is intact when the lesion spreads to the enamel–dentin junction (EDJ). When caries reaches the EDJ, it spreads laterally along this junction. As a result of this spreading, subsurface migration of the healthy enamel occurs. Simultaneously, the caries spreads in a cervical direction along the dentinal tubules and a cone-shaped lesion is created. At this stage of dentinal caries there is no penetration of bacteria into the tissue. In comparison with healthy enamel, the decalcified enamel is extremely porous. Therefore, acids, bacterial toxins, and enzymes can diffuse into the dentin. This process and other chemical attractions lead to a reaction of the pulp–dentin unit, which determines the histology of the sclerotic dentin.

By microscopic investigations, we can differentiate the following zones (Figure 3.8):

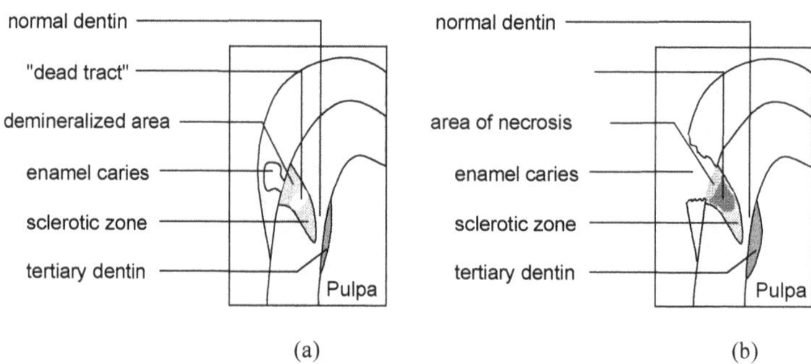

FIGURE 3.8 Schematic description of the structures of dentinal caries at different stages: (a) early lesion, (b) advanced lesion.

- Formation of tertiary dentin
  - The formation of tertiary dentin occurs at the borderline between the pulp and dentin. The tertiary dentin protects the pulp against the infiltration of toxic or irritating liquids. The attached dentin consists of an irregular highly mineralized structure with a low number of small tubules.[82]
- Normal dentin
  - Regular primary and secondary dentin with healthy odontoblasts.
- Sclerotic area
  - Sclerotization is likewise a protection mechanism against caries progression. Because of the accumulation and precipitation of mineral salts, the dentinal tubules are closed and the diffusion of acids and toxic compounds is inhibited. The barrier has to inhibit the migration of enzymes or bacteria along the tubules into the pulp.[81] Normally the carious destruction process is slowed in this way but not completely stopped.[82]
- Zone of "dead tracts"
  - This is the core of the lesion of early dentinal caries. At the superficial part, the peritubular dentin as well as the intertubular dentin are partially decalcified. Dead tracts arise by the closure of the tubules at their pulpal end. The tubules are filled with air. The low refractive index of air leads to a total reflection of light and the zone appears dark.[83]
  - The advanced lesion appears after the cavitation of enamel. From this stage on, the bacteria are able to penetrate the dentin surface. With progressive penetration and as a result of the bacterial activity, additional histological zones become evident.
- Area of penetration
  - At this zone the dentin tubules are penetrated by bacteria. Their metabolism products lead to local restricted swelling of the dentin tubules. Furthermore, a high degree of demineralization is found at the intertubular dentin.[84]
- Area of necrosis
  - Normally the area of necrosis is highly colored and often fragmented and nothing remains of the common dentinal structure. In this area the dentin substrate is completely disturbed by the microbial activity. The penetration of the microorganisms, which was limited to the dentin tubules and their branches, spreads to the entire dentin.

3.2.2 Chemical Composition

From a chemical point of view, teeth are principally formed as a composite of two completely different materials: hydroxyapatite and collagen in combination with water. The composition of these two materials differs over a wide range in the different teeth substrates as shown in Table 3.2.

3.2.3 Structure of Hydroxyapatite

Hydroxyapatite refers to the group of calcium phosphates, under which ceramic materials with different amounts of calcium and phosphorus are classified. The name

TABLE 3.2
Density and Composition of Hard Tissues by Percentage of Volume and Weight

	Bone (%)	Dentin (%)	Enamel (%)
Mineral	41	48	92
(Density, 3000 kg/m^3)	(64)	(69)	(97)
Organic	48	29	2
(Density, 1400 kg/m^3)	(31)	(20)	(1)
Water	11	23	6
(Density, 1000 kg/m^3)	(5)	(11)	(2)

Source: Linde, A. in *Dentine and Dentine Reactions in the Oral Cavity*, Thylstrup, A., Leach, S.A., and Quist, V., Eds., Inform. Print. Ltd., Oxford, 1987, p. 17.
Note: % of weight shown in parentheses

apatite has been given to a group of materials, which is described by the general chemical formula $M_{10}(XO_4)_6Z_2$ with $M^{2+} = Ca^{2+}$ or Ba^{2+}; X = P, V, Cr, Mn; $Z^- =$ OH. Hydroxyapatite $[Ca_{10}(PO_4)_6OH_2]$ is the inorganic component of natural bone and teeth, but it can also be synthesized, for example, by precipitating ammonium phosphate and calcium nitrate from aqueous solutions. However, it is important to note that bone and teeth mineral is characterized by calcium and hydroxyl deficiency, ionic substitution within the apatite lattice, and internal crystal disorder — it is not a direct analog of hydroxyapatite as is commonly believed.

In bone and teeth the hydroxyapatite is produced in solution in the presence of salvia and other complex physiological fluids. Not surprisingly, its calcium ions undergo substitution for many elements including barium, lead, strontium, sodium, or magnesium. Furthermore hydroxyl groups are also reported to be readily exchanged with fluoride, carbonate, or chloride, resulting in a highly complex chemistry.

Substitution of Ca by Mg, Fe, Mn, or Al ions impedes the growth of hydroxyapatite and promotes the formation of tricalcium phosphate. Magnesium in saliva is believed to cause the formation of tricalcium phosphate in dental callus because tricalcium phosphate can have up to 10% of its Ca ions substituted by Mg, which has the effect of decreasing the overall acid dissolution rate.[86]

For the substitution of carbonate into hydroxyapatite, two types of substitution are proposed in the literature, these being the substitution of CO_3^{2-} for OH^- (Type A) and CO_3^{2-} for PO_4^{3-} (Type B). For both types, increasing solubility was observed with increasing carbonate content in the apatite.

In addition to the carbonate substitution, OH^- may also be substituted by chloride and most importantly in dentistry, by fluoride ions. The substitution by fluoride ions results in denser packing between the fluoride and calcium ions, which leads to an increase in crystallinity and a decrease in solubility. Advantage can be taken of this behavior in caries prevention, for example, by applying fluoridated toothpastes and varnishes.

3.2.4 Structure of Collagen

Collagen is the family name of macromolecular proteins, which are important fiber proteins in the human body: About 25% of human protein is composed of collagen. Compared with other proteins, the collagen molecule contains a huge amount of glycine, proline, and hydroxyproline. These amino acid units stabilize the helix structure. Every third amino acid of the triple helix is glycine. The glycine groups are oriented toward the inside of the helix for the formation of lateral cross-linking hydrogen bonds. Type I collagen is quantitatively the predominant type of collagen in dentin, bone, tendon, and skin.

Collagen fibers consist of collagen fibrils (diameter 0.2–0.5 μm), which are built up partly inside the cells at the fibroblasts and partly outside the cells. The formation of procollagen occurs inside the cell. This collagen subunit consists of three left-hand helix polypeptide chains of 1056 amino acids each.[87] They form a fiber of 300 nm in length and 1.5 nm in diameter with high tensile strength. In contrast to tropocollagen, procollagen contains short peptide segments called telopeptides at the N- and C-terminal end groups of the molecule. In contrast to tropocollagen, telopeptides do not contain glycine at every third place in the chain and they do not have a helical structure. The gaps offer places for the formation of intermolecular, chemical cross-links between the collagen molecules.[88]

Outside the cell, telopeptide and tropocollagen are separated by peptidases, while the tropocollagen fibers arrange themselves spontaneously into collagen fibrils. Each tropocollagen molecule is displaced 67 nm laterally from its neighbor. For the whole length of a tropocollagen fiber (300 nm), five of these displacements were used. Because of this, there is a gap of 35 nm between two consecutively arranged tropocollagen fibers (Figure 3.9). Collagen fibrils viewed by electron microscopy show a characteristically periodic banded pattern of 67 nm. This pattern corresponds to the gap overlap structure of the fibrils and can be related to the axial distribution of amino acids in the triple helix.[89]

In bone and also in dentin, it is this gap region between two tropocollagen fibrils, in which mineral is first deposited during the mineralization of dentin.[90] The position of the collagen fibrils relative to each other is adapted to the biological function of the related tissue: parallel orientation in tendons (power transmission), flat shapes for skin, two-dimensional networks for the sclera of the eye (tensile strength), or three-dimensional translucent networks in the case of the vitreous body in the eye (mold stability).

The collagens can be differentiated into 3 main groups:

- The fiber collagens (Type I, II, III, V, and XI)
- The fiber-associated (Type IX and XII)
- The nonfibrillate types (Type IV, VI, VII, VIII and X)[91]

The typical sequence of amino acids in dentinal collagen is glycine-X-Y. X and Y are amino acids except tryptophane, cystine, and tyrosine. Proline and alanine often correspond to the X position, whereas glutamine acid, leucine, and phenylalanine are often found in the Y position. The composition of dentinal collagen is summarized in Table 3.3.[92]

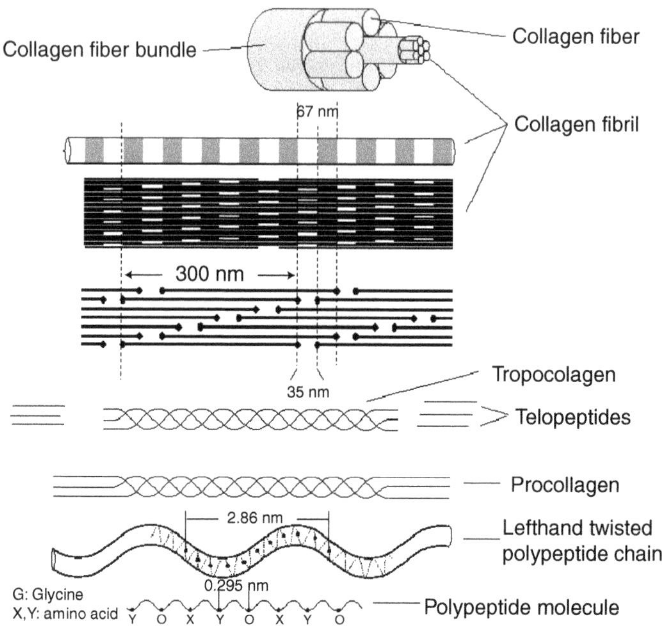

FIGURE 3.9 Structure and chemical composition of collagen fibers.

In mineralized dentin, collagen fibrils are closely packed together and have a diameter of 20–50 nm. Fibrils are also present in the dentin tubules in close relation to the odontoblast processes.

3.2.5 Physical Properties of Enamel and Dentin

It is important for our understanding of the mechanical function of restored teeth to know how the natural materials in teeth — that is, dentin and enamel — behave under the application of an external load. In other words, we need to know which of the various alternative models of their biomechanical characteristics can adequately describe their behavior. The human dentition is replaced once in a lifetime, but during this lifetime, the permanent teeth undergo cyclical loading many times. Any mechanical structure undergoing this kind of repetitive loading can deteriorate, both from stress overload and from the propagation of cracks as a consequence of mechanical fatigue. Thus, it is imperative that stresses be kept to a minimum. To withstand the test of time, teeth must therefore be both tough and resistant to wear. These two properties do not necessarily go hand in hand. Hard structures, which are resistant to wear, are usually brittle and offer little resistance to crack propagation, whereas tough materials tend not to be as wear resistant. The structure of human teeth appears to have evolved so as to incorporate both of these properties. The outer shell of enamel acts as a hard, high-stiffness, wear-resistant shell, which is approximately five times harder than dentin.[93,94] Nevertheless, it is also extremely susceptible to fracture in a direction parallel to the prisms. In contrast, dentin appears to be about four times tougher than enamel[95] and of considerably lower stiffness.

TABLE 3.3
Amino Acid Composition of Dentinal Collagen Chains

Amino Acids	Units/1000 units
Aspartic acid	57
Threonine	19
Serine	38
Glutamic acid	78
Glycine	317
Alanine	110
Valine	26
Cystine	—
Methionine	—
Isoleucine	11
Leucine	26
Tyrosine	4.5
Phenylalanine	15
Histidine	8
Hydroxylysine	9.2
Lysine	25.3
Arginine	49
4-Hydroxyproline	92
Proline	117

Source: Gage, J.P., Francis, M.J.O., and Smith, R., *J. Dent. Res.*, 67, 1097–1102, 1988.

3.2.5.1 Anisotropy of Enamel

Enamel is thought to have highly anisotropic stiffness characteristics because of its prismatic structure (Figure 3.10). It is very likely that enamel is stiffer in the prism direction than in the direction perpendicular to it. The prisms are thought to run approximately perpendicular to the enamel–dentin junction. Several studies have been conducted to gain some understanding of the process of stress dissipation in teeth and how it is affected both by the design of restorations and by the properties using finite element techniques.[96–110] Yettran et al. suggested that since enamel is considerably stiffer than dentin, the masticatory forces tend to flow around the "enamel cap" of the tooth.[96] As a consequence, the enamel near the enamel–cementum junction is highly stressed. It was established that the anisotropic characteristics of enamel had a negligible effect on this stress concentration. Since this result is counterintuitive — the prismatic, anisotropic nature of enamel surely serves some adaptive and presumably mechanical purpose — the effects of the anisotropic nature of enamel on the mode of stress distribution in a tooth under load was reexamined by Spears et al.[102] They showed that the ordered arrangement of enamel prisms serves an important functional purpose. The anisotropy helps to dissipate occlusal loads more effectively. A major function of enamel anisotropy is to reduce tensile

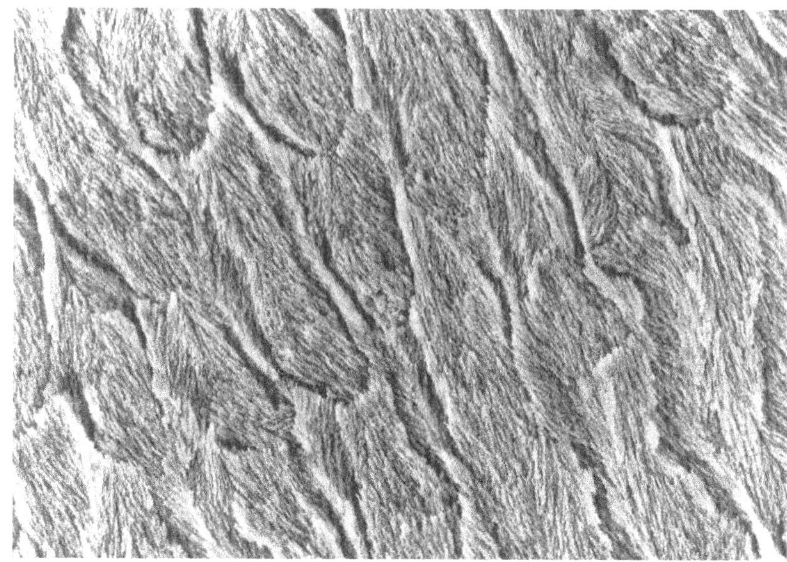

FIGURE 3.10 SEM of the prismatic enamel structure.

and compressive stresses that would otherwise occur in the enamel, thereby reducing the risk of enamel fracture, particularly in the cervical region.

3.2.5.2 Anisotropy of Dentin

The microstructure of dentin, which is dominated by the presence of dentinal tubules, would be expected to impart anisotropic properties to the tissue (Figure 3.11).

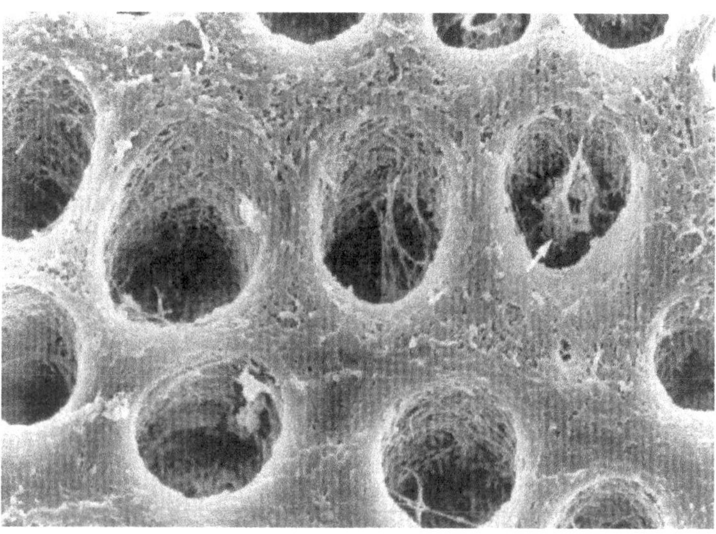

FIGURE 3.11 SEM of the dentin tubular micro structure.

Tubules traverse the entire dentin. The tubule density and diameter decreases from the pulpal surface to the outer dentin. Tubules occupy approximately 10% of the total dentin volume, and they may function hydraulically in stress transfer. The dentin matrix, consisting largely of Type I collagen with embedded apatite crystals, is also oriented with respect to the tubules. Collagen occurs as a compact mass of interwoven fibrils that are arranged perpendicularly to the tubules and are predominantly parallel to the inner dentin surface. Despite the distinctive microstructure, it has been argued that dentinal tubules exert only a minor influence on mechanical properties.[103] Difficulties in the preparation and testing of small samples with precise tubule orientation have hampered systematic studies of human dentin. These difficulties, plus localized structural variations, have led to a wide range of results in the reported mechanical properties of dentin (Table 3.4).[104–106] Isotropic behavior has been reported for a range of mechanical properties including the elastic modulus, propagation limit, and compressive and flexural strength.[94,107,108] Minor anisotropy has been reported in energy of fracture and shear strength.[94,108,109] Lertchirakarn et al. observed a significant effect of tubule orientation on the microtensile bond strength with the greatest strength being achieved when tensile force was applied perpendicular to the dentinal tubules.[110] This result is consistent with previous reports that dentin is easiest to fracture across dentinal tubules and may be explained in relation to collagen and apatite crystal orientation with respect to the tubules. Several authors have suggested that the orientation of collagen fibrils in composite materials, such as bone and dentin, influences strength.[111] Collagen fibrils are interwoven and arranged perpendicular to the tubules, while apatite crystals tend to be positioned parallel with the long axis of the collagen fibrils.[112] Thus, fractures perpendicular to the tubules occur predominantly within the plane of the collagen network, while fractures parallel with the tubules require disruption of the collagen fibrils.

TABLE 3.4
Comparison of Selected Mechanical Properties of Dentin and Enamel

Mechanical Parameter	Dentin	Enamel
Young's modulus (GPa)	10–20	9–90
Flexural modulus (GPa)	12–20	20–100
Tensile strength (MPa)	30–104	8–35
Compressive strength (MPa)	230–370	95–385
Knoop hardness	65–80	320–390
Shear strength (MPa)	36–138	90

Source: Spears, I.R., van Noort, R., Crompton, R.H., Cardew, G.E., and Howard, I.C., *J. Dent Res.*, 72, 1526–1531, 1993; Skinner, E.W. and Phillips, R.W., *The Science of Dental Materials*, 6th ed., Saunders, Philadelphia, 1967; Stanford, J.W., Paffenbarger, G.C., Kampula, J.W., and Sweeny, W.T., *J. Am. Dent. Assoc.*, 57, 487–495, 1958.

TABLE 3.5
Energy of Different Types of Interaction

Type of Interaction	Energy (kJ/mol)	Example
Chemical interaction:		
Covalent bonding	200–800	Polymers, ester or amide bonds
Metallic bonding	100–350	Metals
Physical forces		
Ionic interaction	60–1200	Salt crystals
Van der Waals Interactions	20	Adsorption of nonpolar solvents
Complex interaction	60–1000	Tenside with metal ions
Hydrogen bondings	60	Water adsorption

3.2.5.3 Comparison of Selected Properties of Enamel and Dentin

Dentin possesses a pale yellow color compared to the gray or blue-white of enamel. Because of the low opacity of enamel (21–67%), dentin is responsible for (opacity 50–91%) the color of the crown. The refractive index of dentin (1.56) is smaller than that of the birefringent enamel (1.60–1.62). Dentin is a harder tissue compared with bone or cementum but much softer (more elastic) than enamel. This is clearly shown by the mechanical values in Table 3.5. As a result of its mechanical properties, dentin shows a 25 times higher abrasion compared with enamel.

The mechanical data published in the literature vary widely. It is well known that the mechanical properties depend on many factors, for instance the point of measurement, the humidity of the material, or the age of the individual. Because of the presence of dentin tubules, dentin is much more permeable and the density of dentin (2.7 $g \cdot cm^{-3}$) is much lower than that of enamel (2.8–3.0 $g \cdot cm^{-3}$). The thermal expansion coefficients of dentin (8–9 ppm/K) and enamel (11–12 ppm/K) are also slightly different.[113]

3.2.6 Pretreatment of Enamel and Dentin

3.2.6.1 Adhesion to Enamel

Acid etching of enamel changes a smooth surface to an irregular, retentive one by decalcification and solution processes on the hydroxyapatite crystals. Fluid resin of low viscosity wets this surface and penetrates into the microporosities created by the conditioning through capillary attraction (Figure 3.12). After polymerization, the tags formed by this extension of resin into the microporosities create a strong micromechanical interlocking with the enamel.[37,114–117] In the process, a resin infiltration zone is formed, which is comparable with the hybrid layer.[51]

There have been several attempts, at least in the case of pit and fissure sealants, to improve the resin penetration in the acid-formed surface porosities. To ensure complete penetration of the up to 200-µm-deep etch pattern by a light-curing bonding

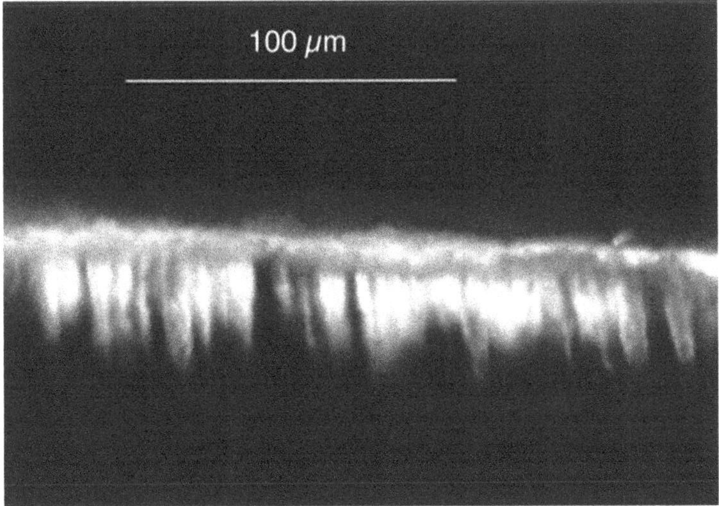

FIGURE 3.12 CLSM image of a resin-infiltrated etched enamel surface.

agent, researchers recommend a contact time of some seconds.[118,119] In addition, the application of ultrasound to the sealant and drying the etched enamel with acetone can improve the quality of the sealing.[120] Because of the enlargement of the surface area by etching, an increase of the surface energy is achieved.[121]

From a microbiological point of view, the tooth surface is disinfected by acid etching. The addition of an antimicrobial agent such as benzalkonium chloride to the etchant showed no increase in the inhibition of bacterial growth.[122]

3.2.6.2 Adhesion to Dentin

Although adhesion to enamel is a predictable and established method in restorative dentistry, an adequate bond to dentin is much more difficult to achieve. In contrast to enamel, dentin is a vital tissue. The permeability of dentin depends on the number and diameter of the dentin tubules. The continuous flow of dentin liquor from the pulp chamber to the prepared dentin surface leads to a permanent modification of the surface and dilution of substances applied on the dentin surface. *In vivo*–prepared, burr-cut dentin surfaces possess what is known as a smear layer (Figure 3.13). This smear layer consists of dentin particles, collagen fibers, residues from the odontoblasts, and bacteria. Morphological studies have demonstrated that the smear layer is deposited on the dentin as a result of cavity instrumentation. Depending on a number of factors, this layer can have a thickness between 0.5 and 5.0 μm.[52] It will prevent intimate contact between the adhesive system and the substrate, thus nullifying a prerequisite for the occurrence of an adhesive reaction. For this reason, pretreatment of the dentin and enamel surface before the application of the adhesives is necessary. For the pretreatment of the tooth surfaces, the following methods have become established over the years.

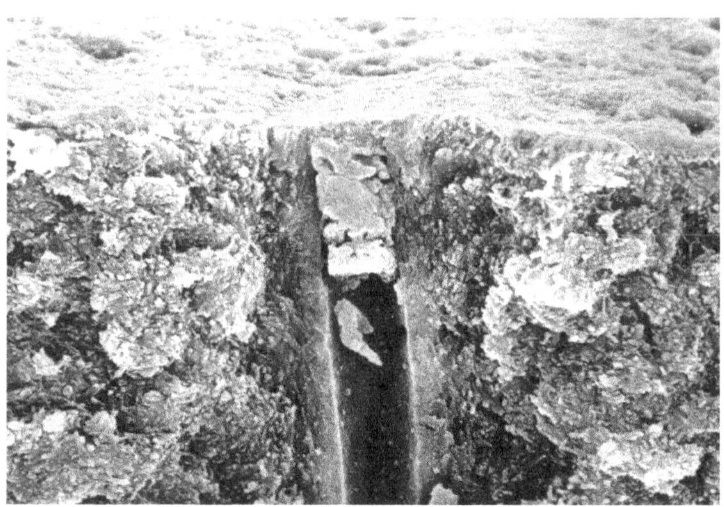

FIGURE 3.13 SEM image of a smear layer on top of dentin.

3.2.6.2.1 Pretreatment with Acid: Total-Etch Bonding

Generally, 35 to 40% phosphoric acid has been preferred for conditioning enamel. Simultaneous conditioning of hard dental tissues appears to be a recent innovation. It is a technique that has been under study for more than two decades.[54] Acid attack of dentin removes the smear layer from the dentin and is responsible for dentinal demineralization to depths of 0.5 to 7.5 μm, depending on the type of concentration, pH value, and viscosity of the acid, and the duration of the application.[123] One disadvantage of acid etching dentin is the increase in the permeability of dentin combined with the higher risk of pulp damage in the case of marginal disintegration.[124]

To interact with the intrinsically moist dentin tissue, an adhesive system has to be capable of reacting under such conditions. Consequently, hydrophilic primers have become a part of numerous adhesive systems, seeking to secure a strong bond to dentin. Thus, most total-etch adhesive systems have incorporated hydrophilic components that are diluted in organic solvents to dislodge moisture from the conditioned dentin and achieve intimate interaction at the demineralized intertubular and peritubular dentin, creating the interdiffusion zone (Figure 3.14 and Figure 3.15). This zone, also called the hybrid layer, seems to be essential for an ideal bond to dentin.[55,124,125] Figure 3.15 shows the penetration of resin into the intertubular and peritubular dentin, the tubules, and even into the lateral branches.

For chemomechanical caries removal, a NaOCl-based gel (Carisolv) is offered on the market.[126] NaOCl removes the collagen structure on the dentin. Some investigators have shown that on surfaces treated in this way conventional adhesive systems produce relatively high bond strength values.[127–129] However, no hybrid layer formation was observed on NaOCl-pretreated dentin surfaces.[129]

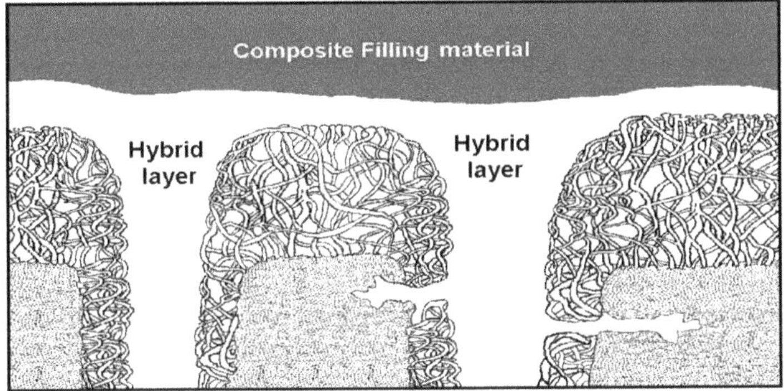

FIGURE 3.14 Schematic drawing of the hybrid layer.

3.2.6.2.2 *Self-Etching Primers*

The concept of "self-etching" adhesives is based on the use of polymerizable acidic monomers that simultaneously condition and prime dentin and enamel. Because the same acidic solution remains after conditioning, the smear layer will incorporate itself into the hybrid layer or at least it will be hybridized. Thus, self-conditioning adhesives offer a simpler clinical application because self-etching primers eliminate

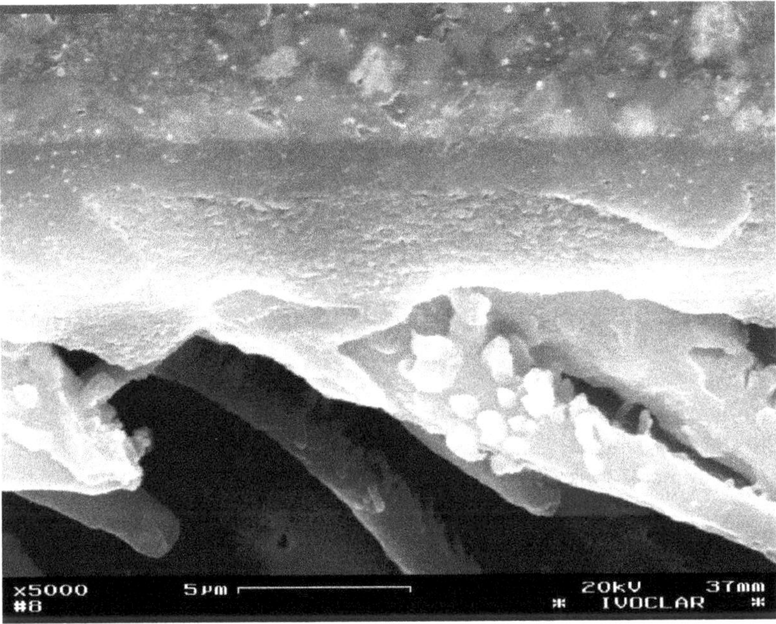

FIGURE 3.15 SEM image of a hybrid layer.

the technique-sensitive rinsing step used in the total-etch systems. In addition, they are capable of conditioning the tooth surface and simultaneously preparing it for adhesion.[130,131] Removal of the etchant becomes unnecessary, imparting greater ease and safety to the procedure, in addition to avoiding critical problems brought about by acid etching. The difficulty in finding the ideal moisture conditions for the dentin is eliminated. Furthermore, possible negative influences on adhesion are dramatically reduced. If acid etching is performed to remove the smear layer completely, superficially demineralizing the dentin in the process, there is the possibility that resin monomers will not diffuse into the depths of the altered dentin, thus weakening the adhesive bond through nanoleakage. This appears not to happen with efficient self-etching primer systems because these acidic primers have a certain quantity of resin monomers that will simultaneously interact with the dentinal tissue. Because of this bonding mechanism, self-etching systems are low in technique sensitivity with regard to the dentin surface conditions (dry, wet, moist etc.), resulting in a very low clinical postoperative sensitivity.

Most of the currently available self-etching primers have the following general composition: acid monomer, comonomer, and water-based solvent with a pH value in the range of 1.5–2.5.[130] Under these strong acidic conditions, esters such as MDP (methacryloyloxydecyl hydrogen phosphate) or HEMA (2-hydroxyethyl methacrylate) are hydrolytically degraded.[132,133] Therefore, hydrolytically stable systems, as previously shown, should be used for self-etching primers to avoid clinical failure.[123,134]

3.3 PHYSICAL AND CHEMICAL ASPECTS OF ADHESION

3.3.1 Basics of Adhesion

An assembly made by the use of an adhesive is called an adhesive joint or an adhesive bond. Solid materials in the adhesive joint, other than the adhesive, are known as the adherents. The phenomenon that allows the adhesive to transfer a load from the adherent to the adhesive joint is called adhesion. Apart from adhesion due to micromechanical interlocking, there is another form of adhesion that is a physical phenomenon resulting from the same attractive forces that bind atoms together that binds molecules together to make liquids and solids. To understand adhesion, we must first understand the forces that exist between atoms or molecules and then apply that knowledge to what occurs at the surface and within the boundary layer.

We can classify the mechanisms and interactions, which are responsible for adhesion into the following groups:

Micromechanical retention
Chemical bonding
Physical interactions

The power of the different forces differs widely depending on the type of interaction between the adherent and adhesive as described in Table 3.5 and Figure 3.16. Obviously, good adhesion based on physical forces depends on the type of interaction between the adhesive and adherent on one hand and the number of physical forces on the other. For the adhesion on dentin and enamel, the formation

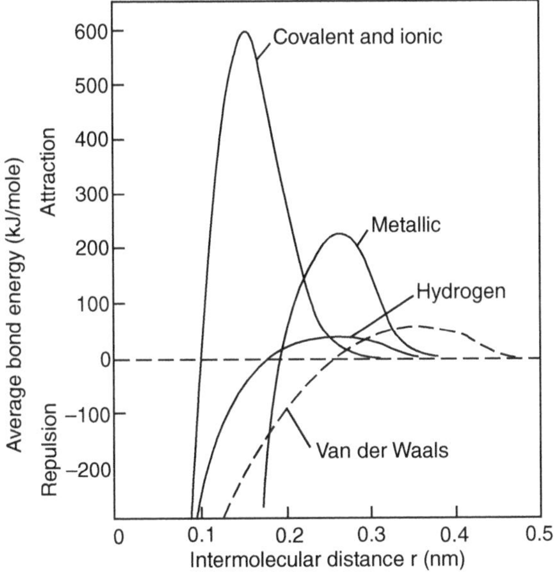

FIGURE 3.16 Energy of different forces in dependence of the intermolecular distance.

of micromechanical retention and chemical forces as described in the following part are the most important processes.

3.3.2 Wetting and Penetration of Dental Substrates

After cavity preparation, enamel and dentin surfaces are covered by a smear layer. Acid etching or treatment with self-etching primers removes the smear layer, leaving clean cavity walls. For reliable adhesion, there must be intimate contact between the tooth structure and the restorative material or adhesive resin, respectively. For this reason, the adhesive resins must be able to wet and penetrate the pretreated surface. There must be good compatibility between the adhesive and surface relative to polarity, wetting, and penetration behavior.

The wetting of a surface by a liquid is characterized by determining the contact angle of a droplet placed on the polished flat surface. If the liquid spreads out completely on the solid surface, the contact angle is zero, i.e., there is complete wetting. The surface tension of the liquid adhesive, therefore, must be less than the surface free energy of the substrate, i.e., enamel and dentin. A freshly acid-etched enamel surface has a surface energy of more than twice that of an unetched enamel surface.[135] Furthermore, it is easily wetted by the monomers used in dental adhesive systems. Because of the high polarity of enamel and especially dentin, monomers containing functional groups that are capable of ionic interactions or the formation of hydrogen bonds are suitable for reliably penetrating dentin and enamel surfaces. Therefore, because of its ability to form hydrogen bonds and its excellent wetting behavior, HEMA is widely used in dental adhesive systems, for example.

3.3.3 Adhesion by Micromechanical Retention

After wetting and penetration of the monomers into the adherent, surface adhesion is performed by different mechanisms. Theoretically, for micromechanical retention to occur, the liquid adhesive has to penetrate into pores or cavities of the rough surface of the adherents. After hardening, the adhesive adheres by mechanical retention like a dowel. The penetration of the adhesive into the rough surface cavities depends on different factors such as the viscosity of the adhesive, the surface energy of the adherent, the surface tension of the adhesive, and the shape, depth, and diameter of the cavities as well as other factors. For adhesion to occur by micromechanical retention, a sufficiently hard substrate and surface roughness is essential. Etched enamel meets these conditions. The conditioning of prepared or unprepared enamel by phosphoric acid or what are known as "self-etching primers" results in a highly roughened surface. The etching pattern after conditioning by phosphoric acid is shown in Figure 3.17 on the left. The rough adhesive surface formed by the penetration of the adhesive into the rough enamel surface and subsequent polymerization is shown on the right. In contrast, adhesion by micromechanical retention on acid-etched dentin is much more questionable. Although dentin bonding appears similar to etched enamel bonding, the strength of the mechanical bond to dentin established in this manner is surprisingly low. To obtain a bond of the desired strength, dentin bonding agents may feature a chemical reaction. The dentin bonding agents with chemical activity may include a methacrylic group for polymerization that is linked by a spacer group capable of bonding to the dentin surface through chemical or physical interactions.

Ionic bonds and complex formation will be established by the electrostatic attraction between, for example, negative charges on the adhesive molecules and the positive charges of the Ca^{2+} ions of the hydroxyapatite. Molecules containing phosphoric, phosphonic, or carboxylic acid groups, for example, EDTA, citric acid, MDP, or 4-META, are capable of this reaction.

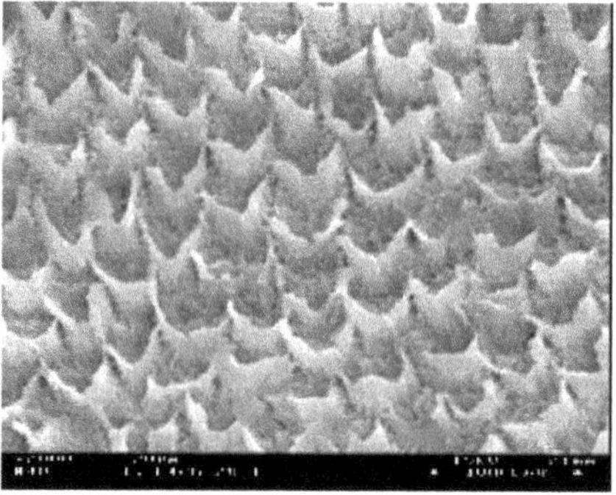

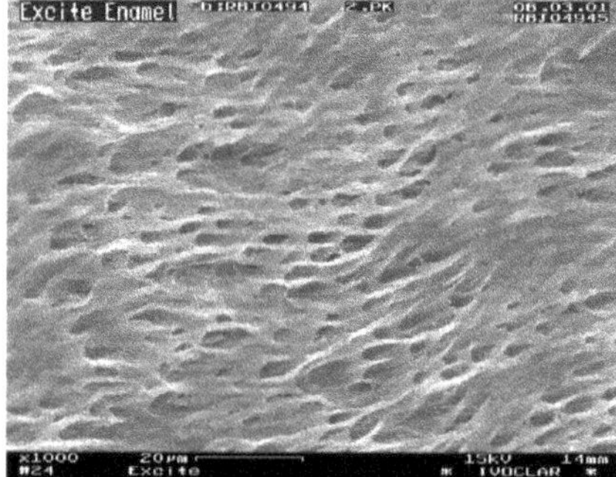

FIGURE 3.17 Left side: Surface of human enamel after conditioning with phosphoric acid. Right side: Adhesive surface after removal of the tooth.

3.3.4 Adhesion by Chemical Bonding and Physical Forces

Adhesion can principally be established by different physical and chemical forces as described below.

Chemical bonds:	Covalent bonding Metallic bonding Ionic interactions Complex interactions
Physical forces:	van der Waals interactions Dipol–dipol interactions Hydrogen bonds

Beside the polymerization of adhesive monomers, the formation of covalent bonds between the adherent and adhesive plays a minor role. The most popular example for the formation of a chemical bond for adhesion on dental substrates is the cross-linking of collagen by glutaraldehyde due to a Schiff base reaction. Glutaraldehyde is a cross-linking reagent capable of bonding to the amine groups of proteins.[137]

Figure 3.18 illustrates how glutaraldehyde forms covalent bonds to two proteins or collagen chains. In this way, highly cross-linked, insoluble protein aggregates are formed. This behavior is used, for example, in desensitizers and dentin adhesives. Ionic interactions combined with hydrogen bonds are the most important forces of adhesion in dentistry. The formation of ionic interactions between the calcium ions of hydroxyapatite and adhesives is a major contributor to adhesion. The adhesive monomers suitable for this purpose are, for example, derivatives of carboxylic acids and phosphoric or phosphonic acids. These groups enable the formation of stable ionic interactions between hydroxyapatite and adhesive monomers as shown in Figure 3.19.[138]

According to this premise, the calcium ions of hydroxyapatite in these compounds will form a complex. Pretreatment with solutions containing Al^{3+} or Fe ions reinforce this effect because they form more stable complexes with phosphoric compounds and carboxylic acids than Ca^{2+} ions do.[139,140]

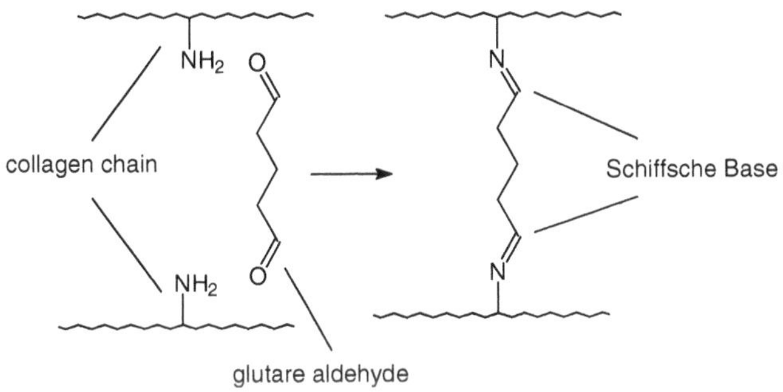

FIGURE 3.18 Reaction of glutaraldehyde with collagen.

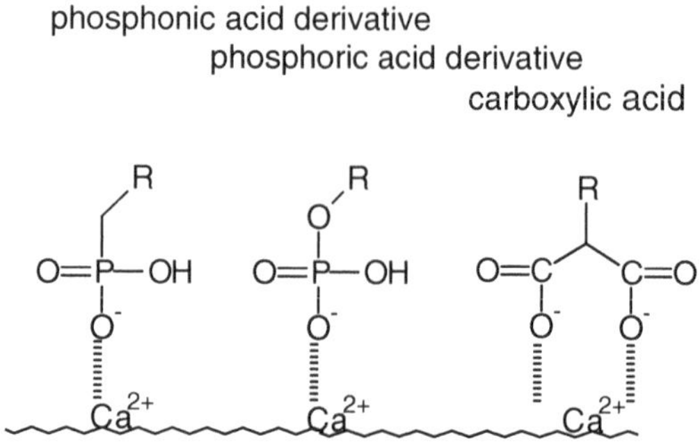

phosphonic acid derivative
phosphoric acid derivative
carboxylic acid

FIGURE 3.19 Groups that enable the formation of stable ionic interactions between hydroxyl apatite and derivatives of carboxylic acids, phosphoric, or phosphonic acids.

Hydrogen bonds form between molecules containing polar groups such as hydroxyl, amine, amide, and carboxyl groups, for example. Because enamel and especially dentin are wet and they are highly polar substrates, hydrogen bonding is important for the penetration and wetting behavior of the adhesive on the one hand and for adhesion on the other. Therefore, monomers that are capable of forming hydrogen bonds, for example, HEMA or GDMA, were used in adhesive formulations.

The previous theoretical considerations regarding adhesion have to be modified in the presence of water. Adhesion can be affected by water in different ways. The formation of a thin film of water on the adherents resulting from water adsorption can weaken the adhesive's strength. Penetration of water into the boundary layer between the adherent and adhesive may result in hydrolytic degradation and/or swelling of the adhesive or adherent because of water adsorption.[141]

An interesting example of an adhesive that functions in an aqueous medium is presented by the mussel adhesives.[141] The following requirements are fulfilled by this adhesive: Low binding layers on the adherent are removed, the surface is wetted by the adhesive, numerous interactions on the interface can build up, and the adhesive layer can be cured. From a chemical point of view, the mussel adhesives consist of poly(phenolic) peptides with a repeating decapeptide structure. For reliable adhesion, these proteins wet the adherent and displace the water layer from the surface. The proteins of mussel adhesives are tailormade for this reason. The decapeptide sequence of the polyphenolic proteins consists of alanine 1×, proline 1×, serine 1×, hydroxyproline 2×, threonine 1×, lysine 2×, tyrosine 1×, and dopa 1×. In contrast to the composition of collagens, the mussel adhesives contain dopa. This constituent enables the formation of hydrogen bonds, the formation of complexes with different elements, and Michael addition with primary amines for strong interactions with the adherent as indicated in Figure 3.20. The proteins themselves are capable of ionic interactions because most of the lysine is deprotonated. The hydroxy groups of serine, threonine, and hydroxyproline are responsible for the water compatibility. The polyphenolic proteins were applied as an emulsion from the mussel foot and were cured by oxidation processes. This example shows that a tailormade adhesive with an optimized composition and structure enables reliable adhesion on a wet surface.

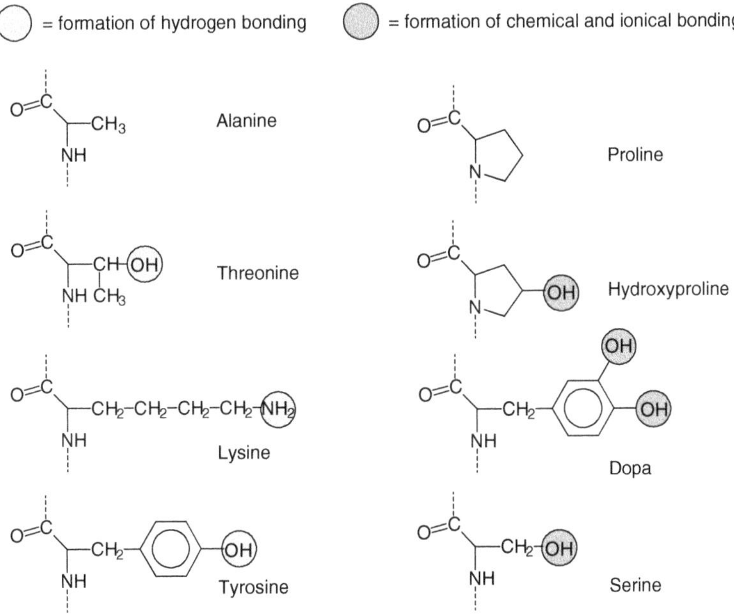

FIGURE 3.20 Adhesion properties of amino acids that are components in mussel adhesives.

3.4 METHODS FOR THE ASSESSMENT OF ENAMEL–DENTIN ADHESION

3.4.1 Bond Strength Measurements

3.4.1.1 Methods and Variables

In 1987, Olio reviewed the debonding tests used in dentin adhesion measurements and divided them into qualitative screening tests and quantitative tests, depending on the expectations of the test.[143] The quality test should be standardized and easy to perform. It can be a shear, tensile, torsion, cleavage, pull or extrusion, or four-point bending test.[143–145] A problem is presented by the lack of standardization of the test methods mainly because of the many variables connected with the substrate itself, the specimen preparation and treatment, and the way in which the debonding test is conducted.[146] Therefore, no ISO standard for dentin adhesives exists; there is just a rough guideline for testing them.[147] The main variables for testing the bond strength are shown in Table 3.6.[145,148,149]

In addition to the multitude of variables, the situation is complicated by the fact that in many publications the chosen test parameters are not listed in detail.[148] The following examples show how influential some of these variables are.

3.4.1.1.1 Substrate

Because of the limited availability and the increased awareness regarding the infection hazards associated with human teeth, bovine teeth have been used in many studies.

TABLE 3.6
Variables Influencing Bond Strength Testing

Substrate	Surface preparation
Human or bovine teeth?	Smear layer formation (diamond burr, sanded surface, grit size)
Tooth selection (molar, premolar, incisor)?	Etching
Superficial, middle or deep dentin?	Priming
Occlusal, proximal, or buccal cut?	Wet, dry, over wet, rewetting
Reuse of teeth?	
Storage conditions/stress simulation	**Primer/adhesive application**
Water, saline, chloramine?	Passive or active application?
Thermal cycling, number of cycles?	Light curing, self curing?
Occlusal load?	
Test performance	
Dentinal liquor stimulation	
Immediate vs. 24 h vs. months	
Crosshead speed	

Bovine coronal dentin possesses larger dentinal tubules but shows bond strength similar to human permanent dentin.[151–153] Bovine root dentin and dentin near the pulp produce different bonding results.[152] Causton stated that living human dentin would be the best substrate.[153] Difficulties with *in vivo* bond strength studies have led some investigators to use vital teeth for the adhesive application and to perform the bond strength tests after tooth extraction.[154]

Decreases in bond strength in deep dentin have been reported by several authors in the past.[155,156] However, as dentin adhesives have become more hydrophilic, the sensitivity of the bond strength in relation to the distance from the pulp has decreased.[157]

Effects of regional variations in tooth structure, such as the orientation of enamel prisms and dentinal tubules and the variability of cavity preparation, are still not completely understood. Different results have been found with regard to the influence of the orientation of the tubules on bond strength. In one investigation, the tensile bond strength of the group with tubules parallel to the bond interface was higher than that of the group with tubules cut perpendicular, independent of the type of adhesive system used (self-etch vs. total-etch).[158] However, Phrukkanon et al. and Watanabe et al., for example, found no influence of tubule orientation on the microtensile bond strength.[159,160]

In the case of enamel, it is well known that cavity preparation should be performed by cutting enamel prism more or less rectangularly (see Figure 3.21) to obtain higher bond strength.[161,162] Recently, Shimada and Tagami found a less pronounced influence of the prism orientation in the case of a self-etching adhesive system.[163]

3.4.1.1.2 Surface Preparation

For clinical cavity preparation, different methods can be selected by the dentist, for example, chemomechanical caries removal, laser ablation, air abrasion, or mechanical

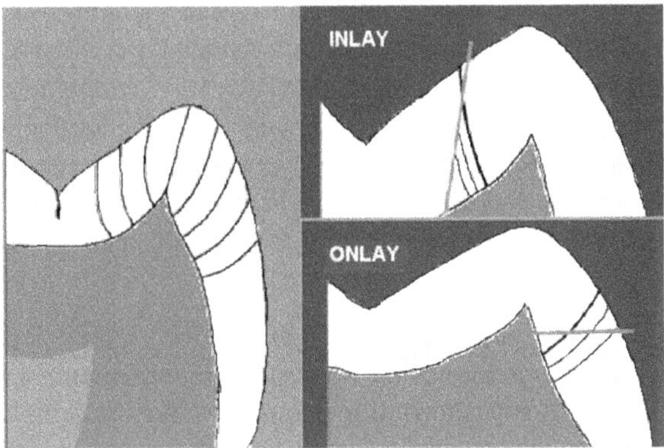

FIGURE 3.21 Recommendation for enamel preparation depending on the type of restoration.

preparation by rotating instruments, which is the most common method.[164–166] Each of these methods has a specific influence on the dentin–enamel surface conditions, which have to be taken in account for the selection of the corresponding adhesion technology and adhesive.[165] Mechanical tooth preparation mainly influences the surface roughness and the thickness of the smear layer formed on dentin. In the lab, tooth surfaces are usually ground with sandpaper of different grit size.

Dentin shear bond strength values are only minimally affected by the type of sandpaper, for example, silicon carbide or aluminum oxide, and the grit size.[166] The thickness of the smear layer, however, is influenced by the grit size of the sandpaper. In the case of total-etch systems, the bond strength is not influenced by the thickness of the smear layer. However, the function of self-etching systems depends very much on the thickness of the smear layer. Some systems do not totally dissolve and hybridize thick smear layers, which results in low bond strength values.[167]

3.4.1.1.3 Storage Conditions/Stress Simulation

In many cases freshly extracted teeth are not available for *in vitro* testing. Therefore, extracted teeth have to be stored over a period of at least a few weeks. To prevent bacterial contamination, researchers store them in disinfecting solutions such as 10% formalin, 70% ethanol, 0.1–1% chloramine, or 0.05–0.1% thymol. Phenolic compounds like thymol can inhibit radical polymerization. Aldehydes such as formalin or glutaraldehyde are known to react with collagen.[138] Retief et al., for example, reported a significant decrease in bond strength values on dentin in teeth stored in 0.05% thymol or 70% ethanol compared with saline or formalin.[168] In contrast, Cooley et al. found a significant increase in the bond strength by storing extracted teeth in 10% formalin over a period of several months.[169]

Reports about the long-term stability of the adhesive joint between adhesive resins and dentin or enamel, although rare, are important for evaluating clinical behavior. Sano et al. carried out a 1-year *in vivo* monkey study to evaluate the durability of resin–dentin bonds in the oral cavity.[170] Over the period of 1 year *vivo,* no decrease in the microtensile bond strength was observed. However, the number of porosities on the hybrid layer and within the adhesive increased over time. In many cases long-term behavior is evaluated by stress tests. The most frequently carried out stress test is thermal cycling.[171,172] In this test the specimens are alternately dipped in a water bath of 5°C and 55–60°C, for about 30–60 s each. The highest stress is created when the coefficient of thermal expansion of the resin (80–120 ppm/K) and the tooth structure (8–12 ppm/K) is very different. In some cases the teeth are also mechanically loaded to simulate chewing forces.[171]

3.4.1.1.4 Test Performance

Apart from the personal influence of the operator, for example, skill, motivation, experience, etc., the performance of the bond strength measurement is very decisive to the test results.[173,174] It was shown that parameters like the sample thickness and crosshead speed influence the results of bond strength measurements.[175–177] A crosshead speed of 0.8–1.0 mm/min is recommended for bond strength measurements.

To simulate *in vivo* conditions, some investigators applied hydrostatic intrapulpal pressure to the extracted teeth.[28,178–180] In many cases water or saline were used as substitutes for the dentinal liquor, which resulted in a decrease in the bond strength because the applied adhesive became diluted.[178,179] However, Nikaido et al. showed that if serum was used as the dentin liquor substitute, no decrease in the bond strength occurred.[28] Because of protein precipitation by the acids in the corresponding primers, dentin permeability decreased. Pameijer and Louw confirmed these results by comparing the adhesion of vital and nonvital teeth.[180] They found no statistically significant difference between the two systems.

Polymerization shrinkage in composite-based restorative materials occurs immediately after initiation of radical polymerization. In the clinical situation the dentist wants to start with finishing immediately after having placed the restoration. Therefore, adequate bond strength between the composite and the tooth structure is already required in this early phase. Usually bond strengths are measured after 24-h storage of the test specimen in water at 37°C.[147] Recently, 10-min values have also been measured.[181,182] It has been shown that there is a direct correlation between bond strength values and C-C double bond conversions and the build up of the mechanical properties of the resin.[181]

3.4.1.2 Shear Bond Strength

The easiest bonding test methods to perform are shear tests. For this purpose a composite cylinder is polymerized on a flat, ground enamel or dentin surface after the adhesive application. Several test setups are shown in Figure 3.22 with the force being applied parallel to the tooth surface. The shear bond strength (SBS), or the stress at failure between the composite and the substrate, is reported as the load of fracture divided by the cross-sectional area of the bonded surface in newtons per square millimeter:

$$\text{SBS} = \frac{\text{Load at fracture (N)}}{\text{Adhesion area (mm}^2\text{)}}$$

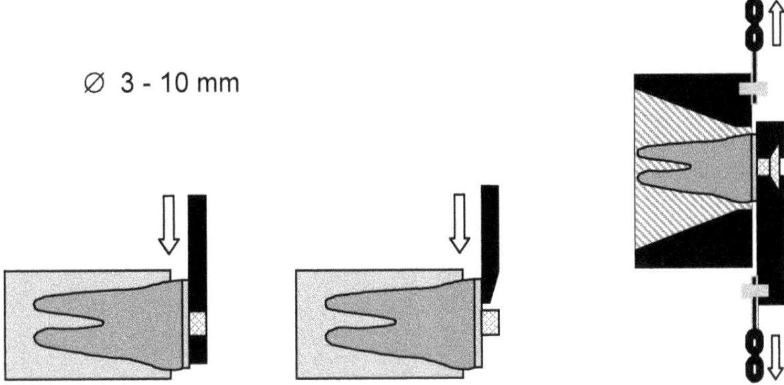

FIGURE 3.22 Schematic drawing of different test set-ups for measuring shear bond strength.

The most important criterion for the shear bond strength test is that the stresses at the interface between the adhesive and the substrate are anything but uniform (bending, tensile) and are highly dependent on the test geometry and loading configuration adopted.[183,184] In any case the mode of failure should be reported in addition to the bond strength values. The failure mode can be adhesive (located in the interface), cohesive (fracture in one of the materials on either side of the interface), or a mixture of both. If there is a cohesive part of failure, the bond strength values are irrelevant because the calculated adhesion area does not correspond to the fractured area. Figure 3.23 shows two currently used setups for measuring shear bond strength: what is known as the "Ultradent method" and the guillotine method.

3.4.1.3 Push Out Test

A test in which shear forces are also applied to the composite is the push out test.[144,186] The test setup is shown in Figure 3.24. An important advantage of the push out test is that marginal adaptation via replica and bond strength can be evaluated with the same test specimen. The test's drawback is that during water storage minor swelling of the composite can significantly increase the friction, which does not directly correspond to the adhesion between the composite and the tooth.

3.4.1.4 Tensile Bond Strength

Tensile bond strength tests (Figure 3.25) are believed to create more uniform stress distributions. However, finite element analysis (FEA) has shown that stress distribution in tensile tests can also be nonuniform, depending on the geometry and dimensions of the test specimen.[183,187] Tensile bond strength measurements with an adhesion surface diameter of 4 mm, as shown in Figure 3.25, are still performed, but nowadays microtensile bond strength measurement are preferred by most of the investigators.[188]

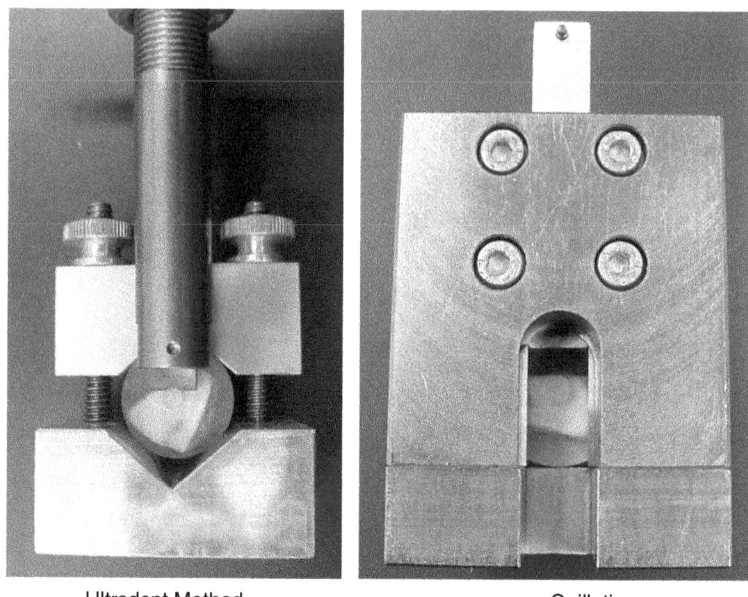

FIGURE 3.23 Ultradent method and the Guillotine — test devices for measuring shear bond strength.

3.4.1.5 Microtensile Bond Strength

One of the main reasons for performing microbond strength tests was to evaluate the influence of local effects on the tooth surface on bond strength. Both the application of tensile and shear force has been used for this purpose.[162,189,190] However, the microtensile bond strength method (μTBS) was more accepted for several reasons.[191,192] The microtensile bond strength method was introduced by Sano et al. in 1994.[189] They found that tensile bond strengths are inversely related

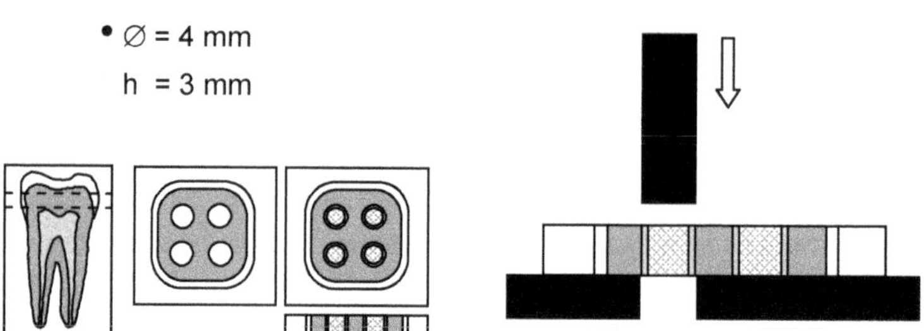

FIGURE 3.24 Test setup of the push out test.

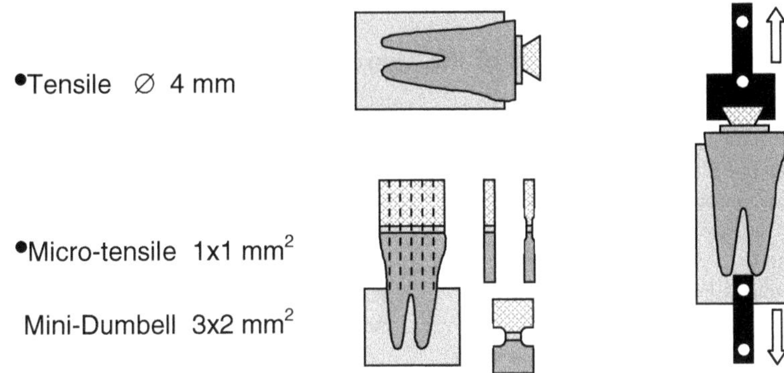

FIGURE 3.25 Test setup for tensile bond strength measurement.

to bonded surface areas using small areas in the range of 0.25–12 mm^2. There was a correlation between the cross-sectional area of the bond specimen and the failure mode. Below 2 mm^2 all the test specimens failed adhesively. In essence, this new bond strength method produces higher bond strength values compared with conventional methods. The results are dependent on the bonded surface area. Furthermore, the new method produces mainly adhesive failures in surface areas below 2 mm

The test specimen preparation is more labor intensive. After curing and storage in water, the test specimen is vertically sectioned in slabs using a low-speed diamond saw (Figure 3.25 and Figure 3.26). The resulting slabs are either additionally sectioned to four-square pins or reduced with an ultrafine burr to a minidumbbell shape.[189,193] For more homogeneous stress distribution, some prefer to trim the test specimen to an hourglass shape, resulting in a cylindrical cross-sectional bond area.[194] The advantages and disadvantages of the microtensile bond strength test are shown in Table 3.7.[146]

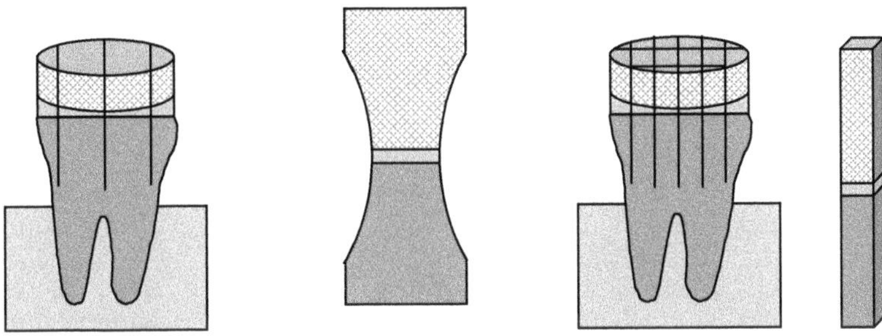

FIGURE 3.26 Schematic of the specimen preparation for the microtensile bond strength method.

TABLE 3.7
Advantages and Disadvantages of the Microtensile Bond Strength Test

Advantages	Disadvantages
More adhesive failures, fewer cohesive failures, higher initial bond strengths	Labor intensive
Permits measurements of regional bond strengths	Technically demanding
Means and variances can be calculated for single teeth	Prestress of the bond by sample preparation; therefore, difficult to measure bond strength <10 MPa
Permits testing of bonds to irregular surfaces	Requires special equipment
Permits testing of very small area	Samples are so small that they dehydrate rapidly
Facilitates SEM examination of the failed bonds because the surface area is approximately 1 mm^2	

3.4.2 Marginal Adaptation

Besides a high bond strength, a good marginal seal at the resin composite–tooth bonded interface is required for clinically successful restorations. Many attempts have been made to find out if there is a correlation between marginal integrity and bond strength.[195–197] Because there was no direct correlation between these two parameters for the assessment of the clinical potential of an adhesive system, both parameters had to be evaluated.

Two methods in principle have been established to quantify *in vitro* marginal integrity of adhesively placed fillings: either marginal analysis by scanning electron microscopy (SEM) (Figure 3.27) or determination of marginal leakage by dye penetration.[198–203] In some cases both methods have been combined.[204,205]

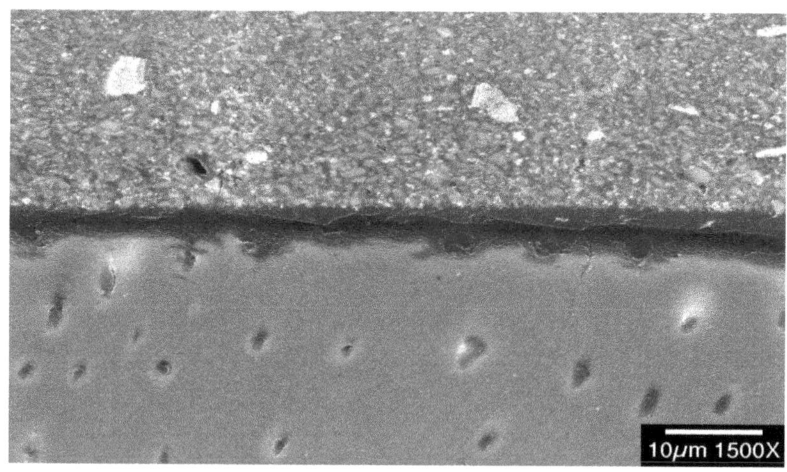

FIGURE 3.27 SEM image of a margin between composite filling material and dentin.

Therefore, after having made the replicas for the SEM analysis, the restored extracted teeth are immersed in a dye solution for about 24 h. Both methods have their disadvantages. In the case of the SEM analysis, only defects directly on the surface can be detected and the examination of the margin is very labor intensive and subjective. For the evaluation of the dye penetration score, the restored tooth is sectioned into three to six slabs. Less than about 2% of the whole margin is visible for quantification.

As is the case in bond strength evaluations, influencing factors such as the storage media of the teeth, penetration of the dye, and simulation of the intrapulpal pressure are tested and discussed. Furthermore, long-term behavior is evaluated by stress tests such as thermal cycling and/or mechanical loading.[206–210]

The advantage of these *in vitro* methods is that the geometric conditions, that is, the C-factors and the related polymerization shrinkage stress at the interface, are very much comparable with those of the clinical situation.[211,212] The C-factor is the ratio of bonded to unbonded surfaces. In the case of bond strength measurement, the C-factor is in the range of 1, which is clinically irrelevant. The disadvantage of the microleakage study is that the diffusion of synthetic dye molecules is not directly correlated to the diffusion of bacteria and the corresponding toxins.[213] This can lead to an overestimation of the results obtained with this method.

3.4.3 Morphology of the Interface

An important indicator for a good adhesive system is the formation of a homogeneous hybrid layer.[214,215] However, there is no direct correlation between the thickness of the hybrid layer and bond strength.[216,217] For the investigation of the micromorphology of the hybrid layer, microscopic methods, for example, SEM, TEM, atomic force microscopy (AFM), and confocal laser scanning microscopy (CLSM) have been used.[124,215,218–227] Figure 3.28 shows the SEM image of a hybrid layer and resin impregnated tubules.

Compared with SEM, TEM (Figure 3.29) AFM (Figure 3.30) and CLSM (Figure 3.31) show a higher resolution for imaging ultrastructural phenomena. However, TEM requires sophisticated sample preparation. TEM is often used for investigating nanoleakage, which in principle involves the decalcified nonhydbridized dentin at the bottom of the hybrid layer.[77,228] In the case of self-etching, water-based adhesives, the formation of what are known as water trees, which occurred as a result of water diffusion through the adhesive layer, was observed by TEM.[229,230]

In most cases, AFM was used to investigate the influence of surface treatment on the underlying dentin micromorphology. Intensive air-drying after removal of the smear layer created with phosphoric acid leads to a collapse of the exposed collagen fibril network.[222,225,231]

An advantage of CLSM is that no vacuum is required. It is still unclear if the monomers of the adhesive systems penetrate into the dentin surface like the fluorescent dyes used in this method to visualize the micromorphology.

3.4.4 Interfacial Chemistry

The following objectives are being pursued for obtaining more information about the interfacial chemistry:

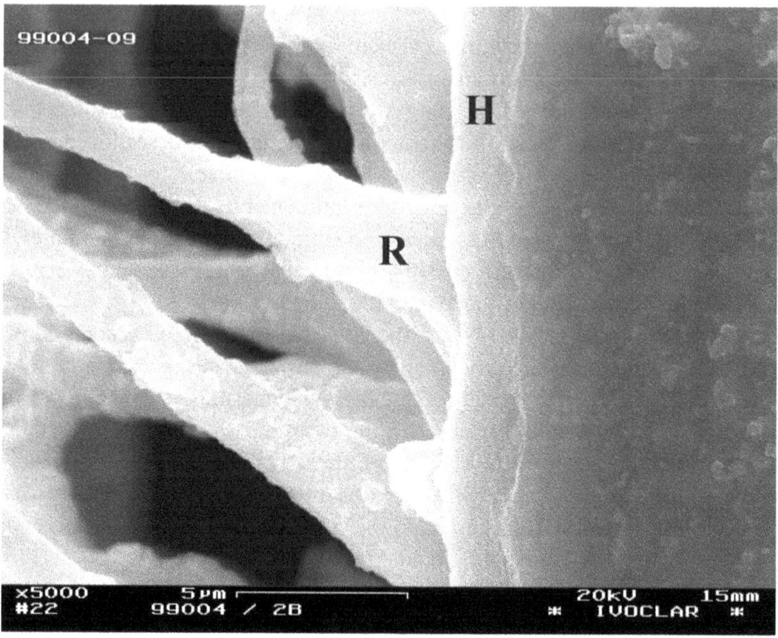

FIGURE 3.28 SEM image of a hybrid layer (H) and resin tags (R).

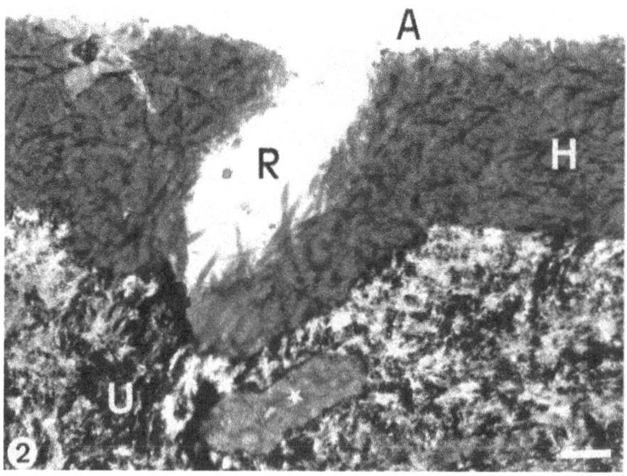

FIGURE 3.29 TEM-image of a hybrid layer (H), dentin tubule filled with polymer (R), the intact dentin (U), and the adhesive layer (A).

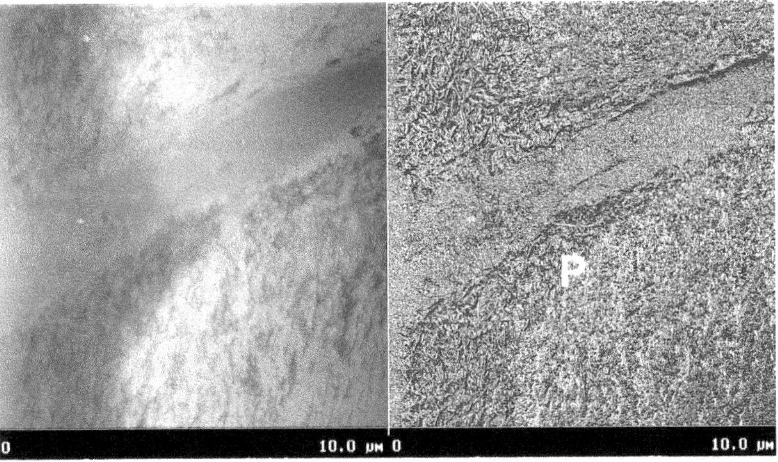

FIGURE 3.30 AFM-image of a hybrid layer at the peritubular region.

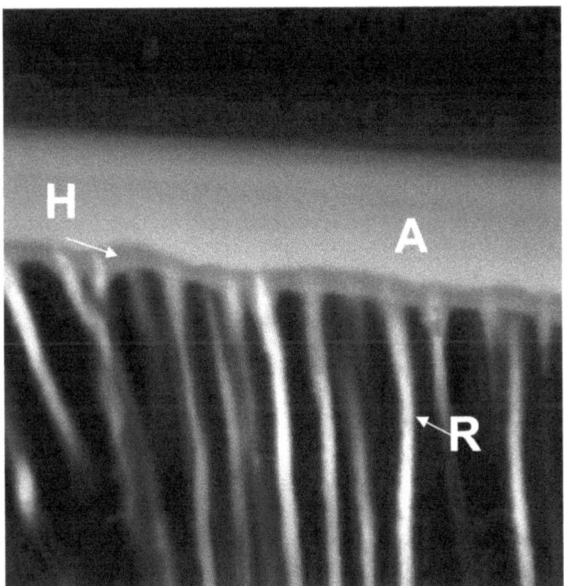

FIGURE 3.31 CLSM-image of a hybrid layer formed by a self-etching adhesive. Hybrid layer (H), dentin tubule filled with polymer (R), and the adhesive layer (A).

Investigation of chemical interactions and reactions between adhesive components and the tooth structure (collagen, hydroxyapatite)
Analysis of the chemical composition of the hybrid layer (monomer penetration)
Characterization of the polymerization kinetics in the interface (double bond conversion)

The following analytical methods have been used for this purpose:

Nuclear magnetic resonance spectroscopy (NMR)[232,233]
X-ray photoelectron spectroscopy (XPS) or electron spectroscopy for chemical analysis (ESCA)[234]
Infrared spectroscopy (IR)[235]
Auger spectroscopy [236]
Raman spectroscopy[237–243]

In the case of NMR and XPS spectroscopy, the interaction with pure collagen and hydroxyapatite was investigated.[232–234] For investigating chemical reactions on dentin, the high water content of dentin in the range of 25% is the limiting factor. ESCA analysis demands ultra high vacuum, and IR spectroscopy is limited by the overlap of the strong water bands.

The chemistry at the interface of the resin and tooth structure has been investigated by Raman spectroscopy relatively frequently. Raman spectroscopy is based on the Raman effect, which is the inelastic scattering of photons by molecules. There is hardly any dependency on the wavelength of incident light. Mainly argon laser (λ = 514.5 nm) was used. Nevertheless, there is a natural fluorescence in this wavelength region. Therefore, laser-emitting light at higher wavelengths, for example, Nd:YAG-laser (λ = 1064 nm) would be preferred. Raman spectroscopy was used, for example, for establishing the chemical composition of the resin–dentin interface and for investigating the polymerization kinetics by measuring the double bond conversion of the corresponding methacrylates.[237–243]

3.5 CHEMISTRY OF ENAMEL AND DENTIN ADHESIVES

3.5.1 Introduction

To achieve a strong bond between the filling material and the natural tooth substance (enamel and dentin), researchers have used a great number of reactive chemical compounds as dental adhesive monomers. In general, these adhesive monomers are bifunctional molecules containing at least, first, a polymerizable group P, which can react with the restorative material by copolymerization; second, an adhesive group AD capable of interacting or reacting with the tooth substance under formation of a chemical bond; and finally, a spacer group R designed to influence, for example, the solubility, flexibility, and wetting properties of the adhesive monomer (Figure 3.32).

Aside from the efficient interaction with both the dental hard tissue and the restorative material, the adhesive monomers should contribute to meeting the following

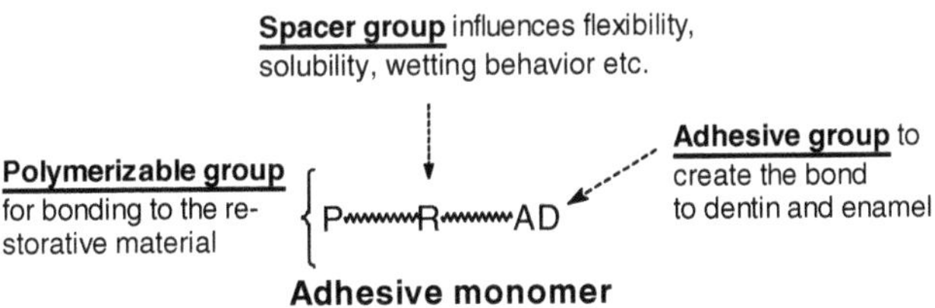

FIGURE 3.32 General structure of an adhesive monomer.

physicochemical requirements, which determine the processing and clinical performance of the dental bonding material:

Solubility in water and polar solvent
Optimal wetting and film-forming behavior on the tooth surface
Ability to penetrate, for example, into the dentinal tubules
Self-etching properties
Fast interaction with the dental hard tissue
High polymerization rate
Hydrolytical stability, both of the monomer and formed adhesive polymer
Sufficient mechanical strength of the adhesive layer
High durability of the hybrid zone and dense sealing of tooth surfaces
Capacity of the adhesive layer to resist shrinkage or thermal stress
Minimal water uptake and low swelling degree of the adhesive layer
Storage stability of the uncured adhesive
Low oral toxicity and cytotoxicity, and no mutagenic or carcinogenic effect

These requirements can be fulfilled by adhesive monomers with a specially designed structure combining appropriately polymerizable groups with optimized spacers.[130,244–246] Presently, the monomer matrix of restorative materials is based on a mixture of radically polymerizable cross-linking monomers. Therefore, a strong bond between the adhesive and the restorative material can be accomplished by copolymerization of the filling composite with adhesive monomers, which contain at least one radically polymerizable group. In this context (meth)acrylate or (meth)acrylamide groups demonstrate sufficient reactivity, whereas vinyl or styryl derivatives are less reactive (Figure 3.33). Moreover, in the case of allyl or 1,2-disubstituted ethylene derivatives, such as maleic acid, polymerization takes place only in the presence of more reactive cross-linking monomers.

The chemical adhesion on the natural tooth hard tissue can be realized by the formation of primary chemical bonds with monomers that contain an appropriate adhesive group (Figure 3.34). Thus, chelating agents such as β-diketones, salicylic acid, or α-amino acids enable the formation of coordinative linkages to the calcium ions of enamel or dentin. Ionic bonds are formed by the reaction of carboxylic and phosphonic acids or acidic phosphates with the inorganic component of the tooth hard tissue. Furthermore, coupling groups can be used to create covalent bonds

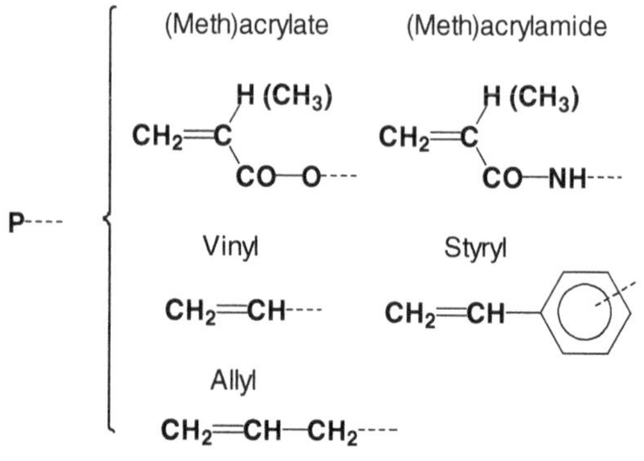

FIGURE 3.33 Polymerizable groups in adhesive monomers.

between the collagen molecules and the adhesive monomer. Because the dentinal collagen contains reactive groups, especially amino or hydroxyl groups, the reaction of dentin with aldehydes, isocyanates, epoxides, or anhydrides can result in the formation of covalent bonds to the collagen fibers under mild conditions. Moreover, secondary valence forces, such as attraction forces of molecular (van der Waals forces) and induced dipoles (London dispersion forces) or attraction forces caused by the formation of hydrogen bridges or charge-transfer interactions may additionally contribute to the adhesion (physical adhesion). Finally, in the case of the formation of a hybrid layer and resin tags, the adhesion mechanism mainly involves mechanical adhesion, while chemical and physical adhesion aspects are more or less relevant.

The structure of the spacer between the polymerizable and the adhesive group (Figure 3.35) influences the solubility, viscosity, and wetting and penetration behavior

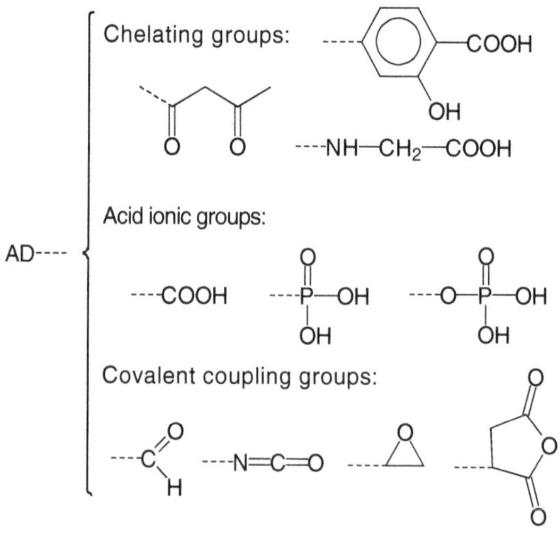

FIGURE 3.34 Adhesive groups enable chemical adhesion to enamel or dentin.

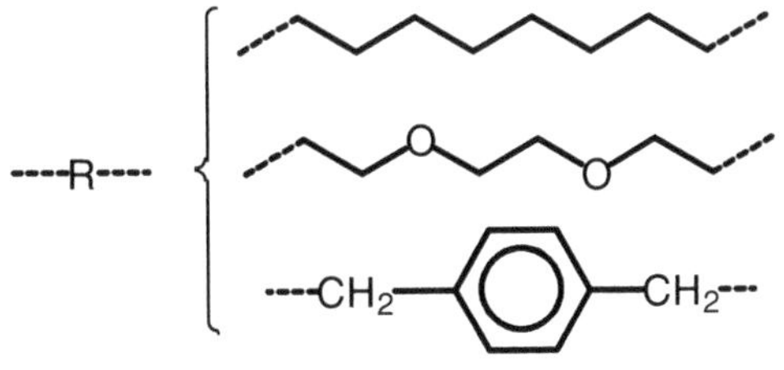

FIGURE 3.35 Spacer groups in adhesive monomers.

of the entire adhesive monomer and the flexibility, water uptake, and swelling behavior or mechanical properties of the formed adhesive polymer. For example, with the increasing chain length of alkylene spacers, the solubility in water or polar solvents of the monomer and the water uptake of the polymer will decrease, whereas the monomer viscosity and polymer flexibility will increase. Therefore, the introduction of oxygen into the spacer chain results in a corresponding increase in the solubility and in the swelling degree of polar solvents, for example, water. Moreover, spacers with a xylylene structure can be used to increase the hydrophobicity of highly water-soluble monomers containing ionic adhesive groups.

3.5.2 Acidic Bonding Agents

3.5.2.1 Phosphorus-Containing Monomers

The glycerol dimethacrylate ester of phosphoric acid (GDMP) was one of the first chemical compounds to be investigated in an effort to improve the bonding to human dentin.[53,247] It was prepared by the reaction of the disodium salt of glycerol 2-phosphate with methacryloyl chloride (Figure 3.36).

In general, phosphorus-containing monomers are capable of etching enamel and dentin. Furthermore, these monomers promote monomer diffusion into the acid-conditioned and underlying intact dentin. Therefore, various methacryloxyalkyl groups containing hydrogen (A) or dihydrogen phosphates (B) or diphosphates (C) (Figure 3.37) have been described in numerous patents in the last 25 years.[248–256] One of the first acidic methacrylate phosphates applied to improve the bond to dentin was the reaction product of phosphorous oxychloride with Bis-GMA.[250,257] Further examples of monomers that are used in practice, such as methacryloyloxyethyl

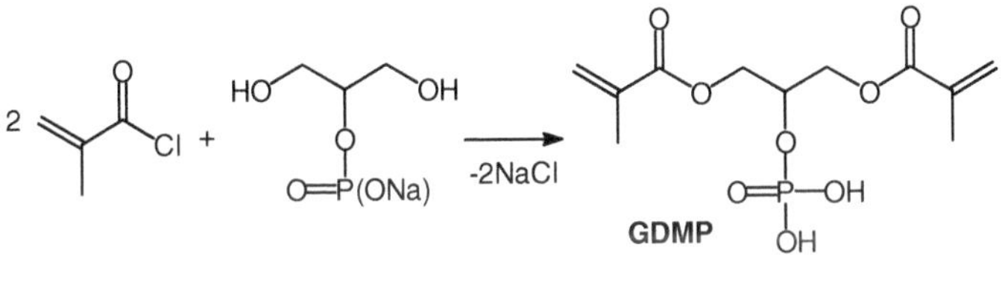

FIGURE 3.36 Reaction scheme of the synthesis of GDMP.

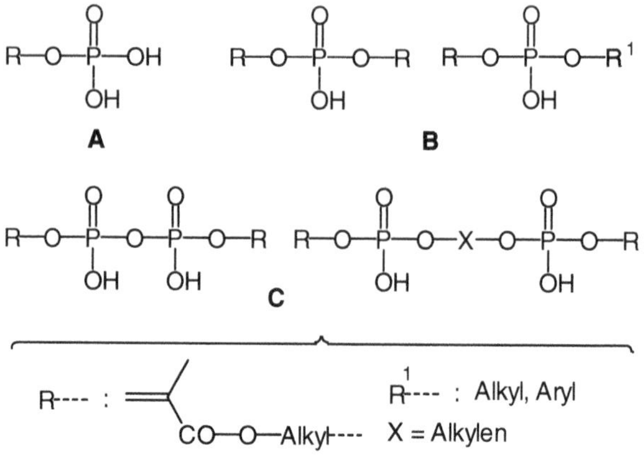

FIGURE 3.37 General formulas of methacryloyloxyalkyl hydrogen phosphates or diphosphates.

phenyl hydrogen phosphate (MEP-P), methacryloyloxydecyl hydrogen phosphate (MDP), methacryloyloxypropyl dihydrogen phosphate (MPP), methacryloyloxyethyl dihydrogen phosphate (MEP), and dipentaerythrolpentaacryloyl dihydrogen phosphate (Penta-P), are summarized in Figure 3.38. The synthesis and dental adhesive application of MEP-P and its *p*-methoxy derivative was first described by Nakabayashi and coworkers.[258,259]

Although the bond strength to enamel was excellent, the bond strength to etched dentin was rather low. Furthermore, it was found that the length of the polymer tags of an MEP-P based adhesive in acid-etched vital dentin was significantly lower than that in nonvital dentin.[260] Similarly to MEP-P, MDP also promotes the diffusion of

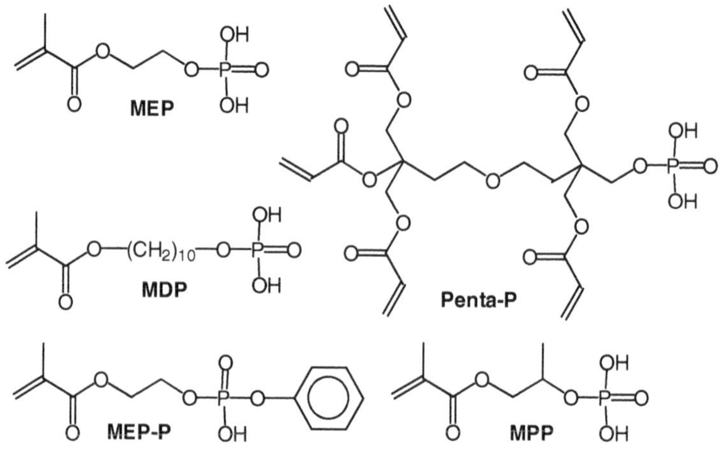

FIGURE 3.38 Examples of polymerizable acidic phosphates used in dental adhesives.

monomers into the dentin and improves the bond strength to dentin and enamel. Many of the polymerizable acidic phosphates shown in Figure 3.38 were first used in dental adhesives of the second generation. Presently, these strong acidic monomers are attracting additional interest because they enable the preparation of self-etching adhesives (adhesives of the fifth generation).[262–264] Thus, Reinhart et al. reevaluated the adhesive potential of GDMP and investigated the dentin adhesion of MPP. They found shear bond strength values of about 27.8 MPa for both monomers without pretreatment of the dentin surface with phosphoric acid. Nevertheless, it must be noted that self-etching adhesives of this kind are mostly used as a water-based solution of the polymerizable acidic phosphates. In the case of all the methacrylate phosphates shown in Figure 3.38, hydrolysis of the methacrylate ester bond will take place in the presence of water and is catalyzed by hydrogen ions of the phosphoric acid group. For MEP, we found both the hydrolysis of the methacrylate and phosphate ester bond under formation of both methacrylic acid (MAA) and 2-hydroxyethyl methacrylate (HEMA), which is illustrated in Figure 3.39.[266,267] general, the hydrolytic stability of the phosphoric acid esters increases in the following order: trialkyl phosphate < dialkyl hydrogen phosphate < monoalkyl dihydrogen phosphate.[268] Therefore, hydrolysis of the phosphate ester bond in the monoester MEP was not expected. Furthermore, we found that in the case of longer alkylene spacers, for example, MDP, the phosphate ester bond is more stable. Nevertheless, aqueous solutions of MDP are also not stable in storage at room temperature and have to be stored in a refrigerator.

The problem with the hydrolytical instability of the methacrylate phosphates can be overcome with monomers containing more hydrolytically stable bonds between the polymerizable group and the strongly acidic phosphorous group. One possibility is the use of phosphonates, which were first patented in 1985.[248] dentistry, organic phosphonates are well known and used in dentifrices to reduce the formation of supragingival dental calculus because they act as calcium sequestrants or as inhibitors of the crystal growth of calcium phosphates.[269] A first

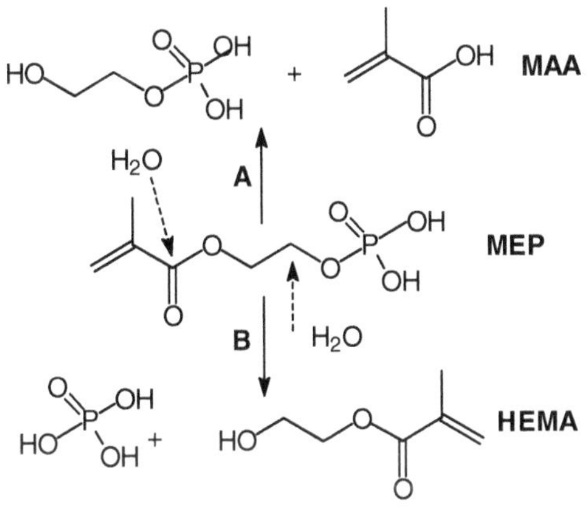

FIGURE 3.39 Hydrolysis of MEP in the presence of water.

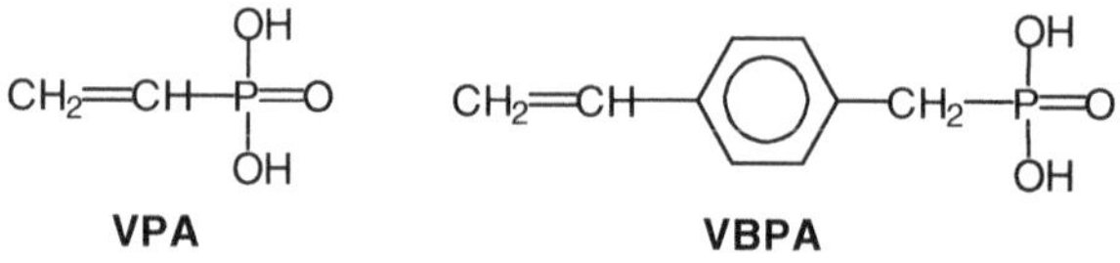

FIGURE 3.40 Structure of the monomeric phosphonic acids VPA and VBPA.

evaluation of polymerizable phosphonates for dental adhesives was carried out by Anbar and coworkers.[270–272] They showed that vinylphosphonic acid (VPA) and 4-vinylbenzylphosphonic acid (VBPA) (Figure 3.40) or corresponding copolymers can improve the adhesion of filling composites on etched enamel and decrease the adsorption of proteins on enamel. Unfortunately, VPA and VBPA are less reactive than methacrylates in radical polymerization. In this context we were able to synthesize a number of hydrolytically stable acrylic phosphonic acids, APA-1 to APA-3, in which the polymerizable methacrylate group and the strong acidic phosphorous group are connected via a hydrolytically stable ether bond (Figure 3.41).[267,273–275] Among these monomers, APA-2 showed the best dentin adhesive properties, whereas the corresponding phosphonic acid half ester APA-2-HE, carboxylic acid APA-2-CA, or the nitrile derivative APA-2-CN (Figure 3.42) exhibited significantly less adhesive action. This could be explained on the basis of, for example, the lower solubility (APA-2-CA) or radical polymerizability (APA-2-CN) of the monomers. Recently, a number of methacrylates of hydroxylalkylphosphonates have been proposed, for example, MAPA-1 or the difunctional monomer MAPA-2 (Figure 3.43).[276,277] However, these monomers are not hydrolytically stable because they undergo hydrolysis in the presence of water under formation of methacrylic acid. In this context, the phosphonic acids DMHD and MAMPA (Figure 3.44) described in a recent patent should be hydrolytically stable.[278] Nevertheless, DMHD is not an appropriate monomer for radical polymerization. Unfortunately, no results of adhesion measurements were presented in the patent.[278]

In summary, the phosphorus-containing monomers are capable of etching enamel and dentin, and promoting the monomer diffusion into the acid-conditioned and underlying intact dentin. Therefore, they can be used for the preparation of

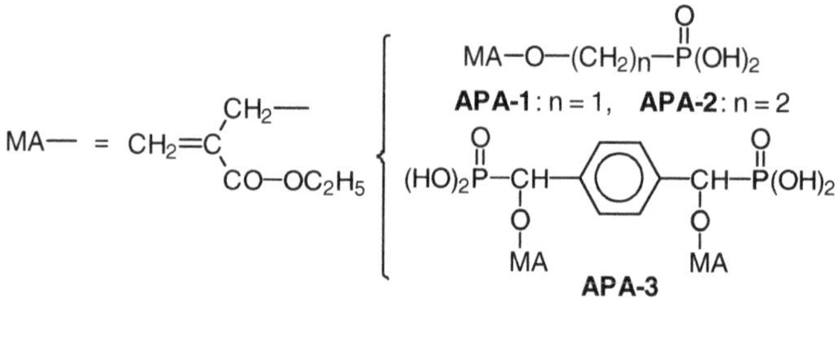

FIGURE 3.41 Structure of hydrolytically stable acrylic phosphonic acids AOA-1 and Tp APA-3.

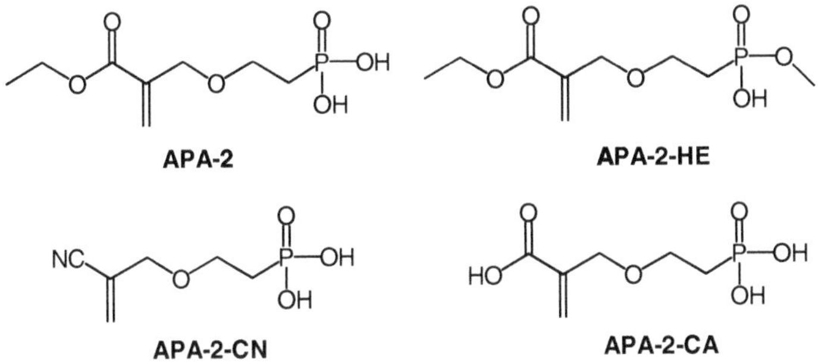

APA-2 APA-2-HE

APA-2-CN APA-2-CA

FIGURE 3.42 Structure of various derivatives of the stable acrylic phosphonic acids APA-2.

self-etching primers. Moreover, the hydrolytically stable acrylic phosphonic acids have enabled the development of one-bottle systems.

3.5.2.2 COOH-Group Containing Monomers and Polymerizable Carboxamides

In 1965, Bowen postulated that surface active comonomers (SAC) could facilitate the bonding of resins to dental surfaces, to walls of dental cavities, and to solid surfaces containing metals or metal ions.[56–69] The SACs, for example, NPG-GMA or NTG-GMA (Figure 3.45), the addition product of *N*-phenylglycine (NPG) or *N*-tolylglycine (NTG) and glycidyl methacrylate (GMA), are reactive monomers that can chelate ions and contain hydrophilic (OH, COOH), hydrophobic (phenyl), and polymerizable (methacrylate) groups. Therefore, the SACs should be both capable of forming a five-atom chelate ring with the surface calcium ions and of copolymerization with a methacrylate-based dental material (Figure 3.46). In fact, it was found that NPG-GMA forms a monolayer on the surface of hydroxyapatite under salt formation and that the chemisorption of NPG on hydroxyapatite was mediated via the oxygen atom of the COOH group and the nitrogen atom of the amino group.[60,279,280] Furthermore, polyfunctional SACs were obtained by the reaction of

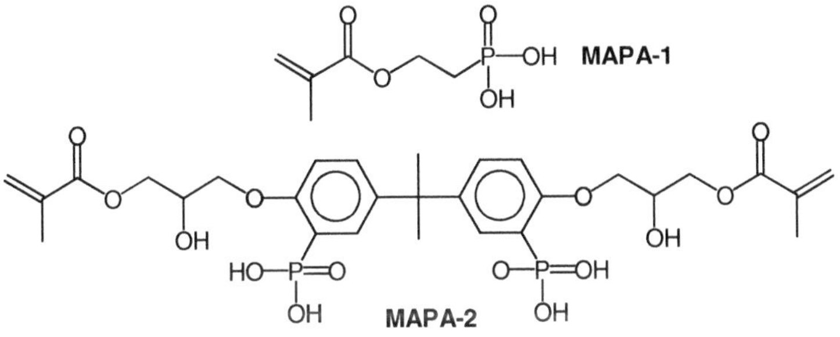

MAPA-1

MAPA-2

FIGURE 3.43 Structure of methacryloyloxyalkylphoshonic acids MAPA-1 and MAPA-2.

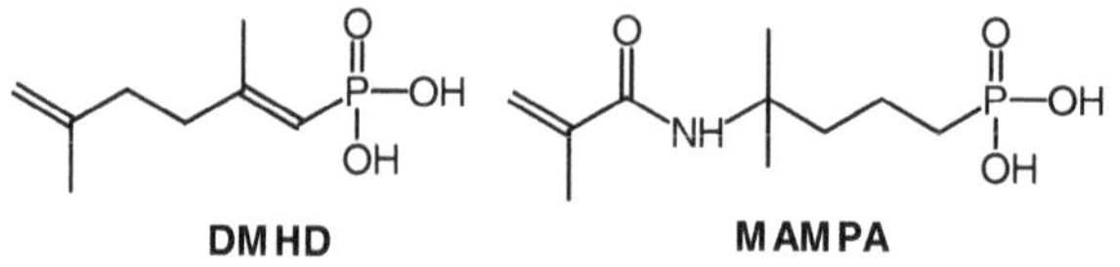

DMHD MAMPA

FIGURE 3.44 Structure of phosphonic acids DMHD and MAMPA.

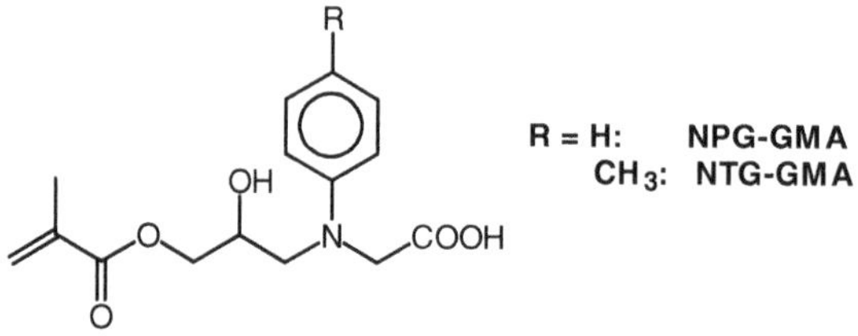

R = H: NPG-GMA
CH_3: NTG-GMA

FIGURE 3.45 Surface active comonomers NPG-GMA and NTG-GMA.

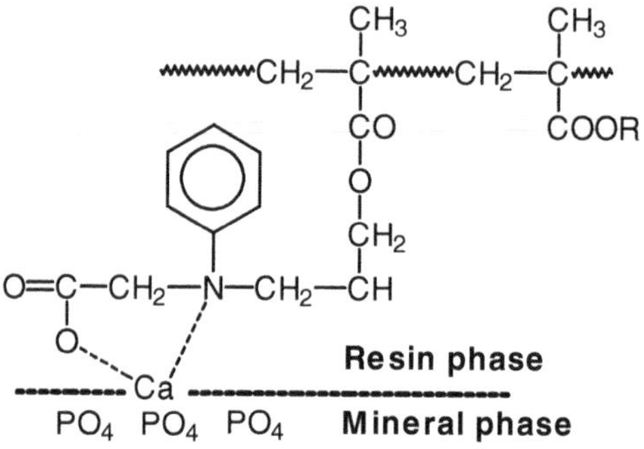

Resin phase
Mineral phase

FIGURE 3.46 Hypothetical bonding mechanism of NPG-GMA.

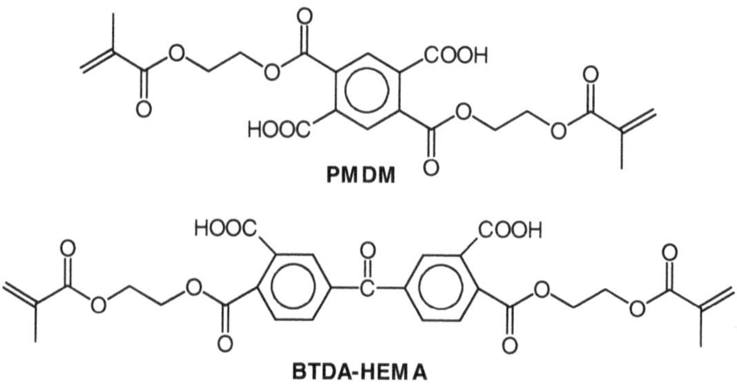

PMDM

BTDA-HEMA

FIGURE 3.47 COOH-group containing dimethacrylates PMDM and BTDA-HEMA.

oligomeric diglycidyl ether of bisphenol A with acrylic acid followed by the reaction with lithium aminobenzoate.[61] An improvement of the quality of the binding sites on the inorganic portion of the dentin and the formation of sites in or on the organic material was achieved by using "mordants." Among the studied ions [Fe(III), Cu(II), Al(III), Zn(II), Co(II)], ferric ions showed the greatest affinity to the hard tooth tissues.[62–73] Based on these results, a new method for obtaining a strong adhesive bond between composites and dentin and enamel was developed by Bowen.[67–70] The bonding mechanism involves the formation of precipitates on the pretreated dentinal substrates and bonding of the adhesive resin via chemical and mechanical interaction. According to this method, the mechanically prepared tooth surface was treated with a 5.3% aqueous solution of ferric oxalate, washed with water, and dried with air. Then, a 10% acetone solution of NTG-GMA was applied and the surface was dried with air. Finally, an acetone solution of, for example, the 1:2-addition product PMDM of pyromellitic acid anhydride and HEMA or the addition reaction product BTDA-HEMA of 3,3,4,4-benzophenonetetracarboxylic dianhydride (BTDA) and HEMA was applied (Figure 3.47). Later, this method was simplified to a two-step technique.[71–73]

In Japan, Nakabayashi and coworkers followed the concept of diffusion and impregnation of monomers into the subsurfaces of pretreated dentinal substrates and their polymerization, creating a hybrid layer of resin reinforced dentin.[55,281–285] The starting MMA resin was developed by Masuhara using the *tri-n*-butyl borane (TBB) in the presence of water and oxygen to initiate the polymerization of MMA and promote the bonding of MMA via graft copolymerization.[286] Furthermore, they used monomers containing hydrophobic and hydrophilic groups, which promoted monomer diffusion into the pretreated dental hard tissues. Adhesive monomers, such as 2-hydroxy-3-phenoxypropyl methacrylate (HPPM) or 2-hydroxy- 3-(2-naphthoxy)-propyl methacrylate (HNPM) (Figure 3.48), which were not reactive with calcium salts, were investigated initially, improving the bonding to the tooth substrate. Nevertheless, it was found that the carboxylic acid monomer 4-methacryloyloxyethyl trimellitate anhydride (4-META), which hydrolyzes into 4-methacryloyloxyethyl trimellitic acid (4-MET), is more effective in promoting monomer diffusion than HNPM. In the proposed procedure for the 4-META/

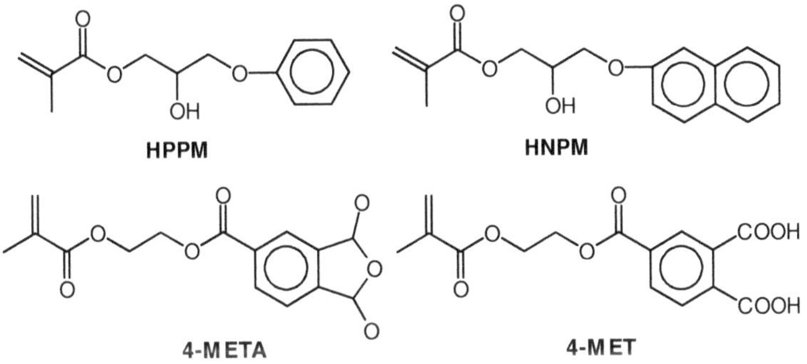

FIGURE 3.48 Diffusion promoting monomers HPPM, HNPM, 4-META, and 4-MET.

MMA/TBB bonding system, 3% ferric chloride in 10% citric acid (10:3 solution) was applied to remove the smear layer and demineralize the underlying intact dentin. Then, a 5% 4-META solution in MMA was used and polymerization was initiated by TBB, producing an excellent hybridized dentin. Raman spectroscopic investigations confirmed that in the case of the 4-META system, the primary bonding mechanism is more likely to be due to micromechanical bonding. Therefore, the function of the 4-MET in the bonding system is to wet the tooth surface through hydrogen bonding, allowing MMA monomers to diffuse and penetrate deeper into the dentin.

A number of additional monomers containing a carboxylic group, which have been described as adhesive monomers in enamel or dentin bonding systems, are summarized in the following list.

Reaction products of cyclic dianhydride with HEMA (Figure 3.49): BTDA-HEMA is fabricated in the same way as the reaction products of HEMA with other cyclic dianhydride or aromatic tetracarboxylic acids for dentin bonding systems described in the patent.[288]

Benzoic acid derivatives (Figure 3.50): 4-Vinylbenzoic acid (VBA) and 4-vinylsalicylic acid (VSA) showed pure radical polymerizability. Nevertheless, they improve the adhesion of dentin bonding systems.[289,290] More reactive in their radical polymerization are the methacrylic acid derivatives, such as *N*-methacryloyl aminosalicylic acid (MASA) and methacryloyloxy benzoic acids (MABA).[290–292]

Naphthalene-tricarboxylic anhydride derivatives (Figure 3.51): The isomeric methacryloyloxyethyloxycarbonyl derivative of naphthalene-1,2,6-, -2,3,6, and -1,4,5-tricarboxylic anhydride derivatives were synthesized by the reaction of the acid monochloride anhydrides with HEMA and improved the adhesion with the MMA-TBB bonding system.[293]

Polymerizable derivatives of aliphatic dicarboxylic acids (Figure 3.52): The application of monomethacryloyloxyethyl oxalate, malonate, and succinate in dental adhesive compositions was first described in 1970.[294] Among the polymerizable derivatives of saturated aliphatic dicarboxylic acids, succinoxy alkylene methacrylates (SAM) and succinoxy methacrylates with further hydrophobic groups (SXM) resulted in adhesives that were effective in

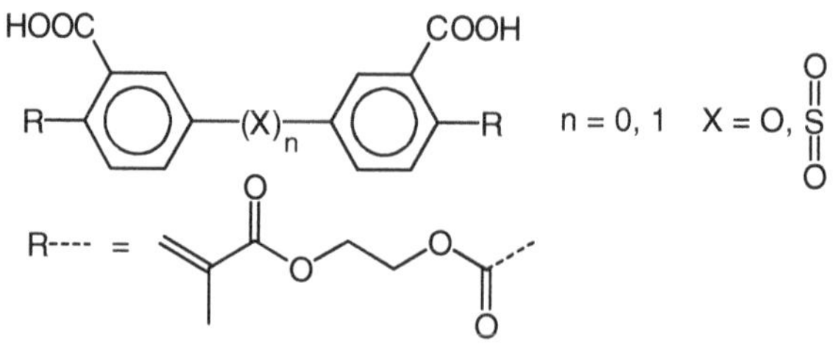

HOOC COOH
R—(X)$_n$—R n = 0, 1 X = O, SO_2
R---- =

FIGURE 3.49 Dimethacrylate dicarbocylic acids based on aromatic cyclic anhydrides.

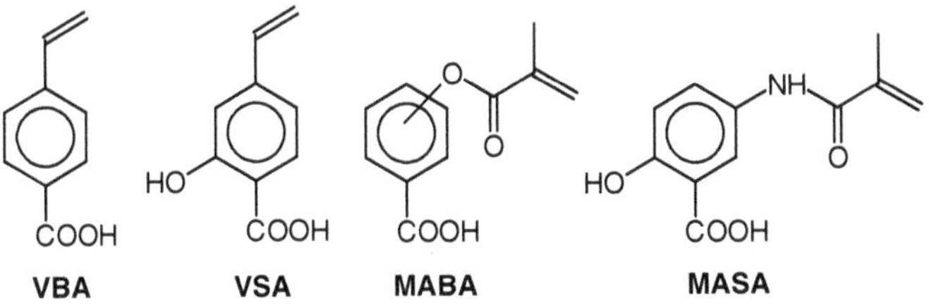

VBA VSA MABA MASA

FIGURE 3.50 Examples of monomeric adhesive benzoic derivatives.

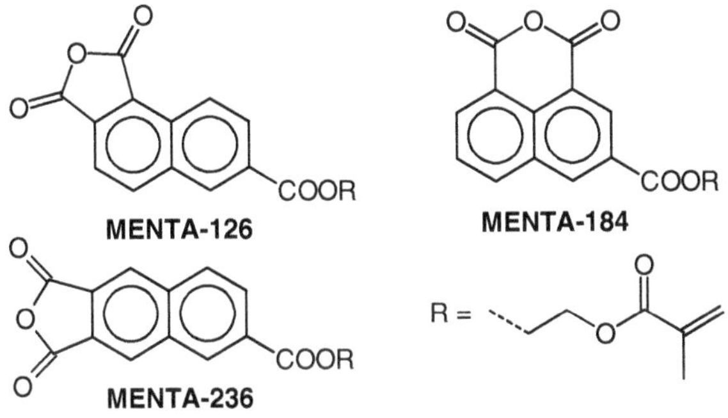

MENTA-126 MENTA-184 MENTA-236

FIGURE 3.51 Polymerizable naphthalene-tricarboxylic anhydride.

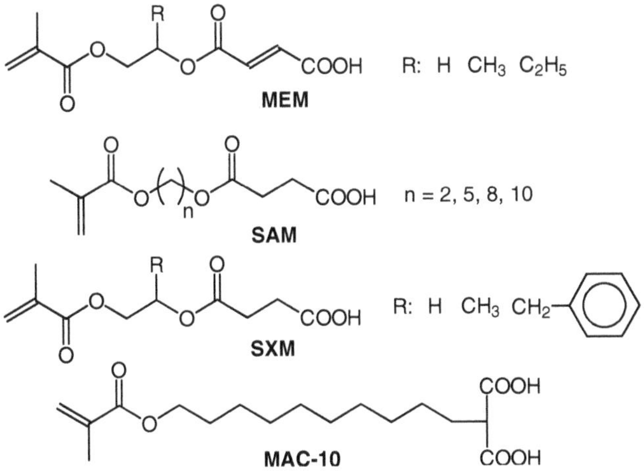

MEM R: H CH_3 C_2H_5

SAM n = 2, 5, 8, 10

SXM R: H CH_3 CH_2–

MAC-10

FIGURE 3.52 Polymerizable derivatives of aliphatic dicarboxylic acids.

adhering to dental hard tissues and alloys.[295–299] Similar to the succinates, methacryloyloxyalkyl hydrogen maleate (MEM) showed high bonding effectiveness to etched dentin.[298] Ferrari and Garcia-Godoy describe the synthesis of the adhesive monomer MAC-10 and 2-methacryloyloxyalkyl-malonic acids.[201]

Polymerizable imino diacids (Figure 3.53): *N*-(Vinylbenzyl)iminodiacetic acid (VBIDIAA) can be easily synthesized by the reaction with chloromethylstyrene with iminodiacetic acid and exhibits good adhesiveness to teeth and dental ceramic.[300,301]

Modified polymeric carboxylic acids: Polycarboxylic acids that bear lateral methacrylate groups (Figure 3.54) can be prepared by polymer analogous reactions of the polycarboxylic acid with glycidyl methacrylate (GMA) or 2-isocyanatoethyl methacrylate (IEMA).[302,303] GMA-modified poly(acrylic acid) (PAA) and a GMA-modified poly(5-norbornene-2,3-endo/exo-dicarbocylic acid) (Figure 3.54) obtained by ring-opening metathesis polymerization were used for the preparation of dentin adhesives.[253,304,305] A bioadhesive composition based on a polymer containing carboxylic groups was described by Müller et al.[306]

A number of new polymerizable amide monomers as components of dental adhesives were patented by Bayer AG, including the *N*-alkyl-*N*(meth) acryloylalkylcarboamides, for example, the trimellitic acid derivative TMAEAH, or (meth)acrylic esters containing formamide groups, such as 3-formamidopropyl methacrylate (FAPMA) or *N*-methacryloyloxyethyl-*N*-methylformamide (MFAEMA), which enables the treatment of collagen-containing substances (Figure 3.55).[306–310] (Meth)acrylic acid esters containing formylpiperazine groups, for example, *N*-formyl-*N*-5-(methacryloyloxyethyl)piperazine FMAEP and alkanediyl-*bis*-carboxamides, such as *N,N*-ethanediyl-*bis*[-(*N*-formyl)amino-ethyl 2-methyl-2-propenoate] (EDFAMA), showed similar reactivity.[309,310]

3.5.2.3 Combinations of Aldehydes and Ketones and Monomers with Active Hydrogen

In 1978, Antonucci described the synthesis of benzaldehyde methacrylates derived from hydroxybenzaldehyde (Figure 3.56).[311] He postulated that these monomers may promote bonding to the dentinal surface via both a Schiff base reaction between primary amino groups of collagen with the aldehyde groups and adhesion of carboxylic groups formed by oxidation of unreacted aldehyde moieties.

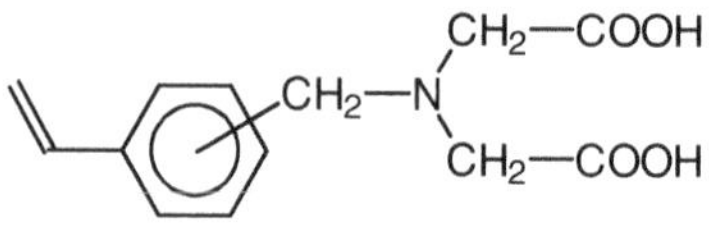

$CH_2-N(CH_2-COOH)_2$ VBIDIAA

FIGURE 3.53 Structure of VBIDIAA.

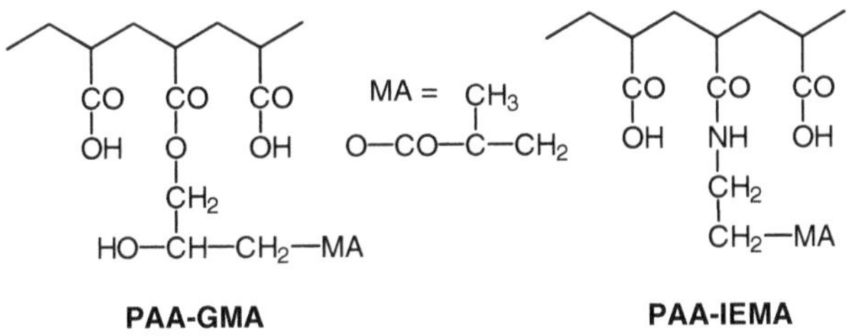

FIGURE 3.54 PAA modified with GMA or IEMA.

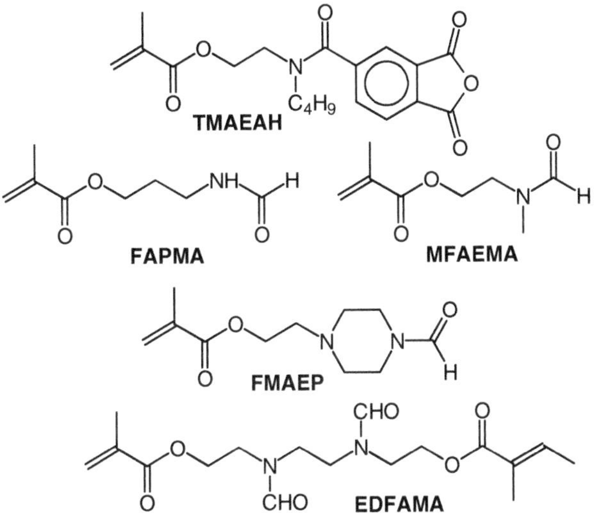

FIGURE 3.55 Adhesive amide monomers.

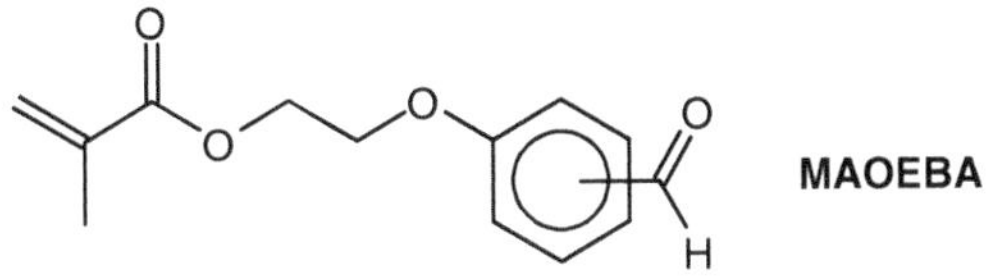

FIGURE 3.56 Structure of benzaldehyde methacrylates.

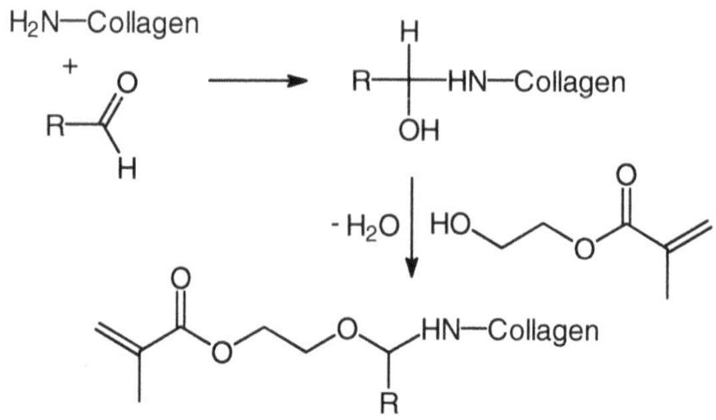

FIGURE 3.57 Proposed mechanism for the interaction of HEMA, an aldehyde, and collagen.

Asmussen and coworkers investigated dentin adhesives, starting on combinations of aldehydes, mainly formaldehyde and glutaraldehyde, with HEMA, which were the basis for a number of patents registered by Bayer AG.[138,312–315] It was suggested that in the first step the glutaraldehyde forms an *N*-(hydroxyalkyl) intermediate, which reacts with HEMA under the formation of water and an *O,N*-acetal bond between HEMA molecules and the collagen–glutaraldehyde reaction complex. Subsequently applied resin would copolymerize with the collagen-linked methacrylate groups (Figure 3.57). In a series of various aliphatic aldehydes, propionaldehyde exhibited the highest tensile bond strength value in the presence of HEMA, while other aromatic and heteroaromatic aldehydes were less reactive.[316,317] In this way, it was shown that the monofunctional aldehyde propanal may also act as cross-linking agent.[318] Furthermore, it was found that the pretreatment acidic solutions of amino acids, for example, glycine, *N*-phenyl-glycine, or lysine increased the tensile bond strengths obtained with Gluma.[319,320]

Because a primer based on HEMA and maleic acid mediated an exceptionally good bond to dentin, maleic anhydride was also combined with propanal in adhesive resin cement.[321–323]

3.5.2.4 Cyanoacrylates, Isocyanates, and Cyanurate

In 1957, alkylesters of cyanoacrylic acid (Figure 3.58) were first patented by Eastman Kodak as a component of high-strength adhesives for bonding all kinds of materials such as glass, metals, plastics, rubber, wood, and cement.[324] Cyanoacrylates are

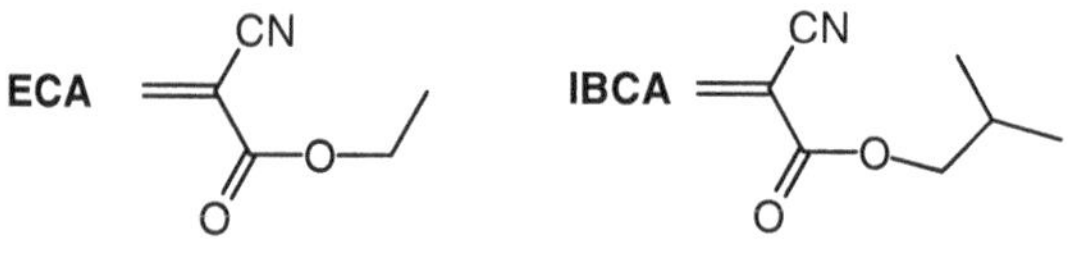

FIGURE 3.58 Structure of alkyl 2-cyanoacrylates tested in dental adhesives.

readily polymerizable, with polymerization being initiated by hydroxyl or amino groups of proteins or water. They should offer a number of advantages in the dental field. In fact, ethyl (ECA) and isobutyl 2-cyanoacrylate (IBCA) achieved very durable bonds to dentin.[325] However, the bonding strength of acrylic resins to dentin with 2-cyanoacrylate esters decreased with prolonged water exposure.[326] Therefore, more hydrophobic hydrolytically stable cyanoacrylates have to be developed.

It is well-known that isocyanates are capable of reacting with hydroxyl or amino and/or carboxylic groups under formation of urethanes or substitution products of urea. The formed polyurethanes show strong adhesion to many substrates. Therefore, as early as 1971, various commercially available diisocyanates such as toluene-2,4-diisocyanate (TDI), hexamethylene diisocyanate (HMDI), or diphenylmethane-4,4diisocyante (MDI) were used as a component in primers, which resulted in improved adhesion to enamel or dentin.[327] Polymerizable isocyanates were prepared by the reaction of diisocyanates with HEMA. They showed adhesion-promoting properties for proteinaceous substrates such as bone and dentin.[328] A bifunctional monomer containing an isocyanate group, a hexamethylene spacer, and a methacrylic moiety has been used in the bonding of restorative resins to dentin. Polymerizable isocyanates for dental adhesive systems are also described in patents, for example, the reaction product of Bis-GMA and HMDI.[328,330,331] The adhesive properties of several oligomers synthesized, for example, from 2-isocyanatoethyl methacrylate (IEMA) or *m*-isopropenyldimethylbenzyl isocyanate (TMI) (Figure 3.59) and various vinyl or methacrylate comonomer were described by Brauer and coworkers.[332–337] Alkyl α-isocyanatoacrylates, for example, ethyl α-cyanatoacrylate (α-EIA) (Figure 3.59), which was also used for the preparation of copolymers for dental adhesives, represent another class of reactive monomers.[338–341] The effect of IEMA on the dentin adhesion of adhesives using tri-*n*-butyl borane oxide as the free radical initiator is described in Taira et al.[342] and Chappelow et al.[343] Finally, it should be mentioned that a series of 4,6-dichloro-1,3,5-triazines (Figure 3.60) were synthesized as adhesive monomers.[333–345] These monomers contain chlorine atoms that can react with the amino or hydroxyl groups of collagen and increase the capability of copolymerization with composite monomers. 4,6-Dichloro-1,3,5-triazines were easily synthesized by the reaction of cyanuric chloride with, for example, allylamine (ADT) or HEMA (MADT).

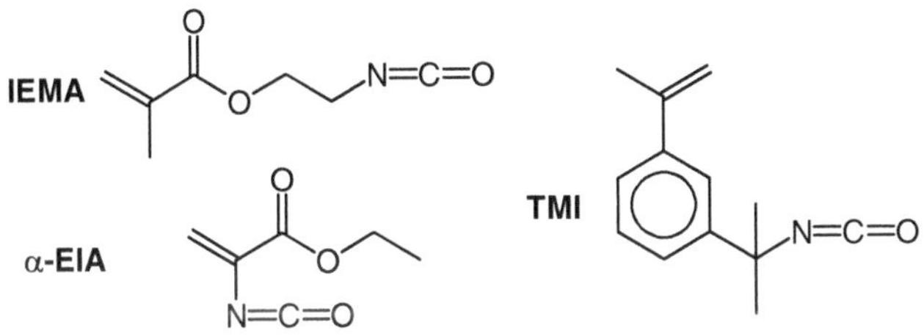

IEMA
α-EIA
TMI

FIGURE 3.59 Structure of polymerizable methacrylates tested in dental adhesives.

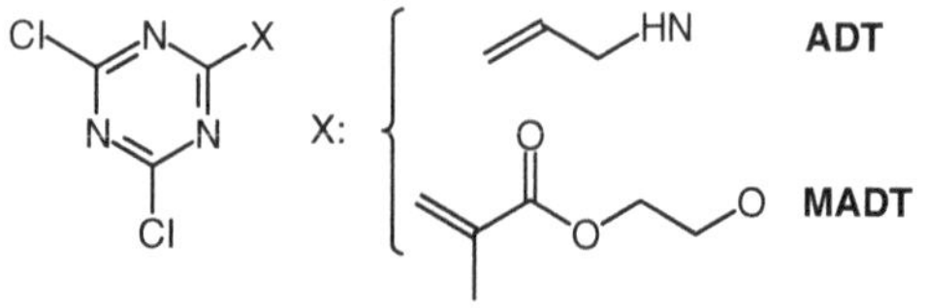

FIGURE 3.60 Structure of 4,6-dichloro-1,3,5-triazines.

3.6 INTERACTIONS INFLUENCING ENAMEL–DENTIN ADHESION

3.6.1 Saliva or Blood Contamination

During cavity preparation and application of the adhesive, there is a risk that blood or saliva could contaminate the bonding area. Therefore, the use of a rubber dam is recommended.[346] Nevertheless, only a minority of the general practitioners uses a rubber dam during the placement of an adhesive restoration.[347] For estimating the risk of blood or saliva contamination on enamel–dentin adhesion, several studies have been conducted.[348–352] Most of the investigations showed that saliva or blood contamination did not cause any or only minor adverse effects, depending on the adhesive used. In most of the cases, the bond strength was regained by reapplying the adhesive. Contamination of the cured adhesive layer, however, should be avoided.[352]

3.6.2 Disinfecting Agents

Disinfection of the tooth or the prepared cavity during restorative measures serves two purposes. First, it is well-known that while dental professionals work with rotating instruments or ultrasonic units like scalers, aerosols spread not only blood and saliva, but also pathogenic bacteria, viruses, and fungi from the oral cavity. By rinsing with a chlorhexidine digluconate solution before the treatment, a drastic germ reduction in the aerosol can be achieved and the risk of infection efficiently minimized.[354] The disinfection of prepared cavities or core preparations is accomplished with the aim of eliminating cariogenic germs to reduce the risk of recurrent caries formation. Second, the smear layer formed by the preparation with rotating instruments contains a lot of cariogenic bacteria.[231] However, there is no clinical proof of a correlation between the initial bacteria colonization and recurrent caries. If the core or the cavity is disinfected, the operator must ensure that this procedure does not have an adverse effect on the enamel-dentin adhesion.

One of the most popular disinfectants in dentistry is chlorhexidine.[355] Initially, it was used for the treatment of gingivitis. In the process, it was also found to demonstrate a high antimicrobial potential against the cariogenic bacteria *Streptococcus mutans*. Therefore, it is now also used for cavity disinfection. Commercial products for this purpose are also available. However, many investigations showed that chlorhexidine has an adverse effect on enamel and dentin adhesion, or microleakage, with the effect being more pronounced on cut enamel.[356–364]

The biocides used to control dental unit waterline bacterial biofilms represent another type of disinfectant used in the dental surgery. A wide range of commercial intermittent and continuous chemical treatments for dental unit waterlines have been developed and marketed. Their chemical composition is very different: Some are peroxide-based, while others contain glutaraldehyde, sodium hypochlorite, or chlorhexidine.[365,366] At least two studies have shown adverse effects of such dental unit waterline disinfectants on enamel and dentin bond strength.[367,368]

Perhaps cavity disinfection is unnecessary because at least some adhesives possess antimicrobial properties.[369,370] Furthermore, polymerizable antimicrobials, which can be part of the adhesive monomer mixture, are being developed (see Figure 3.61).[371]

3.6.3 Temporary Materials

The temporary restoration of prepared teeth prior to the placement of indirect restorations, such as inlays, onlays, crowns, or bridges, is needed for the protection of the pulp and the restoration of the patient's aesthetic and functional needs. In the case of zinc-oxide temporary cements, eugenol-containing cements are preferred because of their sedative effect on the pulp. However, prior to definitive adhesive cementation with a composite luting material and dentin adhesive, the use of eugenol-containing temporary cements has to be considered critical because phenols like eugenol are know to inhibit radical polymerization. The statements regarding the effect of eugenol-containing temporary cements on the function of the subsequent adhesive restoration are contradictory. Yap et al., for example, found an adverse effect of eugenol-containing temporary cements on the bond strength and microleakage.[372,373] Others, however, did not find any adverse effects either on the bond strength or on marginal adaptation.[374–377]

3.6.4 Tooth Bleaching

For aesthetic reasons, teeth whitening is becoming more and more popular. The bleaching agents used are hydrogen peroxide or carbamide peroxide (10–35%), which is decomposed to hydrogen peroxide by water contact.

Recent studies have shown that peroxide bleaching agents adversely affect the bond strength of composites to acid etched enamel, with the contact time and the peroxide concentration exerting the main influence on bond strength.[378–381] The reduction of the bond strength may be caused by structural changes in the surface morphology. Nevertheless, the main reason seems to be polymerization inhibition by oxygen.[379] A period of up to 3 weeks is required before the composite–enamel bond strength returns to values obtained for unbleached enamel.[382] However, if the

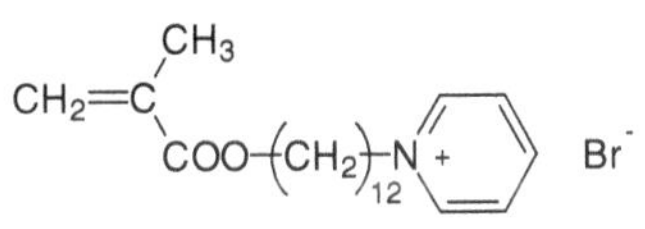

$$CH_2{=}C(CH_3){-}COO{-}(CH_2)_{12}{-}N^{+}C_5H_5 \quad Br^{-}$$

FIGURE 3.61 Antibacterial monomer 12-methacryloyloxydodecylpyridinium bromide.

surface layer of enamel is removed prior to bonding, there is an immediate return of the bond strength values to the range found in unbleached teeth.[383] The compromised bond strength of bleached enamel has been effectively reversed with an antioxidant such as sodium ascorbate.[384]

3.7 CONCLUSION AND PERSPECTIVE ON THE FUTURE

In the last couple of years, the desire of patients for esthetic restorations has significantly increased. Tooth shaded, invisible fillings with invisible filling margins are being demanded, as well as esthetic crowns, inlays, and veneers that are bonded with an invisible composite luting material according to the adhesive technique. For caries prevention, the sealing of fissures with a low-viscosity composite-based fissure sealant has been established for many years. In the process, the fissure sealant is fixed to the tooth structure using the acid-etch technique. A further application of the adhesive technique in dentistry is the bonding of brackets to enamel in orthodontic treatment.

The adhesive restorative technique, which was introduced in 1955, by etching enamel with phosphoric acid to create micromechanical retentions to achieve clinically durable adhesion between the tooth structure and the polymerized methacrylate on top. Today, this procedure is well-established in restorative therapy and is called the acid-etch technique.

For adhesion to dentin, the smear layer produced during cavity preparation has to be removed by acid-etch treatment. In the case of the total-etch technique, this results in the creation of a 3–5 μm deep demineralized zone in the dentin surface. Collagen fibrils are almost completely denuded of hydroxyapatite by acid etching, forming a microretentive interpenetrated polymer network of applied dimethacrylate based resins. "Total-etch" adhesives involve the simultaneous application of acid to enamel and dentin, after which the acid needs to be rinsed off. The concept of "self-etching" adhesives is based on the use of polymerizable acidic monomers that simultaneously condition and prime dentin and enamel.

Human teeth are composed of two different materials: dentin and enamel. Enamel consists mainly of hydroxyapatite crystals, while dentin can be defined as a composite of hydroxyapatite and collagen. Because of the different compositions and anisotropic structures, different adhesion mechanisms are used on both substrates. On enamel, adhesion can be achieved by the formation of microporosities and extension of the resin into the porosities. After curing, adhesion occurs through micromechanical retention. In contrast, the formation of a hybrid layer is the most important mechanism for promoting adhesion on the polar dentin. On the wet and hydrophilic dentin surface, ionic interactions, such as the formation of hydrogen bonds of polar monomers and complex or calcium-salt formation between hydroxyapatite and adhesive monomers, play an important role.

For the qualitative and quantitative assessment of the adhesive performance, bond strength measurements and marginal analyses of fillings placed *in vitro* carried out. Both test methods are very sensitive. They are influenced by variables connected with the substrate itself, specimen preparation and treatment, and the performance of the test. Examinations of the morphology of the interface by SEM,

TEM, AFM, and CLSM produce a lot of information about the bonding mechanism, such as smear layer removal, monomer penetration, hybrid layer formation, nanoleakage, water penetration, and long-term stability of the adhesion.

Information about the interfacial chemistry is gained by the analytical methods commonly used in surface analysis, for example, NMR, XPS/ESCA, IR, and RAMAN spectroscopy. The main focus is the chemical interaction between the adhesive components and the tooth structure, the analysis of the hybrid layer composition, and characterization of the polymerization kinetics at the interface.

The monomers in enamel and dentin adhesives, which may create a strong bond between the filling material and the tooth substance (dentin and enamel), have to fulfill a number of physicochemical requirements to demonstrate efficient processing and clinical performance. To meet these requirements, the following constituents are necessary: suitable adhesive monomers, such as bifunctional molecules containing a polymerizable group for the copolymerization with the restorative material; an adhesive group capable of reacting with the tooth substance; and a spacer designed to influence the hydrophilicity, flexibility, and wetting properties of the adhesive monomer. For self-etching enamel and dentin adhesives, polymerizable carboxylic acid, phosphonic acid, and mono- or dihydrogenphosphate, which show self-etching properties and a high reactivity in the radical polymerization, are currently the most promising adhesive monomers.

Practitioners should be aware of interactions influencing enamel and dentin adhesion to avoid failures. These interactions are very complex and include saliva and blood contamination, disinfectants, bleaching agents, or preused materials for temporary treatments. In many cases the interactions are very technique and adhesive specific.

REFERENCES

1. Lutz, F., Krejci I., and Besek, M., Operative dentistry: the missing clinical standards, *Pract. Period. Aesth. Dent.*, 9, 541–548, 1997.
2. Pitts, N.B., Current methods and criteria for caries diagnosis in Europe, *J. Dent. Educ.*, 57, 409–414, 1993.
3. Peters, M.C. and McLean, M.E., Minimal invasive operative care — I. Minimal intervention and concepts for minimally invasive cavity preparations, *J. Adhes. Dent* 3, 7–16, 2000.
4. Anusavice, K.J., Treatment regimes in preventive and restorative dentistry, *J. Am. Dent. Assoc.*, 126, 727–740, 1995.
5. Anusavice, K.J., Efficacy of non-surgical management of the initial caries lesion, *J. Dent. Educ.*, 61, 895–905, 1997.
6. Black, G.V., *A Work on Operative Dentistry; The Technical Procedures in Filling Teeth*, Medico-Dental Publishing, Chicago, 1908.
7. Sigurjons, H., Extension for prevention: historical development and current status of Black's concept, *Oper. Dent.*, 8, 57–63, 1983.
8. Bryant, R.W., Direct posterior composite resin restorations: a review. 1. Factors influencing case selection, *Aust. Dent. J.*, 37, 81–87, 1992.
9. Summitt, J.B., Della Bona, A., and Burgess, J.O., The strength of class II composite restorations as affected by preparation design, *Quintessence Int.*, 25, 251–257, 1994.

10. Simonsen, R.J., Pit and fissure sealant: review of the literature, *Pediatr. Dent.*, 24, 393–414, 2002.
11. Bayne, S.C., Heymann, H.O., and Swift, E.J., Update on dental composite restorations, *J. Am. Dent. Assoc.*, 125, 687–701, 1994.
12. Brännström, M., The hydrodynamic theory of dentinal pain: sensation in preparations, caries, and the dentinal crack syndrome, *J. Endod.*, 12(10), 453–457, 1986.
13. Brännström, M., Etiology of dentin hypersensitivity, *Proc. Finn. Dent. Soc.*, 88 Suppl 1, 7–13, 1992.
14. Pashley, D.H., Theory of dentin sensitivity, *J. Clin. Dent.*, 5, 65–67, 1994.
15. Nordenvall, K.J., Malmgren, B., and Brännström, M., Desensitization of dentin by resin impregnation: a clinical and light-microscopic investigation. *ASDC J. Dent. Child.*, 51(4), 274–276, 1984.
16. Christensen, G.J., Preventing sensitivity in class II composite resin restorations, *J. Am. Dent. Assoc.*, 129, 1469–1470, 1998.
17. Gangarosa, L.P., Current strategies for dentist-applied treatment in the management of hypersensitive dentine, *Arch. Oral Biol.* (Suppl), 39, 101S–106S, 1994.
18. Pashley, D.H., Dentin permeability, dentin sensitivity, and treatment through tubule occlusion, *J. Endo.*, 12, 465–474, 1986.
19. Kim, S., Hypersensitive teeth: desensitization of pulpal sensory nerves, *J. Endo.*, 12, 482–485, 1986.
20. Pereira, R. and Chava, V.K., Efficacy of a 3% potassium nitrate desensitizing mouthwash in the treatment of dentinal hypersensitivity. *J. Periodontol.*, 72, 1720–1725, 2001.
21. Kishore, A., Mehrotra, K.K., and Saimbi, C.S., Effectiveness of desensitizing agents, *J. Endo.*, 28, 34–35, 2002.
22. Nakabayashi, N. and Pashley, D.H., *Hybridization of Dental Hard Tissues*, Quintessence Publishing, Tokyo, 1998.
23. Turesky, S.S. and Spencer, J.L., Method for Desensitizing Dentin, U.S. Patent No. 5,211,939 (to Gillette Canada Inc.),1993.
24. Schüpbach, P., Lutz, F., and Finger, W.J., Closing of dentinal tubules by Gluma desensitizer, *Eur. J. Oral. Sci.*, 105, 414–421, 1997.
25. Ide, M., Morel, A.D., Wilson, R.F., and Ashley, F.P., 1998. The role of a dentine-bonding agent in reducing cervical dentin sensitivity, *J. Clin. Periodontol.*, 25, 286–290, 1998.
26. Watanabe, T., Sano, M., Itoh, K., and Wakumoto, S., The effects of primers on the sensitivity of dentin, *Dent. Mater.*, 7, 148–150, 1991.
27. Suh, B.I. and Hamer, M., Composition and Method for Desensitizing Dentin, U.S. Patent No. 5,133,957 (to Bisco Inc.), 1992.
28. Nikaido, T., Burrow, M.F., Tagami, J., and Takatsu, T., Effect of pulpal pressure on adhesion of resin composite to dentin: bovine serum versus saline, *Quintessence Int* 26, 221–226, 1995.
29. Brännström M., Mattsson, B., and Torstenson, B., Materials techniques for lining composite resin restorations: a critical approach, *J. Dent.*, 19(2), 71–79, 1991.
30. Handelman, S., Washburn, F., and Wopperer, P., Two-year report of sealant effect on bacteria in dental caries, *J. Am. Dent. Assoc.*, 93, 967–970, 1979.
31. Mjör, I.A, Glass-ionomer cement restorations and secondary caries: a preliminary report, *Quintessence Int.*, 27, 171–174, 1996.
32. Wilson, N.H., Burke, F.J., and Mjör, I.A., Reasons for placement and replacement of restorations of direct restorative materials by a selected group of practitioners in the United Kingdom, *Quintessence Int.*, 28, 245–248, 1997.

33. Mjör, I.A., Moorhead, J.E., and Dahl, J.E., Reasons for replacement of restorations in permanent teeth in general dental practice, *Int. Dent. J.*, 50, 361–366, 2000.
34. Deligeorgi, V., Mjör, I.A., and Wilson, N.H., An overview of reasons for the placement and replacement of restorations, *Prim. Dent. Care*, 8, 5–11, 2001.
35. Mjör, I.A. and Toffenetti, F., Secondary caries: a literature review with case reports, *Quintessence Int.*, 31, 165–179, 2000.
36. Calamia, J.R., High-strength porcelain bonded restorations: anterior and posterior, *Quintessence Int.*, 20, 717–726, 1989.
37. Buonocore, M.G., A simple method of increasing the adhesion of acrylic filling materials to enamel surfaces, *J. Dent. Res.*, 34, 849–853, 1955.
38. Poole, D.F. and Johnson, N.W., The effects of different demineralizing agents on human enamel surfaces studied by scanning electron microscopy, *Arch. Oral. Biol* 12, 1621–1634, 1967.
39. Blosser, R.L., Time dependence on 2.5% nitric acid solution as an etchant on human dentin and enamel, *Dent. Mater.*, 6, 83–87, 1990.
40. Hicks, M.J. and Silverstone, L.M., Internal morphology of surface zones from acid-etched caries-like lesions: scanning electron microscopic study, *J. Dent. Res.*, 64, 1296–1301, 1985.
41. Retief, D.H., Busscher, H.J., de Boer, P., Jongebloed, W.L., and Arends, J., A laboratory evaluation of three etching solutions, *Dent. Mater.*, 2, 202–206, 1986.
42. McLean, J.W., Status report on the glass ionomer cements, *J. Am. Dent. Assoc.*, 99, 221–226, 1979.
43. Abendroth, R. and Bössmann, K., Variationen der Ätzmuster an Schmelzoberflächen nach Behandlung mit verschiedenen Ätzmitteln, *Dtsch. Zahnärztl. Z.*, 34, 181–186, 1979.
44. Swift, E.J. and Cloe, B.C., Shear bond strength of new enamel etchants, *Am. J. Dent.* 6, 162–164, 1993.
45. Gross, J.D., Retief, D.H., and Bradley, E.L., An optimal concentration of phosphoric acid as an etching agent — Part II: Microleakage studies, *J. Prosthet. Dent.*, 52, 786–789, 1984.
46. Shinchi, M.J. Soma, K., and Nakabayashi, N., The effect of phosphoric acid concentration on resin tag length and bond strength of a photo-cured resin to acid-etched enamel, *Dent. Mater.*, 16, 324–329, 2000.
47. Lutz, F., Der Einfluss einer Fluoridapplikation nach der Schmelzätzung auf Adaption und Haftung von Adhäsivfüllungen, *Schweiz. Mschr. Zahnheilk.* 87, 712–723, 1977.
48. Meola, M.T. and Papaccio, G., A scanning electron microscope study of the effect of etching time and mechanical pretreatment on the etch pattern of acid etching on the enamel of primary teeth, *Int. Dent. J.*, 36, 49–53, 1986.
49. Gwinnett, A.J. and Garcia-Godoy, F., Effect of etching time and acid concentration on resin shear bond strength to primary tooth enamel, *Am. J. Dent.*, 5, 237–239, 1992.
50. Retief, D.H., Clinical applications of enamel adhesives, *Oper. Dent. Suppl.* 5, 44–49, 1992.
51. Nygaard, V.K. and Simmelink, J.W., Ultrastructural study of the resin infiltration zone in acid-treated human enamel, *Arch. Oral. Biol.*, 23, 1151–1156, 1978.
52. Gwinnett, J.A., Smear layer: morphological considerations, *Oper. Dent.*, Suppl. 3, 3–12, 1984.
53. Buonocore, G., Wileman, W., and Brudevold, F., A report on a resin composition capable of bonding human dentin surfaces, *J. Dent. Res.*, 35, 846–851, 1956.
54. Fusayama, T., Nakamura, M., Kurosaki, N., and Iwaku, M., Non-pressure adhesion of a new adhesive restorative resin, *J. Dent. Res.*, 58, 1364–1370, 1979.
55. Nakabayashi, N., Kojima, K., and Masuhara, E., The promotion of adhesion by infiltration of monomers into tooth substrates, *J. Biomed. Mater. Res.*, 16, 265–273, 1982.

56. Bowen, R.L., Surface–Active Comonomers and Method of Preparation, U.S. Patent No. 3,200,142, 1963.
57 Bowen, R.L., Adhesive bonding of various materials to hard tooth tissues — II. Bonding to dentin promoted by a surface-active comonomer, *J. Dent. Res.*, 44, 895–902, 1965.
58. Bowen, R.L., Adhesive bonding of various materials to hard tooth tissues — III. Bonding to dentin improved by pre-treatment and the use of surface-active comonomer, *J. Dent. Res.*, 44, 903–905, 1965.
59. Bowen, R.L., Adhesive bonding of various materials to hard tooth tissues — IV. Bonding to dentin, enamel, and fluoroapatite improved by the use of a surface-active comonomer, *J. Dent. Res.*, 44, 906–911, 1965.
60. Misra, D.N. and Bowen, R.L., Adhesive bonding of various materials to hard tooth — XII. Adsorption of *N*-(2-hydroxy-3-methacryloxypropyl)-*N*-phenylglycine (NPG-GMA) on hydroxyapatite, *J. Coll. Interfaces Sci.*, 61,14–20, 1977.
61. Bowen, R.L., Adhesive bonding of various materials to hard tooth tissues — XVII. Synthesis of a polyfunctional surface-active comonomer, *J. Dent. Res.*, 58, 1101–1107, 1979.
62. Misra, D.N., Bowen, R.L., and Wallace, B.M., Adhesive bonding of various materials to hard tooth tissues — VIII. Nickel and copper ions on hydroxyapatite surface, *J. Coll. Interface Sci.*, 51, 36–43, 1974.
63. Misra, D.N. and Bowen, R.L., Adhesive bonding of various materials to hard tooth tissues — X. Initial rates of adsorption of nickel and copper ions on hydroxyapatite surface, *J. Biomed. Mat. Res.*, 12, 505–5615, 1978.
64 Bowen, R.L., Adhesive bonding of various materials to hard tooth tissues. XIV. Enamel mordant selection assisted by ESCA (XPS), *J. Dent. Res.*, 57, 551–556, 1978.
65. Bowen, R.L., McClendon, L.T., and Gills, T.E., Adhesive bonding of various materials to hard tooth tissues — XV. Neutron activation analysis of dentin sorption of mordant salts, *J. Dent. Res.*, 57, 255–260, 1978.
66. Bowen, R.L., McClendon, L.T., and Gills, T.E., Adhesive bonding of various materials to hard tooth tissues — XXII. The effects of a cleaner, mordant, and PolySAC on adhesion between a composite resin and dentin, *J. Dent. Res.*, 59, 809–814, 1980.
67. Bowen, R.L., Method for Obtaining Strong Adhesive Bonding of Composites to Dentin, Enamel and Other Substrates, U.S. Patent No. 4,514,527, 1985.
68. Bowen, R.L., A method for bonding to dentin and enamel, *J. Amer. Dent. Assoc* 107, 734–736, 1983.
69. Bowen, R.L., Cobb E.N., and Rapson, J.E., Adhesive bonding of various materials to hard tooth tissues: improvement in bond strength to dentin, *J. Dent. Res.*, 61, 1070–1076, 1982.
70. Bowen, R.L., Cobb, E.N., and Misra, D.N., Adhesive bonding by surface initiation of polymerization, *Ind. Eng. Chem. Prod. Res. Dev.*, 23, 78–81, 1984.
71. Bowen, R.L., Simplified Method for Obtained Strong Adhesive Bonding of Composites to Dentin, Enamel and Other Substrates, U.S. Patent No. 4,659,751, 1987.
72. Bowen, R.L., Tung, M.S., and Blosser, R.L., Dentin and enamel bonding agents, *Intern. Dent. J.*, 37, 158–161, 1987.
73. Blosser, R.L. and Bowen, R.L., Effects of purified ferric oxalate/nitric acid solutions as a pretreatment for the NTG-GMA and PMDM bonding system, *Dent. Mater.*, 4, 225–231, 1988.

74. Tay, F.R., Gwinnett, J.A., and Wei, S.H., Micromorphological spectrum from overdrying to overwetting acid-conditioned dentin in water-free acetone-based, single-bottle primer/adhesives, *Dent. Mater.*, 12, 236–244, 1996.
75. Takeyama, M., Kashibuchi, N., Nakabayashi, N., and Masuhara, E., Studies on dental self-curing resins: XVII. Adhesion of PMMA with bovine enamel or dental alloys, *J. Jpn. Soc. Dent. Appar. Mater.*, 19, 179–185, 1978.
76. Chang, J.C., Hurst. T.L., Hart, D.A., and Estey, A.W., 4-META use in dentistry: a literature review, *J. Prosthet. Dent.*, 87, 216–224, 2002.
77. Sano, H., Takatsu, T., Ciucchi, B., Horner, J.A., Mathhews, W.G., and Pashley, D.H., Nanoleakage: leakage within the hybrid layer, *Oper. Dent.*, 20, 18–25, 1995.
78. Kugel, G. and Ferrari, M., The science of bonding: from first to sixth generation, *J. Am. Dent. Assoc.*, 131, 208–258, 2000.
79. Waters, N.E., Some mechanical and physical properties of teeth, in *Mechanical Properties of Biological Materials,* Symposia of the Society for Experimental Biology, No. 34, Vincent, J.F.V. and Curey, J.D. Eds., Cambridge University Press, Cambridge, 1980, pp. 99–135.
80. Miller, W., Dental caries, *Am. J. Dent. Sci.*, 17, 77–130, 1883.
81. Hörsted-Bindslev, P. and Mjör, I.A., *Moderne Konzepte in der Zahnerhaltung. Quintessenz,* Verlag GmbH, Berlin, 1994.
82. Pilz, M.E., *Praxis der Zahnerhaltung und oralen Prävention,* Carl Hanser Verlag, München, 1985.
83. Gängler, P., *Klinik der konservierenden Zahnheilkunde*, Verlag Gesundheit GmbH, Berlin, 1987.
84. Hellwig, E., Klimek, J., and Attin, T., *Einführung in die Zahnerhaltung*, Urban & Schwarzenberg, München, 1995.
85. Linde, A. in *Dentine and Dentine Reactions in the Oral Cavity,* Thylstrup, A., Leach, S.A., and Quist, V., Eds., Inform. Print. Ltd., Oxford, 1987, p. 17.
86. Schroeder, H.E., *Orale Strukturbiologie*, Georg Thieme Verlag, Stuttgart, 1987.
87. Gage, J.P., Francis, M.J.O., and Triffitt, J.T., *Collagen and Dental Matrices,* Butterworth, London, UK, 1989.
88. Gebelein, C.G., Collagen biotechnology and its medical applications, in *Biotechnological Polymers*, Technomic, 66–81, 1993.
89. Meadows, R.S., Holmes, D.F., Gilpin, C.J., and Kadler, K.E., Electron cryomicroscopy of fibrilar collagens, *Methods Mol. Biol.*, 139, 95–109, 2000.
90. De Duve, C., *Die Zelle: Expedition in die Grundstruktur des Lebens* [A Guided Tour of the Living Cell], Spektrum Akademischer Verlag, Heidelberg, 1992.
91. Drenckhahn, D. and Zenker, W., *Benninghoff Anatomie*, Urban & Schwarzenberg, München, 1994.
92. Gage, J.P., Francis, M.J.O., and Smith, R., Abnormal amino acid analyses obtained from osteogenesis imperfecta dentin, *J. Dent. Res.*, 67, 1097–1102, 1988.
93. Spears, I.R., van Noort, R., Crompton, R.H., Cardew, G.E., and Howard, I.C., The effects of enamel anisotropy on the distribution of stress in a tooth, *J. Dent. Res.*, 72, 1526–1531, 1993.
94. Craig, R.G. and Peyton, F.A., Elastic and mechanical properties of human dentin, *J. Dent. Res.*, 37, 710–718, 1958.
95. Rasmussen, S.T. and Patchin, R.E., Fracture properties of human enamel and dentin in an aqueous environment, *J. Dent. Res.*, 63, 1362–1368, 1984.
96. Yettram, A.L., Wright, K.W.J., and Pickard, H.M., Finite element stress analysis of the crowns of normal and restored teeth, *J. Dent. Res.*, 55, 1004–1011, 1976.

97. De Vree, J.H.P., Peters, M.C., and Plasschaert, A.J.M., The influence of modification of cavity design on the distribution of stresses in a restored molar. *J. Dent. Res.*, 63, 1217–1220, 1984.
98. Williams, K.R., Edmundsen, J.T., and Rees, J.S., Finite element stress analysis of restored teeth, *Dent. Mater.* 3, 201–206, 1987.
99. Khera, S.C., Goel, U.K., Chen, R.C.S., and Gurusami, S.A., A three dimensional finite element model, *Oper. Dent.*, 13, 128–137, 1988.
100. Morin, D.L., Cross, M., and Voller, V.R., Biophysical stress analysis of restored teeth: modeling and analysis, *Dent. Mater.*, 4, 77–84, 1988.
101 Van Noort, R., Howard, I.C., and Cardew, G.E., A study of the interfacial shear and tensile stresses in a restored molar tooth, *J. Dent.*, 16, 286–293, 1988.
102. Spears, I.R., van Noort, R., Crompton, R.H., Cardew, G.E., and Howard, I.C., The effects of enamel anisotropy on the distribution of stress in a tooth, *J. Dent. Res.*, 72, 1526–1531, 1993.
103. Kinney, J.H., Balooch, M., Marshall, G.W., and Marshall, S.J., A micromechanics model of the elastic properties of human dentine, *Arch. Oral. Biol.*, 44, 813–822, 1999.
104. Waters, N.E., Some mechanical and physical properties of teeth, in *The Mechanical Properties of Biological Materials,* Cambridge University Press, Cambridge, 1980, pp. 99–135.
105. Pashley, D.H., Dynamics of the pulpo-dentine complex, *Crit. Rev. Oral Biol. Med* 7, 104–133. 1996.
106. Marshall, G.W., Jr., Marshall, S.J., Kinney, J.H., and Balooch, M., The dentin substrate: structure and properties related to bonding, *J. Dent.*, 25, 441–458, 1997.
107. Tyldesly, W.R., The mechanical properties of human enamel and dentin, *Br. Dent. J* 106, 169–278, 1959.
108. Stanford, J.W., Weigelm K.V., Paffenbarger, G.C., and Sweeney, W.T., Compressive properties of hard tooth tissues and some restorative materials, *J. Am. Dent. Assoc.* 60, 746–756, 1960.
109. Watanabe, L.G., Marshall, G.W., Jr., and Marshall, S.J., Dentin shear strength: effects of tubule orientation and intratooth location, *Dent. Mater.*, 12, 109–115. 1996.
110. Lertchirakarn, V., Palamara, J.E., and Messer, H.H., Anisotropy of tensile strength of root dentin, *J. Dent. Res.*, 80, 453–456, 2001.
111. Currey, J.D., Brear, K., and Zioupos, P., Dependence of mechanical properties on fibre angle in narwhal tusk, a highly oriented biological composite, *J. Biomech.*, 27, 885–897, 1994.
112. Sögaard-Petersen, B., Boye, H., and Matthiessen, M.E., Scanning electron microscope observations on collagen fibers in human dentin and pulp, *Scand. J. Dent. Res.*, 98, 89–95, 1990.
113. Skinner, E.W. and Phillips, R.W., *The Science of Dental Materials*, 6th ed., Saunders, Philadelphia, 1967.
114. Stanford, J.W., Paffenbarger, G.C., Kampula, J.W., and Sweeny, W.T., Determination of some compressive properties of human enamel and dentine, *J. Am. Dent. Assoc* 57, 487–495, 1958.
115. Marshall, G.W., Marshall, S.J., Kinney, J.H., and Balooch, M., Dentin substrate: structure and properties related to bonding, *J. Dent.*, 25, 441–458, 1997.
116. Buonocore, M.G., Matsui, A., and Gwinnett, A.J., Penetration of resin dental material into enamel surfaces with reference to bonding, *Arch. Oral Biol.*, 13, 61–70, 1968.
117. Gwinnett, A.J. and Matsui, A., A study of enamel adhesives. The physical relationship between enamel and adhesive, *Arch. Oral Biol.*, 12, 1615–1620, 1967.

118. Retief, D.H., Rutland, J.R., and Jamison, H.C., Microleakage of conventional and microfilled composite restorative resins, *J. Biomed. Mater. Res.*, 16, 901–910, 1982.
119. Chosak, A. and Eidelman, E., Effect of time from application until exposure to light on the tag lengths of a visible light-polymerized sealant, *Dent. Mater.*, 4, 302–306, 1988.
120. Kersten, S., Lutz, F., and Schüpbach, P., Fissure sealing: optimization of sealant penetration and sealing properties, *Am. J. Dent.*, 14, 127–131, 2001.
121. Armengol, V., Laboux, O., Weiss, P., Jean, A., and Hamel, H., Effects of Er:YAG and Nd:YAP laser irradiation on the surface roughness and free surface energy of enamel and dentin: an *in vitro* study, *Oper. Dent.*, 28, 67–74, 2003.
122. Settembrini, L., Boylan, R., Strassler, H., and Scherer, W., A comparison of antimicrobial activity of etchants used for a total etch technique, *Oper. Dent.*, 22, 84–88, 1997.
123. Van Meerbeck, B., Inokoshi, S., Braem, M., Lambrechts, P., and Vanherle, G., Morphological aspects of the resin-dentin interdiffusion zone with different dentin adhesive systems, *J. Dent. Res.*, 71, 1530–1540, 1992.
124. Pashley, D.H., Micherlich V., and Kehl, T., Dentin permeability: effects of smear layer removal, *J. Prosthet. Dent.*, 46, 531ñ537, 1981.
125. Nakabayashi, N., Adhesive bonding with 4-META, *Oper. Dent.* (suppl 5), 17, 125–130, 1992.
126. Moran, C., Lynch, E., Petersson, L., and Borsboom, P., Comparison of caries removal using carisolv or a conventional slow-speed rotary instrument, *Caries Res.*, Abstr. 94, 33, 313, 1999.
127. Haak, R., Fritz, U.B., Faber, F.J., and Noack, M.J., Influence of chemical caries removal on dentin bonding, *J. Dent. Res.*, Abstr. 2111, 78, 369, 1999.
128. Saboia, V.P., Rodrigues, A.L., and Pimenta, L.A., Effect of collagen removal on shear bond strength of two single-bottle adhesive systems, *Oper. Dent.*, 25, 395–400, 2000.
129. Ferrari, M., Mason, P.N., Vichi, A., and Davidson, C.L., Role of hybridization on marginal leakage and bond strength, *Am. J. Dent.*, 13, 329–336, 2000.
130. Watanabe, I., Nakabayashi, N., and Pashley, D.H., Bonding to ground dentin by a Phenyl-P self-etching primer, *J. Dent. Res.*, 73, 1212–1220, 1994.
131. Yoshiyama, M., Matsuo, T., Ebisu, S., and Pashley, D., Regional bond strength of self-etching/self-priming adhesive systems, *J. Dent.*, 26, 609–616, 1998.
132. Salz, U., Gianasmidis, A., and Rheinberger, V., *In Vitro* Performance and Storage Stability of a Hydrolytically Stable Self Etching Primer, The First International Congress on Adhesive Dentistry, Tokyo, April 19–21, 2002, O-27, p. 301.
133. Van Dijk-Wolthuis, W.N.E., Van Steenbergen, M.J., Underberg, W.J.M., and Hennink, W.E., Degradation kinetics of methacrylated dextrans in aqueous solution, *J. Pharm. Sci.*, 86, 413–417, 1997.
134. Salz, U., Gianasmidis, A., Moszner, N., and Rheinberger, V., Synthesis and storage stability of a hydrolytically stable self-etching primer, *J. Dent. Res.*, Abstr. 1147, 81 (Special Issue A), A-161, 2002.
135. Jendresen, M.D. and Glantz, P.O., 1981, Microtopography and clinical adhesiveness of an acid etched tooth surface, *Acta. Odontol. Scand.*, 39, 47–53, 1981.
136. Munksgaard, E.C., and Asmussen, E., Bond strength between dentin and restorative resins mediated by mixtures of HEMA and glutaraldehyde, *J. Dent. Res.*, 63, 1087–1089, 1984.
137. Nimni, M.E., Cheung, D., Strates, B., Kodama, M., and Sheikh, K., Chemically modified collagen: A natural biomaterial for tissue replacement, *J. Biomed. Mater. Res.*, 21, 741–771, 1987.

138. Asmussen, E. and Uno, S., Adhesion of restorative resins to dentin: chemical and physicochemical aspects, *Oper. Dent., Suppl.* 5, 68–74, 1992.
139. Jakobasch, H.J. and Freitag, K.H., Zur Adhäsion von Polymeren, *Acta. Polym.*, 30, 453–469, 1979.
140. Bischoff, C. and Possart, W., *Adhäsion*, Akademie-Verlag, Berlin, 1983.
141. Comyn, J., The relationship between joint durability and water diffusion, in *Developments in Adhesives*, Kinloch, A.J., Ed., Vol.2, Applied Science, Barking, UK, 1981, p. 279.
142. Waite, J.H., Nature's underwater adhesive specialist, *Int. J. Adhesion Adhesives*, 7, 9–14, 1987.
143. Olio, G., Adhesion of dental materials to dentin: debonding tests, in *Dentine and Dentine Reactions in the Oral Cavity*, Thylstrup A., Leach S.A., and Qvist, V., Eds. IRL Press, Oxford, 1987, pp. 219–224.
144. Haller, B., Hofmann, N., Klaiber, B., and Pfannkuch, A., Beständigkeit des Komposit-Dentinverbundes bei künstlicher Alterung, *Dtsch Zahnärztl. Z.*, 48, 100–104, 1993.
145. Watanabe, I. and Nakabayashi, N., Measurement methods for adhesion to dentine: the current status in Japan, *J. Dent.*, 22, 67–72, 1994.
146. Pashley, D.H., Sano, H., Ciucchi, B., Yoshiyama, M., and Carvalho, R.M., Adhesion testing of dentin bonding agents: a review, *Dent. Mater.*, 11, 117–125, 1995.
147. ISO (2003). ISO/TR 11405 Dental materials — testing of adhesion to tooth structure.
148. Al-Salehi, K.S. and Burke, F.J.T., Methods used in dentin bonding tests: an analysis of 50 investigations on bond strength, *Quintessence Int.*, 28, 717–723, 1997.
149. Leloup, G., D'Hoore, W., Bouter, D., Degrange, M., and Vreven, J., Meta-analytical review of factors involved in dentin adherence, *J. Dent. Res.*, 80, 1605–1614, 2001.
150. Rueggeberg, F.A., Substrate for adhesion testing to tooth structure — review of the literature, *Dent. Mater.*, 7, 2–10, 1991.
151. Nakamichi, I., Iwaku, M., and Fusayama, T., Bovine teeth as possible substitutes in the adhesion test, *J. Dent. Res.*, 62, 1076–1081, 1983.
152. Schilke, R., Bauss, O., Lisson, J.A., Schuckar, M., and Geurtsen, W., Bovine dentin as a substitute for human dentin in shear bond strength measurements, *Am. J. Dent* 12, 92–96, 1999.
153. Causton, B.E. and Johnson, N.W., Changes in the dentine of human teeth following extraction and their implication for *in-vitro* studies of adhesion to tooth substance, *Arch. Oral. Biol.*, 24, 229–232, 1979.
154. Nakabayashi, N., Watanabe, A., and Ikeda, W., Intra-oral bonding of 4-META/MMA-TBB resin to vital human dentin, *Am. J. Dent.*, 8, 37–42, 1995.
155. Tao, L. and Pashley, D.H., Shear bond strength to dentin: effects of surface treatments, depth and position, *Dent. Mater.*, 73, 371–378, 1988.
156. Konishi, N., Watanabe, L.G., Hilton, J.F., Marshall, G.W., Marshall, S.J., and Staninec, M., Dentin shear strength: effect of distance from the pulp, *Dent. Mater.*, 18, 516–20, 2002.
157. Prati, C. and Pashley, D.H., Dentin wetness, permeability, thickness and bond strength of bonding systems, *Am. J. Dent.*, 5, 33–38, 1992.
158. Ogata, M, Okuda, M, Nakajima, M, Pereira, P.N., Sano, H., and Tagami, J., Influence of the direction of tubules on bond strength to dentin, *Oper. Dent.*, 26, 27–35, 2001.
159. Phrukkanon, S., Burrow, M.F., and Tyas, M.J., The effect of dentine location and tubule orientation on the bond strengths between resin and dentine, *J. Dent.*, 27, 265–274, 1999.
160. Watanabe, L.G., Marshall, G.W., and Marshall, S.J., Dentin shear strength: effects of tubule orientation and intratooth location, *Dent. Mater.*, 12, 109–115, 1996.

161. Munechika, T., Suzuki, K., Nishiyama, M., Ohashi, M., and Horie, K., A comparison of the tensile bond strengths of composite resins to longitudinal and transverse sections of enamel prisms in human teeth, *J. Dent. Res.*, 63, 1079–1082, 1984.
162. Ikeda, T., Uno, S., Tanaka, T., Kawakami, S., Komatsu, H., and Sano, H., Relation of enamel prism orientation to microtensile bond strength, *Am. J. Dent.*, 15, 109–113, 2002.
163. Shimada, Y. and Tagami, J., Effects of regional enamel and prism orientation on resin bonding, *Oper. Dent.*, 28, 20–27, 2003.
164. Maragakis, G.M., Hahn, P., and Hellwig, E., Chemomechanical caries removal: a comprehensive review of the literature, *Int. Dent. J.*, 51:291–299, 2001.
165. Yazici, A.R., Ozgunaltay, G., and Dayangac, B., A scanning electron microscopic study of different caries removal techniques on human dentin, *Oper. Dent.*, 27, 360–366, 2002.
166. McInnes, P.M., Wendt, S.L., Retief, D.H., and Weinberg, R., Effect of dentin surface roughness on shear bond strength, *Dent. Mater.*, 6, 204–207, 1990.
167. Koibuchi, H., Yasuda, N., and Nakabayashi, N., Bonding to dentin with self-etching primer: the effect of smear layers, *Dent. Mater.*, 17, 122–126, 2001.
168. Retief, D.H., Wendt, S.L., Bradley, E.L., and Denys, F.R., The effect of storage media and duration of storage of extracted teeth on shear bonds strength of Scotchbond 2/Silux to dentin, *Am. J. Dent.*, 2, 269–273, 1989.
169. Cooley, R.L. and Dodge, W.W., Bond strength of three dentinal adhesives on recently extracted versus aged teeth, *Quintessence Int.*, 20, 513–516, 1989.
170. Sano, H., Yoshikawa, T., Pereira, P.N.R., Kanemura, N., Morigami, M., Tagami, J., and Pashley, D.H., Long-term durability of dentin bonds made with self-etching primer, *in vivo*, *J. Dent. Res.*, 78, 906–911, 1999.
171. Nikaido, T., Kunzelmann, K.H., Chen, H., Ogata, M., Harada, N., Yamaguchi, S., Cox, C.F., Hickel, R., and Tagami, J., Evaluation of thermal cycling and mechanical loading on bond strength of a self-etching primer system to dentin, *Dent. Mater.*, 18, 269–275, 2002.
172. Miyazaki, M., Sato, M., Onose, H., and Moore, B.K., Influence of thermal cycling on dentin bond strength of two-step bonding systems, *Am. J. Dent.*, 11, 118–122, 1998.
173. Miyazaki, M., Onose, H., and Moore, B.K., Effects of operator variability on dentin bond strength of two-step bonding systems, *Am. J. Dent.*, 13, 101–104, 2000.
174. Ciucchi, B., Bouillaguet, S., Holz, J., and Roh, S., The battle of the bonds 1995, *Schweiz Monatsschr Zahnmed.*, 107, 37–39, 1997.
175. Takemori, T, Chigira, H., Itoh, K., Hisamitsu, H., and Wakumoto, S., Factors affecting tensile bond strength of composite to dentin, *Dent. Mater.*, 9, 136–138, 1993.
176. Hara, A.T., Pimenta, L.A., and Rodrigues, A.L., Influence of cross-head speed on resin-dentin shear bond strength, *Dent. Mater.*, 17, 165–169, 2001.
177. Oshida, Y. and Miyazaki, M., Dentin bonding system. Part II: Effect of crosshead speed, *Biomed. Mater. Eng.*, 6, 87–100, 1996.
178. Prati, C., Pashley, D.H., and Montanari, G., Hydrostatic intrapulpal pressure and bond strength of bonding systems, *Dent Mater.*, 7, 54–58, 1991.
179. Pioch, T., Staehle, H.J., Schneider, H., Duschner, H., and Dorfer, C.E., Effect of intrapulpal pressure simulation *in vitro* on shear bond strengths and hybrid layer formation, *Am. J. Dent.*, 14, 319–323, 2001.
180. Pameijer, C.H., and Louw, N.P., Significance of pulpal pressure during clinical bonding procedures, *Am. J. Dent.*, 10, 214–218, 1997.
181. Yanagawa, T. and Finger, W.J., Relationship between degree of polymerization of resin composite and bond strength to Gluma-treated dentin, *Am. J. Dent.*, 7, 157–160, 1994.

182. Burrow, M.F., Nikaido, T., Satoh, M., and Tagami, J., Early bonding of resin cements to dentin — effect of bonding environment, *Oper. Dent.*, 21, 196–202, 1996.
183. Van Noort, R., Noroozi, S., Howard, I.C., and Cardew, G., A critique of bond strength measurements, *J. Dent.*, 17, 61–67, 1989.
184. Sudsangiam, S. and Van Noort, R., Do dentin bond strength tests serve a useful purpose? *J. Adhes. Dent.*, 1, 57–67, 1999.
185. Jessop, N.T., Testing Shear Bond Strength, U.S. Patent No. 6,324,916 (to Ultradent), 2001.
186. Wakefield, C.W., Draughn, R.A., Sneed, W.D., and Davis, T.N., Shear bond strength of six bonding systems using the pushout method of *in vitro* testing, *Oper. Dent.*, 23, 69–76, 1998.
187. Van Noort, R., Cardew, G.E., Howard, I.C., and Noroozi, S., The effect of local geometry on the measurement of the tensile bond strength to dentin, *J. Dent. Res* 70, 889–893, 1991.
188. Mota, C.S., Demarco, F.F., Camacho, G.B., and Powers, J.M., Tensile bond strength of four resin luting agents bonded to bovine enamel and dentin. *J. Prosthet. Dent* 89, 558–564, 2003.
189. Sano, H., Shono, T., Sonoda, H., Takatsu, T., Ciucchi, B., Cavallo, R., and Pashley, D.H., Relationship between surface area for adhesion and tensile bond strength — evaluation of a micro-tensile bond test, *Dent. Mater.*, 10, 236–240, 1994.
190. Shono, Y., Ogawa, T., Terracita, M., Carvalho, R.M., Pashley, E.L., and Pashley, D.H., Regional measurement of resin-dentin bonding as an array, *J. Dent. Res.*, 78, 699–705, 1999.
191. Pashley, D.H., Carvalho, R.M., Sano, H., Nakajima, M., Yoshiyama, M., Shono, Y., Fernandes, C.A., and Tay, F., The microtensile bond test: a review, *J. Adhes. Dent* 1, 299–309, 1999.
192. Inoue, S., Vargas, M.A., Abe, Y., Yoshida, Y., Lambrechts, P., Vanherle, G., Sano, H., and Van Meerbeek, B., Microtensile bond strength of eleven contemporary adhesives to dentin, *J. Adhes. Dent.*, 3, 237–245, 2001.
193. Nakabayashi, N., Watanabe, A., and Arao, T., A tensile test to facilitate identification of defects in dentine bonded specimens, *J. Dent.*, 26, 379–385, 1998.
194. Ibarra, G., Vargas, M.A., Armstrong, S.R., and Cobb, D.S., Microtensile bond strength of self-etching adhesives to ground and unground enamel, *J. Adhes. Dent.*, 4, 115–124, 2002.
195. Prati, C., Simpson, M., Mitchem, J., Tao, L., and Pashley, D.H., Relationship between bond strength and microleakage measured in the same class I restorations, *Dent. Mater.*, 8, 37–41, 1992.
196. Retief, D.H., Mandras, R.S., and Russell, C.M., Shear bond strength required to prevent microleakage at the dentin/restoration interface, *Am. J. Dent.*, 7, 44–46, 1994.
197. Pereira, P.N.R., Okuda, M., Nakajima, M., Sano, H., Tagami, J., and Pashley, D.H., Relationship between bond strengths and nanoleakage: evaluation of a new assessment method, *Am. J. Dent.*, 14, 100–104, 2001.
198. Roulet, J.F., Reich, T., Blunck, U., and Noack, M., Quantitative margin analysis in the scanning electron microscope, *Scanning Microsc.*, 3, 147–158, 1989.
199. Blunck, U. and Roulet, J.F., Marginal adaptation of compomer Class V restorations *in vitro*, *J. Adhes. Dent.*, 1, 143–151, 1999.
200. Krejci, I., Besek, M., and Lutz, F., Clinical and SEM study of Tetric resin composite in posterior teeth: 12-month results, *Am J Dent.*, 7, 27–30, 1999.
201. Ferrari, M. and Garcia-Godoy, F., Sealing ability of new generation adhesive-restorative materials placed on vital teeth, *Am. J. Dent.*, 15, 117–128, 2002.

202. Tay, F., Pang, K.M., Gwinnett, A.J., and Wei, S.H., A method for microleakage evaluation along the dentin/restorative interface, *Am. J. Dent.*, 8, 105–108, 1995.
203. Bedran de Castro, A.K., Pimenta, L.A., Amaral, C.M., and Ambrosano, G.M., Evaluation of microleakage in cervical margins of various posterior restorative systems, *J. Esthet. Restor. Dent.*, 14, 107–114, 2002.
204. Dietrich, T., Kraemer, M., Losche, G.M., and Roulet, J.F., Marginal integrity of large compomer class 2 restorations with cervical margins in dentine, *J. Dent.*, 28, 399–405, 2000.
205. Manhart, J., Chen, H.Y., Mehl, A., Weber, K., and Hickel, R., Marginal quality and microleakage of adhesive class 5 restorations, *J. Dent.*, 29, 123–130, 2001.
206. Haller, B., Hofmann, N., Klaiber, B., and Bloching, U., Effect of storage media on microleakage of five dentin bonding agents, *Dent. Mater.*, 9, 191–197, 1993.
207. Ahlberg, K.M., Assavanop, P., and Tay, W.M., A comparison of the apical dye penetration patterns shown by methylene blue and India ink in root-filled teeth, *Int. Endod. J.*, 28, 30–34,1995.
208. Spahr, A., Schon, F., and Haller, B., Effect of gingival fluid on marginal adaptation of Class II resin-based composite restorations, *Am. J. Dent.*, 13, 261–266, 2000.
209. Mathew, M., Parameswaran Nair, E.K., and Krishnan, K., Bonding agent is a decisive factor in determining the marginal leakage of dental composites subjected to thermal cycling: an *in vitro* study, *J. Oral. Rehabil.*, 28, 68–77, 2001.
210. da cunha Mello, F.S., Feilzer, A.J., de Gee, A.J., and Davidson, C.L., Sealing ability of eight resin bonding systems in a class II restoration after mechanical fatiguing, *Dent. Mater.*, 13, 372–376, 1997.
211. Feilzer, A.J., de Gee, A.J., and Davidson, C.L., Setting stress in composite resin in relation to configuration of the restoration, *J Dent. Res.*, 66, 1636–1639, 1987.
212. Yoshikawa, T., Burrow, M.F., and Tagami, J., The effect of bonding system and light curing method on reducing stress of different c-factor cavities, *J. Adhes. Dent.*, 3, 177–183, 2001.
213. Hanks, C.T., Wataha, J.C., Parsell, R.R., Strawn, S.E., and Fat, J.C., Permeability of biological and synthetic molecules through dentine, *J. Oral Rehabil.*, 21, 475–487, 1994.
214. Van Meerbeek, B., Vargas, M., Inoue, S., Yoshida, Y., Perdigao, J., Lambrechts, P., and Vanherle, G., Microscopy investigations. Technique, results, limitations, *Am. J. Dent.*, special issue. 13, 3D–18D, 2000.
215. Van Meerbeek, B., Vargas, M., Inoue, S., Yoshida, Y., Peumans, M., Lambrechts, P., and Vanherle, G., Adhesives and cements to promote preservation dentistry, *Oper. Dent.*, Suppl. 6, 119–144, 2001.
216. Harada, N., Yamada, T., Inokoshi, S., and Tagami, J., Tensile bond strengths and adhesive interface of ten dentin bonding systems, *J. Med. Dent. Sci.*, 45, 85–96, 1998.
217. Nakajima, M., Sano, H., Burrow, M.F., Tagami, J., Ebisu, S., Ciucchi, B., Russell C.M., and Pashley, D.H., Tensile bond strength and SEM evaluation of caries-affected dentin using dentin adhesives, *J. Dent. Res.*, 74, 1679–1688, 1995.
218. Perdigao, J. and Swift, E.J., Analysis of dental adhesive systems using scanning electron microscopy, *Int. Dent. J.*, 44, 349–359, 1994.
219. Piemjai, M. and Nakabayashi, N., Effect of dentin conditioners on wet bonding of 4-META/MMA-TBB resin, *J. Adhes. Dent.*, 3, 325–331, 2001.
220. Hashimoto, M., Ohno, H., Sano, H., Kaga, M., and Oguchi, H., *In vitro* degradation of resin-dentin bonds analyzed by microtensile bond test, scanning and transmission electron microscopy, *Biomaterials*, S24, 3795–3803, 2003.

221. Nakajima, M., Kanemura, N., Pereira, P.N., Tagami, J., and Pashley, D.H., Comparative microtensile bond strength and SEM analysis of bonding to wet and dry dentin, *Am. J. Dent.*, 13, 324–328, 2000.
222. Van Meerbeek, B., Yoshida, Y., Snauwaert, J., Hellemans, L., Lambrechts, P., Vanherle, G., Wakasa, K., and Pashley, D.H., Hybridization effectiveness of a two-step versus a three-step smear layer removing adhesive system examined correlatively by TEM and AFM, *J. Adhes. Dent.*, 1, 7–23, 1999.
223. Tay, F.R., Moulding, K.M., and Pashley, D.H., Distribution of nanofillers from a simplified-step adhesive in acid-conditioned dentin, *J. Adhes. Dent.*, 1, 103–117, 1999.
224. Yoshida, Y., Van Meerbeek, B., Snauwaert, J., Hellemans, L., Lambrechts P., Vanherle, G., Wakasa, K., and Pashley, D.H., A novel approach to AFM characterization of adhesive tooth-biomaterial interfaces, *J. Biomed. Mater. Res.*, 47, 85–90, 1999.
225. El Feninat, F., Ellis, T.H., Sacher, E., and Stangel, I., A tapping mode AFM study of collapse and denaturation in dentinal collagen, *Dent. Mater.*, 17, 284–288, 2001.
226. Watson, T.F., Applications of confocal scanning optical microscopy to dentistry, *Br. Dent. J.*, 171, 287–291, 1991.
227. Pioch, T., Staehle, H.J., Wurst, M., Duschner, H., and Dorfer, C., The nanoleakage phenomenon: influence of moist vs dry bonding, *J. Adhes. Dent.*, 4, 23–30, 2002.
228. Tay, F.R., King, N.M., Chan, K.M., and Pashley, D.H., How can nanoleakage occur in self-etching adhesive systems that demineralise and infiltrate simultaneously? *J. Adhes. Dent.*, 4, 255–269, 2002.
229. Tay, F.R. and Pashley, D.H., Water treeing — a potential mechanism for degradation of dentin adhesives, *Am. J. Dent.*, 16, 6–12, 2003.
230. Tay, F.R., Pashley, D.H., Yiu, C.K., Sanares, A.M., and Wei, S.H., Factors contributing to the incompatibility between simplified-step adhesives and chemically-cured or dual-cured composites. Part I. Single-step self-etching adhesive, *J. Adhes. Dent.* 27–40, 2003.
231. Pashley, D.H., Ciucchi, B., and Sano, H., Dentin as a bonding substrate, *Dtsch. Zahnärztl. Z.*, 49, 760–763, 1994.
232. Nishiyama, N., Suzuki, K., Komatsu, K., Yasuda, S., and Nemoto, K., A ^{13}C NMR study on the adsorption characteristics of HEMA to dentinal collagen, *J. Dent. Res* 81, 9–471, 2002.
233. Nishiyama, N., Suzuki, K., Asakura, T., Komatsu, K., and Nemoto, K., Adhesion of *N*-methacryloyl-omega-amino acid primers to collagen analyzed by ^{13}C NMR, *J. Dent. Res.*, 80, 855–859, 2001.
234. Yoshida, Y., Van Meerbeek, B., Nakayama, Y., Snauwaert, J., Hellemans, L., Lambrechts, P., Vanherle, G., and Wakasa, K., Evidence of chemical bonding at biomaterial-hard tissue interfaces, *J. Dent. Res.*, 79, 709–714, 2000.
235. Spencer, P., Byerley, T.J., Eick, J.D., and Witt, J.D., Chemical characterization of the dentin/adhesive interface by Fourier-transform infrared photoacoustic spectroscopy, *Dent. Mater.*, 8, 10–15, 1992.
236. Eick, J.D., Miller, R.G., Robinson, S.J., Bowles, C.Q., Gutshall, P.L., and Chappelow, C.C., Quantitative analysis of the dentin adhesive interface by auger spectroscopy, *J. Dent. Res.*, 75, 1027–1033, 1996.
237. Spencer, P., Wang, Y., Walker, M.P., Wieliczka, D.M., and Swafford, J.R., Interfacial chemistry of the dentin/adhesive bond, *J. Dent. Res.*, 79, 1458–1463, 2000.
238. Van Meerbeek, B., Mohrbacher, H., Celis, J.P., Roos, J.R., Braem, M., Lambrechts, P., and Vanherle, G., Chemical characterization of the resin-dentin interface by micro-Raman spectroscopy, *J. Dent. Res.*, 72, 1423–1428, 1993.

239. Miyazaki, M., Onose, H., and Moore, B.K., Analysis of the dentin-resin interface by use of laser Raman spectroscopy, *Dent. Mater.*, 18, 576–580, 2002.
240. Wang, Y. and Spencer, P., Hybridization efficiency of the adhesive/dentin interface with wet bonding, *J. Dent. Res.*, 82:141–145, 2003.
241. Xu, J., Stangel, I., Butler, I.S., and Gilson, D.F., An FT-Raman spectroscopic investigation of dentin and collagen surfaces modified by 2-hydroxyethylmethacrylate, *J. Dent. Res.*, 76, 596–601, 1997.
242. Stangel, I., Sacher, E., Ellis, T., and Bertrand, L., Chemical characterization of the resin-dentin interface by micro-Raman spectroscopy, *J. Dent. Res.*, 72, 1423–1428, 1993.
243. Jessop, J.L.P., Armstrong, S.R., and Zou, Y., Raman spectroscopy of adhesive resin in dental composites bonded to dentin, *Polym. Mater. Sci. Engin.*, 88, 243–244, 2003.
244. Asmussen, E. and Uno, S., Chemische und physikalische Aspekte des Dentinbondings, *Phillip J.*, 11, 143–147, 1994.
245. Ruyter, I.E., The chemistry of adhesive agents, *Oper. Dent.*, Suppl. 5, 32–43. 1992.
246. Ruyter, I.E. and Oeysaed, H., Die chemischen Grundlagen dentaler Adhäsivsysteme, *Phillip J.*, 12, 481–488, 1995.
247. Hagger, O., Unsaturated Esters, GB Patent No. 687,299 (to De Trey AG), 1953.
248. Yamauchi, J, Masuhara, E., Nakabayashi, N., Shibatani, K., and Wada, T., Method of Filling a Tooth Cavity, U.S. Patent No. 4,259,075 (to Kuraray Co.), 1981.
249. Omura, I., Yamauchi, J., Nagase, Y., and Uemura, F., Adhesive Composition, U.S. Patent No. 4.539,382 (to Kuraray Co.), 1985.
250. Bunker, J.E., Dentin and Enamel Adhesive, European Patent No. 58,483 B1 (to 3M Company), 1982.
251. Bunker, J.E., Dentin and Enamel Adhesive, European Patent No. 61,240 A2 (to 3M Company), 1983.
252. Bunker, J.E., Dentin and Enamel Adhesive, European Patent No. 84,407 A2 (to 3M Company), 1983.
253. Billington, R.W., Blackwell, G.B., and Prodger, T.E., Adhesion Promoters, European Patent No. 88,527 B1 (to Dentsply Corporation), 1983.
254. Huang, C.-T. and Jefferies, S.R., Adhese Composition Which Bonds to Collagen and Calcium, European Patent No. 321,683 B1 (to Dentsply Corporation), 1989.
255. Nemcek, J. and Roberts, T.A., Polymerisable Composition, European Patent No. 132.929 B1 (to ICI), 1989.
256. Janda, R., Photopolymerisierbarer phosphathaltiger dentaler Haftvermittler-Lack, German Patent No. 3,414,163 C2 (to Kulzer & Co. GmbH), 1987.
257. Ruse, N.D. and Smith, D.C., Adhesion to bovine dentin–surface characterization, *J. Dent. Res.* 70, 1002–1008, 1991.
258. Yamauchi, J., Nakabayashi, N., and Masuhara, E., Adhesive agents for hard tissue containing phosphoric acid monomers, ACS, Div. Polym. Chem., *Polym. Prepr* 20(1), 594–595, 1979.
259. Nikaido, T. and Nakabayashi, N., Photocurable bonding liner for teeth. Part II. Effect of 2-methacryloxyethyl *p*-methoxyphenyl phosphoric acid on bond strength to dentin, *Jpn. J. Dent. Mat.*, 6, 690–694, 1987.
260. Iwaku, M., Nakamichi, I., Nakamura, K., Horie, K., Suizu S., and Fusayama, T., Tags penetrating dentin of a new adhesive resin, *Bull. Tokyo Med. Dent. Univ.*, 28, 45–51, 1981.
261. Wand, T., Nikaido, T., and Nakabayashi, N., Photocure bonding agent containing phosphoric methacrylate, *Dent. Mat.*, 7, 59–62, 1991.
262. Stefan, K.-P., Adhäsivsystem für dentale Zwecke, European Patent No. 878,183 A2, (to ESPE Dental AG), 1998.

263. Rheinhardt, K.-J., Primer for Preparing a Tooth Cavity for a Composite Filling, U.S. Patent No. 5,919,836 (to Ernst Mühlbauer KG), 1999.
264. Klee, J.E. and Walz, U., Self-Adhesive Polymerizable Monomer and Dental/Medical Compositions Therefrom, WO Patent No. 00/67701 (to Dentsply International Inc.), 2000.
265. Rheinhardt, K.-J. and Rüter, W., Einsatz von Phosphorsäureestern als Dentinhaftvermittler, *Phillip J.*, 11–12, 333–342, 1998.
266. Salz, U., Burtscher, P., Vogel, K., Moszner, N., and Rheinberger, V. New adhesive monomers for dental application, *Polym. Prepr.* 38(2), 143, 1997.
267. Moszner, N., Zeuner, F., Rumphorst, A., Salz, U., and Rheinberger, V., Hydrolysestabile Phosphonsäuremonomere als Dentinhaftvermittler, *Dental-Praxis*, 18, 105–112, 2001.
268. Heathcook, I. and Clayton, H., *Introduction to Organic Chemistry*, Macmillan, New York, 1976, p. 503.
269. Francis, M.D., Russel, R.G.G., and Fleisch, H., Diphosphonates inhibit formation of calcium phospahte crystals *in vitro* and pathological calcification *in vivo*, *Science* 165, 1264–1266, 1969.
270. Anbar, M., St. John, G.A., and Scott, A.C., Organic polymeric polyphosphonates as potential preventive agents of dental caries: *in vitro* experiments, *J. Dent. Res.*, 53, 867–878, 1974.
271. Anbar, M. and Farley, E.P., Potential use of organic polyphosphonates as adhesive in the restoration of teeth, *J. Dent. Res.*, 53, 879–888, 1974.
272. Farley, E.P., Johnes, R.L., and Anbar, M., Improved adhesion of acrylic restorative materials to dental enamel by precoating with monomers containing phosphonate groups, *J. Dent. Res.*, 56, 943–952, 1977.
273. Moszner, N., Zeuner, F., Fischer, U.K., and Rheinberger, V., Monomers for adhesive polymers, 2. Synthesis and radical polymerisation of hydrolytically stable acrylic phosphonic acids, *Macromol. Chem. Phys.*, 200, 1062–1067, 1999.
274. Moszner, N., Zeuner, F., and Rheinberger, V., Hydrolysis-Stable and Polymerizable Acrylicphosphonic Acids, U.S. Patent No. 6,172,131 B1 (to Ivoclar AG), 2001.
275. Moszner, N., Zeuner, F., Fischer, U.K., and Rheinberger, V., Monomers for adhesive polymers, 3. Synthesis, radical polymerisation and adhesive properties of hydrolytically stable acrylic phosphonic acid monomers, *Macromol. Mater. Eng.*, 286, 225–231, 2001.
276. Löhden, G., Dorn, K., and Albert, P., Dentalwerkstoff mit polymerisierbaren Phosphonsäuren, German Patent No. 199,18,974 A1 (to Degussa-Hüls AG), 1999.
277. Mou, L., Singh, G., and Nicholson, J.W., 2000, Synthesis of a hydrophilic phosphonic acid monomer for dental materials, *Chem. Commun.*, 5, 345–346, 2000.
278. Mühlbauer, W. and Neffgen, S., Phosphonsäuren enthaltendes Dentalmaterial, European Patent No. 1.169,996 A1 (to Ernst Mühlbauer KG), 2000.
279. Alexieva, C., Character of the hard tooth tissue-polymer bond. I. Study of the interaction of calcium phosphate with *N*-phenylglycine and with *N*-phenylglycine-glycidyl methacrylate adduct, *J. Dent. Res.*, 58, 1879–1883, 1979.
280. Alexieva, C., Character of the hard tooth tissue-polymer bond. II. Study of the interaction of human tooth enamel and dentin with *N*-phenylglycine-glycidyl methacrylate adduct, *J. Dent. Res.*, 58, 1884–1886, 1979.
281. Takeyama, M., Kashibuchi, N., Nakabayashi, N., and Masuhara, E., Studies on dental self-curing resins. Adhesion of PMMA with bovine enamel or dental alloys, *J. J Soc. Dent. Appar. Mat.*, 19, 179–185, 1978.

282. Nakabayashi, N., Masuhara, E., Mochida, E., and Ohmori, I., Development of adhesive pit and fissure sealants using a MMA resin initiated by a tri-*n*-butyl borane derivative, *J. Biomed. Mater. Res.*, 12, 149–165, 1978.
283. Tanaka, T., Nagata, K., Takeyama, M., Atsuta, M., Nakabayashi, N., and Masuhara, E., 4-META opaque resin — A new resin strongly adhesive to nickel-chromium alloy, *J. Dent. Res.*, 60, 1697–1706, 1981.
284. Nakabayashi, N. and Masuhara, E., Preparation of hard tissue compatible materials: dental polymers, in *Polymeric Materials and Pharmaceuticals for Biomedical Use* (Symposium Proceedings), Goldberg, E.P. and Nakajima, A., Eds., Academic Press, New York, 1980, pp. 85–111.
285. Nakabayashi, N., Adhesive bonding with 4-META, *Oper. Dent. Suppl.*, 5, 125–130, 1992.
286. Masuhara, E., Über die Chemie eines neuen haftfähigen Kunststoff-Füllungsmaterials, *Dtsch. Zahnärztl. Z.*, 24, 620–628, 1969.
287. Leung, Y. and Morris, M.D., Characterization of the chemical interactions between 4-MET and enamel by Raman spectroscopy, *Dent. Mat.*, 11, 191–195, 1995.
288. Suh, B. and Hammer, M., Dentin Bonding System, U.S. Patent No. 5,348,988 (to Bisco Inc.), 1964.
289. Iwakura, Y., Uno, K., Nakabayashi, N., and Kojima, T., Reactive monomers derived from p-vinylbenzoic acid, *Bull. Chem. Soc. Japan*, 41,186–191, 1968.
290. Kasashima, Y., Miyata, A., Akutsu, F., Naruchi, K., Miura, M., and Nakabayashi, N., Effectiveness of 4-vinylsalicylic acid and 4-vinylacetylsalicylic acid on adhesion to dentin, *Kobunshi Ronbunshu*, 51, 193–199, 1994.
291. Tagami, J., Hosoda, H., Imai, Y., and Masujara, E., Evaluation of a new adhesive liner as an adhesive promoter and a desensitizer on hypersensitive dentin, *Dent. Mater. J.,* 6,201–208, 1987.
292. Hirasawa, T. and Hirashima, I., (Meth)acrylsäureester und deren Verwendung, German Patent No. 3,736,554 C2 (to G-C Dental Ind. Corp.), 1993.
293. Hirashima, I, Hirasawa, T., Tomiaka, K., and Okada, J., Adhesion to tooth substrates and dental alloys by methacrylates having a naphthalic anhydride structure, *Dent. Mater. J.*, 7, 141–150, 1988.
294. Masuhara, E., Kojima, K., Tarumi, N., and Hotta, H., Adhesive Compositions, U.S. Patent No. 3,527,737 (to GC), 1970.
295. Chigira, H., Koike, T., Hasegawa, T., Itoh, K., Wakumoto, S., and Hayakawa, T., Effect of the self etching dentin primers on the bonding efficacy of a dentin adhesive, *Dent. Mater. J.*, 8, 86–92, 1989.
296. Fukushima, T., Ferracane, J.L., Horibe, T., and Okabe, T., Bonding of various succinoxy methacrylates to dental alloys, *Dent. Mater. J.*, 7, 1–12, 1988.
297. Fukushima, T., Kawaguchi, I.Y., Miyazaki, K., and Horibe, T., Application of functional monomers for dental use (9). Syntheses of succinoxy methacrylates and their adhesion to polished and etched tooth surfaces, *Dent. Mater. J.*, 4, 33–99, 1985.
298. Fukushima, T. and Horibe, T., A scanning electron microscopic investigation of bonding of methacryloyl hydrogen maleate to etched dentin, *J. Dent. Res.*, 69, 46–50, 1989.
299 Iwamoto, O., Kunimoto, S., Kusumoto, K., and Fujisawa, O., Acrylate Compound and Composition Containing the Same, U.S. Patent No. 4,755,620 (to Tokuyama Soda), 1988.
300. Suzuki, K., Kiyahara, T., and Kitoh, S., Dental Adhesive Composition, European Patent No. 284,275 B1 (to Lion Corp.), 1992.

301. Kitoh, S., Suzuki, K., Kiyahara, T., and Kurita, K., Adhesive monomers to dental ceramics. III. Influence of surface treatment on effective adhesion of calcium metaphosphate ceramic with *N*-(vinylbenzyl)iminodiacetic acid, *J. Appl. Polym. Sci.*, 60, 1821–1825, 1996.
302. Jandourek, H., Composition and Method for Improving Adherence of Polymeric Materials to Substrates, U.S. Patent No. 3,872,047, 1975.
303. Mitra, B.N., Curable cements based on poly(alkenoates)/ion-leachable glass hybrid systems, *Polym. Prep.*, 32, 517–518, 1991.
304. Rheinberger, V., Moszner, N., Stelzer, F., Schitter, R., and Zeuner, F., Funktionalisiertes und polymerisierbares Polymer, German Patent No. 196,16,183 A1 (to Ivoclar AG), 1997.
305. Chaudhuri, R.K., Haldar, R.K., and Gangadharan, B., Bioadhesive Composition, U.S. Patent No. 5,055,046 (to ISC Investments), 1991.
306. Müller, M., Podszun, W., Finger, W., and Winkel, J., *N*-Alkyl-*N*-(meth)acryloyloxyalkylcarboxamide aromatischer Carbonsäuren und aromatischer Carbonsäureanhydride sowie Adhäsive enthaltend diese Verbindungen, European Patent No. 471,252 B1 (to Bayer AG), 1994.
307. Müller, M., Finger, W., Podszun, W., and Winkel, J., Dentaladhäsive, European Patent No. 499,923 B1 (to Bayer AG), 1992.
308. Müller, M. Podszun, W., and Alker, B., Adhäsivkomponente zur Behandlung kollagenhaltiger Materialien, European Patent No. 355,562 B1 (to Bayer AG), 1994.
309. Müller, M. and Podszun, W., Formylpiperazinyl-(Meth)Acrylic Acid Derivatives for Treatment of Collagen, U.S. Patent No. 5,068,264 (to Bayer AG), 1991.
310. Müller, M. and Podszun, W., Adhesive Components Containing Alkanediyl-*bis*-Carboxamides for Treatment of Collagen, U.S. Patent No. 5,071,933 (to Bayer AG), 1991.
311. Antonucci, J.M., Aldehyde methacrylates derived from hydroxybenzaldehydes, *J. Dent. Res.*, 57, 500–505, 1978.
312. Asmussen, E. and Munksgaard, E.C., Formaldehyde as bonding agent between dentin and restorative resins, *Scand. J. Dent. Res.*, 92, 480–483, 1984.
313. Munksgaard, E.C. and Asmussen, E., Dentin-polymer bond mediated by glutaraldehyde/HEMA, *Scand. J. Dent. Res.*, 93, 463–486, 1985.
314. Asmussen, E. and Munksgaard, E.C., Adhesion Promoting Agent, Process for Its Preparation and Use Thereof on Collagenous Material, European Patent No. 141,324 B1 (to Bayer AG), 1988.
315. Asmussen, E. and Munksgaard, E.C., Coating Agent for Collagen-Containing Materials, U.S. Patent No. 5,183,832 (to Bayer AG), 1993.
316 Asmussen, E. and Munksgaard, E.C., Bonding of restorative resins to dentine promoted by aqueous mixtures of aldehydes and active monomers, *Intern. Dent. J.*, 35, 160–165, 1985.
317. Munksgaard, E.C., Irie M., and Asmussen, E., Dentin-polymer bond promoted by Gluma and various resins, *J. Dent. Res.*, 64, 1409–1411, 1985.
318. Peutzfeldt, A. and Asmussen, E., Influence of aldehydes on selected mechanical properties of resin composites, *J. Dent. Res.*, 71, 1522–1524, 1992.
319. Asmussen, E. and Bowen, R.L., Adhesion to dentin mediated by Gluma: effect of pretreatment with various amino acids, *Scand. J. Dent. Res.*, 95, 521–525, 1987.
320. Asmussen, E. and Bowen, R.L., Effect of acidic pretreatment on adhesion to dentin mediated by Gluma, *J. Dent. Res.*, 66, 1386–1388, 1987.
321. Causton, B.E. and Sefton, J., Some bonding characteristics of a HEMA/maleic acid adhesion promoter, *Br. Dent. J.*, 167, 308–311, 1989.
322. Camps, J., Saradell, J.M., Dejou, J., Pignoly, C., and Jacquot, B., Influence of concentration and application time of maleic acid on dentin permeability, *Dent. Mater.*,11, 177–181, 1995.

323. Asmussen, E. and Peutzfeldt, A., The role of maleic anhydride in adhesive resin cements, *Eur. J. Oral Sci.*, 106, 882–886, 1998.
324. Coover, H.W. and Shearer, N.H., Adhesive Compositions Containing Alkyl Esters of Cyanoacrylic Acid, U.S. Patent No. 2,794,788 (to Eastman Kodak Company), 1957.
325. Beech, D.R., Bonding of alkyl 2-cyanoacrylates to human dentin and enamel, *J. Dent. Res.*, 51, 1438–1442, 1971.
326. Brauer, G.M., Jackson, J.A., and Termini, D.J., Bonding of acrylic resins to dentin with 2-cyanoacrylates esters, *J. Dent. Res.*, 58, 1900–1907, 1979.
327. Lee, H.L., Cupples, A.L., Schubert, R.J., and Swartz, M.L., An adhesive dental restorative material, *J. Dent. Res.,* 50,125–132, 1970.
328. Antonucci, J.M., Brauer, G.M., and Termini, D.J., Isocyanato urethane methacrylates derived from hydroxyethyl methacrylate, *J. Dent. Res.*, 59, 35–43, 1978.
329. Asmussen, E. and Munksgaard, E.C., Bonding of restorative resins to dentin by means of methacryloyl chloride and methacryloyl-R-isocyanate, *Scand. J. Dent. Res.*, 91, 153–155, 1983.
330. Bennett, R., Dental Adhesive System, European Patent No. 064,834 B1 (to Dentsplsy Intern), 1987.
331. Mukai, N., Ige, H., Makino, T., and Atarashi, J., Dental Adhesive Composition, European Patent No. 347,771 A2 (to Mitsubishi Rayon Co.), 1989.
332. Brauer, G.M. and Lee, C.H., Methacrylate oligomers with pendant isocyanate groups as tissue adhesives, *Polym. Mater. Sci. Eng.*, 59, 397–401, 1988.
333. Brauer, G.M., Lee, C.H., and Stansbury, J.W., Copolymers of 2-isocyanatoethyl methacrylate or *m*-isopropenyl-α,α-dimethylbenzyl isocyanate: synthesis and adhesives properties, *J. Dent. Res.*, 65, 827, 1986.
334. Brauer, G.M. and Lee, C.H., Oligomers with pendant isocyanate groups as tissue adhesives. I. Synthesis and characterization, *J. Biomed. Mater. Res.*, 23, 295–309, 1989.
335. Brauer, G.M. and Lee, C.H., Oligomers with pendant isocyanate groups as tissue adhesives. II. Adhesion to bone and other tissue and characterization, *J. Biomed. Mater. Res.*, 23, 753–763, 1989.
336. Brauer, G.M. and Lee, C.H., Effect of isocyanate content and molecular weight of adhesive on bonding, *J. Dent. Res.*, 68, 959, 1989.
337. Lee, C.H. and Brauer, G.M., Oligomers with pendant isocyanate groups as adhesives for dentin and other tissues, *J. Dent. Res.*, 68, 484–488, 1989.
338. Byerley, T.J., Franska, C.B., and Eick, J.D., Isocyanatoacrylates: a new multifunctional adhesive: monomer synthesis and polymerization, *J. Dent. Res.*, 69, 116, 1990.
339. Byerley, T.J., Chappelow, C.C., Chappell, R.P, Millich, F., and Eick, J.D., Isoatoacrylates: a new class of dental adhesives, *J. Dent. Res.*, 70, 363, 1991.
340. Chappelow, C.C., Byerley, T.J., Millich, F., Pinzino, C.S., and Eick, J.D., Design and development of isocyanatoacrylates as dental adhesives, *J. Dent. Res.*, 72, 282, 1993.
341. Chappelow, C.C., Byerley, T.J., Pinzino, C.S., Millich, F., and Eick, J.D., Design and development of isocyanatoacrylates as dental adhesives, *J. Dent. Res.* 75, 761–767, 1996.
342. Taira, Y., Matsumara, H., and Atsuta, A., Use of 2-isocyanatoethyl methacrylate and iron(II) perchlorate for bonding tri-*n*-butylborane-initiated luting agents to dentin, *Eur. J. Oral. Sci.*, 106, 887–891, 1998.
343. Chappelow, C., Power, M.D., Bowles, C.Q., Miller, R.G., Pinzino C.S., and Eick, J.D., Novel priming and crosslinking systems for use with isocyanatomethacrylate dental adhesives, *Dent. Mater.*, 16, 396–405, 2000.
344. Smith, D.C., Maric, B., and Vougiouklagis, G., Bonding of dichlorotriazines to dentine, *Dent. Res.*, Abstr. No 673, 58 (Spec. Iss. A), 1979.

345. Lee, C.H., Liu, X.Q., and Gong, X.Q., Triazine monomers and their adhesion to dentin, *J. Dent. Res.*, 65, 1402–1405, 1986.
346. Christensen, G.J., Using rubber dams to boost quality, quantity of restorative services, *J. Am. Dent. Assoc.*, 125, 81–82, 1994.
347. Liebenberg, W.H., Extending the use of rubber dam isolation: alternative procedures. Part I, *Quintessence Int.*, 23, 657–665, 1992.
348. Taskonak, B. and Sertgoz, A., Shear bond strengths of saliva contaminated 'one-bottle' adhesives, *J. Oral. Rehabil.*, 29, 559–564, 2002.
349. Kaneshima, T., Yatani, H., Kasai, T., Watanabe, E.K., and Yamashita, A., The influence of blood contamination on bond strengths between dentin and an adhesive resin cement, *Oper. Dent.*, 25, 195–201, 2000.
350. Hitmi, L., Attal, J.P., and Degrange, M., Influence of the time-point of salivary contamination on dentin shear bond strength of 3 dentin adhesive systems, *J. Adhes. Dent.*, 1, 219–232, 1999.
351. Abdalla, A.I. and Davidson, C.L., Bonding efficiency and interfacial morphology of one-bottle adhesives to contaminated dentin surfaces, *Am. J. Dent.*, 11, 281–285, 1998.
352. Fritz, U.B., Finger, W.J., and Stean, H., Salivary contamination during bonding procedures with a one-bottle adhesive system, *Quintessence Int.*, 29, 567–572, 1998.
353. Bennett, A.M., Fulford, M.R., Walker, J.T., Bradshaw, D.J., Martin, M.V., and Marsh, P.D., Microbial aerosols in general dental practice, *Br. Dent. J.*, 189, 664–667, 2000.
354. Eschmann-Speer, C., Lange, D.E., and Müller, R.F., Reduktion des Keimgehalts behandlungsbedingter zahnärztlicher Aerosole, *Dtsch. Zahnärztl. Z.*, 52, 436–438, 1997.
355. Jones, C.G., Chlorhexidine: is it still the gold standard? *Periodontol.*, 15, 55–62, 1997.
356. Tulunoglu, O., Ayhan, H., Olmez, A., and Bodur, H., The effect of cavity disinfectants on microleakage in dentin bonding systems, *J. Clin. Pediatr. Dent.*, 22, 299–305, 1998.
357. Vieira Rde, S. and da Silva, I.A., Jr., Bond strength to primary tooth dentin following disinfection with a chlorhexidine solution: an *in vitro* study, *Pediatr. Dent.*, 25, 49–52, 2003.
358. Bishara, S.E., Vonwald, L., Zamtua, J., and Damon, P.L., Effects of various methods of chlorhexidine application on shear bond strength, *Am. J. Orthod. Dentofacial Orthop.*, 114, 150–153, 1998.
359. Damon, P.L., Bishara, S.E., Olsen, M.E., and Jakobsen, J.R., Bond strength following the application of chlorhexidine on etched enamel, *Angle. Orthod.*, 67, 169–172, 1997.
360. Bishara, S.E., Damon, P.L., Olsen, M.E., and Jakobsen, J.R., Effect of applying chlorhexidine antibacterial agent on the shear bond strength of orthodontic brackets, *Angle. Orthod.*, 66, 313–316, 1996.
361. Filler, S.J., Lazarchik, D.A., Givan, D.A., Retief, D.H., and Heaven, T.J., Shear bond strengths of composite to chlorhexidine-treated enamel, *Am. J. Dent.*, 7, 85–88, 1994.
362. Meiers, J.C. and Shook, L.W., Effect of disinfectants on the bond strength of composite to dentin, *Am. J. Dent.*, 9, 11–14, 1996.
363. Meiers, J.C. and Kresin, J.C., Cavity disinfectants and dentin bonding, *Oper. Dent* 21, 153–159, 1996.
364. Perdigao, J., Denehy, G.E., and Swift, E.J., Effects of chlorhexidine on dentin surfaces and shear bond strengths, *Am. J. Dent.*, 7, 81–84, 1994.
365. Tuttlebee, C.M., O'Donnell, M.J., Keane, C.T., Russell, R.J., Sullivan, D.J., Falkiner, F., and Coleman, D.C., Effective control of dental chair unit waterline biofilm and marked reduction of bacterial contamination of output water using two peroxide-based disinfectants, *J. Hosp. Infect.*, 52, 192–205, 2002.

366. Meiller, T.F., Kelley, J.I., Baqui, A.A., and DePaola, L.G., Laboratory evaluation of anti-biofilm agents for use in dental unit waterlines, *J Clin Dent.*, 12(4), 97–103, 2001.
367. Roberts, H.W., Karpay, R.I., and Mills, S.E., Dental unit waterline antimicrobial agents' effect on dentin bond strength, *J. Am. Dent. Assoc.*, 131, 179–183, 2000.
368. Taylor-Hardy, T.L., Leonard, R.H., Mauriello, S.M., and Swift, E.J., Effect of dental unit waterline biocides on enamel bond strengths, *Gen. Dent.*, 49, 421–425, 2001.
369. Prati, C., Fava, F., Di Gioia, D., Selighini, M., and Pashley, D.H., Antibacterial effectiveness of dentin bonding systems, *Dent. Mater.*, 9, 338–343, 1993.
370. Ohmori, K., Maeda, N., and Kohno, A., Evaluation of antibacterial activity of three dentin primers using an *in vitro* tooth model, *Oper. Dent.*, 24, 279–285, 1999.
371. Imazato, S., Torii, M., Tsuchitani, Y., Nishida, K., and Yamauchi, J., Antimicrobial Polymerizable Composition, the Polymer and Article Obtained from the Same, European Patent No. 537,774 B1 (to Kuraray Company), 1998.
372. Yap, A.U., Shah, K.C., Loh, E.T., Sim, S.S., and Tan, C.C., Influence of eugenol-containing temporary restorations on bond strength of composite to dentin, *Oper. Dent.*, 26, 556–561, 2001.
373. Yap, A.U., Shah, K.C., Loh, E.T., Sim, S.S., and Tan, C.C., Influence of ZOE temporary restorations on microleakage in composite restorations, *Oper. Dent.*, 27, 142–146, 2002.
374. Peutzfeld, A. and Asmussen, E., Influence of eugenol-containing temporary cement on efficacy of dentin-bonding systems, *Eur. J. Oral Sci.*, 107, 65–69, 1999.
375. Ganss, C. and Jung, M., Effect of eugenol-containing temporary cement on bond strength of composite to dentin, *Oper. Dent.*, 23, 55–62, 1998.
376. Jung, M., Ganss, C., and Senger, S., Effect of eugenol-containing temporary cement on bond strength of composite to enamel, *Oper. Dent.*, 23, 63–68, 1998.
377. Peters, O., Goehring, T.N., and Lutz, F., Effect of eugenol-containing sealer on marginal adaptation of dentin-bonded resin fillings, *Int. Endod. J.*, 33, 53–59, 2000.
378. Sung, E.C., Chan, S.M., Mito, R., and Caputo, A.A., Effect of carbamide peroxide bleaching on the shear bond strength of composite to dental bonding agent enhanced enamel, *J. Prosthet. Dent.*, 82, 595–599, 1999.
379. Dishman, M.V., Covey, D.A., and Baughan, L.W., The effect of peroxide bleaching on composite to enamel bond strength, *Dent. Mater.*, 9, 33–36, 1994.
380. Titley, K.C., Torneck, C.D., and Ruse, N.D., The effect of carbamide-peroxide gel on the shear bond strength of a microfilresin to bovine enamel, *J. Dent. Res.*, 71, 20–24, 1992.
381. Torneck, C.D., Titley, K.C., Smith, D.C., and Adibfar, A., The influence of time of hydrogen peroxide exposure on the adhesion of composite resin to bleached bovine enamel, *J. Endod.* 16, 123–128, 1990.
382. Cavalli, V., Reis, A.F., Giannini, M., and Ambrosano, G.M., The effect of elapsed time following bleaching on enamel bond strength of resin composite, *Oper. Dent* 26, 597–602, 2001.
383. Cvitko, E., Denehy, G.E., Swift, E.J., and Pires, J.A., Bond strength of composite resin to enamel bleached with carbamide peroxide, *J. Esthet. Dent.*, 3(3), 100–102, 1991.
384. Lai, S.C., Tay, F.R., Cheung, G.S., Mak, Y.F., Carvalho, R.M., Wei, S.H., Toledano, M., Osorio, R., and Pashley, D.H., Reversal of compromised bonding in bleached enamel, *J. Dent. Res.*, 81, 477–481, 2002.

4 Application of Polymers in the Therapy for Gingivitis, Periodontitis, and Treatment of Dry Socket

Shalaby W. Shalaby and Ulrich Salz

CONTENTS

4.1 INTRODUCTION

Gingivitis and periodontitis are the two major forms of inflammatory diseases affecting the gingiva and periodontal attachment apparatus of the teeth. By definition (1) gingivitis is inflammation of the gingiva and (2) periodontitis is inflammation of the supporting structures of the teeth, including bone and periodontal ligament. Inflammation of the periodontium can be caused by many factors, yet most forms of gingivitis and periodontitis result directly from growth and accumulation of oral microorganisms. Failure to treat gingivitis and periodontitis leads eventually to loss of teeth and deterioration of the adjacent soft and bony tissues. Apart from gingivitis and periodontitis, but somewhat related to them, are the traumatic events associated with tooth extraction, which can result in delayed healing and infection at the respective site. This leads to the so-called dry socket. Failure to treat dry socket in a timely fashion can cause bone resorption.

4.2 GENERAL APPROACHES TO THE THERAPY FOR GINGIVITIS AND PERIODONTITIS

Therapy for gingivitis is aimed primarily at the reduction of etiologic factors to allow the reparative processes of the body to respond and the gingival tissue to heal. On the other hand, the therapeutic approaches to periodontitis are more elaborate and fall into two main categories: (1) those designed to stop the progression of periodontal attachment loss and (2) those designed to regenerate structures destroyed by a previous disease process.

4.2.1 General Approaches to the Therapy for Gingivitis

Associated with gingivitis as an inflammatory disease affecting the gingival tissues that will be addressed in this section are mainly (1) chronic gingivitis, (2) acute gingival diseases, and (3) gingival overgrowth.

4.2.1.1 Chronic Gingivitis

Therapy for individuals with chronic gingivitis (CG) is initially directed toward the reduction of oral bacteria and associated calcified tissues. Patients with chronic gingivitis and no significant calcified deposits, alteration in gingival morphology, or systemic diseases that affect oral health may respond to a therapeutic regimen consisting of improved personal plaque control alone.[1] However, it has been suggested that a self-administered plaque control program without periodic professional reinforcement is not consistently successful in providing long-term reversal of gingivitis.

Many patients with gingivitis have calculus, which interferes with their ability to remove bacterial plaque. For these patients, an effective therapy entails professionally performed scaling and root planing to remove plaque and calculus, thus creating an environment that allows the patient to use a plaque control approach to reducing the oral bacterial count below the threshold capable of initiating inflammation.

Successful therapy for gingivitis in some patients is based on the use of antibacterial rinses to assist in the reduction of the bacterial plaque. Two commonly accepted products are used in this way to reduce bacterial plaque and gingival inflammation. The active ingredients of one product are thymol, menthol, eucalyptol, and methyl salicylate. The active ingredient in the second product is chlorhexidine digluconate.

4.2.1.1 Acute Gingival Diseases

A major acute form of gingivitis is herpes gingivitis, which is associated with the oral manifestation of a primary herpes simplex virus type. In healthy patients, treatment of herpes gingivitis consists of palliation and hydration. However, for immunocompromised patients with herpes gingivitis, systemic antiviral therapy with acyclovir would be appropriate.[4] Another major gingival disease is acute necrotizing ulcerative gingivitis, which is the result of specific bacterial accumulations occurring in individuals with lowered host resistance. It responds to therapy that reduces oral bacteria by a combination of personal plaque control and professional debridement.

4.2.1.3 Gingival Overgrowth

This results from chronic gingival inflammation and may be exaggerated in patients with generic or drug-related system factors.[5] A combination of personal plaque control and scaling or planing can be used in treating gingival overgrowth because it leads to reduction of the tissue mass and improvement of the periodontal architecture.[6] In some patients with gingival overgrowth, the modification of tissue contours by surgical means may be necessary.[7]

4.2.1.4 Role of Polymers in the Therapy for Gingivitis

To date, most commonly used approaches to the therapy of gingivitis do not involve the use of polymeric material. However, as seen later in Section 4.3.1, polymers are used experimentally as drug carriers to control the release of antibacterial and other bioactive agents with established efficacy as single-dose preparations in the therapy for gingivitis.

4.2.2 General Approaches to Therapy for Periodontitis

Periodontitis destroys tissues at the level of periodontal attachment and results in the creation of a periodontal pocket. Strategies for periodontitis therapy entail halting the progression of the active disease process and stabilizing periodontal attachment. The therapy for periodontitis is aimed at reducing the level of etiologic factors at the site of disease below the threshold capable of producing continuing breakdown, to allow the repair of the affected site. Key approaches to achieving this aim include scaling and root planing, surgical therapy, pharmacological therapy, and periodontal regeneration. It is to be noted that appropriate therapy for patients with periodontitis varies with the extent and pattern of attachment loss, local anatomical variations of the affected area, and type of periodontal disease.

4.2.2.1 Scaling and Root Planing

Scaling and root planing coupled with personal plaque control in the treatment of periodontitis can lead to (1) reduction of clinical inflammation, (2) positive alteration in the subgingival microflora; (3) reduction of the probing depth, and (4) gain of clinical attachment.[8–10] However, root planing efficacy is diminished at sites with deep probing depth and in the furcation region.[11,12]

4.2.2.2 Surgical Therapy

This approach to the treatment of periodontitis is pursued to (1) provide an easy access for removal of etiologic factors, (2) create a posttherapy architecture suitable for adequate personal plaque control to prevent reinitiation of inflammation, and (3) allow the placement of an agent capable of stimulating the regeneration of the periodontium lost structure. Longitudinal evaluation of healing has shown that procedures, including surgical access, result in greater posttherapy reduction of probing depth as compared with nonsurgical debridement.[13]

4.2.2.3 Pharmacological Therapy

This approach was (1) acknowledged by early investigators as having an adjunctive role in the management of periodontitis using nonpharmacological treatment protocols, (2) not recommended by conservative investigators who consider that using drugs, such as antibiotics, can be associated with undesirable side effects such as the development of resistant bacterial strains, and (3) described by contemporary investigators as being highly effective in treating periodontitis when the drug is administered using controlled release formulations as described in Section 4.3.[14–18] Meanwhile, for patients who do not respond to mechanical debridement procedures or other specific types of periodontitis, as in juvenile periodontitis, the adjunctive use of antibiotics was indicated.[19,20] A list of antibiotic systems and structure of active ingredients for local periodontitis is provided in Table 4.1 and Figure 4.1, respectively.

4.2.2.4 Periodontal Regeneration

In patients who have lost a significant amount of periodontal attachment, the regeneration of lost tissue is the most logical goal. And this cannot be achieved adequately by a combination of root debridement with plaque control since these procedures alone have not been shown to produce significant amounts of new connective tissue attachment, although bone fill may occur in selected sites.[21–24] Restoration of new attachment can be enhanced by the use of adjunctive materials and techniques, which include (1) the use of chemical agents to condition the root surface while promoting new attachment, (2) bone grafting, (3) guided tissue regeneration techniques with or without bone graft augmentation, and (4) the use of biologically engineered soft and hard tissue inductive proteins to stimulate periodontal regeneration.[25–32]

4.2.2.5 Role of Polymers in the Therapy for Periodontitis

Polymers do have an important role in the therapy for periodontitis, which is expected to become more significant with the advancement in the technology of (1) local controlled release of bioactive agents, including the antimicrobial and tissue growth

TABLE 4.1
Antibiotic Systems for Local Periodontitis Therapy

System	Composition	Absorption (time)	Release Rate
Tetracycline fiber[a]	Ethylene–vinyl acetate copolymer; tetracycline	No	Controlled over a longer period of time
Metronidazole gel[b]	Sesame oil; metronidazole	Yes (1 day)	Short
Chlorhexidine chip[c]	Gelatin matrix; chlorhexidine	Yes (8 days)	Controlled over a longer period of time
Minocycline gel[d]	Lipid gel; minocycline	Yes (1 day)	Short
Doxycycline gel[e]	Lactide–glycolide copolymer; doxycycline	Yes (27 days)	Controlled over a longer period of time

Source: Data from Greenstein, G. and Polson, A.M., *J. Periodontol.*, 69, 507, 1998.
[a] Actisite (Alza); [b]Elyzol (Dumex); [c]Periochip (Perio Products); [d]Dentomycin (Cyanamid); [e]Atridox (Atrix Lab)

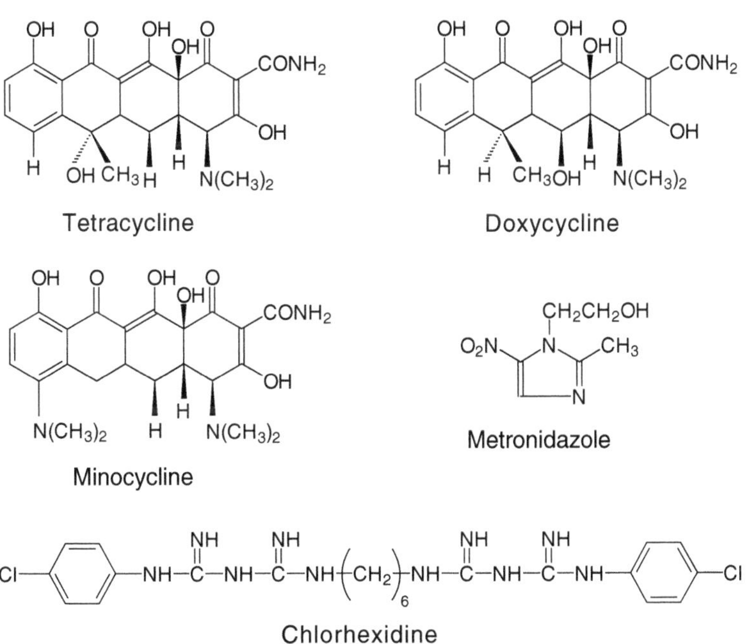

FIGURE 4.1 Active ingredients already used for local periodontitis therapy.

promoting types as they relate to the pharmacological and periodontal regeneration approaches to the therapy of periodontitis, respectively, and (2) tissue engineering as it relates to periodontal regeneration and replacement of lost tissue.[31–34]

4.3 EVOLUTION OF POLYMER APPLICATIONS IN THE THERAPY FOR GINGIVITIS AND PERIODONTITIS

The applications of polymers in the therapy for gingivitis and periodontitis have evolved quite differently in these two areas, depending on the advancement made in the area of drug and polymer development and changes in patient populations and needs. The advancements that are most pertinent to polymers dealt with (1) their use as carriers for the controlled delivery of bioactive agents and particularly antimicrobials, (2) their use in conjunction with tissue regeneration and healing, and (3) factors pertinent to the effectiveness of implemented therapies. Accordingly, this section primarily addresses these topics.

4.3.1 Polymers for Controlled Drug Delivery

The majority of the early work on controlled delivery systems (CDS) dealt with the administration of antimicrobials for the treatment of periodontitis and to a lesser extent, gingivitis. Early CDS placed in or near the periodontal pocket or in the vicinity of a compromised gingival tissue consisted of (1) a reservoir-type device with a cellulose acetate dialysis tube (or hollow fiber) loaded with tetracycline, (2) monolithic fibers of ethylene vinyl acetate (EVA) copolymer and tetracycline — the monolithic tetracycline fiber (Actisite®) was approved for use in humans and is still being used, (3) a cellulose acetate dialysis tube containing chlorhexidine, (4) acrylic strips containing metronidazole, chlorhexidine, or tetracycline, (5) an ethyl cellulose matrix containing chlorhexidine, (6) a collagen film containing chlorhexidine, (7) an injectable, white petroleum gel loaded with tetracycline, chlorhexidine, or stannous fluoride, (8) chlorhexidine or tetracycline in hydroxypropyl cellulose, and (9) tetracycline or metronidazole in polyhydroxy butyric acid.[33–44]

Phenomenal growth in the area of absorbable polymers over the past two decades affected significantly the dental community's approach to controlled drug delivery systems for use in the therapy for gingivitis and periodontitis. Absorbable polymers containing copolymers of lactide and glycolide, and segmented copolymers of these monomers have played a key role in the development of several controlled drug delivery systems. The scheme for the synthesis and degradation of a typical copolymer is shown in Figure 4.2. The documented uses of absorbable polymers include a combination of sanguinarine and a lactide/glycolide copolymer solution in *n*-methyl pyrrollidone, which precipitated into a solid after injection into the periodontal pocket.[45] Drug concentration was reported to be sustained at therapeutic levels ranging from 100 to 260μL/mL in crevicular fluid for up to 12 days. Microbial data obtained with DNA probes for select pathogens indicated that subgingival sanguinarine reduced the bacterial population in a comparable manner to scaling and root planing.[47] It was also reported that clinical results obtained in a 3-month split mouth trial indicated that subgingival sanguinarine is equivalent or

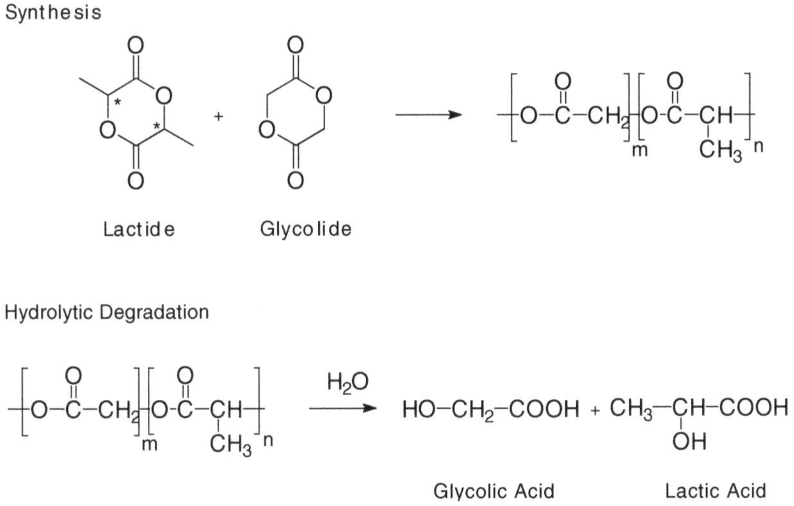

Synthesis

Lactide + Glycolide → $-[O-C(=O)-CH_2]_m-[O-C(=O)-CH(CH_3)]_n-$

Hydrolytic Degradation

$-[O-C(=O)-CH_2]_m-[O-C(=O)-CH(CH_3)]_n- \xrightarrow{H_2O} HO-CH_2-COOH + CH_3-CH(OH)-COOH$

Glycolic Acid   Lactic Acid

FIGURE 4.2 Synthesis and hydrolytic degradation of lactide–glycolide copolymer.

superior to scaling and root planing in terms of pocket depth reduction.[48] Major clinical drawbacks of the solid-forming, injectable solution containing sanguinarine are (1) it is a two-part formulation, (2) its use of tissue irritating solvent, and (3) the possible biomechanical incompatibility of the *in situ* formed solid in the periodontal pocket. Nonetheless, the same carrier was used in preparing a patented, two-part injectable doxycycline formulation that was described as being effective in treating periodontitis.[49] In spite of the success of these absorbable, solid-forming controlled release systems, the clinically disconcerting issue cited above and recent availability of absorbable liquid gel-forming carriers, which have been evaluated successfully in several controlled release systems, prompted Shalaby and coworkers to use such gel formers as carriers to control the release of doxycycline for treating periodontitis.[18,50–53] The absorbable gel-forming liquid used as carrier for doxycycline consists of liquid segmented copolymers of polyethylene glycol end-grafted with mixtures of glycolide and *dl*-lactide. The liquid carrier also contains a small amount of an absorbable microparticulate cation exchanger.[50] The doxycycline gel-forming formulation has been the subject of a successful clinical study in Germany, which reflected higher efficacy in treating periodontitis compared with earlier approaches. The clinical study was designed using the results of an extensive *in vitro* study on selected formulations. Accordingly, absorbable gel-forming liquids comprising copolymers of polyethylene glycol grafted with a mixture of *dl*-lactide and glycolide were prepared as described earlier by Shalaby.[50] The liquid gel former is mixed with polyglycolic acid microparticles and doxycycline hydrochloride (DOX) at about 15–20% and 12–17%, respectively, to produce the controlled release formulation. The release profile was monitored for over 200 h using a continuous flow system where a phosphate buffer at pH 7.4 and 27°C contacts tangentially at 40–100 mg mass of the formulation at a flow rate of about 30–60 μL/h. Samples of the effluent buffer

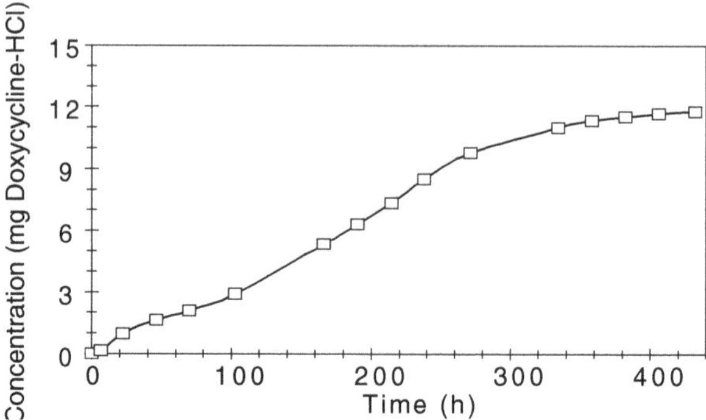

FIGURE 4.3 Cumulative *in vitro* relase profile of 15% w/w doxycycline-HCl from periodontal gel-forming formulation.

solution were collected in vials placed at 4°C. Analysis for doxycycline in periodically collected samples was conducted using HPLC. Release profile of a representative controlled release formulation containing 15% doxycycline-HCl is shown in Figure 4.3. The release profile represents an average of three separate sets of experiments. The cumulative release profile of this formulation demonstrates a sustained release over at least 200 h and gives the amount of doxycycline released over 200 h under conditions simulating the intended application in the periodontal pocket. Results also indicate that the antibiotic can be available at concentrations well above the expected effective level.

Recent investigations dealing with the development of new drug delivery systems using polymeric materials as carriers are outlined as follows.

In a study using tetracycline-loaded fibers to evaluate the clinical, radiological, and microbiological response to the local delivery of tetracycline to sites with persistent periodontal lesions, a split-mouth design was used.[54] And 19 patients with at least four bilateral pockets of 4–5 mm and bleeding on probing were treated with scaling and root planing plus tetracycline fibers (test sites) or with scaling and root planing alone (control sites). Clinical and radiological measurements were taken at baseline, 6 months, and 12 months postoperatively. Subgingival plaque samples were collected at baseline, when the fibers were removed, and at 6 and 12 months following treatment, and were analyzed by polymerase chain reaction. Results of the study indicated that both treatments yielded a statistically significant reduction of probing depth (2.05 and 1.21 mm), gain of clinical attachment level (1.71 and 0.53) and reduction of bleeding on probing scores (23.68 and 57.89%) for the tetracycline and scaling and root planing groups, respectively, when comparing 12-month data with baseline. The differences between the two groups were significant. The prevalence of *T-denticola* and *B-forsythus* decreased after therapy in both groups; in the test site, *A-actinomycetemcomitans* and *P-intermedia* were not yield detected. The pathogens could be eliminated from 5 periodontal pockets by scaling and root planing alone, while 21 tetracycline sites were not recolonized at 12 months. This allowed the investigators to conclude that scaling and root planing plus tetracycline fibers gave the greatest advantage in the treatment of periodontal persistent lesions at least 12 months following treatment.

This was consistent with the results of an earlier study designed to evaluate the effects of tetracycline fibers as an adjunct to scaling and root planing in the treatment of generalized, aggressive periodontitis and to compare the effects with mechanical treatment only in 10 patients, 24–39 years old.[55] In this study, a split-mouth experimental design was used. Measurements of bleeding on probing, pocket depth, and clinical attachment level were performed at 12 sites, randomly selected. Clinical recordings were made at baseline, 2 and 6 months, and after treatment. Subgingival plaque samples were taken for microbiological analysis using the "checkerboard" DNA–DNA hybridization technique at baseline, immediately after treatment, and after 2 and 6 months. Full-mouth scaling and root planing were performed, with the exception of two preselected sites, which served as controls. Tetracycline fibers were applied in five pockets located in the same half mouth. Analysis of clinical findings showed that mechanical instrumentation in combination with tetracycline fiber application led to a greater improvement in clinical parameters than scaling and root planing only. Microbial analysis showed a statistically significant greater reduction in the percentages of detection for *B. forsythus*, *P. nigrescens*, and *A. naeslundii genospecies* II in pockets where tetracycline fibers were applied.

In another earlier trial, tetracycline free base was used to prepare a semisolid, injectable formulation using a bioerodible poly(orthoester) (POES) as a matrix and was directly injectable in the periodontal pocket.[56] It showed sustained and almost constant *in vitro* release in phosphate buffer, pH 7.4 at 37°C, for up to 14 days. Total polymer degradation concomitant with drug release was obtained. Synthesis and hydrolytic degradation of polyorthoesters are illustrated in Figure 4.4. Formulations containing 10 or 20% (wt/wt) tetracycline were evaluated in a panel of 12 patients suffering from severe and recurrent periodontitis. In the first trial including six patients, single-rooted teeth and molar teeth with furcations were treated immediately

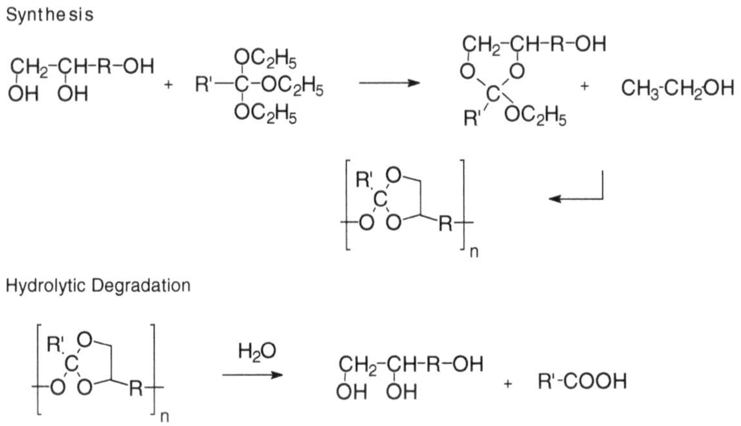

Synthesis

Hydrolytic Degradation

FIGURE 4.4 Synthesis and hydrolytic degradation of polyorthoesters.

after scaling and root planing. Patients tolerated both formulations well, experienced no pain during application, and showed no signs of irritation or discomfort during the observation period. An improved clinical protocol followed in the second study (stopping bleeding after scaling and root planing) prolonged the retention of the formulations in the inflamed periodontal pockets. For up to 11 days, tetracycline concentrations in the gingival cervicular fluid were higher than the minimum inhibitory concentration of tetracycline against most periodontal pathogens.

A novel drug delivery system using tetracycline as the active agent for the treatment of periodontitis was developed using two components.[57] The first was tetracycline free base loaded into the microtubular excipient halloysite, which was coated with chitosan to further retard drug release. The second component developed was a vehicle for the drug-loaded, coated halloysite, which was primarily based on the thermoresponsive polymer, poloxamer 407. A selected formulation was prepared, which consisted of 200 mg of halloysite double loaded with tetracycline base and coated with chitosan suspended in 1 mL of poloxamer 407, 20% (w/w), PEG 20,000, 0.5% (w/w), octyl cyanoacrylate, 1.0% (w/w), water to 100%, adjusted to pH 4. The syringeability of this formulation at various temperatures was evaluated to ensure ease of delivery to the periodontal pocket. This formulation offered ease of delivery to the periodontal pocket and sustained release of the antibiotic for up to 6 weeks. The formulation had preliminary *in vivo* testing performed in dogs to determine levels of drug release, antimicrobial activity, and retentive ability of the product. A wound pocket creation model was developed for the purposes of the trial. Results showed that the product was retained in the pocket for up to 6 weeks with effective tetracycline levels released locally over this period, which achieved good antibacterial activity.

Other developments in the use of controlled delivery systems for treating periodontitis include: (1) a new chitosan/PLGA film delivery system for lipophilic drugs such as ipriflavone, (2) bioadhesive gel formations containing metronidazole and a combination of hydroxyethyl cellulose, polyvinyl pyrrolidone, and carbopol, (3) sparfloxacin in a diethylphthalate-plasticized chip containing ethyl cellulose and polyethylene glycol 4000, and (4) povidone-iodine (polyvinyl pyrrolidone-iodine complex) as a periodontal pocket disinfectant.[58–61]

4.3.2 Use of Polymers in Conjunction with Tissue Regeneration

It is well established that progressive periodontitis leads to tooth loss through destruction of the tooth attachment apparatus. In teeth where continued function requires additional periodontal support, controlling the periodontal infection as discussed in Section 4.3.1 is not sufficient, and regeneration of the lost periodontium is needed. Procedures used in the treatment of periodontal disease to achieve replacement or reconstitution of lost periodontal tissue have evolved over the past few decades and are denoted as regenerative therapy.[62] Accordingly, periodontal regeneration is defined as restoration of lost supporting tissue, including new alveolar bone, cementum, and periodontal ligament. New connective tissue attachment deals with the development of a new connective tissue with a root surface that has been deprived of its periodontal ligament, through the formation of new cementum by inserting collagen fibers.[62] A clinical restoration of bone tissue in previously treated periodontal defects is called bone fill. Guided tissue regeneration describes procedures designed to manipulate cells that repopulate the wound healing site leading to tissue regeneration.[62] Earlier, as well as current, implementation of these procedures entailed the use of the following procedures.

1. Extra-oral and intra-oral autogenous bone grafts.
2. Allogenic bone grafts, with and without an antimicrobial agent. Histological analysis following these graft procedures indicates that partial periodontal regeneration may occur; however, the presence of clinical bone fill does not necessarily indicate periodontal regeneration.
3. Flap management, where the sequences of wound healing events that include fibrin, clot formation between the flap margin and the root surface, followed the replacement of the fibrin clot by a connective tissue matrix attached to the root surface.
4. Bone substitutes and alloplasts, which are commercially available as non-porous hydroxyapatite, porous hydroxyapatite (replaminoform), beta tri-calcium phosphate, and HTR polymer (a calcium layered polymeric system of polymethyl methacrylate and polyhydroxyethyl methacrylate). When used as grafts for mandibular defects, all the alloplasts materials produce improved clinical conditions, but induce little or no bone fill and very limited or no periodontal regeneration.
5. Root surface demineralization using citric acid to modify the root surface and expose collagen fibrils in the cementum or dentin. This treatment provided no significant clinical improvement.
6. Matrix derived proteins and/or growth factors to expand the amount of predictable regeneration. This area became the subject of more recent studies, and the controlled release of growth factors is a challenge that is currently addressed by contemporary investigators; and
7. Guided cell repopulation or guided tissue regeneration using nonabsorbable and absorbable polymeric membranes or autogenous connective tissue grafts as membranes.[63–79]

Apart from using collagen in conjunction with the autogenous and allogenic grafts, the guided tissue regeneration and bone substitutes or allografts are unique in terms of using polymeric materials, which are free of the safety issues associated with biological materials, in the respective protocols. Accordingly, this section was designed to provide a more detailed treatment, focusing on advances in tissue regeneration and healing associated with the use of polymers as outlined in the following sections. The choice to focus on guided tissue regeneration is consistent with the analysis contained in a systematic review of guided tissue regeneration for the treatment of periodontal, intrabony furcation defects.[80]

Application of polymeric membranes in guided tissue regeneration evolved from the early use of Millipore filters to expanded tetrafluoroethylene membranes and recently to absorbable membranes or meshes.[75–81] The recent interest in using absorbable or biodegradable membranes was justified since their nonabsorbable counterparts require a second surgical procedure for their removal. In a clinical study using an absorbable copolyester barrier in polymer-assisted regeneration therapy in periodontal intrabony therapy, 40 periodontal osseous defects were treated with two types of absorbable barrier materials (Atrisorb and Resolut XT).[82] In this study, 30 patients suffering from moderate to advance periodontitis were randomly assigned to receive either Atrisorb barrier or Resolut XT barrier therapy. Periodontal phase I treatment and oral hygiene instruction were performed before periodontal surgery. Papillary preservation, partial thickness flap, citric acid root conditioning, and decortication procedures were applied during the operation. Bone defects were filled with a mixture of demineralized freeze-dried bone allograft and minocycline (4:1 ratio). Postoperative care included 0.10% chlorhexidine rinse daily and antibiotic medication for 2 weeks. Clinical assessments, including probing depth, clinical attachment level, gingival recession, plaque index, gingival index, and radiographic examinations were taken at the baseline, preoperatively, and at 3- and 6-months after regenerative surgery. Results of the study showed that 6 months following therapy, both Atrisorb and Resolut XT groups had achieved comparable clinical improvement in pocket reduction (3.9 vs. 4.4 mm), attachment tissue gain (clinical attachment gain: 3.5 vs. 3.6 mm), and reduction in the gingival and plaque indices. Within-group comparisons showed significant attachment gain and pocket reduction between baseline data and both 3- and 6-months postoperatively.

To test the hypothesis that guided tissue regeneration procedures provide predictable reconstruction of periodontal tissues in the treatment of furcation involvements in animals and humans, Cetiner et al. studied the long-term effectiveness of two different types of polylactic acid membranes on periodontal regeneration in surgically created class II furcation defects in dogs.[83] In the study, a full thickness mucoperiosteal flap was raised on the buccal aspects of the experimental teeth and class II furcation defects having 5 mm vertical dimensions were created on mandibular premolars III and IV in each quadrant. The exposed root surfaces were thoroughly planed, and polylactic acid membranes were placed over the experimental defects on both sites. Liquid polymer membrane was applied to one site, and resorbable periodontal mesh membranes were applied to the other. The animals were sacrificed 7 months after surgery, and the specimens were processed for histological evaluation. The results of the study indicated that the average length of new attachment formed on the treated roots in both groups ranged from 3.02 mm to 4.5 mm. Complete bone filling was observed at the furcation sites. No statistically significant differences were found between the two membranes in any of the parameters. The favorable regenerative outcomes of the study led to the suggestion that the two different types of polylactic acid membranes can be used as alternatives to guided tissue regeneration.

Recognizing that predictable periodontal regeneration following periodontal disease is a major goal of therapy led to the design of a study using a copolymeric glycolide/lactide (PLGA) sponge to evaluate the ability of cementoblasts and dental follicle cells to promote periodontal regeneration in a rodent periodontal fenestration model.[84] In the study, the buccal aspect of the distal root of the first mandibular molar was denuded of its periodontal ligament, cementum, and superficial dentin through a bony window created bilaterally in 12 athymic rats. Treated defects were divided into three groups: (1) carrier alone (PLGA polymer sponges); (2) carrier plus follicle cells; and (3) carrier plus cementoblasts. Cultured murine primary follicle cells and immortalized cementoblasts were delivered to the defects via biodegradable PLGA polymer sponges, and mandibulae were retrieved 3 and 6 weeks postoperatively for histological evaluation. *In situ* hybridization for gene expression of bone sialoprotein, osteocalcin, and histomorphometric analysis were further done on 3-week specimens. Results of the study indicated that 3 weeks after surgery, histology studies of defects treated with carrier alone indicated PLGA particles, fibrous tissue, and newly formed bone scattered within the defect area. Defects treated with carrier plus follicle cells had a similar appearance, but with less formation of bone. In contrast, in defects treated with carrier plus cementoblasts, mineralized tissues were noted at the healing site with extension toward the root surface, periodontal ligament region, and laterally beyond the buccal plate envelope of bone. No periodontal ligament–bone fibrous attachment was observed in any of the groups. *In situ* hybridization showed that the mineralized tissue formed by cementoblasts gave strong signals for both bone sialoprotein and osteocalcin genes, confirming its nature as cementum or bone. The changes noted at 3 weeks were also observed at 6 weeks. Cementoblast-treated and carrier alone–treated defects exhibited complete bone bridging and periodontal ligament formation, whereas follicle cell-treated defects showed minimal evidence of osteogenesis. No new cementum was formed along the root surface in these two groups. Cementoblast-treated defects were filled with trabeculated mineralized tissue similar to, but more mature than, that seen at 3 weeks. In addition, the periodontal ligament region was maintained with well-organized collagen fibers connecting the adjacent bone to a thin layer of cementumlike tissue observed on the root surface. Neoplastic changes were observed at the superficial portions of the implants at two of the 6-week cementoblast-treated specimens, possibly due, in part, to the SV40-transformed nature of the implanted cell line. It was concluded that cementoblasts have a marked ability to induce mineralization in periodontal wounds when delivered via polymer sponges, while implanted dental follicle cells seem to inhibit periodontal healing. The results also confirm the selective behaviors of different cell types *in vivo* and support the role of cementoblasts as a tool to better understand periodontal regeneration and cementogenisis.

As noted earlier, interest in bone growth promoters has grown considerably over the past few years. And the use of recombinant human bone morphogenetic protein-2 (rhBMP-2) technologies were shown to significantly support efforts directed to alveolar bone formation. Biomaterial limitations, however, have restricted the biologic potential for onlay indications. To this end, a study was pursued to evaluate regeneration of alveolar bone and periodontal attachment, and biomaterials reaction following surgical implantation of a space-providing, bioabsorbable, macroporous, polyglycolic acid–trimethylene carbonate (PGA-TMC) membrane combined with a rhBMP-2 construct in a discriminating onlay defect model.[85] In the study, routing supra-alveolar periodontal defects were created at the mandibular premolar teeth in nine beagle dogs. Contralateral jaw quadrants in subsequent animals were randomly assigned to receive the dome-shaped PGA-TMC (100- to 120-μm pores) membrane with rhBMP-2 (0.2 mg/mL) in a bioresorbable hyaluronan carrier or the PGA-TMC membrane with hyaluronan alone (control). The gingival flaps were advanced to submerge the membranes and teeth and then sutured. Animals were euthanized at 8 and 24 weeks postoperatively for histology observations. Results of the study revealed that jaw quadrants receiving the PGA-TMC membrane alone experienced exposures at various times throughout the study. Jaw quadrants receiving the PGA-TMC/rhBMP-2 combination remained intact, although one site experienced a late minor exposure. Newly formed alveolar bone approached and became incorporated into the macroporous PGA-TMC membrane in sites receiving rhBMP-2. The PGA-TMC biomaterial was occasionally associated with a limited inflammatory reaction. Residual PGA-TMC could not be observed 24 weeks postoperatively. Residual hyaluronan could not be observed at any time interval. Regeneration of alveolar bone height was significantly increased in sites receiving the PGA-TMC/rhBMP-2 combination compared with the control (3.8 vs. 0.7 mm at 8 weeks and 4.6 vs. 2.1 mm at 14 weeks). Limited cementum regeneration was observed for PGA-TMC/rhBMP-2 and PGA-TMC control sites. Ankylosis compromised regeneration in sites receiving PGA-TMC/rhBMP-2. Results of this study led to the conclusion that (1) a bioabsorbable, space-providing, macroporous PGA-TMC membrane appears to be a compatible biomaterial for bone augmentation procedures, and (2) rhBMP-2 significantly enhances alveolar bone augmentation and soft tissue healing when combined with the PGA-TMC membrane.

Adjunct to the advances in tissue regeneration discussed in some detail previously, there have been several supplementary investigations pertaining to (1) the effect of different bioactive agents including antimicrobials on the tissue regeneration, (2) the degradation of absorbable polymers used as barrier membranes, (3) the use of injectable gels, and (4) role of ligature-induced periodontitis.[86–93] Specific illustrations of these investigations include:

- Barrier membrane and systemic antibiotics in the treatment of intra-osseous defects
- Attachment of periodontal ligament cells to chlorhexidine-loaded guided tissue regeneration membranes
- Effect of polylactide/glycolide membrane loaded with metronidazole on periodontal regeneration following guided tissue regeneration in dogs
- Effects of simvastatin gels on murine calvarial bone growth
- Use of chitin-based gel as injectable materials in periodontal surgery
- Susceptibility of guided tissue regeneration–regenerated periodontal attachment to ligature-induced periodontitis
- Spectroscopic study of the enzymatic degradation of biodegradable composite periodontal membrane
- Long-term results of guided tissue regeneration therapy with nonabsorbable and bioabsorbable barriers relative to intrabony defects.[86–93]

Other studies focusing primarily on the use of absorbable polymers and expanded polytetrafluoroethylene in conjunction with guided tissue regeneration include:

Treatment of human class II furcation defects using connective tissue grafts, bioabsorbable membrane, and resorbable hydroxyapatite
Combined use of enamel matrix proteins and a tetracycline-coated expanded polytetrafluoroethylene barrier membrane in the treatment of intra-osseous defects
Clinical performance of a regenerative strategy for intrabony defects using e-PTFE and bioabsorbable membrane.[94–96]

4.3.3 Pertinent Factors to the Effectiveness of Implemented Therapies

The degree of effectiveness of implemented therapies for gingivitis and periodontitis discussed in Sections 4.3.1 and 4.3.2 may depend on events taking place in the vicinity of the treated sites. These events can be typically associated with the use of dentifrices and dental restoratives. To address the effect of dentifrices, a study was conducted to determine whether a fluoridated liquid product with added triclosan and a vinyl methyl ether–maleic acid copolymer (PVM-MA) copolymer delivery system is efficacious for the control of supragingival plaque and gingivitis.[97] For this, a 6-month, double-blind, parallel stratified clinical study was conducted in accordance with American Dental Association guidelines for the clinical evaluation of antiplaque–antigingivitis products. Subjects who qualified with a suitable amount of existing plaque and gingivitis were given one of two dentifrices: an experimental liquid dentifrice containing 0.3% triclosan, 2.0% PVM/MA copolymer, and 0.243% sodium fluoride (NaF) in a silica base, or a placebo dentifrice containing 0.243% NaF in a silica base. The subjects' plaque and gingival index scores were collected at baseline and at 3- and 6-month intervals. Results of the study indicate that the use of the experimental liquid dentifrice provided a significant reduction in existing levels of plaque and gingivitis as compared with the placebo standard dentifrice. At 6 months, the experimental group demonstrated a 34.9% reduction in plaque formation and a 25.7% reduction in gingivitis as compared with the placebo group. It was concluded that (1) the experimental dentifrice had a significantly better ability to reduce plaque and gingivitis as compared with the placebo, (2) the new form of dentifrice achieved results comparable in efficacy to those of traditional dentifrice pastes with matching active ingredients, and (3) a liquid dentifrice containing a triclosan/PVM/MA copolymer/NaF delivery system is clinically efficacious in its ability to reduce existing plaque and gingivitis.

The relationship between subgingival dental restoration and periodontal health has been the subject of several investigations. However, longitudinal data on the subgingival microflora features after placement of well-finished subgingival restorations were nonexistent. This led to a study to compare the short-term clinical and microbiological features occurring in the gingival after the completion of different subgingival restorations.[98] In the study, 16 systemically healthy subjects (mean age 39.35 years) who were nonsmokers and were positive for the presence of three crevical abrasion or erosion defects to be restored in three different adjacent teeth were enrolled. The defects were each restored by using one of three different materials: amalgam, glass ionomer cement, or composite resin. Immediately before class V cavity preparations and restorations (baseline), clinical monitoring and subgingival plaque sampling were performed in the midbuccal aspect of each experimental restored tooth and in one adjacent sound, nontreated control tooth. These procedures were repeated every 4 months over the following year. Acquired results show that throughout the study, the clinical parameters recorded did not change significantly in the experimental group and no differences were detected among them at each clinical session. Over this time, no significant changes in the composition of the subgingival microflora were observed in amalgam, glass ionomer cement, and control groups. Conversely, in the composite resin group, there was a significant increase in the total bacterial counts, and a significant decrease in Gram-positive aerobic bacteria, which was associated with a significant increase in the Gram-negative, anaerobic microbiota. This led to the conclusion that over a 1-year observation period, amalgam, glass ionomer cement, and composite resin subgingival restorations do not significantly affect the clinical parameters recorded. However, composite resin restorations may have some negative effects on the quality and quantity of subgingival plaque.

4.4 DRY SOCKET AND USE OF POLYMERIC SYSTEMS IN ITS TREATMENT

Traumatic events associated with tooth extraction can result in delayed healing and infection at the respective sites and, in turn, lead to so-called dry socket. Failure to treat dry socket in a timely fashion can cause bone resorption. Until recently, practically all clinical protocols used to treat dry socket, with limited success, relied on single-time treatments, which usually entail the use of antimicrobial agents. Incidents of dry socket are more frequent and can lead to more serious complications in compromised geriatric and diabetic patients, and particularly those with periodontitis. This and the successful use of a doxycycline-based absorbable, gel-forming, controlled release system in treating periodontitis prompted the pursuit of a comparative study of a similar doxycycline formulation containing the antiinflammatory drug naproxen and a second formulation containing clindamycin as a potent antibiotic for treating oral infections.[18,99] In the study, two antibiotic, controlled release formulations (DF and CF) were used.[99] One of the formulations, DF, contained a small amount of a nonsteroidal antiinflammatory drug, which was intended to reduce the inflammation at the surgical site, which may in turn increase the effectiveness of the antimicrobial drug. This formulation DF was prepared using doxycycline hydrochloride, naproxen sodium, an acid-terminated microparticulate polyglycolide, and a liquid gel-forming polyethylene glycol copolymerized with glycolide and *dl*-lactide as described earlier, at 12, 3, 20, and 65%, respectively.[18] The second formulation, CF, was prepared using 25.6% cleocin (to provide about 12% active clindamycin), 9.4% carboxyl-terminated microparticulate polyglycolide, and 65% of the gel-forming PEG-copolyester.

Searching the literature for a suitable animal model to conduct the study was fruitless. This led to the development of an animal use protocol that was approved by the Animal Research Committee at Clemson University using a beagle dry socket for the animal model. All surgical procedures were conducted according to the approved AAALAC accredited animal housing facility. The protocol consisted of phases I and II: phase I dealt with the development of the infected dry socket model; phase II addressed the treatment of the infected socket with the antibiotic controlled release formulations (CF and DF). For phase I, two beagles were purchased and used in the study. Animal A was a retired female breeder, 4 years old, weighing about 16 lbs. Animal B was a retired female breeder, 5 years old, weighing 27 lbs. Both animals arrived in good general health. Each displayed a significant amount of tartar build up and inflamed, irritated gums, which were most likely associated with periodontitis.

Toward pursuing phase I of the protocol, the mouths of the dogs were swabbed preoperatively along the gum line proximal to the upper canine tooth. A blood sample was taken from each animal for a complete blood count (CBC). The animals were then sedated with acepromazine (a tranquilizer and sedative administered at 0.05 mg/kg), glycopyrrolate (an anticholinergic given to decrease salivary secretions administered at 0.01 mg/kg), and butorphanol (an opioid analgesic administered at 0.4 mg/kg). The animals were anesthetized by inhalation with isofluorane. The animals were then dosed with carprofen (a nonsteroidal antiinflammatory drug) administered at 4 mg/kg). A veterinary oral surgeon removed the upper canines. The mouths were swabbed with small piece of sterile gauze. The gauze was packed into the socket and sutured in place with a 3-0 PDS II suture. One suture knot was made on each side of the tooth socket. Two additional sutures were used to close the incision that had been made in the gum to remove the canine. This procedure was repeated to remove the other upper canine. One socket from each animal was swabbed. These animals were closely monitored for body temperature and activity; and blood was taken for a CBC. After 3 days, the animals were anesthetized as described above. The gums were inspected for infection. The gauze sutured into each socket was removed and retained for microbial investigation. The sockets had no blood clot, there was severe swelling and redness in the gums, and an extremely fetid odor.

For treating the infected socket as planned in phase II of the protocol, the antibiotic-loaded gel formers were administered into the socket of each animal. An attempt to suture the sockets closed was made with variable results because of the friable condition of the gums. These animals were closely monitored for body temperature and activity; and a CBC done. All swabs were used to investigate the microbial communities associated with the mouth and the infection. Colony counts were made, and the predominant microbes were identified. The treatment scheme of the beagles with the antibiotic formulations, DF and CF, and controls D and C (containing 0.25% doxycycline and clindamycin in saline, respectively) are outlined in Table 4.2.

Results of the colony counts and CBC for both beagles showed clearly that infection can be induced using the developed phase I protocol. At 3 days following the treatment with the antibiotics formulations, some reduction in the infecting microorganism was evident. Most sites treated with the antibiotics in a gel formulation were found to be practically free of infection at 11 days. However, the infections at the control site treated with the saline formulation were minimally affected.

TABLE 4.2
Gum Treatment Scheme with Formulations

Animal	Side	Teeth Extracted	Formulation Used
A	Right	Lower premolar	DF
	Left	None	Control D
B	Right	Upper molar, Lower incisor (2) Lower premolar	CF
	Left	Upper premolar	Control C

Results also indicate that gel-forming formulations CF and CD were equally effective. This led to the conclusion that an animal model for studying dry socket was developed. Results of the colony counts and CBC for both beagles showed clearly that infection can be induced using the phase I protocol. At 3 days following the treatment with the antibiotic gel-forming formulations CF and CD, some reduction in the infecting microorganisms was evident. Most of these sites were found to be practically free of infection at 11 days.

4.5 CONCLUSION AND PERSPECTIVE ON THE FUTURE

By contrasting the limited use of polymers in therapy for gingivitis and periodontitis prior to the 1990s with their more extensive applications in recent years, we clearly see the unprecedented appreciation of the dental community for the significant role of the recently uncovered, fast-growing technology of polymers, and particularly the absorbable types, because they pertain to advances in the controlled delivery and localized administration of bioactive agents, including antimicrobials and tissue growth promoters. These observations, in concert with the distinct increase in the population of geriatric and diabetic patients, permit one to forecast future emphasis on:

The use of bioactive formulation-based absorbable polymers and particularly those which can easily be injected into the periodontal pocket to undergo instant gelation to provide a sustained release of selected active agents for at least 2 weeks

The search and use of new antimicrobials, such as peptides that do not lead to drug-resistant bacteria

The development of antimicrobial and polymeric formulations that are also capable of reducing the inflammation at the treatment sites

The use of guided tissue regeneration to develop new, effective means for *in situ* tissue engineering using novel forms of absorbable polymers

The development of reliable animal models for evaluating new formulations for treating periodontitis and dry socket

The development of a better understanding of the relationship between periodontitis and other pathological and surgical events and restorative treatments that can be encountered in the oral cavity

REFERENCES

1. Loe, H., Theilade, E., and Jensen, S.B., Experimental gingivitis in man, *J. Periodontol.* 15, 485, 1988.
2. Listgarten, M.A., Schifter, C.C., and Lister, L., Three-year longitudinal study of the periodontal status of an adult population with gingivitis, *J. Clin. Periodontol.*, 12, 225, 1985.
3. Gordon, J.M., Lamster, I.B., and Seiger, M.C., Efficiency of Listerine antiseptic in inhibiting the development of plaque and gingivitis, *J. Clin. Periodontol.*, 12, 697, 1985.
4. Redding, S.W. and Montgomery, M.T., Acyclovir prophylaxis for oral herpes simplex infection in patients with bone marrow implants, *Oral Surg. Oral Med. Oral Pathol.* 67, 680, 1989.
5. Butler, R.T., Kalkwarf, K.L., and Kaldahl, W.B., Drug induced gingival plaque hyperplasia: phenytoin, cyclosporine and nifedipine, *J. Am. Dent. Assoc.*, 114, 56, 1987.
6. Tagge, D. L., O'Leary, T.J., and El-Kafrawy, A.H., The clinical and histological response of periodontal pockets to root planing and oral hygiene, *J. Periodontol.*, 46, 527, 1975.
7. Schluger, S., Yuodelis, R.A., Page, R.C., and Johnson, R.H., *Periodontal Diseases* Lea & Febiger, Philadelphia, PA, 1990, p. 453.
8. Mosques, T., Listgarten, M.A., and Phillips, R.A., Effect of scaling and root planing on the composition of human subgingival microbial flora, *J. Periodont. Res.*, 15, 144, 1980.
9. Badersten, A., Neiveus, R., and Egelberg, J., Effect of non-surgical periodontal therapy I. Moderately advanced periodontitis, *J. Clin. Peridontol.*, 8, 57, 1981.
10. Kaldahl, W., Kalkwarf, K., Patil, K., Dyer, J., and Bates, R., Jr., Evaluation of four modalities of periodontal therapy: mean probing depth, probing attachment level and recession changes, *J. Periodontol.*, 59, 783, 1988.
11. Rabbani, G.M., Ash, M.M., and Caffesse, R.G., The effectiveness of subgingival scaling and root planing in calculus removal, *J. Periodontol.*, 13, 119, 1981.
12. Fleischer, H.C., Mellonig, J.T., Brayer, W.K., Gray, J.L., and Barnett, J.D., Scaling and root planing in multirooted teeth, *J. Periodontol.*, 60, 402, 1989.
13. Ramfjord, S.P., Knowles, J.W., Nissle, R.R., Schick, R.A., and Burgett, F.G., Longitudinal study of periodontal therapy, *J. Periodontol.*, 44, 66, 1973.
14. Korman, K.S. and Karl, E.H., The effect of long-term low-dose tetracycline therapy on subgingival microflora refractory adult periodontitis, *J. Periodontol.*, 53, 604, 1982.
15. Haffajee, A.D., Dzink, J.L., and Socransky, S.S., Effect of modified Widman flap surgery and systemic tetracycline on subgingival microbiota of periodontal lesions, *J. Clin. Periodontol.*, 15, 255, 1988.
16. Howell, T.H., Chemotherapeutic agents as adjuncts in the treatment of periodontal disease, *Curr. Opin. Dent.*, 1(1), 81, 1991.
17. Okuda, K., Wolff, L., and Oliver, R., Minocycline slow-release formulation effect on subgingival bacteria, *J. Periodontol.*, 63, 73, 1992.
18. Salz, U., Bolis, C., Radl, A., Rheinberger, V.V., Carpenter, K.A., and Shalaby, S.W., Absorbable gel-forming doxycycline controlled system for non-surgical periodontal therapy, *Trans. Soc. Biomater.*, 24, 294, 2001.
19. Magnusson, I., Clark, W.B., Low, S.B., Maruniak, J., Mark, R.G., and Walker, C.B., Effect of non-surgical periodontal surgery combined with adjunctive antibiotics with refractory periodontal disease, *J. Clin. Periodontol.*, 16, 647, 1989.

20. Korman, K.S. and Robertson, P.B., Clinical and microbiological evaluation of therapy for juvenile periodontitis, *J. Periodontol.*, 56, 443, 1983.
21. Caton, J. and Zander, H., The attachment between tooth and gingival tissues after periodic root planing and soft tissue curettage, *J. Periodontol.*, 50, 462, 1979.
22. Caton, J. and Nyman, S. Histometric evaluation of periodontal surgery II. Connective tissue attachment levels after four regenerative procedures, *J. Clin. Periodontol.* 224, 1980.
23. Froum, S.J., Coran, J., Thaller, B., Kushner, L, Scopp, I.W., and Stahl, S.S., Periodontal healing following open debridement procedure. I. Clinical assessment of soft tissue and osseous repair, *J. Periodontol.*, 53, 8, 1982.
24. Isidor, F. Attstrom, R., and Karring, T., Regeneration of alveolar bone following surgical and non-surgical periodontal treatment, *J. Clin. Periodontol.*, 12, 687, 1985.
25. Albair, W.B., Cobb, C.M., and Killoy, W.J., Connective tissue attachment to periodontally diseased roots after citric acid demineralization, *J. Periodontol.*, 53, 515, 1982.
26. Wikesjö, UME, Baker, P.J., Christersson, L.A., Genco, R.J., Lyall, R.M., Hic, S., DiFlorio, R.M., and Terranova, V.P., A biochemical approach to periodontal regeneration: tetracycline treatment conditions on dentin surfaces, *J. Periodont. Res.*, 21, 322, 1986.
27. Dragoo, M.R. and Sullivan, H.C., A clinical and histologic evaluation of autogenous iliac bone grafts in humans: part 1. Wound healing 2 to 8 months, *J. Periodontol.* 44, 599, 1973.
28. Rummelhart, J.M., Mellonig, J.T., Gray, J.L., and Towle, H.J., Comparison of freeze-dried bone allograft in human periodontal osseous defects, *J. Periodontol.*, 60, 655, 1989.
29. Gottlow, J., Nyman, S., Karring, T., and Lindhe, J., New attachment formation as the result of controlled tissue regeneration, *J. Clin. Periodontol.*, 11, 494, 1984.
30. Schallhorn, R.G. and McClain, P.H., Combined osseous composite grafting, root conditioning, and guided tissue regeneration, *Int. J. Peridontics Restorative Dent.* 8(4), 9, 1988.
31. Seyedin, S.M., Osteoinduction: A report on the discovery and research of unique protein growth factors mediating bone development, *Oral Surg. Oral Med. Oral Pathol.*, 66, 527, 1989.
32. Lynch, S.E., Williams, R.C., and Polson, A.M. et al., A combination of platelet-derived and insulin-like growth factors enhances periodontal regeneration, *J. Clin. Periodontol.*, 16, 545, 1989.
33. Eckles, T.A., Reinhardt, R A., Dyer, J.K., Tussing, C.J., Szydlowski, W.M., and DuBois, L.M., Intracrevicular application of tetracycline in white petrolatum for treatment of periodontal disease, *J. Clin. Periodontol.*, 17, 454, 1990.
34. Goodson, J.M., Offenbacher, S., Farr, D.H., and Hogan, P.E., Periodontal disease treatment by local drug delivery, *J. Periodontol.*, 56, 265, 1985.
35. Goodson, J.M., Haffajee, A.D., and Socransky, S.S., Periodontal therapy by local delivery of tetracycline, *J. Clin. Periodontol.*, 6, 83, 1979.
36. Coventry, J.F. and Newman, H.N., Experimental use of a slow release device employing chlorhexidine gluconate in areas of acute periodontal inflammation, *J. Clin. Periodontol.*, 9, 129, 1982.
37. Addy, M., Rawle, L., Handley, R., Newman, H.N., and Coventry, J.F., The development and *in vitro* evaluation of acrylic strips and dialysis tubing for local drug delivery, *J. Clin. Periodontol.*, 11, 467, 1984.

38. Addy, M. and Langerouidi, M., Comparison of the immediate effects on the subgingival microflora of acrylic strips containing 40% chlorhexidine, metronidazole, or tetracycline, *J. Clin. Periodontol.*, 11, 379, 1984.
39. Soskoline A., Golomb, G., Friedman, M., and Sela, M., New sustained release dosage form of chlorhexidine for dental use. Use in periodontal therapy, *J. Periodontic Res.* 18, 330, 1983.
40. Minabe, M., Takeuchi, K., Tamura, T., Hori, T., and Umemoto, T., Subgingival administration of tetracycline on a collagen film, *J. Periodontol.*, 60, 552, 1989.
41. Oosterwall, P.J. M., Mikx, F.H.M., van Hoff, M.A., and Renggli, H.H., Comparison of the antimicrobial effect of the application of chlorhexidine gel, amine fluoride gel and stannous fluoride in debrided periodontal pockets, *J. Clin. Periodontol.*, 18, 245, 1991.
42. Noguchi, T., Izumizawa, K., Fukuda, M., Kitamura, S., Suzuki, Y., and Ikura, H., New method for local drug delivery using resorbable base material in periodontal therapy, *Bull. Tokyo Med. Dent. Univ.*, 31, 145, 1984.
43. Noguchi, T., Fukuda, M., and Ishikawa, I., Periodontal treatment by local drug delivery using resorbable base material, *Adv. Dent. Res.*, 2, 401, 1988.
44. Deasy, P., Collins, A., MacCarthy, D., and Russell, R., Use of strips containing tetracycline hydrochloride or metronidazole for the treatment of advanced periodontal disease, *J. Pharm. Pharmacol.*, 41, 695, 1989.
45. Dunn, R., Tipton, A., and Harkrader, R., et al., Pharmacokinetics of a biodegradable subgingival delivery system for sanguinarine, *J. Dent. Res.*, 70 (special issue), 323 (Abstract), 1991.
46. Godowski, K, Wolff, E., Sherman, R., Dunn, R., and Thompson, D., Microflora effects of subgingival sanguinarine delivered by a biodegradable system, *J. Dent. Res.*, 70 (special issue), 324 (Abstract), 191.
47. Polson, A., Southard, G., Dunn, R., Laster, L., Jones, B., and Stoller, N., Periodontal pocket treatment with subgingival sanguinarine from a biodegradable system, *J. Dent. Res.*, 70 (special issue), 374 (Abstract), 191.
48. Williams, R.C., Medical progress. Periodontal disease, *N. Engl. J. Med.*, 322, 373, 1990.
49. Dunn, R.L., English, J.P., Cowsar, D.R., and Vanderbilt, D.P., Biodegradable *In Situ*-Forming Implants and Methods of Producing the Same, U.S. Patent No. 4,938,763, 1990.
50. Shalaby, S.W., Hydrogel-Forming, Self-Solvating Absorbable Polyester Copolymers and Methods for Use Thereof (Composition), U.S. Patent No. 5,612,052, 1997.
51. Corbett, J.T., Martin, C., Fulton, L., Jerome, J.E., Kline, J.D., Allan, J.M., and Shalaby, S.W., Controlled release of ganciclovir from an intravitreal polymeric absorbable gel-former for treating cytomegalovirus retinitis, *Trans. Soc. Biomater.*, 21, 203, 1998.
52. Corbett, J.T., Martin, C., Farris, H., Jerome, J.E., Kline, J.D., Allan, J.M., and Shalaby, S.W., Intravitreal controlled release of cyclosporin A, *Proc. Int. Symp. Control. Rel. Bioact. Mater.*, 25, 39, 1998.
53. Corbett, J.T., Jerome, J.E., Allan, J.M., Kelley, W., Kline, M., Farris, H., Fulton, L., and Shalaby, S.W., *In vitro* and *in vivo* release of vancomycin and gentamicin from an injectable absorbable gel-forming matrix for treating osteomyelitis, *Proc. Mater. Res. Soc.*, 1997, p. 351.
54. Aimetti, M., Romano, F., Torta, I., Cirillo, D., Caposio, P., and Romagnoli, R., Debridement and local application of tetracycline-loaded fibres in the management of persistent periodontitis: results after 12 months, *J. Clin. Periodontol.*, 31(3), 166, 2004.

55. Sakellari, D, Vouros, I., and Konstantinidis, A., The use of tetracycline fibres in the treatment of generalized aggressive periodontitis: clinical and microbiological findings, *J. Int. Acad. Periodontol.*, 5(2), 52, 2003.
56. Schwach-Abdellaoui, K., Loup, P.J., Vivien-Castioni, N., Mombelli, A., Baehni, P., Barr, J., Heller, J., and Gurny, R., Bioerodible injectable poly(ortho ester) for tetracycline controlled delivery to periodontal pockets: preliminary trial in humans, *AAPS, Pharm. Sci.*, 4(4), 20, 2002.
57. Kelly, H.M., Deasy, P.B., Ziaka, E., and Claffey, N., Formulation and preliminary *vivo* dog studies of a novel drug delivery system for the treatment of periodontitis, *Int. J. Pharm.*, 274(1–2), 167, 2004.
58. Perugini, P., Genta, I., Conti, B., Modena, T., and Pavanetto, F., Periodontal delivery of ipriflavone: new chitosan/PLGA film delivery system for a lipophilic drug, *Int. J. Pharm.* 252(1–2), 1, 2003.
59. Varshosaz, J., Tavakoli, N., and Saidian, S., Development and physical characterization of a periodontal bioadhesive gel of metronidazole, *Drug Delivery*, 9(2), 127, 2002.
60. Pathasarathy, V., Manavalan, R., Mythili, R., Siby, C.T., and Jeya, M., Ethyl cellulose and polyethylene glycol-based sustained-release sparfloxacin chip: an alternative therapy for advanced periodontitis, *Drug Dev. Ind. Pharm.*, 28(7), 849, 2002.
61. Hoang, T., Jorgensen, M.G., Keim, R.G., Pattison, A.M., and Slots, J., Providone-iodine as a periodontal pocket disinfectant, *J. Periodontal Res.*, 38(3), 311, 2003.
62. American Academy of Periodontology, *Glossary of Periodontic Terms*, 3rd ed., 1992.
63. Schallhorn, R.G., Hiatt, W.H., and Boyce, W., Iliac transplants in periodontal therapy, *J. Periodontol.*, 41, 566, 1970.
64. Hiatt, W.H. and Schallhorn, R.G., Intraoral transplants of cancellous bone and marrow in periodontal lesions, *J. Periodontol.*, 44, 194, 1973.
65. Nabers, C.L. and O'Leary, T.J., Autogenous bone transplants in the treatment of osseous defects, *J. Periodontol.*, 36, 5, 1965.
66. Altiere, E.T., Reeve, G.M., and Sheridan, P.J., Lyophilized bone allografts in periodontal intraosseous defects, *J. Periodontol.*, 50, 510, 1979.
67. Evans, G.H., Yukna, R.A., and Sepe, W.W., et al., Effect of various graft materials with tetracycline in localized juvenile periodontitis, *J. Periodontol.*, 60, 491, 1989.
68. Polson, A.M. and Proye, M.P., Fibrin linkage: a precursor for new attachment, *J. Periodontol.*, 54, 141, 1983.
69. Yukna, R.A., Harrison, B.G., and Caudill, R., et al., Evaluation of durapatite ceramic as an alloplastic implant in periodontal osseous defects. II. Twelve month reentry results, *J. Periodontol.*, 56, 540, 1985.
70. Meffert, R.M., Thomas, J.R., Hamilton, K.M., and Brownstein, C.N., Hyrroxylapatite as an alloplastic graft in the treatment of human periodontal osseous defects, *J. Periodontol.*, 56, 63, 1985.
71. Register, A.A. and Burdick, F.A., Accelerated reattachment with cementogenisis to dentin, demineralized *in situ*: I. Optimum range, *J. Periodontol.*, 46, 646, 1975.
72. Caffesse, R.G., Kerry, G.J., Chaves, E.S., et al., Clinical evaluation of the use of citric acid and autologous fibronectin in periodontal surgery, *J. Periodontol.*, 59, 565, 1988.
73. Bowers, G., Felton, F., and Middleton, C., et al., Histologic comparison of regeneration in human intrabony defects when osteogenin is combined with demineralized freeze-dried bone allograft and with purified bovine collagen, *J. Periodontol.*, 62, 690, 1991.
74. Melcher, A.H., On the repair potential of periodontal tissues, *J. Periodontol.*, 47, 256, 1976.

75. Gottlow, J., Nyman, S., and Karring, T., Maintenance of new attachment gained through guided tissue regeneration, *J. Clin. Periodontol.*, 19, 315, 1992.
76. Handelsman, J., Davarpanah, M., and Celletti, R., Guided tissue regeneration with and without citric acid treatment in vertical osseous defects, *Int. J. Periodontics Restorative Dent.*, 11(5), 350, 1991.
77. Schultz, A.J. and Gager, A.H., Guided tissue regeneration using an absorbable membrane (polyglactin 910) and osseous grafting, *Int. J. Periodontics Restorative Dent.* 10(1), 8, 1990.
78. Wasserman, D., Shalaby, S.W., and Bousma, O.J., Improved Dental Periodontal Disease, U.S. Patent No. 5,191,148, 1992.
79. Lekovic, V., Kenney, E.B., Carranza, F.A., and Massimiliano, M., The use of autogenous periosteal grafts as barriers for the treatment of class II furcation involvments in lower molars, *J. Periodontol.*, 61, 775, 1991.
80. Murphy, K.G. and Gunsolley, J.C., Guided tissue regeneration for the treatment of periodontal intrabony and furcation defects. A systematic review, *Ann. Periodontol.* 8(1), 266, 2003.
81. Nyman, S., Lindhe, J., Karring, T., and Rylander, H., New attachment following surgical treatment of human periodontal disease, *J. Clin. Periodontol.*, 9, 290, 1982.
82. Hou, L.T., Yan, J.J., Tsai, A.Y., Lao, C.S., Lin, S.J., and Liu, C.M., Polymer-assisted regeneration therapy with Atrisorb barriers in human periodontal intrabony defects, *J. Clin. Periodontol.*, 31(1), 68, 2004.
83. Cetiner, D., Unsal, B., Parlar, A., Gultekin, E., and Kurtis, B., Evaluation of periodontal healing in class II furcation defects following guided tissue regeneration with two different types of polylactic acid membranes, *Chin. Med. J. (English)*, 117(2), 270, 2004.
84. Zhao, M., Jin, Q., Berry, J.E., Nociti, F.H., Jr., Giannobile, W.V., and Somerman, M.J., Cementoblast delivery for periodontal tissue engineering, *J. Periodontol.*, 75(1), 154, 2004.
85. Wikesjo, U.M., Lim, W.H., Thomson, R.C., Cook, A.D., Wozney, J.M., and Hardwick, W.R., Periodontal repair in dogs: Evaluation of a bioabsorbable space-providing macroporous membrane with recombinant human bone morphogenetic protein-2, *J. Periodontol.*, 74(5), 635, 2003.
86. Loos, B.G., Louwerse, P.H., Van Winkelhoff, A.J., Burger, W., Gilijamse, M., Hart, A., and van der Velden, U., Use of barrier membranes and systemic antibiotics in the treatment of intraosseous defects, *J. Clin. Periodontol.*, 29(10), 910, 2002.
87. Chen, Y.T., Hung, S.L., Lin, L.W., Chi, L.Y., and Ling, I.J., Attachment of periodontal ligament cells to chlorhexidine-loaded guided tissue regeneration membranes, *Periodontol.*, 74(11), 1652, 2003.
88. Kurtis, B., Unsal, B., Cetiner, D., Gultekin, E., Ozcan, G., Celebi, N., and Ocak, O., Effect of polylactide/glycolide (PLGA) membranes loaded with metronidazole on periodontal regeneration following guided tissue regeneration in dogs, *J. Periodontol.*, 73(7), 694, 2002.
89. Thylin, M.R., McConnell, J.C., Schmid, M.J., Reckling, R.R., Ojha, J., Bhatacharyya, I., Marx, D.B., and Reinhardt, R.A., Effects of simvastatin gels on murine calvarial bone, *J. Periodontol.*, 73(1), 1141, 2002.
90. Gerentes, P., Vachoud, L., Dory, J., and Domard, A., Study of a chitin-based gel as injectable material in periodontal surgery, *Biomaterials*, 23(5), 1295, 2002.
91. Kostopoulos, L. and Karring, T., Susceptibility of GTR-regenerated periodontal attachment to ligature-induced periodontitis, *J. Clin. Periodontol.*, 31(5), 336, 2004.

92. Reggiani, M., Taddei, P, Tinti, A., and Fagnano, C., Spectroscopic study on the enzymatic degradation of a biodegradable composite periodontal membrane, *Biopolymers* 74(1–2), 146, 2004.
93. Kim, T.S., Holle, R., Hausmann, E., and Eickholz, P., Long-term results of guided tissue regeneration therapy with non-resorbable and bioabsorbable barriers. II. A case series of intrabony defects, *J. Periodontol.*, 73(4), 450, 2002.
94. Belal, M.H., Al-Noamany, F.A., El-Tonsy, M.M., El-Guindy, H.M., and Ishikawa, I., Treatment of human class II furcation defects using connective tissue grafts, bioabsorbable membrane, and resorbable hydroxyapatite: A comparative study, *J. Int. Acad. Periodontol.*, 7(4), 114, 2005.
95. Sipos, P.M., Loos, B.G., Abbas, F., Timmerman, M.F., and van der Velden, W., The combined use of enamel matrix proteins and a tetracycline-coated expanded polytetrafluoroethylene barrier membrane in the treatment of intra-osseous defects, *J. Clin. Periodontol.*, 32(7), 765, 2005.
96. Cortellini, P. and Tonetti, M.S., Clinical performance of a regenerative strategy for intrabony defects: scientific evidence and clinical experience, *J. Periodontol.*, 76(3), 341, 2005.
97. Triratana, T., Rustogi, K.N., Volpe, A.R., DeVizio, W., Petrone, M., and Giniger, M., Clinical effect of a new liquid dentifrice containing triclosan/copolymer on existing plaque and gingivitis, *J. Am. Dent. Assoc.*, 13(2), 219, 2002.
98. Paolantonio, M., D'ercole, S., Perinetti, G., Tripodi, D., Catamo, G., Serra, E., Brue, C., and Piccolomini, R., Clinical and microbiological effects of different restorative materials on the periodontal tissues adjacent to subgingival class V restorations, *J. Clin. Periodontol.*, 31(3), 200, 2004.
99. Corbett, J.T., Fulton, L.K., Heintze, S.D., Bolis, C., Rheinberger, V.M., and Shalaby, S.W., Absorbable gel-forming antibiotic formulations for treating dry socket: a pilot study, *Trans. Soc. Biomater.*, 26, 580, 2003.

5 Maxillofacial Bone Augmentation and Replacement

Guigen Zhang

CONTENTS

5.1 INTRODUCTION

Bone is a connective tissue with mineralized matrix, and it functions to provide mechanical support and physical forms for the human skeleton and to provide a vast storage of calcium for homeostasis. Osseous defects in the maxillofacial bone can cause severe functional abnormalities and aesthetic deformities. They can occur as a result of congenital abnormalities, ablative surgery, or traumatic avulsion. These defects may or may not be healed automatically by the body, depending on the size and nature of the defects. Small defects can be healed efficiently via the body's regeneration process, but large defects cannot be healed without some assistive measures. In many cases, these measures require the use of bone grafts or other synthetic substitutes to fill the bony deficits. In this chapter, methods and synthetic materials used for maxillofacial bone augmentation and replacement are discussed.

5.2 BONE RECONSTRUCTION AND HEALING

When injured, bone has the unique ability to heal and to restore its full function without scarring or deformity through a process similar to that seen during embryonic bone development. Such striking similarities between the mechanisms of embryogenesis and wound healing are mainly due to progenitor cells and bone morphogenetic proteins that play crucial roles in both processes. This regenerative healing process, however, is effective only for healing small bony defects. For many maxillofacial defects, reconstructive procedures are necessary in which substitutive materials or devices such as bone grafts or implants are often used to restore form and function. While both are used for bone augmentation or replacement purposes, a graft is a transferable material that contains living cells whereas an implant is a reconstructive device that contains no living cells.

Many factors influence the bone healing process, including bone metabolism, changes in hormonal balance, and other external conditions. In the case of a bone graft reconstruction, angiogenesis and revascularization are mandatory for bone formation because these newly formed blood vessels are essential for transporting oxygen, nutrients, and hormonal substances to the graft so that it can be slowly remodeled and replaced.[1] Cancellous bone allows easy penetration for revascularization whereas cortical bone is more difficult for capillaries to penetrate.

For an autogenous bone graft, the initial regenerative process begins within hours of the grafting procedure. Entrapped platelets degranulate, releasing potent growth factors such as platelet-derived growth factor (PDGF) from their alpha granules and transforming growth factor (TGF-1).[2] Endothelial cells initiate capillary ingrowth as they bind to PDGF. Next, endosteal osteoblasts and hematopoiteic cells are stimulated to initiate mitosis to increase their numbers, which then lead to the production of osteoid.[3] This process is mediated by the binding of TGF-1 to cell receptors. After about 3 days, the influence of the growth factors is replaced by the action of locally induced macrophages. They efficiently synthesize growth factors to regulate bone healing from this point on. By the end of the second week, the graft will demonstrate complete revascularization. Endosteal osteoblasts from the transplanted bone will begin laying down osteoid, and hematopoiteic cells will begin differentiating into osteoblasts, thus leading to the formation of islands of bone within the graft.

This initially formed bone is referred to as first phase bone, or woven bone. It is extremely cellular and disorganized and does not demonstrate any structural strength. During the second phase of healing, bone will undergo a remodeling process, often referred to as lamellar compaction. The resultant lamellar bone is less cellular, more mineralized, and is highly organized structurally. As with all bones, this newly formed matrix will then remodel in response to the physical and mechanical demands placed upon it.[4]

Osseous healing is achieved by direct osteogenesis via osteoinduction and osteoconduction. Osteoinduction describes a process in which new bone is produced in a nonbone region. This is achieved by the osteoinductive materials that stimulate the differentiation of osteogenic cells from mesenchymal or hematopoiteic cells. Osteoconduction, on the other hand, describes bone formation by the process of ingrowth of capillaries and osteoprogenitor cells from the recipient bed into or around a graft or implant. The graft or implant acts as a scaffold for new bone formation. Unlike osteoinduction, this process occurs in an already bone-containing environment.

5.3 OSSEOUS DEFECTS IN THE MAXILLOFACIAL BONE

Bony defects in the maxillofacial skeleton can arise from congenital abnormalities (e.g., cleft lip and palate), ablative surgery (e.g., segments of bones are excised to treat tumors), or trauma (e.g., osseous tissue is traumatically avulsed), among others. Besides the traumatically or surgically caused bony defects, most common defects in maxillofacial bone include alveolar ridge and sinus floor atrophies. The cause for resorption of alveolar bone can range from disuse (e.g., tooth loss) atrophy, decreased blood supply, to localized inflammation. Because alveolar bone forms the primary support for the teeth, these defects will lead to inadequate amount of bone for the support and anchorage of dental implants.

The first line of defense for avoiding alveolar bone loss is to prevent its occurrence. To do that, several methods have been developed. These methods include the retention of tooth roots, autotransplantation of teeth, and orthodontic space closure. These procedures are effective at slowing down the process of alveolar ridge resorption, but for these prevention procedures to be successful, their timing is very important. In many situations, such alveolar bone loss is often too late to be prevented. Thus, other reconstructive procedures, such as using bone grafts or other substitute materials, are necessary to fill the bony deficits.

5.4 METHODS FOR MAXILLOFACIAL BONE AUGMENTATION

When bone atrophy in the maxillofacial skeleton cannot be prevented, reconstructive procedures become necessary; minor surgical procedures and bone grafts are very common ones. These procedures have the advantage of not needing a donor bone, but they are most effective for alveolar ridge augmentation in the maxilla. For more severe augmentation needs, however, bone grafts are commonly used. For example, bone grafts have been used to augment severely atrophic edentulous alveolar ridges, to reconstruct alveolar defects in cleft palate patients, and to bridge defects that are the result of ablative surgery or trauma. Traditionally, bone grafts have been categorized into three major types: autografts, allografts, and xenografts. Autografts refer to tissue transplanted from one site to another within the same individual. Allografts are obtained from cadavers or living individuals of the same species. Xenografts are composed of tissues taken from an animal source. Autogenous bone grafting has been used to restore maxillofacial defects for over a century,[6] and even to this date, the use of autogenous bone grafts is still the standard in reconstructive oral and maxillofacial surgery.

5.4.1 Procedures for Minor Maxillofacial Bone Augmentation

There are a number of techniques available that allow the surgeon to reconstruct the bone in the maxillofacial skeleton without harvesting a bone graft. Osteocondensation is one such technique. It can help reshape the alveolar bone in the maxilla to better house a dental implant and provide needed stability. This technique mainly creates an implant bed with either minimal drilling or no bone removal,[7] and uses osteotomes and sometimes a press-fit fixture to compress the bone.[8,9] Many experiments have been reported using osteocondensation to increase the width of alveolar bone, facilitate sinus floor elevation, widen the alveolar ridge laterally, and increase the density of cancellous bone.[9,10] Alveolar ridges can also be widened using the crestal split technique with osteotomes and chisels. Lateral widening by completely exposing the labial cortex has also been introduced.[11] Crestal widening allows the thin alveolar bone to be utilized to support implants without grafting.[12]

Guided bone regeneration has also been used for minor augmentation procedures in the maxillofacial skeleton prior to dental implantations.[13] With this technique, bone growth is enhanced by preventing soft tissue ingrowth into the area desired for bone growth by using absorbable or nonabsorbable membranes. Of course, the use of membranes is controversial, and it is considered to be highly technique sensitive.[14] Absorbable membranes may cause inflammation, and nonabsorbable membranes may require a second operation for their removal.[15] Nevertheless, good results with augmentation procedures using membranes have been achieved,[13,16] and vertical increase of a narrow alveolar crest is possible with the guided bone regeneration procedure.[15]

5.4.2 Autogenous Bone Grafts

Autogenous bone grafts are commonly used for severe augmentation needs in the maxillofacial skeleton. There are three types of bone sources for autogenous bone grafts: cortical, cancellous, or combined corticocancellous bones. The combined type is probably the one most often used in reconstructive oral and maxillofacial surgery. Cancellous grafts can be revascularized more rapidly than cortical grafts, and they tend to heal completely over time, whereas cortical grafts are likely to remain as a mixture of necrotic and viable bone.[17]

Although cortical grafts are able to provide mechanical strength, they take more time for revascularization to occur. Thus, cortical grafts have very limited application. Common sites for harvesting cortical grafts are the cranial vault, ribs, and the posterior iliac crest as well as the mandibular symphysis.[18,19]

Cancellous grafts, by contrast, have more widespread applications, and they can be revascularized more rapidly. Autogenous cancellous bone grafts can produce successful and predictable results.[4] Although cancellous bone lacks the mechanical strength because of its porous structure, the very structure allows for rapid revascularization, cellular ingrowth and differentiation, and subsequent remodeling. Cancellous grafts are commonly used in oral and maxillofacial surgery to fill bony defects such as alveolar clefts and maxillary sinus floor augmentations.[20] The most common donor sites for autogenous cancellous grafts are the anterior or posterior iliac crest or the tibial plateau.

Corticocancellous grafts usually produce the best results by combining the benefits of both the cortical and cancellous grafts. Corticocancellous grafts provide mechanical strength while at the same time allow for rapid revascularization. They are often used for the restoration of continuity defects in the jaws. Typical donor sites are rib, iliac crest, fibula, or radius, whereas oral sites include the chin, the retromolar area, and the mandibular body.

Although autogenous bones are the best materials available for grafting purpose because of their nonimmunogenic characteristic and their ability to retain viability immediately after grafting, the major disadvantages of autogenous grafts include the limited availability of donor tissues, the need for a second surgical site, and donor site morbidity. To overcome these drawbacks, we need less invasive harvesting methods or substitutes for autologous bones.

5.4.3 Allogenic Bone Grafts

The primary forms of allogenic bone are from fresh frozen, freeze-dried, and demineralized freeze-dried and irradiated bone. Fresh frozen bone is rarely used today because of concerns of transmission of viral diseases.[17] A freeze-dried procedure is often used to treat the bone to minimize possible immunogenic problems. Other methods such as deproteination and demineralization are also used to deal with immunogenicity.[17] Freeze-dried bone is a good grafting material for onlay application.[4] While osteoconductive, a freeze-dried allogenic bone has no osteogenic or osteoinductive capabilities. Thus freeze-dried allogenic bones are usually placed in conjunction with autogenous grafts in the reconstruction of maxillofacial defects. Since these allografts are not osteogenic, bone formation takes longer and results in less volume as compared with autogenous grafts. Furthermore, in the highly vascular area of the maxillofacial skeleton, the revascularization process of the allograft bones may pose a potential problem for antigen transmission, which could lead to the rejection of the bone grafts.

Demineralized freeze-dried and irradiated bone presents a very low risk for transmitting viral diseases such as HIV or AIDS.[21] The process of demineralizing the freeze-dried bone will lead to a reduction in the mechanical strength of the bony matrix, but it may help retain some osteoinductive properties.[22] Removal of the mineral content from the bone matrix will help expose native proteins (e.g., the bone morphogenetic protein). For easy delivery, demineralized bone has been incorporated into various carriers such as collagen or selected polymers to make them more malleable. These substitutes can be used in the treatment of periodontal defects, alveolar ridge reconstruction, bone reconstruction associated with dental implant placement, and bony defects of the jaws.[23,24] Although more readily available, one big concern in the use of allografts for bony reconstruction is its implication in disease transmission; thus it is seldom used in clinic practice.

5.4.4 Xenogenic Bone Grafts

Xenogenic bone grafts are often derived from mammalian bones, including bovine, porcine, and marine bones; bovine derived bones are most commonly used for xenografts,[25] especially the deproteinized bovine derived bone matrix.[26] This inorganic bone mineral matrix has the structure of bone and is osteoconductive.

Its structure consists of a wide interconnective pore system that can easily be invaded by blood vessels for promoting osteoblastic migration. It has high porosity (70 to 75%), which is higher than other available synthetic materials.[27] Bovine bone mineral matrix is often thermally and chemically treated for extracting organic constituents to minimize its antigenicity and potential inflammatory response.[28]

Xenografts have been used for the filling of defects or extraction sites in the alveolus prior to dental implantation.[29] Xenogenic bones should be eventually replaced by the host tissue. Resorption of bovine derived bone has been observed in animal studies, but this result is not consistent with human clinical trials.[29] While bovine xenografts will help reduce donor site morbidity by eliminating the need for a donor bone as required in autogenous bone grafts, their disadvantage includes the possibility of future bovine spongiform encephalopathy due to potentially slow virus transmission into the bovine-derived matrices.[30]

5.5 SYNTHETIC MATERIALS FOR MAXILLOFACIAL BONE AUGMENTATION AND REPLACEMENT

Considering the benefits and drawbacks of bone grafting procedures and materials, an ideal solution for maxillofacial bone augmentation should be to use synthetic substitutes that are biologically inert, readily available, easily adaptable to the site in terms of size and shape, biodegradable, and replaceable by host bone.[31] For this purpose, many synthetic materials consisting of biocompatible substances for the filling of the osseous defects have been developed for alleviating or minimizing the need for autogenous bone grafts as well as the immunogenic and viral transmission problems.

5.5.1 Tricalcium Phosphate and Hydroxyapatite

Sintered calcium phosphates such as tricalcium phosphate (TCP) or hydroxyapatite (HA) are two common inorganic matrix materials that have been extensively used for bone grafting. These osteoconductive minerals have been used for a variety of bone augmentations such as periodontal defects,[32] alveolar clefts,[33] facial contour corrections,[34] and alveolar ridges,[35] although they lack the capacity to bridge critical sized maxillofacial defects.[36]

Both TCP and HA materials are available as solid or porous block, chips, or granules. They have different physical and degradation properties. In general, TCP degrades and absorbs rapidly (in days or weeks after implantation), whereas HA degrades and absorbs slowly (in years) because of its crystalline structure. TCP often degrades faster than it can be replaced by the newly formed bone, while HA degrades too slowly with respect to the characteristic time span for bone regeneration. The porous form of HA allows rapid fibrovascular tissue ingrowth, which will help not only to accelerate the healing of the bony defects but also to stabilize the graft and resist micromotion. HA has been used for the filling of bony defects, the retention of alveolar ridge following tooth extraction, and a bone expander during ridge augmentation and maxillary sinus floor augmentation procedures.[37] While the structure of HA resembles closely that of bone matrix, thus representing a better scaffold material for bone ingrowth than TCP, the slow degradation of HA may pose a stress-shielding threat to the bone formed within its porous network because of the high mechanical strength of HA. This could hinder the bone remodeling process. Studies have shown that HA does not ossify completely but rather becomes encapsulated with fibrous tissue.[34] The tendency for granular migration and incomplete resorption of the HA matrix may pose a long-term problem.[34,38]

5.5.2 Active Glass Ceramics

Bioactive glasses with silicophosphate chains have been used in dentistry as glass ionomer cement. They are composed of calcium salts and phosphates in similar proportions as in bone and tooth, along with sodium salts and silicates, which are essential for bone mineralization. They have the ability to chemically bond to the bone.[20] These ceramics are available in either amorphous or crystalline forms. Amorphous ceramics show more favorable properties than crystalline ones because the former degrades faster under the influence of tissue fluids by physical-chemical reactions. These bioactive glass ceramics are not porous, so ingrowth of blood vessels and other tissue components into the ceramics is very difficult. Bioactive glasses are osteoconductive, and they have been used to treat periodontal bony defects[39,40] to preserve alveolar ridge after tooth loss, and to heal preimplant mandibular osseous defects.[41,42]

5.5.3 Coral Derived Granules

Another hydroxyapatite structure that can be used as bony matrix is derived directly from the exoskeletons of corals from relatively unpolluted waters.[43] Corals from contaminated waters may contain petrochemical impurities. These calcium-carbonate rich and osteoconductive mineral materials once grafted in maxillofacial skeleton are quickly incorporated into the human bony skeleton and replaced by human bone within 18 months.[44] One of the major disadvantages of coral derived granules is its low initial mechanical strength (55% of cancellous bone strength)[45] and the difficulty in handling it. This thus excludes its use in cases where initial mechanical strength is desired. With the ingrowth of bone after implantation, the mechanical properties of coralline implants will be dramatically improved. For example, in 6 months its mechanical strength can reach up to three times that of a cancellous autograft.[46]

Coral derived granules exhibit some unique characteristics such as being completely absorbable and replaceable by host bone.[31,43,44] The process of coral resorption is believed to be due to the action of carbonic anhydrase,[47] an enzyme contained in osteoclasts, on the calcium carbonate in the coral skeleton. Implanted coral is well tolerated in a variety of animal models[48] and in humans.[49] Because coral derived matrix gives rise to natural bone formation, it could help alleviate donor site morbidity in maxillofacial osseous reconstruction by eliminating the need for grafting bone while accomplishing a satisfactory reconstructive result. Of course, for this to happen, we would need a vast supply of unpolluted corals, which are often not limitless and hard to find.

5.5.4 Tissue Engineering Approaches Using Synthetic Materials

To overcome these limitations, researchers have developed new therapeutic approaches for facilitating the healing of bony defects. Various tissue engineering strategies for the replacement of tissue lost to injury and disease have been clinically tested in the past decades. Polymers, especially absorbable polymers, have played many significant roles in this fast growing field of tissue engineering. Tissue engineering procedures offer significant advantages for maxillofacial bony augmentations as compared with the conventional grafting approaches because there is no need for donor bones and no consequence of donor site morbidity.

Tissue engineering procedures, which combine scaffolds of absorbable polymers with biological cells (e.g., autogenous mesenchymal stem cells) and osteoinductive agents (e.g., bone morphogenetic proteins), are being applied to maxillofacial bone regeneration. One major class of these absorbable polymers is the copolymers of polyglycolic acid (PGA) and polylactic acid (PLA), or PLGA, which have been used in the form of sutures and scaffolds as well as biodegradable fixation materials.[37,50] PLGA based scaffolds have been used to reconstruct mandibular defects and preserve alveolar ridges. But the incomplete degradation of the PLA component may impair the later placement of dental implants in the case of alveolar ridge augmentation.

Lately, the development of tissue-engineered materials aims at providing materials with better mechanical properties than those currently used. Intensive experimentation is taking place to create tissue-engineered hard tissue components like bones. In using polymeric materials to create a bone regenerative scaffold, it is important that the scaffold has adequate permeability rather than just porosity. Porosity describes the presence, but not the spatial localization, of a void structure, while permeability describes the ability of fluid to move freely through such a void structure. Porosity does not reveal whether the voids are interconnected, but permeability provides a quantitative measure of the ability of a liquid to flow through a porous network. Thus, obtaining adequate permeability in the design of polymeric scaffolds is very important for osteoinduction and osteoconduction applications. Polymeric materials hold the promise and potential to be fashioned into scaffolds with desired permeability and porosity for bone regeneration applications.

To provide the desired mechanical properties to the synthetic materials, researchers have explored the development of composite materials. Using composite materials will surely enable us to take advantage of their amenable tailoring characteristics to derive materials with desired mechanical properties. It may also help reduce the amount of autogenous bone needed for osseous augmentation in the maxillofacial skeleton. For example, the use of autogenous bone grafts for maxillofacial bone augmentations will result a high demand for donor bones, but the amount of autogenous bones suitable for harvesting is so limited. Thus, a composite approach that mixes autogenous bone or cells with other synthetic materials, sometimes referred to as an alloplast, could lead to the reduction of the volume of autogenous bone required to accommodate the reconstruction of the bony defects.

The term "composite graft" refers to grafts that are composed of materials from different origins, such as synthetic materials incorporated with autogenous bones or bone cells and osteoactive agents[53] For instance, to minimize the amount of autogenous bone needed and to accelerate the healing process, autogenous cancellous bone is mixed with synthetic materials along with growth factors[54] or platelet-rich plasma.

The synthetic components of these composite materials can be either polymers or ceramics. With polymers, the latest development is to use absorbable polymer scaffolds that contain transplanted cells along with desired growth factors such as bone morphogenetic protein (e.g., MBP-2, BMP-4, BMP-7) and transforming growth factors (e.g., TGF-1 and TGF-2). The reasons for using absorbable polymers include avoidance of a surgical operation for their removal and the eventual degradation of the scaffolds to make room for bone regeneration. These benefits can only be had with absorbable polymers, and not with nonabsorbable polymers such as high molecular weight polyethylene and poly(etheretherketone) that are often used for permanent replacement applications. Poly(-hydroxy esters) (e.g., PLLA, PGA, PLA, or PLGA), poly(-caprolactone), and poly(-hydroxybutyrate) are few examples of these absorbable polymers.

When used alone, these polymers do not have the mechanical properties needed for bone fracture fixation. For this reason, poly(-hydroxy esters) are sometimes reinforced with nonsintered bioresorbable HA for hard tissue augmentation applications. In the case of poly(-caprolactone) (PCL) to be used in maxillofacial bone replacement, it is reinforced with high modulus and degradable phosphate glass fibers. With such reinforcement, a PCL based composite can be tailored to possess the desired mechanical properties. Furthermore, since both the matrix and filler of such a composite degrade via hydrolysis, this composite material presents the advantage of not needing follow-up surgery for its removal after the bone reconstruction procedure.

With ceramics, autogenous cancellous or corticocancellous bones filled with particles of bioceramic materials such as TCP and HA make good grafting composite materials. These filler particles will enhance the bone binding property and osteoconduction, improve the mechanical behavior, and shorten the solidification process of the grafts.[56] For example, a composite of HA, autogenous corticocancellous bone, collagen fibrils, blood, and antibiotics has been successfully used in cleft alveolus surgery in children and young adults between the ages of 6 and 21 years.[53]

To make these composite materials more osteoinductive, researchers have often added many osteogenic factors such as recombinant human bone morphogenetic proteins, transforming growth factor, and autogenous platelet derived growth factors. Such composites are good alternatives to autogenous bone grafts in osseous reconstructive procedures because they help circumvent the limitation of donor bone supply and the consequence of donor site morbidity. Results show that addition of osteoinductive agents such as bone morphogenetic protein, platelet-rich plasma, and transforming growth factor to the composites will present the greatest potential for regeneration of bony defects.[57] One of the greatest benefits of using composite materials for maxillofacial bone augmentations is that the mechanical properties and the degradation processes of these composites can be tailored for the intended application.[58,59]

Another class of such composite materials is injectable bone substitutes. When a bony defect is in a difficult-to-reach site, injectable bone substitute materials may be preferred. These injectable materials can be made, for example, by dispersing a ceramic matrix in polymeric viscous gels. When a polymer is incorporated into a ceramic matrix, the resultant material will possess the flexibility provided by the polymer and the strength provided by the ceramic. Calcium phosphate cement (CPC), which will set to form HA *in vivo*, is one of such attractive ceramics that are commonly used as bone tissue substitutes. Injectable CPC can be delivered by the addition of viscous gels such as gelatin, sodium alginate, or chitosan. Recently, an injectable bone substitute developed based on biphasic calcium phosphate cement (BCPC) and a hydrosoluble polymer (i.e., methylhydroxypropyl cellulose) has been used for healing osseous defects. Despite of its initial weak mechanical properties, this injectable substitute has produced promising results of bony ingrowth and BCPC resorption simultaneously.[60]

5.6 OTHER METHODS FOR MAXILLOFACIAL BONE AUGMENTATION

5.6.1 Distraction Osteogenesis

Distraction osteogenesis of the long bones in growing children has been used for several decades to gradually lengthen osteotomized bones without a bone graft. The osteotomized gap is initially filled with callus, which later matures into bone. Correction of maxillofacial deformities using distraction osteogenesis technique, however, requires the use of mechanical devices different from those used for long bones. Recently, with the development of special devices and implants, distraction osteogenesis has begun to be applied for the healing of maxillofacial deformities involving bones with divergent geometry in growth, development, and configuration.[62,63]

Maxillofacial distraction osteogenesis is based on the biological process of new bone formation between the surfaces of two divided bone segments under the influence of traction forces. The gap between the bone segments is initially filled with a collagen mesh in which callus begins to form. The process of managed bone formation is initiated by the application of distraction to the soft callus tissue. The generated tension stimulates new bone formation in the direction of distraction. This procedure has been used to treat patients with various maxillofacial deformities, such as cleft palate, different forms of malocclusion, mandibular discontinuity, and obstructed upper airways.[62] One major benefit of distraction osteogenesis is the elimination of donor site morbidity that results from harvesting bone grafts. But its drawbacks range from needing a second surgery to remove and perhaps replace the hardware, enduring the inconvenience of wearing a cumbersome hardware for a long period by the patient, to losing the osteogenetic effect because of the reduction in the distraction force caused by the nonlinear behavior of the hardware.[64]

5.6.2 Ultrasonic Treatment

A substantial part of maxillofacial surgery practice deals with maxillofacial bone healing. Because low-intensity ultrasound treatment has been shown to reduce the healing time of fresh fractures of the extremities and help heal delayed and nonexistent unions, it is believed that ultrasound will be able to stimulate maxillofacial bone healing as well, assuming that the process of bone healing in the extremities and maxillofacial skeleton follows the same mechanism. Although there is limited evidence available to support the susceptibility of maxillofacial bone to the ultrasound signal, ultrasound could be beneficial in the treatment of delayed unions, in callus maturation after distraction, and in the treatment of osteoradionecrosis.

For example, in the treatment of mandibular osteoradionecrosis, ultrasound induced beneficial effects.[65] However, in another attempt to stimulate mandibular defect healing, low-intensity pulsed ultrasound (30 mW/cm^2) failed to stimulate the healing of 5-mm-diameter circular mandibular defect in the rat.[66] Given the successes in the stimulation of bone healing in other parts of the body, it seems that more efforts in this area may lead to promising results, which will determine the feasibility and potential of ultrasound treatment in maxillofacial surgery.

5.7 CONCLUSION AND PERSPECTIVE ON THE FUTURE

Many bony defects in maxillofacial skeleton commonly seen clinically are large defects. They often require reconstructive procedures to restore form and function. These reconstructive procedures include the use of bone grafts or synthetic materials to fill the bony deficits and to facilitate bone regeneration and remodeling. Of the three bone graft techniques (i.e., autograft, allograft, and xenograft), autograft transplantation is the clinically preferred treatment option today because of the concerns of disease or virus transmission with allografts and xenografts, but autografts also suffer from limited bone supply and donor site morbidity. Therefore, an ideal solution would be to use synthetic materials that are readily available, easily shaped or adapted to the defect site, mechanically tailored, biocompatible and biodegradable, porous and permeable, quickly revascularized, and replaced by host bone. Polymer matrix composites have the advantage of being versatile, allowing for the tailoring of the mechanical properties and structural permeability of its final products. Composites made of synthetic materials such as polymers and ceramics hold the promise of providing such an ideal solution. Composites can be designed and produced to meet specific requirements by using a wide range of polymeric and ceramic matrices, reinforcements, osteogenic proteins, and processing methods.

In light of the significant progress made in the past decades in this area, future challenges in the development of synthetic substitute materials for maxillofacial bone augmentation and replacement lie in the following areas. First, these synthetic materials should be of composite nature so that their mechanical properties, both initially and long term, can be tailored to meet the need not only for providing physical form but also for transferring physiological-level mechanical loads from the surrounding tissue to the substitute to promote normal remodeling of the regenerated bone. Second, these substitutes should possess a controllable degradation profile and adequate porosity and permeability for allowing fast angiogenesis and vascularization, and proper bone formation throughout the substitutes. Third, the composite substitutes should be used in conjunction with proper osteogenic proteins and pluripotent cells for achieving not only bone cell differentiation but also sufficient vasculature. Fourth, all these characteristics, including the mechanical properties, permeability, degradation profile, as well as cells and proteins delivery, should be controllable during the entire course of bone reconstruction and regeneration. It is anticipated that these challenges can be overcome by developing and constructing novel synthetic composites with new inputs from the fields of nanotechnology, nanobiotechnology, biomimetics, and tissue engineering.

REFERENCES

1. Lee, A. and Langer, R., Shark cartilage contains inhibitors of tumor angiogenesis, *Science*, 221(4616), 1185–1187, 1983.
2. Caplan, A.I., The mesengenic process: bone heal and regeneration, *Clin. Plast. Surg* 21, 429–435, 1995.
3. Friedenstein, A.J., Platelzky-Shaprio, I.I., and Petchovo, K.V., Osteogenesis in transplants of bone marrow during placement of marrow cancellous bone grafts, *J. Embryol. Exp. Morphol.*, 16, 381–390, 1996.
4. Marx, R.E., Clinical application of bone biology to mandibular and reconstruction, *Clin. Plast. Surg.*, 21, 377, 1994.
5. Marx, R.E., Shellenberger, T., Wimsatt, J., and Correa, P., Severely resorbed mandible: predictable reconstruction with soft tissue matrix expansion (tent pole) grafts, *J. Oral Maxillofac. Surg.*, 60, 878–888, 2002.
6. Muller, W., Zur Frange der tempoaren Schadel an Stelle Der Trepanation, *Zentralbl. Chir.*, 17: 65–68, 1890.
7. Sykaras, N., Iacopino, A.M., Marker, V.A., Triplett, R.G. and Woody, R.D., Implant materials, design and surface topographies: their effect on osseointegration, *Int. J. Oral Maxillofac. Implants*, 15, 675–690, 2000.
8. Valen, M. and Locante, W.M., LaminOss immediate-load implants: II. Introducing osteocompression in dentistry, *J. Oral Implantol.*, 26, 177–184, 2000.
9. de Wijs, F.L.J.A. and Cune, M.S., Immediate labial contour restoration for improved aesthetics: a radiographic study on bone splitting in anterior single-tooth replacement, *Int. J. Oral Maxillofac. Implants*, 12, 686–696, 1997.
10. Summers, R.B., The osteotome technique: Part 4 — Future site development, *Compend. Contin. Educ. Dent.*, 16, 1090–1098, 1995.
11. Duncan, J.M. and Westwood, R.M., Ridge widening for the thin maxilla: a clinical report, *Int. J. Oral Maxillofac. Implants*, 12, 224–227, 1997.
12. Oikarinen, K.S., Sandor, G.K.B., Kainulainen, V.T., and Salonen-Kemppi, M., Augmentation of the narrow traumatized anterior alveolar ridge to facilitate dental implant placement, *Dental Traumatol.*, 19, 19–29, 2003.
13. Simion, M., Jovanovic, S.A., Tinti, C., and Benfenati, S.P., Long-term evaluation of osseointegrated implants inserted at the time or after vertical ridge augmentation. A retrospective study on 123 implants with 1-5 year follow-up, *Clin. Oral Implants Res.*, 12, 35–45, 2001.
14. Chiapasco, M., Abati, S., Romeo, E., and Vogel, G., Clinical outcome of autogenous bone blocks or guided bone regeneration with e-PTFE membranes for the reconstruction of narrow edentulous ridges, *Clin. Oral Implants Res.*, 10, 278–288, 1999.
15. von Arx, T., Hardt, N., and Wallkamm, B., The TIME technique: a new method for localized alveolar ridge augmentation prior to placement of dental implants, *Int. J. Oral Maxillofac. Implants*, 11, 387–394, 1996.
16. Lekovic, V., Camargo, P.M., Klokkevold, P.R., Weinlaender, M., Kenney, E.B., Dimitrijevic, B., and Nedic, M., Preservation of alveolar bone in extraction sockets using bioabsorbable membranes, *J. Periodontol.*, 69, 1044–1049, 1998.
17. Buchardt, H., The biology of bone graft heal, *Clinical Orthop.*, 174, 28–42, 1983.
18. Kainulainen, V.T., Sandor, G.K.B., Clokie, C.M.L., and Oikarinen, K.S., Intraoral bone harvesting in oral and maxillofacial surgery, *Suomen Hammaslaakarilehti* 5, 216–222, 2002.

19. Kainulainen, V.T., Sandor, G.K.B., Caminiti, M.F., Clokie, C.M.L., and Oikarinen, K.S., Extraoral bone harvesting sites for oral and maxillofacial surgery, *Suomen Hammaslaakarilehti*, 10–11, 570–576, 2002.
20. Merkx, M.A.W., Maltha, T.C., and Stoelinga, P.J.W., Assesment of the valve of anorganic bone additives in sinus floor augmentation: a review of clinical reports, *Int. J. Oral Maxillofac. Surg.*, 32, 1–6, 2003.
21. Mellonig, J.T., Prewett, A.B., and Moyer, M.P., HIV inactivation in bone allograft, *J. Periodontol.*, 63, 979–983, 1992.
22. Zhang, M., Powers, R.M., Jr., and Wolfinbarger, L., Jr., Effect(s) of the demineralization process on the osteoinductivity of demineralized bone matrix, *J. Periodontol* 68, 1085–1092, 1997.
23. Caplanis, N., Lee, M.B., Zimmerman, G.J., Selvig, K.A., and Wikesjo, U.M., Effect of allogeneic freeze-dried demineralized bone matrix on regeneration of alveolar bone and periodontal attachment in dogs, *J. Clin. Periodontol.*, 25, 801–806, 1998.
24. Rosenberg, E. and Rose, L.F., Biologic and clinical considerations for autografts and allografts in periodontal regeneration therapy, *Dent. Clin. North Am.*, 42, 467–490, 1998.
25. Jensen, S.S., Aaboe, M., Pinholt, E.M., Hjorting-Hansen, E., Melsen, F., and Ruyter, I.E., Tissue reaction and material characteristics of four bone substitutes, *Int. J. Oral Maxillofac. Impl.*, 11, 55–66, 1996.
26. Iwamoto, Y., Sugioka, Y., Chuman, H., Masuda, S., Hotokebuchi, T., Kawai, S., and Yamamoto, M., Nationwide survey of bone grafting performed from 1980 through 1989, *Japan. Clin. Orthop. Rel. Res.*, 335, 292–297, 1997.
27. Peetz, M., Characterisation of xenogeneic bone material, in *Osseous Reconstruction of the Maxilla and Mandible: Surgical Techniques Using Titanium Mesh and Bone Mineral*, Boyne P.J., Ed., Quintessence Publishing, Carol Stream, IL, 1997, pp. 87–100.
28. Cohen, R.E., Mullarky, R.H., Noble, B., Comeau, R.L., and Neiders, M.E., Phenotypic characterisation of mononuclear cells following anorganic bovine bone implantation in rats, *J. Periodontol.*, 65, 1008–1015, 1994.
29. Valentini, P., Abensur, D., Densari, D., Graziani, J.N., and Hammerle, C., Histological evaluation of Bio-Oss in a 2-stage sinus floor elevation and implantation procedure. A human case report, *Clin. Oral Implants Res.*, 9, 59–64, 1998.
30. Hunter, N., Laboratory studies of bovine spongiform encephalopathy, *Lancet*, 360, 488–489, 2002.
31. Bajpai, P., Biodegradable scaffolds in orthopaedics, oral and maxillofacial surgery, in *Biomaterials in Reconstructive Surgery*, Rubin L.R., Ed., C.V. Mosby, St Louis, 1983, pp. 312–328.
32. Bowen, J.A., Mellonig, J.T., Gray, J.L., and Towle, H.T., Comparison of decalcified freeze-dried bone allograft and porous particulate hydroxyapatite in human periodontal osseous defects, *J. Periodontol.*, 60, 647–654, 1989.
33. El Deeb, M. and Holmes, R.E., Tissue response to facial contour augmentation with dense and porous hydroxyapatite in rhesus monkeys, *J. Oral Maxillofac. Surg.*, 47, 1282–1289, 1989.
34. Rosen, H.M. and McFarland, M.M., The biologic behaviour of hydroxyapatite implanted into the maxillofacial skeleton, *Plast. Reconstr. Surg.*, 85, 718–723, 1990.
35. Mercier, P., Failures in ridge reconstruction with hydroxyapatite. Analysis of cases and methods for surgical revision, *Oral. Surg. Oral Med. Oral Path. Oral Radiol. Endod.*, 81, 376–384, 1996.

36. Boyne, P.J., Advances in preprosthetic surgery and implantation, *Curr. Opin.Dent* 1, 277–278, 1991.
37. Haas, R., Mailath, G., Dortbudak, O., and Watzek, G., Bovine hydroxyapatite for maxillary sinus augmentation: analysis of interfacial bond strength of dental implants using pull-out tests, *Clin. Oral Implants Res.*, 9, 117–122, 1998.
38. Prousaefs, P., Lozada, J., Valencia, G., and Rohrer, M.D., Histologic evaluation of a hydroxyapatite onlay bone graft retrieved after 9 years: a clinical report, *J. Prosthet. Dent.*, 87, 481–484, 2002.
39. Lovelace, T.B., Mellonig, J.T., Meffert, R.M., Jones, A.A., Nummokoski P.V., and Cochran, D.L., Clinical evaluation of bioactive glass in the treatment of periodontal osseous defects in humans, *J. Periodontol.*, 69, 1027–1035, 1998.
40. Yukna, R.A., Evans, G.H., Aichelmann-Reddy, M.B., and Mayer, E.T., Clinical comparison of bioactive glass bone replacement graft material and expanded polytetraflouroethylene barrier membrane in treating human mandibular molar class II furcations, *J. Periodontol.*, 72, 125–133, 2001.
41. Schepers, E., Barbier, L., and Ducheyne, P., Implant placement enhanced by bioactive glass particles of narrow size range, *Int. J. Oral Maxillofac. Implants*, 13, 655–665, 1998.
42. Hall, E.E., Meffert, R.M., Hermann, J.S., Mellonig, J.T., and Cochran, D.L., Comparison of bioactive glass to demineralized freeze-dried bone allograft in the treatment of intrabony defects around implants in the canine mandible, *J. Periodontol.*, 70, 526–535, 1999.
43. Guillemin, G., Patat, J.L., Fournie, J., and Chetail, M., The use of coral as a bone graft substitute, *J. Biomed. Mater. Res.*, 21, 557–567, 1987.
44. Roux, F.X., Brasnu, D., Loty, B., George, B., and Guillemin, G., Madreporic coral: a new bone graft substitute for cranial surgery, *J. Neurosurg.*, 69, 510–513, 1988.
45. Murphy, M.D., Sartoris, D.J., and Bramble, J.M., Radiographic assessment of bone grafts, in *Bone Grafts and Bone Substitutes*, Habal, M.B. and Reddi, A.H., Eds., Saunders, Philadelphia, 1992, pp. 9–36.
46. Bucholz, R.W., Carlton, A., and Holmes, R.E., Hydroxyapatite and tricalcium phosphate bone graft substitutes, *Orthop. Clin. North Am.*, 18, 323–334, 1987.
47. Chetail, M. and Fournie, J., Shell-boring mechanism of the Gastropod Purpura (Thais) lapillus: A physiological demonstration of the role of carbonic anhydrase in the dissolution of $CaCO_3$, *Am. Zoologist*, 9, 983–990, 1969.
48. Shabana, A., Ouhayoun, J.P., Boulekache, H., Sautier, J.M., and Forest, N., Ultra structural study of the effects of coral skeleton on cultured human gingival fibroblasts, *J. Mater. Sci.*, 2, 162–167, 1991.
49. Souyris, F., Pellequer, C., Payrot, C., and Servera, C., Coral, a new biomedical material, *J. Maxillofac. Surg.*, 13, 64–69, 1985.
50. Shalaby, S.W., Bioabsorbable polymers in *Encyclopedia of Pharmaceutical Technology*, Boyan, J.C. and Swarbrick, J., Eds., Marcel Dekker, New York, 1988, pp. 37–39.
51. Suhonen, J. and Meyer, B., Polylactic acid (PLA) root replica in ridge maintenance after loss of a vertically fractured incisor, *Endod. Dent. Traumatol.*, 12, 155–160, 1996.
52. Forest, C.R., What's new in plastic and maxillofacial surgery, *J. Am. Coll. Surg* 200, 399–408. 2005.
53. Habal, M.B., Bone-ceramic composite for enhancement of bone graft regeneration, *J. Craniofac. Surg.*, 2, 27–32, 1991.

54. Ripamonti, U., The induction of bone in osteogenic composites of bone matrix and porous hydroxyapatite replicas: an experimental study on the baboon (*Papio ursinus J. Oral Maxillofac. Surg.*, 49, 817–830, 1991.
55. Marx, R.E., Carlson, E.R., Eichstaedt, R.M., Schimmele, S.R., Strauss, J.E., and Georgeff, K.R., Platelet-rich plasma: growth factor enhancement for bone grafts, *Oral Surg. Oral Med. Oral Pathol. Oral Radiol. Endod.*, 85, 638–646, 1998.
56. Vanassche, B.J., Stoelinga, P.J., De Koomen, H.A., Blijdorp, P.A., and Schoenaers, J.H., Reconstruction of the severely resorbed mandible with interposed bone grafts and hydroxylapatite. A 2-3 year follow-up, *Int. J. Oral Maxillofac. Surg.*, 157–160, 1988.
57. Damien, C.J., Parsons, C.J., Benedict, J.J., and Weisman, D.S., Investigation of a hydroxyapatite and calcium sulfate composite supplemented with an osteoinductive factor, *J. Biomed. Mater. Res.*, 24, 639–654, 1990.
58. Zhang, G., Latour, R.A., Jr., Kennedy, J.M., Del Schutte, H., Jr., and Friedman, R.J., Long-term compressive property durability of carbon fiber-reinforced polyetherether-ketone composite in physiological saline, *Biomaterials*, 17, 781–789, 1996.
59. Mano, J.F., Sousa, R.A., Boesel, L.F., Neves, N.M., and Reis, R.L., Bioinert, biodegradable and injectable polymeric matrix composites for hard tissue replacement: state of the art and recent development, *Comp. Sci. Tech.*, 64, 789–817, 2004.
60. Daculsi, G., Weiss, P., Bouler, J.M., Gauthier, O., Millot, F., and Aguado, E., Biphasic calcium phosphate/hydrosoluble polymer composites: a new concept for bone and dental substitution biomaterials, *Bone*, 25(2), Supplement, 59S–61S, 1999.
61. Ilizarov, G.A., The tension-stress effect on the genesis and growth of tissues. Part I: The influence of stability of fixation and soft tissue preservation, *Clin. Orthop.*, 238, 249–281, 1989.
62. Chin, M. and Toth, B.A., Distraction osteogenesis in maxillofacial surgery using internal devices. Review of five cases, *J. Oral Maxillofac. Surg.*, 54, 45–52, 1996.
63. Watzek, G., Zechner, W., Crismani, A., and Zauza, K., A distraction abutment system for 3-dimentional distraction osteogenesis of the alveolar process: technical note, *Int. J. Oral Maxillofac. Implants*, 15, 731–737, 2000.
64. Zhang, G., Avoiding the material nonlinearity in an external fixation device, *Clinical Biomechanics*, 19, 746-750, 2004.
65. Schortinghuis, J., Stegenga, B., Raghoebar, G.M., and de Bont, L.G.M., Ultrasound stimulation of maxillofacial bone healing, *Crit. Rev. Oral Biol. Med.*, 14(1), 63–74, 2003.
66. Schortinghuis, J., Ruben, J.L., Raghoebar, G.M., and Stegenga, B., Defect healing: a placebo-controlled single-blind study in rats, *J. Oral Maxillofac. Surg.*, 62, 194–201, 2004.

6 Polymeric Biomaterials for Articulating Joint Repair and Total Joint Replacement

Shalaby W. Shalaby, Sheila D. Nagatomi, and Shawn J. Peniston

CONTENTS

6.1 INTRODUCTION

The *Webster Medical Dictionary* defines the term joint as "the point of contact between elements of an animal skeleton, whether movable or rigidly fixed together with parts (such as membranes, tendons, ligaments) that surround and support it, and articulating as to become united or connected by or as if by a joint." Articulations in the body are joints between bones.[1] They perform two seemingly contradictory functions. Articulations hold bones firmly bound to each other, and yet they also perform movement between them.[1] Joints are classified into three types according to the degree of movement they permit, namely, synarthroses (or immovable fibrous joints), amphiarthroses (or slightly movable joints), and diarthroses (or freely movable, synovial joints).[1] The discussion in this chapter is limited to the diarthroses (or freely movable, synovial joints), which are not only the body's most mobile, but also its most numerous, complex, and likely-to-be-compromised joints. Thus, diarthroses are prime candidates for repair or replacement. The diarthrotic, or freely movable, joints are characterized by six structures consisting of:

1. Joint capsule — sleevelike extension of the periosteum of each of the articulating bones and forms a complete casing around the ends of these bones, thereby binding them to each other
2. Synovial membrane — moist, slippery membrane that lines the inner surface of the joint capsule
3. Articular cartilage — thin layer of hyaline cartilage covering and cushioning the articular surface of bones
4. Joint cavity — small space between the articulating surfaces of the two bones
5. Menisci (articular disks) — pads of fibrocartilage located between the articulating ends of bones in some diarthroses
6. Ligaments — strong cords of dense fibrous tissue at most synovial joints, which grow between the bones, lashing them even more firmly together than possible with the joint capsule[1]

Consistent with the tenets of this chapter, one should acknowledge that knowledge of joint-articulating surface motion is essential for design of prostheses, or repair devices, to restore compromised functions in assessment of joint wear, stability, degeneration, and determination of proper diagnosis and surgical treatments of joint disease.[2] The joint-articulating surface motion for the ankle, knee, hip, shoulder, elbow, wrist, and hand were discussed in an excellent review by Kaufman and An.[2] The discussion covered the geometry of the articulating surfaces, joint contact, and axes of rotation. Equally important to the designing bioengineer is the knowledge of the types of movements as in diarthroses (or freely movable joints), which depend on the shape of the articulating surfaces of the bones and positions of joints, ligaments, and nearby muscles and tendons.[1] All diarthroses, however, permit one or more of the following movements: angular, circular, gliding, and special movements. Angular movements change the size of the angle between articulating bones, as in the flexion and extension of the thigh at the hip joint, and the flexion and extension of the upper arm at the shoulder joint. Circular movements are rotation, circumduction, supination, and pronation. Rotation consists of pivoting a bone on its own axis, as in the atlantoaxial joint movements associated with moving the head from side to side. Circumduction, as in the glenohumeral joint movement associated with the arm as it moves a part of its distal end describing a circle and the rest of the arm describing a cone. Supination rotates the forearm outward, thereby turning the hand forward. Pronation rotates the arm inward, thereby turning the back of the hand forward. Gliding movements are simplest of all movements; they take place when the articular surface of one bone barely moves over the articular surface of another without any angular or circular movement. The gliding movements can occur between the carpal bones and between the tarsals. Special movements consist of (1) inversion, turning the sole of the foot inward, while eversion is turning it outward,

(2) protraction, moving the part forward, whereas retraction is moving it backward, and (3) elevation moves a part up, as in closing the mouth, whereas depression moves the part in the opposite direction.

In designing prosthetic joints or components, it is important to determine whether the joints are (1) uniaxial — permit movement around only one axis and only one plane, as in a hinge (of the elbow) and pivot (of the vertebra) joints, (2) biaxial — permit movements around two perpendicular axes in two perpendicular planes as in saddle (the thumbs) and condyloid (ellipsoidal, of the neck) joints, and (3) multiaxial joints — permit movement around three or more axes and three or more planes, as in the ball and socket joints (spheroid joints) of the hip and shoulder and gliding joints associated with flat articulating surfaces.

This discussion of the anatomical, biomechanical aspects of articulating joints would not be viewed as essential to traditional scientists, engineers, and clinicians who were interested in the use of polymers relevant to diseased or malfunctioning joints prior to the 1990s. This is because the use of polymers in this area then pertained mostly to bone cement and sutures. However, for contemporary professionals interested in articulating joints, a discussion of their anatomical and biomechanical aspects is expected to be more than welcomed. This is because of the growing interest in polymers and their use in (1) prosthetic ligaments and tendons, (2) absorbable and nonabsorbable devices for repairing components of articulating joint systems, (3) controlled drug delivery of antibiotics for treating bone infection, (4) carriers for administering medicaments or lubricants into the joint capsule, (5) designing and producing new prosthetic components for total joint replacement, and (6) cartilage and bone tissue engineering. Accordingly, this chapter is designed to review briefly the evolution in the use of polymers relative to articulating joints, provide up-to-date accounts of new clinical and experimental breakthroughs in the area of articulating joints, and document the authors' overall assessments of ongoing and future research activities pertinent to the articulating joints.

6.2 EVOLUTION IN ARTICULATING JOINT REPAIR AND TOTAL REPLACEMENT

Early applications of polymers relevant to articulating joints dealt primarily with their use as (1) articulating joint components, (2) cement interface between implant components and bone tissue, and (3) sutures for repairing ligaments and tendons.

For use as articulating surface components, polymers are selected to have a low coefficient of friction and low wear rate when they are in contact with the opposing surfaces, which are traditionally made of metals or ceramics. Teflon® was the first to be used for the acetabular component in total hip arthroplasty. However, accelerated creep and poor wear resistance (or stress corrosion) of early forms of Teflon directed the attention of early investigators to the use of ultrahigh molecular weight polyethylene (UHMW-PE) as a more effective alternative. And UHMW-PE has been the standard material for a few decades in spite of a number of complications associated with its long-term use. These include creep and formation of wear particles. Attempts to address these complications are discussed in this chapter.

For the use of polymers as a structural interface between the implant component and bone tissue, polymethyl methacrylate (PMMA) bone cement has been the material of choice since its early introduction in 1970. And PMMA bone cement retains its dominance regardless of persistent clinical complaints associated with site infection, poor long-term fatigue resistance, and implant loosening. In an effort to understand the root causes of the complications relative to joint repair and replacement and, specifically in total hip arthroplasty, contemporary investigators recognized that (1) bone cement is used primarily as a grouting material to fix both the stem of the femoral component and the acetabular component in place and distribute the loads more uniformly from the implant to the bone, and (2) the high interfacial stresses result from the accommodation of a high modulus prosthesis within the much lower modulus bone, which can cause the cement to creep and compromise its ability to transfer the loads uniformily.[3] Accordingly, new approaches to address the PMMA bone cement shortcomings have been explored in recent years and are discussed in this chapter.

The early use of polymers as sutures for repairing support structures, such as tendons and ligaments, focused primarily on the clinical application of nonabsorbable sutures and similar constructs in repairing these support structures. More recent efforts on using absorbable and nonabsorbable synthetic fiber constructs, with or without incorporation of natural polymers, are also discussed here.

Fast-growing use of absorbable polymers as devices in surgical procedures led to the genesis of extensive applications of these polymers in several orthopedic areas, including those associated with articulating joints. And accounts of recent developments pertinent to the use of absorbable polymers in the latter area are provided in Section 6.2.2.

6.2.1 Nonabsorbable Polymers, Composites, and Their Applications

As noted previously, PMMA bone cement was one of the systems used earlier and continues to be widely used in conjunction with total hip arthroplasty in spite of its poor fatigue performance, which is related to its amorphous nature, high T_g, and less-than-optimum uniformity. Additionally, the presence of porosity and other stress concentration sites introduced during application contribute further to the weakness of PMMA bone cement. In fact, fatigue fracturing has been found to be one of the main causes for implant loosening and cement fragmentation during the long-term use of the traditional PMMA bone cement. Although a few techniques have been used to address the shortcomings associated with the PMMA, long-term cement fatigue is yet to be circumvented.

To improve the mechanical properties of PMMA bone cement, in general, researchers have explored certain aspects of the composite technology. For example, fibers made of carbon, steel, Kevlar, UHMW-PE, and titanium have been incorporated into the PMMA matrix as reinforcing fillers to improve its mechanical properties. Although these composites did show some improvement in mechanical properties, such as fracture toughness and fatigue resistance, the incompatibility between fibers and matrix posted possible weak interfacial bonding. To overcome the problems with the traditional composites, researchers have developed a new composite technology that uses PMMA fibers as a filler to produce the self-reinforced PMMA composites. While commercial PMMA in bulk form has a strength of about 50 MPa and a breaking elongation of about 5%, PMMA fibers having a strength of 220 MPa, a modulus of 8 GPa, and a breaking elongation of 25% were successfully prepared by melt extrusion and drawing.[4] Such fibers are highly oriented. Because of the increased elongation at break, the PMMA fibers resulted in a significant improvement in ductility of the self-reinforced composites compared with single-component polymers. Using PMMA fibers, Gilbert et al. prepared self-reinforced PMMA composites with a 60% fiber fraction and tested their mechanical properties.[5] The results indicated that although the modulus of composites showed a limited increase in comparison to pure PMMA, the ultimate elongation increased significantly, suggesting high toughness for the self-reinforced PMMA composites. The single edge notched tests showed an increase of almost 100% in fracture toughness for composites. The study of failure mechanisms revealed that the composites absorbed much energy before fracture. Fatigue experimental results showed that the composites had significant fatigue strength improvement over that of bulk PMMA. It was claimed that the fiber-matrix bond in self-reinforced PMMA composites is uniform and continuous through the bulk of the individual composite.

A key factor contributing to bone cement nonuniformity is associated with the radiopacifiers that are used — those which are added to the dry component of a bone cement system in a sufficient amount to give the resulting cement the necessary radiopacity for examination by X-rays. Unfortunately, radiopacifiers, such as barium salts and certain metal oxides, when added to bone cement tend to reduce the mechanical properties of the cement. Radiopacifiers, which have higher density and polarity than the polymeric material they are mixed with, tend to clump or agglomerate in the bone cement. The resulting agglomerates have been shown to act as stress concentration sites and to decrease the ultimate flexural strength, intrinsic tensile strength, fatigue strength, as well as the fracture toughness of the cement.

In a successful effort by Damien and coworkers to prevent agglomeration of the radiopacifier, barium sulfate particles, a common radiopacifier, were microencapsulated with a bone cement compatible material.[6–8] When combined with the liquid monomer, the bone cement compatible material dissolves, releasing the radiopacified particles into the bone cement matrix. By being microencapsulated, the radiopacifier is prevented from agglomerating in the cement. Instead, the radiopacifier particles become dispersed through the bone cement matrix, which not only creates a radiopaque cement but also increases the fatigue life of the cement.[6–8] their study, these investigators also compared both radiopaque and radiolucent Surgical Simplex-P Bone Cement (Howmedica, Rutherford, New Jersey) with their experimental bone cement based on a radiolucent Simplex-P form and barium sulfate particles microencapsulated in PMMA.[7] Comparative mechanical property data based on identically prepared standard test specimens are outlined in Table 6.1 and show that (1) the ultimate breaking strength (UTS) of the commercial radiolucent (Radiolucent) was greater than either the commercial radiopaque (labeled Radiopaque) and the experimental one containing the microencapsulated barium sulfate (labeled Experimental), (2) Young's moduli of the radiolucent and

TABLE 6.1
Tensile and Fatigue Properties of Commercial and Experimental Bone Cements

Tested Properties	Radiolucent	Radiopaque	Experimental
Tensile Properties			
Number of samples	6	24	6
UTS, mPa, mean ± 95% C.I, std. deviation	60.4 ± 3.8	54.7 ± 1.6	53.2 ± 2.6
Modulus, mPa, mean ± 95% C.I., std. deviation	3621.3 ± 107.8	3446.4 ± 70.8	3320 ± 101.01
Fatigue Properties			
Number of samples	12	23	17
Mean log of cycle to failure	4.64	4.84	5.31
Median log of cycles to failure	4.65	5.02	5.30
Standard deviation	0.14	0.60	0.30

experimental cements were similar but lower than that of the radiopaque, which can be associated with the improved toughness of the experimental cement compared with the radiopaque, and (3) the fatigue resistance [measured in terms of log of cycles (*N*) to failure] of the experimental cement exceeded both the radiolucent and radiopaque counterparts, which supports the thesis that uniform dispersion of the radiopacifier particles is needed to improve the fatigue properties of commercially available bone cement. Examination of the fatigue fracture surface of the radiopaque and experimental test specimens using scanning electron microscopy (SEM) reflected the absence of particle agglomeration in the experimental cement compared with the frequent presence of agglomeration and nonuniformity in the radiopaque cement. Further verification of the minimized porosity of the experimental compared with the radiopaque cement was realized upon evaluation of the bulk properties of the respective fatigue specimens using nondestructive C-mode scanning acoustical microscopy (C-SAM).[7,8]

Since its early use in low friction arthroplasty in the 1960s, UHMW-PE has enjoyed prominence in a wide range of applications as a load-bearing material for joint endoprostheses in combination with metal or ceramic articulating counterparts, mostly in aging patients. However, its extended use beyond 10 years, particularly in heavy and/or young, active patients, unveiled the polymer's clinical limitations. These are manifested as wear, creep, and fatigue fractures, which were associated with serious clinical complications. These have led to the failure of implant components resulting from (1) UHMW-PE creep and improper load transfer through bone cement leading to fatigue fractures, (2) formation of UHMW-PE bioincompatible wear micro- or nanoparticles, which over time lead to infection, and (3) loosening of the implant.[9–13] Accordingly, over the past two decades, a great many studies have been conducted toward improving the clinical performance of UHMW-PE.[14–19] few of these studies dealt with reinforcing UHMW-PE and are discussed in Chapter 8 of this text. Other approaches were tried.

1. Radiation-induced crosslinking to increase its creep resistance. Unfortunately, depending on the irradiation and environmental conditions, crosslinking was also associated with chain degradation and loss of strength.[14,15]
2. Reinforcement with carbon fiber to increase its creep resistance. This was subsequently shown to compromise the articulating surface friction coefficient and wear resistance.[12]
3. Self-reinforcement with UHMW-PE high tenacity fibers. This led to substantial improvement in the polymer at exceptionally low fiber loading (5%) (see Figure 6.1).[16]
4. Radiation-induced crosslinking in different gas environments using different irradiation doses. Deng and coworkers have shown that it can be used to minimize the polymer deformability, particularly at 2.5 Mrad in the presence of acetylene (Figure 6.2). The long-term effect of mere radiation sterilization was verified by the same investigators to be detrimental to the polymer mechanical properties.[14]
5. Solid-state orientation using the orthogonal solid-state orientation (OSSO) method was shown by Deng to improve creep resistance.[17]

In a new approach to wear reduction of orthopedic-bearing surfaces, such as that of UHMW-PE, Pavoor et al. investigated the use of conformal polyelectrolyte multilayer (PEM) coatings.[20] In this investigation, PEM films, only a few hundred nanometers thick, were assembled by sequential adsorption of poly(acrylic acid) and poly(allylamine hydrochloride). The wear-reducing capacity of these coatings in the presence of bovine calf serum lubricant solution was established for a commonly used metal–UHMW-PE system over 500,000 cycles of bidirectional motion in a macroscale pin-on-disk test. Pertinent results indicated that the use of the films reduced UHMW-PE wear by up to 33% when compared with the uncoated control.

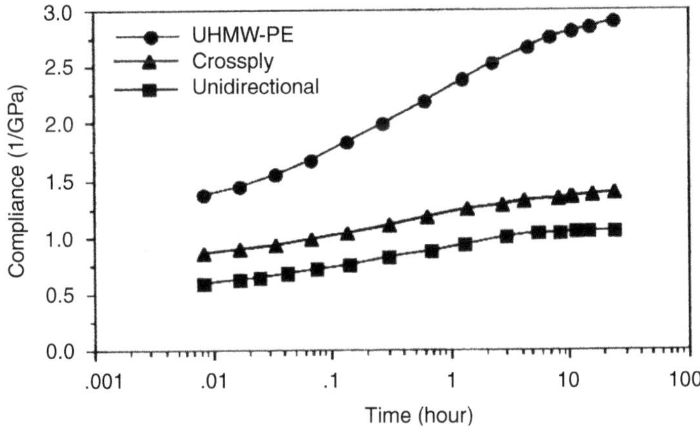

FIGURE 6.1 Tensile creep results of plain UHMW-PE and self-reinforced composites at room temperature and 5 MPa. $W_f = 5\%$ for the composites.

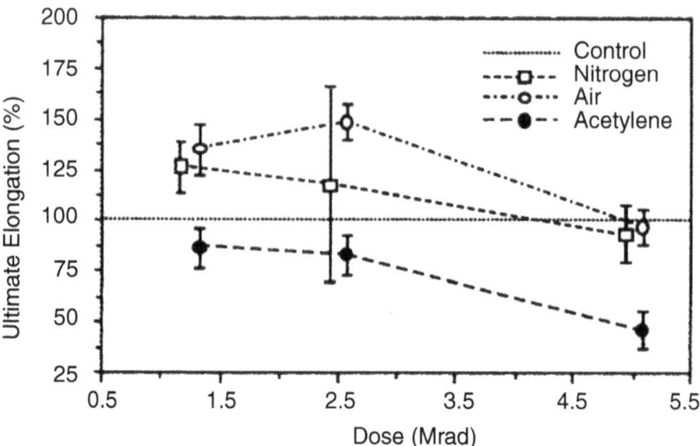

FIGURE 6.2 Effects of gamma irradiation on ultimate elongation of compression-molded UHMW-PE sheets. Control = nonirradiated samples. Nitrogen, air, and acetylene = samples irradiated in nitrogen, air, and acetylene, respectively.

This was suggested to be the first clinically relevant laboratory demonstration of the wear-reducing ability of the PEM films.[20]

Among the growing applications of nonabsorbable polymers in the area of articulating joints are those that pertain to the knee meniscal function. And the treatment for meniscus injury has been changing from resection to repair. However, depending on the type of injury, meniscectomy cannot be avoided. In a preliminary, 1-year study of polyvinyl alcohol–hydrogel (PVA-H) as an artificial meniscus, Kobayashi and coworkers performed animal experiments using rabbits and PVA-H with high water content.[21] In these experiments, the lateral meniscus of both knees on one side were replaced with an artificial meniscus and lateral meniscectomy was performed on the knees of the other side. In the knees having artificial meniscus, regressive changes were initially observed but did not progress after a certain period, and the articular cartilage state was good even after 1 year. In addition, neither wear nor breakage of PVA-H was observed. These results led the investigators to suggest that an artificial meniscus using PVA-H with high water content compensates for meniscus function and is clinically applicable. This work was associated with a study on the effect of water content in PVA-H gel on its mechanical properties to determine the optimum content for use as an artificial meniscus in active athletes with several severe meniscus injuries.[22] For this, the PVA-H candidates were tested for compression and stress relaxation. And PVA-H, having a water content of about 90%, displayed viscoelastic behavior similar to that of a human meniscus.[23] As a follow-up of the preliminary 1-year study using rabbits discussed previously, Kobayashi et al. completed a 2-year study using PVA-H in a rabbit knee model.[21,23] The results of the study showed that the articular cartilage state of the knee joint implanted with the PVA-H meniscus was good even at 2 years, while osteoarthrosis changes progressed in the meniscectomy knee joint. It was also noted that neither wear nor breakage of the PVA-H was observed. This led to the conclusion that the artificial meniscus using PVA-H can compensate for meniscal function and might be clinically applicable.

A new technique for repairing acute rupture of the Achilles tendon was developed by Jennings and coworkers using a polyester tape.[24] The new method requires no postoperative splintage and allows earlier mobilization and prompt return to work and sport. In the study, 30 patients participated and were reviewed prospectively and at a mean of 3 years. The average return to work, full weight-bearing, and driving was 40 days, 45 days, and 49 days, respectively. The average time for return to sport was 122 days. Three patients required further surgery, two for infected wounds and one for scar release. There was one sural nerve injury. Twenty-two patients regained a normal range of ankle and subtalar movement, with the mean power of plantar flexion 84% of the opposite side. Of the 22 patients who played sport, 14 were still performing at the same or a higher level. There were no reruptures over this period.

Kahn and coworkers investigated a biomedical polycarbonate urethane as the acetabular-bearing material in a novel total replacement hip joint.[25,26] In the first segment of their study, the investigators assessed the *in vitro* resistance of the polycarbonate urethane, Corethane 80A, to the main degradation mechanisms observed in polyurethanes (PUs): hydrolysis, environmental stress cracking, metal ion oxidation, and calcification. The performance of Corethane 80A was assessed alongside three other commercially available biomedical PUs: polyether PUs, Pellethane 2363-80A (Dow Chemical), and PHMO-PU ChronoFlex AL-80A (CardioTech). Chemical and structural variables that affect the properties of the materials were analyzed with particular attention to the nature of the material's hard and soft segments. PU degradation was probed using a range of analytical tools and physical testing methods, including mechanical testing, differential scanning calorimetry, Fourier transform infrared spectroscopy, and environmental scanning microscopy. Corethane 80A displayed the best overall resistance to hydrolysis, environmental stress cracking, metal ion oxidation, and calcification, followed by ChronoFlex 80A and PHMO-PU. Pellethane 80A was the least stable. The investigators noted that this study provides compelling evidence for the biostability and effectiveness of Corethane 80A and points to its suitability for use as a compliant bearing layer in hip arthroplasty. In the second segment of the study, Corethane 80A was assessed in a fully functioning ovine total hip arthroplasty model for its *in vivo* performance as a load-bearing surface in a prototype compliant layer, acetabular cup. PU degradation in the retrieved cups was analyzed using a range of analytical and physical testing methods as described above in the first segment of the study. The Corethane 80A functioned well in the total hip arthroplasty model, with the bearing surfaces of the retrieved hip cups showing no significant evidence of biodegradation or wear damage after 3 years *in vivo*. The investigators noted that the findings in this study provide compelling evidence of the biostability and effectiveness of acetabular cups incorporating a Corethane 80A compliant bearing layer.

The use of polymer composites as alternative to metals in hip prostheses has been the goal of many investigators. Accounts of a few moderately successful and promising attempts are outlined in the following paragraphs. DeSantis et al. prepared composite hip prostheses using poly(ether-imide) reinforced with carbon and glass fibers and investigated the effect of fiber organization on the mechanical properties of composite femoral implants in comparison with bone.[27] In their study, the investigators used a stacking sequence of drop-off plies of carbon or glass fibers reinforcing poly(ether-imide), which constitutes a symmetrical and balanced composite hip prosthesis. The hip was manufactured according to the finite element modeling design and using the compression molding and water-jet technologies. The measured stress–strain data according to tensile, flexural, and torsional tests showed agreement with the numerical calculation. Young's modulus and the strength in tension are uniform along the stem axis (40 GPa and 600 MPa, respectively), while the elastic modulus in bending varies from 10 to 60 GPa in the tip-head direction. The composite stem showed a linear load-displacement relation up to 4500 N without breaking. Mechanical behavior of the composite hip prosthesis was found to be comparable with that of a canine femur. Comparison with metal prostheses has also been undertaken. Results of the study reflect the promising properties of the examined composites as alternatives to metals for hip implants.

Among the key applications of polymer composites are those dealing with spinal implants. This is an area of growing importance because of the fast-growing percentage of elderly patients. For a better understanding of the significance of spinal implants, it is to be noted that lower back and neck pain is oftentimes attributed to the rupture or degeneration of intervertebral discs due to degenerative disc disease, spondylolisthesis, deformative disorders, trauma, tumors, and the like. This pain typically results from the compression of spinal nerve roots by damaged discs between the vertebra, the collapse of the disc, or the resulting adverse effects of bearing the patient's body weight through a damaged, unstable vertebral joint. To remedy this, spinal implants have been inserted between the vertebral bodies to restore the joint to its previous height and stabilize the motion at that spinal segment. Surgical treatments to restore the vertebral height typically involve excision of the ruptured soft disc between the vertebrae, often with subsequent insertion of a spinal implant or interbody fusion device to fuse and stabilize the segment. In a recent disclosure, a novel bioactive spinal implant composite material was reported to have the necessary properties for this particular use.[28] The spinal implant material was reported to have a radiopacity similar to bone for facilitating radiographic assessment of fusion. The implant materials of the subject disclosure were also described as being capable of withstanding physiologic, dynamic, compressive loads while remaining bioactive and biocompatible. As defined in the disclosure, bioactive relates to (1) the chemical formation of a calcium phosphate layer via ion exchange between surrounding fluid and the implant materials and (2) materials that elicit a reaction that leads to bone formation, attachment into or adjacent to implants, or bone apposition directly to the implants usually without intervening fibrous tissue. More specifically, the spinal implant was reported to consist of a synthetic, bioactive material having a (1) bisphenol-A–glycidyl methacrylate polymerized resin matrix comprising about 10–60% by weight of the total composition of the implant material — the polymerized resin matrix containing diurethane dimethacrylate and triethylene glycol dimethacrylate resins and the resin matrix further containing silane-treated borosilicate filler, (2) a range of radiopacity from about 30 to about 55, and (3) a range of stiffness from about 6 to about 20 GPa.

Because of certain unique properties of silicon-based materials, silicone rubbers and hydroxyapatite were among the biomaterials used in a number of early orthopedic applications, including intervertebral discs and artificial lumbar.

However, reports suggesting that silicone rubber may cause synovitis directed many investigators away from these materials for a number of years.[30–32] Nonetheless, revived interest was piqued by two relatively recent studies relevant to articulating joints. In one of these studies, Wang and Yu investigated the use of silicone rubber in repairing articular cartilage defects.[29] In this study silicone rubber implants were used to fill full-thickness articular cartilage in the trochlea area of the rabbit knee joint to determine the long-term effects of these implants on surrounding articular tissue. Forty-eight weeks after surgery, the silicone rubbers were still fitted tightly into the defects; surrounding cartilage showed mild degeneration, which was better than the control group. This led to the conclusion that silicone rubber implantation for repairing local articular cartilage defects can effectively delay the pathogenic progression of osteoarthritis. The second of these new studies pertained to incorporating alkoxysilanes and calcium salt in PMMA-based bone cement to impart bioactivity and bonding to bony tissues when used with prosthetic joint implants.[33] this study, PMMA bone cement was modified with 20 mass % of different alkoxysilanes and calcium salts, and its apatite-forming ability was evaluated in Kokubo solution. The apatite formation was observed on the surface of the modified cements containing 20 mass % $CaCl_2$, irrespective of the alkoxysilane used. Meanwhile, the apatite formation was observed on the cement containing $CaCl_2$, $Ca(CH_3COO)_2$, or $Ca(OH)_2$, but not on the cement containing $CaCO_3$ or β-$Ca_3(PO_4)_2$, even when the cement contains 3-methacryloxypropyltrimethoxysilane. These results led to the conclusion that modification with alkoxysilane and calcium salts showing high water solubility is effective for providing PMMA bone cement with bioactivity.

6.2.2 Absorbable Polymers, Composites, and Their Applications

Although this topic has been the subject of many reviews covering orthopedic applications over the past four decades, only a few have been published since 2002.[34–37] Advances made in the absorbable polymers technology in the past decade were paralleled by an impressive growth in the use of these polymers in diverse areas of orthopedic devices, and particularly those pertaining to improved performance, repair, and replacement of components of articulating joints. And this section provides accounts of those applications relevant in general to (1) meniscus repair, (2) internal bone fracture fixation, (3) interference screws and allied anchoring devices, and (4) spinal devices. Specific applications of absorbable polymers are addressed in Sections 6.3 and 6.4 of this chapter.

In a study by Shin et al. on the potential use of electrospun PLGA nanofiber scaffolds for articular cartilage reconstruction, three types of copolymeric scaffolds were prepared and tested for their mechanical properties, stability, degradation, and cellular responses under mechanical stimulation *in vitro*.[38] The electrospun fibers were made from 75/25 and 50/50 *l*-lactide/glycolide (PLGA) copolymers or blends thereof, and were shown to have slightly lower tensile modulus and ultimate tensile stress and elongation than those of human cartilage. The degradation of the scaffolds was dependent on the L/G ratio in the copolymers. Cellular responses were evaluated by examining toxicity, cell proliferation, and extracellular matrix formation using freshly isolated chondrocytes from porcine articular cartilage. The scaffolds were nontoxic, and cell proliferation and extracellular matrix formation in nanofiber scaffolds were superior to those in membrane-type scaffolds. Intermittent hydrostatic pressure applied to cell-seeded nanofiber led to the conclusion that nanofiber-based PLGA scaffolds have the potential to be used for cartilage reconstruction.

One of the uncommon procedures in articulating joints is the reconstruction of rheumatoid wrists. Until recently, the Darrach reconstructive procedure, entailing resectioning of the distal end of the ulna, was used in patients with dislocation or subluxation of the ulna head causing a limitation of the forearm supination and pain during this motion.[39,40] However, this was noted to give rise to abnormal postoperative carpal subluxation, ulnar deviation, or ulnar translation, and the Suave–Kapandji (S-K) procedure has been recommended for use as a preferred alternative to the Darrach procedure for the past two decades.[41] The S-K procedure has been used successfully for rheumatoid patients with pain on motion of the distal radioulnar joint and limited external rotation of the forearm with or without ruptured extensor tendons. The development of absorbable, high modulus PLLA screws based on solid-state orientation in the compressive or preferably in the tensile mode prompted their use instead of metal screws by contemporary academic investigators and clinicians.[42,43] And the usefulness of absorbable PLLA screws, based on solid-state oriented polymer, for rheumatoidal wrist reconstruction in the S-K procedure was evaluated by Nakamura and coworkers.[43] Based on the results of their study, these investigators believed that the PLLA screws were absorbed naturally and that the distal ulnar head regained its original strength. They also concluded that the absorbable PLLA screws are more useful than metal screws in the S-K procedure for rheumatoid patients.

The use of high modulus, absorbable PLLA screws in a number of orthopedic procedures has been quite successful for about two decades. However, the clinical experience with the reliability of absorbable screws in hip surgery is limited. This led Ito et al. to pursue a study on the use of poly-L-lactic acid (PLLA) acid screws for the fixation in hip osteotomy.[44] In this study, the investigators evaluated 68 consecutive hip osteotomies in 61 patients using absorbable PLLA screws for fixation; 47 hips underwent a rotational acetabular osteotomy, 17 hips Chiari's pelvic osteotomy, and 4 hips transtrochanteric rotational osteotomy. Cortical screws were used to transfix the osteotomized acetabulum, and cancellous screws to reattach the intraoperatively osteotomized greater trochanter. All the osteotomized acetabulums united well, but 4 of 54 trochanteric osteotomies failed to unite. Results of the study led to the conclusion that PLLA screws are best for transfixing an osteotomized acetabulum in rotational acetabular osteotomy. However, they may break if used in femoral trochanteric osteotomy and are probably not suitable for reattaching the intraoperatively osteotomized greater trochanter.

A second strategy for increasing the modulus of absorbable screws to match those of bone tissues is based on fiber self-reinforcement. Following this strategy, Viljanen et al. conducted a study to compare the tissue response to absorbable self-reinforced PLLA screws with metal screws in the fixation of cancellous osteotomies using a femoral rabbit model.[45] Based on the results of the study associated with a 48-week follow-up period, these investigators reported that (1) no signs of degradation of the self-reinforced PLLA implant and only a mild foreign-body reaction with no accumulations of inflammatory cells to either self-reinforced PLLA or metallic screws were observed during the follow-up period; (2) both types of screws seemed to induce an osteostimulatory response around their threads — this phenomenon was transient for metallic screws but lasted for at least 48 weeks for self-reinforced PLLA screws, (3) the PLLA screws do not seem to cause osteopenia at the implantation site, and (4) the fixation properties of both self-reinforced PLLA screws and metallic screws appear to be sufficient for the fixation of small fragments of cancellous bone.

Toward increasing the modulus of polylactide-based implants, Prokop et al. used a mixture of poly(L,DL-lactide) and 10% -tricalcium phosphate to produce new composite pin (Polypin-C) implants for clinical use in therapy for radial head fractures. For this, a total of 34 patients underwent a clinical and conventional radiological follow-up examination after an average of 38.2 months. In 29 cases, a computerized tomography (CT) scan was also carried out. Between 18 and 24 months, two cases of grade 1 osteolysis were observed around the pin head. No trace of osteolysis was observed at the final examination in either case. After 24 months, the pins were no longer visible on a conventional X-ray. A CT evaluation showed a density similar to that of spongioid bone in the original pin cavities after 3 years. These results led to the conclusion that the composite pin (Polypin-C) is suitable for treating dislocated radial head fractures.

Since the development of the stainless-steel lumbar interbody cage device in the late 1980s as an adjunct to spinal arthrodesis and interbody fusion, spinal cages have been shown to be clinically effective in relieving patients suffering from various degenerative disorders of the lumbar spine.[47–52] Spinal fusion cages were developed to correct spinal deformation, provide mechanical stability, and create an optimal environment for spinal arthrodesis with limited mobility, without contending with disadvantages associated with the use of autogenous or donor bone alone (insufficient mechanical strength, risk of graft resorption, and pseudoarthrosis of the motion segment).[51,52] Until recently, cages were made of stainless-steel, titanium, or carbon-fiber–reinforced polymer composites in the form of horizontal cylinders, vertical rings, and open boxes packed with bone graft to induce interbody fusion. For the same reasons cited earlier in this book for substituting metals for absorbable polymers as orthopedic implants, Dijk and coworkers prepared and investigated the *in vitro* and *in vivo* degradation of bioabsorbable PLLA spinal fusion cages. In the *in vivo* study, the PLLA cages were packed with bone graft and implanted in the L3-L4 spinal motion segment of 18 Dutch milk goats. At 12, 26, and 52 weeks, the motion segments were isolated and PLLA samples retrieved. The implanted cages showed an advanced decline in inherent viscosity compared with the cages subjected to *in vitro* degradation experiments using a phosphate buffered solution at pH 7.4 and 37°C. At 6 months of implantation, the geometrical shape and original height of 10 mm was maintained. At 12 months, the cage disintegrated into multiple fragments with signs of absorption. Despite the high load bearing conditions, the PLLA cage allowed interbody fusion to occur without collapse of the cage.

6.2.3 Injectable, Intra-articular Polymeric Systems and Their Applications

It is well accepted that the joint capsular environment and the absence of surface physicochemical and biomechanical irregularities of articulating components are most relevant to the functional performance of articulating joints. Contributing to the normal tribological properties of joint surfaces in the capsular environment is hyaluronic acid. It plays a key role in the maintenance of the structural and functional characteristics of the joint. Hyaluronic acid (Ha) is produced by the synoviocytes and determines the viscoelastic properties of the synovial fluid. There is a major component of the extracellular matrix in the cartilage hyaluronan that helps in the formation of an amorphous layer (0.6 μ thick) and covers the articular surface of the cartilage, contributing to the boundary lubrication mechanism in conditions of extreme loading and partially protecting the tissue from penetration of the inflammatory cells and lytic enzymes.[54] Pathological processes, such as osteoarthritis encountered in more than 70% of Americans over the age of 75, can result in the reduction in the molecular weight and concentration of Ha in the synovial fluid because of accumulation in the joint cavity of liquid derived from the inflamed synovial vessel.[55] This leads to a reduction in the viscoelasticity of the fluid and increased susceptibility of the cartilage to break down. Pain is the primary symptom of osteoarthritis, which is due to joint capsule distension, stretching of periosteal nerve endings, and possibly synovial inflammation. Multiple medications are available to relieve pain and improve functions.[56,57] Early efforts to counteract this process were based on the use of intra-articular injections of exogenous Ha. Promising results of this therapeutic strategy prompted the pursuit of a number of studies using Ha, crosslinked with other gels, or gel-forming systems with and without the incorporation of bioactive agents, particularly the anti-inflammatory types.[59,60] Nonsteroidal inflammatory drugs (NSAIDs), such as ibuprofen, have analgesic and anti-inflammatory properties. Ibuprofen is reported to inhibit articular chondrocytes apoptosis and dedifferentiation.[61,62]

Barbucci et al. used an Ha-based hydrogel with a cross-linking degree of 50% in the treatment of chondral defects in rabbit knee.[59] Pertinent results showed that these injections improved chondrocytes density and matrix appearance without evidence of tissue reaction or inflammation. Furthermore, the permanence *in situ* the hydrogel was longer than that of the linear Ha, reducing the number of injections and, consequently, the possibility of infection. More recently these investigators used the same system loaded with an anti-inflammatory drug (ibuprofen-lysine) for local administration in an osteoarthritic knee.[60] The kinetics of drug release were studied *in vitro* using a continuous flow system. The release was studied at three different rates (0.375, 0.073, and 0.005 mL/s), and for the slowest one a period of 8 days was necessary to achieve complete release of the drug. A chondral defect was caused in the right femoral medial condyle of 24 rabbits. Twelve animals were treated with the active Ha gel and 12 with the placebo gel by percutaneous injection. The treatments were repeated every 10 days. A significant difference was observed in bone mineral density of the total tibia of rabbits treated by the active Ha gel (containing ibuprofen-lysine) in comparison with those treated only by the placebo. The positive effects of the active gel on chondral lesions were maintained with the adjunctive effect of increased limb usage.

Paclitaxel is a chemotherapeutic agent that suppresses cellular proliferation and angiogenesis as well as proliferative synovitis in animal models. Bragdon et al. studied early changes induced by intra-articular injection of paclitaxel-impregnated

50 ng in 50/50 poly-(D,L-lactide coglycolide) microspheres.[63] Paclitaxel was released and caused minimal inflammatory response and joint fluid filtration in the first 3 h after injection. Alterations in transsynovial fluid flow and permeability were identified, most notably as increased synovial fluid production and capillary pore size. In a related study on the intra-articular treatment of arthritis with microphase formulations of paclitaxel based on different lactide/glycolide copolymers (PLGA), polylactic acid (PLA) and polycaprolactone (PCL), Liggins et al. found that polymeric microspheres in the 35–105 μm size range were biocompatible whereas smaller microspheres (1–30 μm) produced an inflammatory response. Efficacy studies showed that injection of 20% paclitaxel-loaded PLA microspheres significantly reduced all measures of inflammation in the antigen arthritis rabbit model. This led to the conclusion that paclitaxel-loaded PLA microspheres in the 35–105 μm range released paclitaxel in a controlled manner over several weeks, reflecting the potential of this formulation for the intra-articular treatment of inflammation in arthritic conditions.[64]

In addition to osteoarthritis, which was just discussed, rheumatoid arthritis is a serious disease that compromises the normal function of articulating joints. Rheumatoid arthritis is a chronic inflammatory disease of unknown etiology and complex multifactorial pathogenesis. Rheumatoid arthritis is characterized by progressive and irreversible damage of the synovial-lined joints, leading to loss of joint space, decrease in joint function, and eventual deformity.[65] Although rheumatoid arthritis is commonly treated with NSAIDs, contemporary clinicians prefer early use of slow-acting, disease modifying antirheumatic drugs (DMARDs) because they have the potential to prevent or reduce the joint damage. Most preferred treatments of rheumatoid arthritis entail the use of DMARDs no later than 3 months after commencement of the NSAID treatment.[66,67] Recognition of methotrexate (MTX) as one of the most frequently used DMARDs in the treatment of rheumatoid arthritis and its preferred administration from a controlled delivery system, led Liang and coworkers to pursue a study on the use of MTX-loaded poly-*l*-lactide (PLLA) microspheres for intra-articular delivery of the drug to the joint.[68] The study was intended to develop and characterize MTX-loaded PLLA microspheres and evaluate *in vivo* tolerability and MTX plasma concentrations following intra-articular injection into healthy rabbits. Accordingly, MTX-loaded PLLA (2 kg/mole) microspheres were prepared using the solvent evaporation method. Biocompatibility was evaluated by observing the swelling of the joints of the rabbits and histological analysis following the injection of the microspheres. MTX concentrations in the plasma and urine samples of rabbits were evaluated and showed that MTX-loaded microspheres exhibit a rapid burst phase followed by a slow-release phase. MTX-loaded and control microspheres were found to be biocompatible, and plasma concentrations of MTX were determined to be 10-fold higher in rabbits injected intra-articularly with free MTX than MTX microspheres. Results of the study led these investigators to note the promise of the controlled release system and its potential optimization by using higher molecular weight PLLA or *l*-lactide–glycolide copolymers.

Pertinent to the use of injectable active polymer formulations for treating osteoarthritis or rheumatoid arthritis are methods used in evaluating the effectiveness of such treatments. Lee et al. pursued a study to determine whether magnetic resonance imaging (MRI) can be used to demonstrate the effect of radiation synovectomy after the intra-articular injection of holmium-166–chitosan complex for the treatment of rheumatoid arthritis of the knee.[69] A criterion for inclusion in the study was the absence of observable improvement after 3 or more months of treatment of the knee with DMARDs. MRI images were acquired both prior to and 4 months after treatment. Clinical evaluation included the use of visual analogue scales to assess pain, and the circumference of the knee and its range of motion were also determined. MRI evaluation included measurement of the volume of synovial enhancement and wall thickness, the amount of joint effusion, and quantifiable scoring of bone erosion, bone edema, and lymph nodes. Results of the study showed that visual analogue scale readings decreased significantly after radiation synovectomy. MRI showed that joint effusion decreased significantly and that the volume of synovial enhancement tended to decrease, but to an insignificant extent. This led to the conclusion that the decreased joint effusion noted at the 4-month follow-up resulted from radiation synovectomy of the rheumatoid knee by means of intra-articular injection of holmium-166–chitosan complex. From a second perspective, a histological study of articular cartilage in experimental rat knee arthritis induced by intracapsular injection of cationic polyethyleneimine (PEI) was conducted to elucidate the mechanism of osteoarthritic development in this animal model.[70] Results of the study led to the conclusion that the functional impairment of anionic sites after injecting cationic PEI into rat knee joints induced pathological changes in the rat knee joints, resembling those in osteoarthritic-like animal models.

6.2.4 Tissue Engineering

In a recent review of tissue engineering, Marra discussed the use of biodegradable polymers and microspheres with a focus on (1) the types of polymeric scaffolds in bone, neuronal, and skin tissue engineering, (2) scaffold fabrication, and (3) polymer microspheres and growth factor delivery.[71] Even though the genesis of now traditional tissue engineering technology was an outcome of the impressive development in the absorbable and/or biodegradable polymer technology, there remains a role for nonabsorbable polymers in the field of tissue engineering and particularly the so-called *in situ* type. Because Marra's review and previous reviews did not address, primarily, tissue engineering as it relates to articulating joints, the use of both absorbable and nonabsorbable polymers has prompted the preparation of this section. A justification for not ignoring the nonabsorbable polymers is illustrated by the work of deGroot on the use of nonabsorbable polyurethane (PU) as a scaffold for meniscal tissue regeneration.[72] In discussing the rationale for using PU, deGroot noted that a previously developed collagen meniscus implant (CMI) based on a collagen scaffold made of bovine tendon has not been used extensively.[73,74] This was attributed to the tendency of the CMI to tear under wet conditions. It was also noted that an implant needs to survive until the tissue ingrowth is complete in spite of the prevailing high stresses in the knee, even if the patient is partially immobilized.[72] This led deGroot to investigate a synthetic nonabsorbable PU with enhanced mechanical properties as a preferred alternative to CMI.[75] Accordingly, previously prepared polyurethane-ureas were processed into porous meniscal implants, which were tested in the knees of dogs. The first fibrous tissue ingrowth observed was determined to contain mainly collagen. After a 12- to 20-week induction time, the tissue transformed to fibrocartilagenous meniscuslike tissue, which contained collagen type II and proteoglycans. The compression behavior of the newly formed tissue resembled that of native meniscus tissue. This led to the suggestion that with such an implant, the protection of the articular cartilage in humans is possible. In a second application of nonabsorbable polymers in tissue engineering, Neves and coworkers used a polyethylene terephthalate (PET) scaffold to study the influence of stirring-induced mixing on cell proliferation and extracellular matrix deposition in meniscal cartilage constructs. In this study, PET scaffolds were seeded with meniscal fibrochondrocytes from 6-month-old sheep and cultured under a variety of stirring regimes for 28 days. Stirring-induced mixing increased up to sevenfold the deposition of glucosaminoglycans and up to threefold the deposition of collagen as compared with static cultures. High and medium intensity stirring induced rapid cell proliferation with maximal cell densities achieved within the first 7 days of cultivation. Under these conditions, collagen and glucosaminoglycan deposition occurred predominantly in association with cell proliferation; the specific deposition rate of these biopolymers decreased markedly after 7 days of cultivation as the cell number reached a plateau. Constructs exposed to the highest intensity stirring had the highest levels of collagen and glucosaminoglycans, and a more homogeneous cell distribution. Because the success of the integration at a repair site in the knee of a meniscal construct appeared to be dependent on the cellular activity of the construct, this led to the suggestion that cultivation of meniscal cartilage constructs, under the noted conditions, should not extend for more than 7 days.

While alluding to the role of nonabsorbable polymers in tissue engineering technology, as discussed previously, it must be emphasized that absorbable polymers are most essential to major advancements in tissue engineering. And this has been the consistent view of key investigators in this field who have pointed out the need for developing new biodegradable materials that do not induce scar tissue and have noted that solid absorbable polymer scaffolds need to meet certain physicochemical and morphological requirements to allow for a timely and sufficient tissue ingrowth.[77–79] These requirements included having a certain surface microtexture associated with scaffold inhibiting, continuous, three-dimensional open cells that promote cell attachment and growth and transport of nutrients to the implanted cells while permitting the removal of metabolic by-products.[79] Practically all the solid scaffolds investigated to date are made from absorbable polymers based on one or more of the following monomers: glycolide, lactide, trimethylene carbonate, caprolactone, and *p*-dioxanone. In addition to the biodegradable fermentation products, polyhydroxyalkanoates are being promoted for their potential use in tissue engineering for a number of attributes as reviewed by Chen and Wu.[80] Meanwhile, an increasing number of investigators advocate the use of absorbable and or biodegradable, injectable, gel-forming matrices to provide preferred substrates for certain types of tissue engineering over the well-accepted porous scaffolds.[81–86] This is mostly because an injectable, gel-forming matrix may offer several advantages over preformed solid scaffolds because they are[81–83]:

Flowable materials that can fill a defect of any shape
Suitable for incorporating various bioactive agents (e.g., growth promoters)
Easy-to-prepare by simple mixing without the need for organic solvents
Minimally invasive without requiring surgical procedures for placement
Optimal media for the transport of nutrients as well as metabolic by-products

Among the key examples cited in a review by Gutowska et al. and discussed by the respective investigators are alginate, hyaluronan, and chitosan gels.[81,84–86] While these natural or biosynthetic polymers showed some promise, their effectiveness as tissue engineering matrices may have been compromised by their solubility in water. This led to a new focus on dealing with synthetic, injectable, amphiphilic, gel-forming liquids, such as the absorbable polyether-esters disclosed by Shalaby.[82,83] The effective application of these polyether-esters as matrices for tissue engineering is yet to be determined. Other polymeric gels, which were reviewed by Gutowska and coworkers and have been investigated and may be worth further consideration as matrices for tissue engineering are the (1) thermo-reversible gels made primarily of block copolymers of ethylene oxide and propylene oxide, (2) ionically crosslinked gels that are based on calcium alginate, (3) polyethylene oxide gels having a molecular weight of 20–100 kDa, and (4) poly(*N*-isopropyl acrylamide-co-acrylic acid) gels as matrices for chondrocytes.[87–90] As in the case of natural polymers just described, the water-solubility of most of these synthetic polymers may hinder their broad applicability in tissue engineering applications where a prolonged residence time at the biological site is critical.

Two of the most interesting applications of tissue engineering, which hold a great deal of promise, are those dealing with cartilage and ligaments as discussed in this section. First, recognizing that biological restoration of osteochondral defects requires suitable subchondral support material that also allows the induction of hyaline cartilage tissue, prompted Wang et al. to pursue an *in vitro* study on the tissue engineering of biphasic cartilage constructs using various biodegradable scaffolds.[91] In this study, the investigators explored a number of candidate biodegradable support materials onto which neocartilage was produced *in vitro*. Porcine chondrocytes were seeded in a closed and static bioreactor with a base of biomaterial consisting of either poly-L-lactide (PLLA), poly-D,L-lactide (PDLLA), or collagen-hydroxyapatite and were cultured for 15 weeks. Viable neocartilage was produced on each biomaterial with differing amounts of cellular colonization. PDLLA degradation was more rapid and uneven among the three biomaterials, leading to constructs of irregular shape. And little or no discernable polymer degradation or chondrocyte colonization was reported in the case of PLLA. Collagen–hydroxyapatite constructs were superior in terms of viability, implant morphology, and integration between neocartilage and biomaterial. These results led to the suggestion that the reported system has a potential for producing biphasic implants that may be adequate for repairing osteochondral defects. Choosing a more absorbable scaffold, Uematsu and coworkers studied the generation of cartilage using mesenchymal stem cells (MSCs) and a novel three-dimensional poly(lactic-glycolic acid) (PLGA) scaffold.[92] In the study, PLGA scaffolds seeded with MSCs were transplanted into large defects in rabbit knees and analyzed histologically 4 and 12 weeks postoperatively. It was found that in the engineered cartilage with the PLGA scaffold, the defects were filled with smooth shiny white tissue, macroscopically, and hyaline-like cartilage, histologically, at 12 weeks after the transplantation. This led the investigators to note that the structure of the novel PLGA scaffolds provided architectural support for the differentiation of progenitor cells and demonstrated successful induction of *in vivo* chondrogenesis. In a more elaborate approach to tissue engineered cartilage, Kose and coworkers used matrices made of poly(3-hydroxybutyric acid-co-3-hydroxyvaleric acid) (PHBV), or collagen-containing calcium phosphate (CaP-Gelfix foams.[93] These matrices were characterized for surface chemistry and morphology as well as porosity. Chondrocytes were isolated from the proximal humerus of 22-week-old albino rabbits. The foams were seeded with 1×10^6 chondrocytes and histological examinations were carried out to assess cell-matrix interaction. Macroscopic examination showed that PHBV (with or without chondrocytes) maintained its integrity for 21 days, while CaP-Gelfix® was deformed and degraded within 15 days. Cell-containing and cell-free matrices were implanted into full thickness cartilage defects at the knees of rabbits. Results at 8 and 20 weeks with chondrocyte-seeded PHBV matrices presented early cartilage formation resembling normal articular cartilage and revealed minimal foreign body reaction. In CaP-Gelfix matrices, fibrocartilage formation and bone invasion was noted at 20 weeks. Cells maintained their phenotype in both matrices. PHBV had better healing response than CaP-Gelfix. These results led to the conclusion that both matrices were effective in cartilage regeneration and have great potential for use in the repair of joint cartilage.

The second most interesting type of application of tissue engineering was reviewed by Laurencin and Freeman as an evolutionary material science approach to solving the problem of the anterior cruciate ligament (ACL), the most commonly injured ligament of the knee with over 200,000 patients diagnosed annually with ACL disruption.[94] These and earlier authors noted that (1) the ACL is the major intra-articular ligament of the knee and is critical to its normal kinematic and stability, (2) because of poor vascularization, the ACL has inferior healing capability and is usually replaced after significant damage has occurred, and (3) currently available replacements have a host of limitations, prompting the search for tissue engineered solutions for ACL repair.[94–96] In their discussion of tissue engineered ACL using different types of scaffolds, the authors reported or indirectly indicated that (1) presently investigated scaffolds range from twisted fiber architectures composed of silk fiber to complex three-dimensional, braided structures composed of multifilament yarn based on absorbable polyesters, such as those made of glycolide and *l*-lactide, and (2) the purpose of the sought tissue engineered constructs is to apply approaches, such as the use of porous scaffolds, use of cells, and the application of growth factors, to promote ligament tissue regeneration while providing mechanical properties similar to natural ligament.

6.3 EVOLUTION OF SUPPORT STRUCTURES

Discussion in the previous section focused on the repair and replacement of the primary bony and cartilaginous component of the articulating joints. However, the motion of these components, in tandem with the surrounding tissue, is controlled by support structures, most important of which are tendons and ligaments. Pertinent aspects of the latter as they relate to the use of polymers and means of joint stabilization, as in the case of suture anchors, are the focus of the present section.

6.3.1 Ligaments and Tendons

Repairing ligaments and tendons, the support components to the function of articulating joints, has always been the subject of many studies since the development of surgical sutures. However, recent developments in absorbable and nonabsorbable polymers and newly acquired knowledge pertaining to the control of many biological events such as wound healing and tissue regeneration have propelled scientific, engineering, and clinical investigations on ligaments and tendons to an impressive new level. Accounts of the most recent developments in this area are the subject of this section.

The anterior cruciate ligament (ACL) is a commonly injured ligament of the knee, and its function is crucial to stabilizing the joint. In recent years, there have been several attempts to repair or replace the ACL using various polymers. The tissue engineering approach to designing artificial ligaments strives to create a scaffold that provides mechanical stability and simultaneously promotes the growth of cells, thus creating an ideal environment for ligament tissue regeneration. The Leeds–Keio artificial ligament demonstrated a polyester implant that had a residual tensile strength of 1700 N, which was comparable with that of the ACL (1730 N) in young individuals.[97,98] Tissue induction was observed around the artificial ligament and eventually resulted in the alignment of collagen fibers in the longitudinal direction. Laurencin et al. highlighted recent attempts to tissue engineer the ACL using polyurethane urea, poly desaminotyrosyl-tyrosine ethyl carbonate, polydioxanone, type I collagen, silk, or poly L-lactic acid.[94] The key features that were emphasized as being critical for a successful implant included reinforced scaffold architecture, interconnected pores, and cell adhesion–promoting coatings. With these considerations in mind, Cooper et al. developed a porous, tissue-engineered ligament scaffold based on polylactide-co-glycolide fibers, which was fabricated with three-dimensional braiding technology. The resulting system exhibited three architectural regions to control porosity, where the two attachment sites had a high angle fiber orientation and the intra-articular region had a lower angle fiber orientation. The complexity of the architecture in these scaffolds shows the progress that has taken place in this field.

Another related and notable development is the use of interference screws composed of absorbable polymers, such as polyglycolic acid, for ACL graft fixation. Histologic examination of a high-molecular-weight PLLA screw after 30 months *vivo* showed new bone formation adjacent to the screw and the graft with no significant inflammatory reaction.[101] In another study, MRI showed that interference screws composed of polyglycolic acid and trimethylene carbonate were partially resorbed at 6 months and totally resorbed at 1 year with no substantial inflammatory response.[101] Such findings demonstrate the safety of absorbable interference screws used for ACL fixation.

Absorbable screws have also been used for tendon graft fixation using ACL reconstruction techniques. However, Klein et al. reported that using a bioabsorbable tenodesis screw in an additional tunnel site provided better graft security than using the interference screw alone.[102] As a result, the samples with supplemental tenodesis screw fixation had twice the load to failure compared with those with only the interference screw.[102] Results such as these suggest that further progress can be made to improve the fixation of tendons and ligaments to bone. By examining and incorporating the work that has been completed to date in both tissue engineering and graft fixation, researchers in this area may soon achieve ideal graft substitutes for ligaments and tendons.

6.3.2 Suture Anchor and Allied Devices

Of the advances made over the past two decades on the use of absorbable and nonabsorbable polymers in orthopedic applications, those dealing with suture anchors and allied devices are perhaps the most impressive. Accounts of the most recent accomplishments are the subject of this section.

Metallic anchors machined from titanium or stainless steel still account for over 50% of the total suture anchor market with the balance made up of primarily absorbable materials. However, as the reliability, strength, and absorption characteristics from the use of absorbable copolymers have improved, the market share of absorbable anchors has grown.

PLLA pioneered the absorbable suture anchor market and still accounts for the majority of suture anchors and allied devices. Recently, glycolide–lactide copolymers combined with 30% tricalcium phosphate have been introduced under the name Biocryl Rapide (DePuy Mitek, Raynham, Massachusetts). It is reported that Biocryl Rapide has 70% faster resorption than PLLA. Animal studies completed by Mitek indicate a marked resorption at 18 months with bone formation within the implant profile at 36 months. In contrast, a PLLA implant control was used in the study and showed minimal resorption and bone formation at 36 months.

Although not yet FDA approved, the use of tyrosine-derived degradable polymers for use in orthopedic applications may prove to be of clinical interest. This family of polymers is based on the amino acid tyrosine; they are totally amorphous, and do not degrade to acid by-products as is the case with PLLA or PLGA. The most popular form is a tyrosine-derived polycarbonate that has a characteristic alkyl pendent group that can be varied to modulate properties. Tyrosine-derived polycarbonate structures have been shown to be resistant to radiation and ethylene oxide sterilization and possess similar mechanical properties to PLLA.[103] Steady bone ingrowth in a canine animal model out to 48 weeks has been reported. In the same study using PLLA as a control, bone ingrowth was reported to increase steadily up to 14 weeks, when it peaked and then dropped by half at the 48-week point.[104]

As the orthopedic field has moved to less invasive arthroscopic surgical techniques for performing common surgeries, the need for arthroscopic friendly techniques have developed. One example is the use of knotless suture anchor techniques to avoid the challenge of tying consistent, good quality arthroscopic knots. Arthroscopic Bankart repair is one procedure where the use of a unique knotless suture anchor for soft tissue repair to bone has been used. This technique claims to produce secure, low-profile fixation with increased suture functional strength, generally the weakest link in the fixation device, due to the double suture configuration that is created with the knotless suture anchor loop.[105]

To test the hypothesis that anchors that directly fix the rotator cuff to bone without using sutures may simplify the challenge associated with arthroscopic rotator cuff repair, Lee and coworkers completed a biomechanical comparison of bioabsorbable PLLA sutureless screw anchor versus suture anchor fixation using 12-week fresh-frozen bovine shoulders.[106] Results of this comparative study led to the conclusion that the PLLA anchor provides low-profile fixation of the rotator cuff and eliminates suture placement and knot tying during arthroscopic and mini–open cuff repair. However, it was noted that these data suggest that this anchor may not perform adequately under cyclic loading conditions in patients during postoperative rehabilitation. It was also noted that the bioabsorbable anchor may not provide sufficient fixation for rotator cuff repair in humans. Dejong and coworkers conducted a comparative study on the performance of a metal versus bioabsorbable polylactic acid suture anchor using a goat knee model to determine the difference in the load to failure.[107] Results of this study led to the conclusion that the absorbable polylactic acid suture anchor construct, tested in an *in vivo*, intra-articular model, had strength over a 12-week period of implantation similar to that of a comparable metal anchor construct. The absorbable suture anchor offers a reasonable alternative to metal anchors with comparable strength and function with the advantage of being absorbable.

Acknowledging that repair of a torn rotator cuff should have sufficient initial strength to permit a timely and appropriate rehabilitation, prompted Koh and coworkers to explore the hypothesis that augmentation with a woven polylactic acid (PLA) scaffold strengthens repairs of the rotator cuff.[108] Accordingly, in the suture anchor model, these investigators detached 10 pairs of sheep infraspinatus tendons and repaired them with suture anchors. In half of the specimens, the repair was reinforced with a woven PLA scaffold repaired with the tendon to bone. In the bone-bridge model, sutures were passed through a trough and over a bone bridge distal to the greater tuberosity; half were reinforced by the scaffold. The repairs were then tested to failure. Results of the study indicated that the mean ultimate strength of suture-anchor repairs augmented with the scaffold was significantly greater than that of nonaugmented fixation. Failure occurred when the tendon pulled through the sutures. Scaffold reinforcement of the bone bridge significantly increased the ultimate strength, and the scaffold remained intact in 8 of 10 specimens. The overall experimental data led to the conclusion that the scaffold significantly increased the initial strength of rotator cuff repair by approximately 25%.

Relevant to the suture anchor technology is meniscal repair using absorbable implants. Among the issues of concern is implant migration to the surface of the meniscus, which can cause abrasion of the cartilage on the humeral head of the femur. Suture techniques are still the gold standard, but they are difficult to perform. On the other hand, knotless anchor technologies allow a broader spectrum of surgeons to perform a variety of procedures.

6.4 CONCLUSION AND PROSPECTIVE ON THE FUTURE

Applications of polymeric biomaterials in articulating joints have evolved at uneven rates in the different segments of this area. However, future growth in each individual segment is not expected to follow a simple extrapolation of the present status.

An example is the use of polymers as components of prosthetic joints and bone cement. There have been limited changes over the past four decades. However, major future changes are anticipated which may include the use of

Advanced high modulus polymeric composites as low density alternatives to metals for the production of prosthetic joint components.

Absorbable bone cements and fillers having an exceptionally high impact strength and biomechanical compatibility with bone tissue to allow osseointegration. They are expected to be clinically preferred alternatives in certain applications to PMMA bone cement.

Antimicrobial, uniquely designed composite PMMA bone cement that will replace the existing system, which require antibiotic-bearing PMMA beads.

New forms of high T_g thermoplastics or self-reinforced, chemically crosslinked UHMW-PE as alternatives to existing forms of UHMW-PE.

Totally synthetic meniscal implants to provide a long-term functional performance of the natural meniscus.

In a second totally different situation, the use of absorbable polymers has grown significantly in applications dealing with support structures needed for the normal movements of articulating joints, and yet the use of the polymers in the internal bone fixation witnessed limited progress. Analysis of new development in the polymer and composite technologies allows one to project that (1) there will be a major increase in the use of absorbables in internal bone fixation, and particularly in the spine area, and (2) the use of absorbables in support structures will shift dramatically toward the repair and replacement of natural tendons and ligaments. In a third instance, random and yet fast growth in tissue engineering research relative to the use of absorbables is expected to undergo substantial streamlining to focus on the clinically tangible application of the so-called *in situ* tissue engineering — this is based primarily on placing a cell-free scaffold at the defect site and allowing or promoting it to integrate into the site. The fourth instance deals with the use of injectable formulations, which show some promise in the (1) treatment of infection, (2) intracapsular administration of bioactive agents for treating joint diseases and abnormalities, and, to a limited extent, (3) tissue engineering relative to meniscal implants. Fast growth is foreseen in the area of absorbable injectable formulations that may contain microporous microparticles and/or osteoblasts and chondrocytes.

REFERENCES

1. Anthony, C.P. and Thibodeau, G.A., *Textbook of Anatomy and Physiology*, 11th ed., C.V. Mosby, St. Louis, MO, 1983, chap. 6.
2. Kaufman, K.R. and An, K-N., Joint articulating surface motion, in *The Biomedical Engineering Handbook*, Bronzino, J.D., Ed., CRC Press, Boca Raton, FL, 1995, chap. 22.
3. Katz, J.L., Orthopedic applications, in *Biomaterials Science*, Ratner, B.D., Hoffman, A.A., Schoen, F.J., and Lemons, T.S., Eds., Academic Press, New York, 1996, chap. 77, p. 342.
4. Buckley, C.A., Gilbert, J.L., and Lautenschlager, E.P., Thermomechanical processing of PMMA into high strength fibers, *J. Appl. Polym. Sci.*, 44, 1321, 1992.

5. Gilbert, J.L., Ney, D.S., and Lautenschlager, E.P., Self-reinforced composite poly(methyl methacrylate): static and fatigue properties, *Biomaterials*, 16, 1043, 1995.
6. Demian, H.W. and Shalaby, S.W., Bone Cement Composition Containing Microencapsulated Radiopacifier and Methods of Making Same, U.S. Patent No. 5,795,922, 1998.
7. Demian, H.W., Wey, A.C., and Shalaby, S.W., Bone cement with exceptionally uniform dispersion of radiopacifier, *Trans. Soc. Biomater.*, 18, 368, 1995.
8. Demian, H.W. and Shalaby, S.W., Microencapsulated radiopacifier for bone cements to improve fatigue properties, *Proc. Fifth World Biomater. Cong.*, Toronto, Canada, 1996, vol. 1, p. 912.
9. Kurth, M., Eyerer, P., Ascherl, R., Dittel, K., and Holz, U., An evaluation of retrieved UHMW-PE hip-joint cups, in *Ultra High Molecular Weight Polyethylene as Biomaterial in Orthopedic Surgery*, Willert, H.G., Buchhorn, G.H., and Eyerer, P, Eds., Hogrefe & Huber Publishers, Toronto, 1991, p. 208.
10. Leininger, R.I., Changes in properties of plastics during implantation. *Trans. Am. Soc. Artif. Int. Organs*, 10, 320, 1964.
11. Streicher, R.M., The behavior of UHMW-PE when subjected to sterilization by ionizing radiation, in *Ultra-High Molecular Weight Polyethylene as Biomaterials in Orthopedic Surgery*, Willert, H.G., Buchhorn, G.H., and Eyerer, P., Eds., Hogrefe & Huber Publishers, Toronto, 1991, p. 66.
12. Wright, M., Fubayashi, T., and Burnstein, A.H., The effect of carbon reinforcement on contact area, contact pressure and time dependent deformation in polyethylene tibial components, *J. Biomed. Mater. Res.*, 15, 719, 1981.
13. Wright, T.M. and Rimnac, C.J., Analysis of retrieved polyethylene components from total joint replacements, in *Ultra High Molecular Weight Polyethylene as Biomaterials in Orthopedic Surgery*, Willert, H.G., Buchhorn, G.H., and Eyerer, P., Eds., Hogrefe & Huber Publishers, Toronto, 1991, p. 202.
14. Deng, M., Effect of Reinforcement and Irradiation on Thermal and Mechanical Properties of Ultrahigh Molecular Weight Polyethylene, Ph.D. Dissertation, Clemson University, Clemson, SC, 1995.
15. Deng, M. and Shalaby, S.W., Long-term γ irradiation effects on ultrahigh molecular weight polyethylene, *J. Biomed. Mater. Res.*, 54, 428, 2001.
16. Deng, M. and Shalaby, S.W., Properties of self-reinforced ultrahigh molecular weight polyethylene composites, *Trans. Soc. Biomater.*, 20, 219, 1997.
17. Deng, M. and Shalaby, S.W., Unidirectional orientation of ultrahigh molecular weight polyethylene using solid state process, *Trans. Soc. Biomater.*, 20, 215, 1997.
18. Deng, M., Latour, R.A., Ogale, A.A., and Shalaby, S.W., Study of creep behavior of ultrahigh molecular weight polyethylene systems, *J. Biomed. Mater. Res.*, 40, 214, 1998.
19. Deng, M. and Shalaby, S.W., A 5.5 year-post-irradiation aging study on ultrahigh molecular weight polyethylene, *Trans. Soc. Biomater., Sixth World Biomaterials Congress,* I, 2000, p. 37.
20. Pavoor, P.V., Gearing, B.P., Muratoglu, O., Cohen, R.E., and Bellare, A., Wear reduction of orthopedic bearing surfaces using polyelectrolyte multilayer nanocoating, *Biomaterials*, 27, 1527, 2006.
21. Kobayashi, M., Toguchida, J., and Oka, M., Preliminary study of polyvinyl alcohol-hydrogel (PVA-H) artificial meniscus, *Biomaterials*, 24, 639, 2003.
22. Kobayashi, M., Toguchida, J., and Oka, M., Development of an artificial meniscus using polyvinyl alcohol-hydrogel for early return to, and continuance of, athletic life in sportspersons with severe meniscus injury. I: mechanical evaluation, *The Knee* 10, 47, 2003.

23. Kobayashi, M., Chang, Y-S., and Oka, M., A two year in vivo study of polyvinyl alcohol-hydrogel (PPVA-H) artificial meniscus, *Biomaterials*, 26, 3242, 2005.
24. Jennings, A.G., Sefton, G.K., and Newman, R.J., Repair of acute rupture of the Achilles tendon — a new technique using polyester tape without external splintage, *Ann. R. Coll. Surg. Engl.*, 86(6), 445, 2004.
25. Kahn, I., Smith, N., Jones, E., Finch, D.S., and Cameron, R.E., Analysis and evaluation of a biomedical polycarbonate urethane tested in an *in vitro* study and an ovine arthroplasty model. Part I: Material selection, *Biomaterials*, 26(6), 621, 2005.
26. Kahn, I., Smith, N., Jones, E., Finch, D.S., and Cameron, R.E., Analysis and evaluation of a biomedical polycarbonate urethane tested in an *in vitro* study and an ovine arthroplasty model. Part II: *In vivo* investigation, *Biomaterials*, 26(6), 633, 2005.
27. DeSantis, R., Ambrosio, L., and Nicolais, L., Polymer-based hip prosthesis, *J. Inorg. Biochem.*, 79, 97, 2000.
28. Erbe, E.M., Murphy, J.P., and Pomrink, G.J., Bioactive Spinal Implant Material and Method of Manufacture Thereof, U.S. Patent 6,987,136, 2006.
29. Wang, J. and Yu, C., Silicone rubber: an alternative for repair of articular cartilage defects, *Knee Surg. Sports Traumatol. Arthrosc.*, 12, 556, 2004.
30. Christie, A.J., Weinberger, K.A., and Dietrich, M., Silicone lymphadenopathy and synovitis. Complications of silicone elastomer finger joint prostheses., *J.A.M.A.*, 237 1463, 1977.
31. Oka, Y. and Ikada M., Silastic interposition arthroplasty for osteoarthrosis of the carpometacarpal joint of the thumb, *Tokai. J. Exp. Clin. Med.*, 25, 15, 2000.
32. Perlman, M.D., Schor, A.D., and Gold, M.L., Implant failure with particulate silicone synovitis (detritic synovitis), *J. Foot Surg.*, 29, 584, 1990.
33. Ohtsuki, C., Miyazaki, T., Kyomoto, M., Tanihara, M., and Osaka, A, Development of bioactive PMMA-based cement by modification with alkoxysilane and calcium salt, *J. Mater. Sci. Mater. Med.*, 12, 895, 2001.
34. Shalaby, S.W. and Burg, K.J.K., Eds., *Absorbable/Biodegradable Polymers*, CRC Press, Boca Raton, FL, 2004.
35. Hollinger, J.O., Shalaby, S.W., and Jamiolkowski, D.D., Bone repair, a unique class of biodegradable polymers in *Biomedical Applications of Synthetic Biodegradable Polymers,* Hollinger, J.O., Ed., CRC Press, Boca Raton, FL, 1995, p. 197.
36. Middleston, J.C. and Tipton, A.J., Synthetic biodegradable polymers as orthopedic devices, *Biomaterials*, 21, 2335, 2000.
37 Rokkanen, P.U., Bostman, O., Hirvensalo, E., Antero Makela, E., Partio, E.K., Patiala, H., Vainionpaa, S., Vihtonen, K., and Tormala, P., Bioabsorbable fixation in orthopaedic surgery and traumatology, *Biomaterials*, 21, 2607, 2000.
38. Shin, H.J., Lee, C.H., Cho, I.H., Kim, Y.J., Lee, Y.J., Kim, I.A., Park, K.D., Yui, N., and Shin, J.W., Electrospun PLGA nanofiber scaffolds for articular cartilage reconstruction: mechanical stability, degradation and cellular responses under mechanical stimulation *in vitro*, *J. Biomater. Sci. Polym. Ed.*, 17(1–2), 103, 2006.
39. Darrach, W., Anterior dislocation of the head of the ulna, *Ann. Surg.*, 56, 802, 1912.
40. Darrach, W., Partial excision of the lower shaft of the ulna for deformity following Colles' fracture, *Ann. Surg.*, 57, 764, 1913.
41. Della Santa, D. and Chamay, A., Radiological evolution of the rheumatoid wrist after radio-lunate arthrodesis, *J. Hand Surg.*, 20B, 146, 1995.
42. Matsusue, Y., Yamamuro, T., Yoshii, S., Oka, M., Ikeda, Y., Hyon S.H., and Shikinami, Y., Biodegradable screw fixation of rabbit tibia proximal osteotomies, *J. Appl. Biomater.*, 2, 1, 1991.

43. Nakamura, K., Oda, H., Tanaka, S., Kuga, Y., Yamamoto, M., Nishikawa, T., Juju, T., and Shimizu, M., Usefulness of absorbable screws in the Sauve-Kapandji procedure for rheumatoid wrist reconstruction, *Mod. Rheumatol.*, 12, 144, 2002.
44. Ito, H., Minami, A., Tanino, H., and Matsuno, T., Fixation with poly-l-lactic acid screws in hip osteotomy, *Acta Orthop. Scand.*, 73(1), 60, 2002.
45. Viljanen, J.T., Pihlajamaki, H.K., Tormala, P.O., and Rokkanen, P.U., Comparison of the tissue response to absorbable self-reinforced polylactide screws and metallic screws in the fixation of cancellous bone osteotomies: an experimental study on the rabbit distal femur, *J. Ortho. Res.*, 15(3), 398, 2005.
46. Prokop, A., Jubel, A., Helling, H.J., Udomkaewkanjana, B., Brochhagen, H.G., and Rehm, K.E., New biodegradable polylactide implants (Polypin-C) in therapy for radial head fractures, *Chirurgie*, 73(10), 997, 2002.
47. Bagby, G.W., Arthrodesis by the distraction-compression method using a stainless steel implant, *Orthopedics*, 11, 931, 1988.
48. Agazzi, S., Reverdin, A., and May, D., Posterior lumbar interbody fusion with cages: an independent review of 71 cases, *J. Neurosurg.*, 91, 186, 1999.
49. Kuslich, S.D., Ulstrom, C.L., Griffith, S.L., Ahern, J.W., and Dowdle, J.D., The Bagby and Kuslich method of lumbar interbody fusion. History, techniques, and 2-year follow-up results of a United States prospective multicenter trial, *Spine*, 23, 1267, 1998.
50. Brantigan, J.W., Cunningham, B.W., Warden, K., McAfee, P.C., and Steffee, A.D., Compression strength of donor bone for posterior lumbar interbody fusion, *Spine*, 18, 1213, 1993.
51. Weiner, B.K. and Fraser, R.D., Spine update. Lumbar interbody cages, *Spine*, 23, 634, 1998.
52. McAfee, P.C., Interbody fusion cages in reconstructive operations on the spine, *J. Bone Joint Surg. Am.*, 81, 859, 1999.
53. van Dijk, M., Tunc, D.C., Smit, T.H., Higham, P., Burger, E.H., and Wuisman, P.I.J.M., *In vitro* and *in vivo* degradation of bioabsorbable PLLA spinal fusion cages, *Biomed. Mater. Res. Appl. Biomater.*, 63, 752, 2002.
54. Guerra, D, Frizziero, L., Losi, M., Bacchelli, B., Mezzadri, G., and Pasquali Ronchetti, I., Ultrastructural identification of a membrane-like structure on the surface of normal articular cartilage, *J. Submicrosc. Cytol. Pathol.*, 28, 385, 1996.
55. Dahl, L.B., Dahl, I.M., Enstrom-Laurent, A., and Granath, K., Concentration and molecular weight of sodium hyaluronate in synovial fluid from patients with rheumatoid arthritis and other anthropathies, *Ann. Rheum. Dis.*, 44, 817, 1985.
56. Hinton, R.H., Moody, R.L., Davis, A.W., and Thomas, S.F., Osteoarthritis: diagnosis and therapeutic considerations, *Am. Fam. Physician*, 65, 841, 2002.
57. Oddis, C.V., New perspectives on osteoarthritis, *Am. J. Med.*, 100, 10S, 1996.
58. Peyron, J.G. and Balazs, E.A., Preliminary clinical assessment of Na-hyaluronate injection in human arthritic joint. *Pathol. Biol.*, 22, 7131, 1974.
59. Barbucci, R., Lamponi, S., Borzachiello, A., Ambrosio, L., Fini, M., Torricelli, P., and Giardino, R., Hyaluronic acid hydrogel in the treatment of osteoarthritis, *Biomaterials*, 23, 4503, 2002.
60. Barbucci, R., Fini, M., Giavaresi, G., Torricelli, P., Giardino, R., Lamponi, S., and Leone, G., Hyaluronic acid hydrogel added with ibuprofen-lysine for the local treatment of chondral lesions in the knee: *in vitro* and *in vivo* investigations, *J. Biomed. Mater. Res., Appl. Biomater.*, 75B, 42, 2005.

61. Yoon, J.B., Kim, S.G., Hwang, S.G., Chang, S., Kang, S.S., and Chun, J.S., Nonsteroidal anti-inflammatory drugs inhibit nitric oxide-induced apoptosis and dedifferentiation of articular chondrocytes independent cyclooxygenase activity, *J. Biol. Chem.*, 278, 15319, 2003.
62. Mukherjee, P., Rachita, C., Aisen, P.S., and Pasinetti, G.M., Non-steroidal anti-inflammatory drugs against chondrocytes apoptotic death, *Clin. Exp. Rheumatol.* 19, S7, 2001.
63. Bragdon, B., Bertone, A.L., Hardy, J, Simmons, E.J., and Weisbrode, S.E., Use of an isolated joint model to detect early changes induced by intra-articular injection of paclitaxel-impregnated polymeric microspheres, *J. Invest. Surg.*, 14, 169, 2001.
64. Liggins, R.T., Cruz, T., Min, W., Liang, L., Hunter, W.L., and Burt, H.M., Intra-articular treatment of arthritis with microsphere formulations of paclitaxel: biocompatibility and efficacy determinations in rabbits, *Inflamm. Res.*, 53, 363, 2004.
65. Grassi, W., De Angelis, R., Lamanna, G., and Cervini, C., The clinical features of rheumatoid arthritis, *Eur. J. Radiol.*, 27(Suppl. 1), S18, 1998.
66. Ryan, L. and Brooks, P., Disease-modifying anti-rheumatic drugs, *Curr. Opin. Rheumatol.*, 11, 161, 1999.
67. Theodore, P., O'Dell, J.R., and Kremer, J.M., Combination therapy with multiple disease-modifying antirheumatic drugs in rheumatoid arthritis: a preventive strategy, *Ann. Int. Med.*, 131, 768, 1999.
68. Liang, L.S., Jackson, J., Min, W., Risovic, V., Wassan, K.M., and Burt, H.M., Methotrexate loaded poly(L-lactic acid) microspheres for intra-articular delivery of methotrexate to the joint, *J. Pharm. Sci.*, 93(4), 943, 2004.
69. Lee, S.H., Suh, J.-S., Kim, H., S., Lee, J.D., Song, J., and Lee, S.K., MR evaluation of radiation synovectomy of the knee by means of intra-articular injection of holmium-166-chitosan complex in patients with rheumatoid arthritis: Results at 4-month follow-up, *Korean J. Radiol.*, 4, 170, 2003.
70. Sakano, Y., Terada, N., Ueda, H., Fujii, Y., Hamada, Y., Akamatsu, N., and Ohno, S., Histological study of articular cartilage in experimental rat knee arthritis induced by intracapsular injection of cationic polyethyleneimine, *Med. Electron Microsc.*, 33, 246, 2000.
71. Marra, K.G., Biodegradable polymers and microspheres, in *Bone Tissue Engineering*, Hollinger, J.O., Einhorn, T.A., Doll, B.A., and Sfeir, C., Eds., CRC Press, Boca Raton, FL, 2005, chap. 6.
72. deGroot, J.H., Polyurethane scaffolds for meniscal tissue regeneration (Materials), *Med. Dev. Tech.*, 16/17, 18, 2005.
73. Rodkey, W.G., Steadman, J.R., and Shu-Tung, L., Clinical study of collagen meniscus implant to restore the injured meniscus, *Clin. Orthop.*, S367, 281, 1999.
74. Steadman, J.R., and Rodkey, W.G., Tissue-engineering collagen meniscus implants: 5- to 6-year feasibility study results, *Arthroscopy*, 21(5), 515, 2005.
75. deGroot, J.H., deVrijer, R., Wildeboer, B.S., Spaans, C.S., and Pennings, A.J., New biomedical polyurethane-ureas with high tear strength, *Polym. Bull.*, 38, 211, 1997.
76. Neves, A.A., Medcalf, N., and Brindle, K.M., Influence of stirring-induced mixing on cell proliferation and extracellular matrix deposition in meniscal cartilage constructs based on polyethylene terephthalate scaffolds, *Biomaterials*, 26, 4828, 2005.
77. Cima, L.G., Vacanti, J.P., Vacanti, C.A., Ingber, D., Mooney, D., and Langer, R., Tissue engineering by cell transplantation using degradable polymer substrates, *Biomech. Eng.*, 113, 143, 1991.

78. Vacanti, C.A., Langer, R., Schloo, B., and Vacanti, J.P., Synthetic polymers seeded with chondrocytes provide a template for new cartilage formation, *Plast. Recon. Surg.*, 88, 753, 1991.
79. Langer, R. and Vacanti, J.P., Tissue engineering: the challenges ahead, *Sci. Am.*, 280, 62, 1997.
80. Chen, G.Q. and Wu, Q., The application of polyhydroxyalkanoates as tissue engineering materials, *Biomaterials*, 26, 6565, 2005.
81. Gutowska, A., Jeong, B., and Jasionowski, M., Injectable gels for tissue engineering, *Anal. Rec.*, 263, 342, 2001.
82. Shalaby, S.W., Hydrogel-Forming, Self-Solvating Absorbable Polyester Copolymers, and Methods for Use Thereof, U.S. Patent (Composition) 5,612,052, 1997.
83. Shalaby, S.W., Hydrogel-Forming, Self-Solvating Absorbable Polyester Copolymers, and Methods for Use Thereof, U.S. Patent (Uses) 5,714,159, 1998.
84. Paige, K.T., Cima, L.G., Yaremchuk, M.J., Vacanti, J.P., and Vacanti, C.A., Injectable cartilage, *Plast. Recon. Surg.*, 96, 1390, 1995.
85. Elson, M.L., Soft tissue augmentation. A review, *Dermatol. Surg.*, 21, 491, 1995.
86. Klokkevold, P.R., Vandemark, L., Kenny, E.B., and Bernard, G.W., Osseogenesis enhanced by chitosan poly(*N*-acetyl glucosaminoglycan) *in vitro*, *J. Periodontol* 67, 1170, 1996.
87. Mortensen, K., and Pedersen, S., Structural study on micelle formation of poly(ethylene oxide)-poly(propylene oxide)-poly(ethylene oxide) triblock copolymers in aqueous solution, *Macromolecules*, 26, 805, 1993.
88. Martinsen, A., Skjak-Braek, G., and Smidsrod, O., Alginate as immobilization material I. Correlation between chemical and physical properties of alginate gel beads, *Biotech. Bioeng.*, 33, 79, 1989.
89. Sims, C.D., Butler, P., Casanova, R., Lee, B.T., Randolph, M.A., Lee, A., Vacanti, C.A., and Yaremchuk, M.J., Injectable cartilage using polyethylene oxide polymer substrates, *Plast. Recon. Surg.*, 95, 843, 1996.
90. Web, D., An, Y.H., Gutowska, A., Mironov, V.A., and Friedman, R.J., Propagation of chondrocytes using thermosensitive polymer gel culture, *Orthoped. J. Musc. Orthoped. Surg.*, 3, 18, 2000.
91. Wang, X., Grogan, S.P., Rieser, F., Winkelmann, V., Maquet, V., LaBerge, M., and Maini-Varlet, P., Tissue engineering of Biphasic cartilage constructs using various biodegradable scaffolds: an *in vitro* study, *Biomaterials*, 25, 3681, 2004.
92. Uematsu, K., Hattori, K., Ishimoto, Y., Yamauchi, J., Habata, T., Takakura, Y., Ohgushi, H., Fukuchi, T., and Sato, M., Cartilage regeneration using mesenchymal stem cells and a three-dimensional poly-lactic-glycolic acid (PLGA) scaffold, *Biomaterials*, 26, 4273, 2005.
93. Kose, G.T., Korkusuz, F., Ozkul, A., Soysal, Y., Ozdemir, T., Yildiz, C., and Hasirci, V., Tissue engineered cartilage on collagen and PHBV matrices, *Biomaterials*, 26, 5187, 2005.
94. Laurencin, C. and Freeman, J.W., Ligament tissue engineering: an evolutionary materials science approach, *Biomaterials*, 26, 7530, 2005.
95. Beynnon, B.D. and Fleming, B.D., Anterior cruciate ligament strain *in vivo*: a review of previous work, *J. Biomech.*, 31, 519, 1998.
96. Pennisi, E., Tending tender tendons, *Science*, 295, 1011, 2002.
97. Matsumoto, H. and Fujikawa, K., Leeds-Keio artificial ligament: A new concept for the anterior cruciate ligament reconstruction of the knee, *Keio. J. Med.*, 50(3), 161, 2001.

98. Noyes, F.R., Butler, D.L., Paulos, L.E., and Grood, E.S., Intra-articular cruciate reconstruction. I: perspectives on graft strength, vascularization, and immediate motion after replacement, *Clin. Orthop. Relat. Res.*, 172, 71, 1983.
99. Cooper, J.A., Lu, H.H., Ko, F.K., Freeman, J.W., and Laurencin, C.T., Fiber-based tissue-engineered scaffold for ligament replacement: design considerations and *vitro* evaluation, *Biomaterials*, 26(13), 1523, 2005.
100. Bach, F.D., Carlier, R.Y., Elis, J.B., Mompoint, D.M., Feydy, A., Judet, O., Beaufils, P., and Vallee, C., Anterior cruciate ligament reconstruction with bioabsorbable polyglycolic acid interference screws: MR imaging follow-up, *Radiology*, 225(2), 541, 2002.
101. Morgan, C.D., Gehrmann, R.M., Jayo, M.J., and Johnson, C.S., Histologic findings with a bioabsorbable anterior cruciate ligament interference screw explant after 2.5 years in vivo, *Arthroscopy*, 18(9), E47, 2002.
102. Klein, S.A., Nyland, J., Kocabey, Y., Wozniak, T., Nawab, A., and Caborn, D.N., Tendon graft fixation in ACL reconstruction: *in vitro* evaluation of bioabsorbable tenodesis screw, *Acta Orthop. Scand.*, 75(1), 84, 2004.
103. Hooper, K., Cox, J., and Kohn, J., Comparison of the effect of ethylene oxide and γ-irradiation on selected tyrosine-derived polycarbonates and poly(L-lactic acid), *J. Appl. Polym. Sci.*, 63, 1499, 1997.
104. Choueka, J., Charvet, J., Koval, K., Alexander, H., James, K., Hooper, K., and Kohn, J., Canine bone response to tyrosine-derived polycarbonates and poly(L-lactic acid), *J. Biomater. Res.*, 31, 35–41, 1996.
105. Thal, R., A knotless suture anchor, *Am. J. Sports Med.*, 29, 646, 2001.
106. Lee, S., Mahar, A., Bynum, K., and Pedowitz, R., Biomechanical comparison of bioabsorbable sutureless screw anchor versus suture anchor fixation for rotator cuff repair, *Arthroscopy*, 21(1), 43, 2005.
107. Dejong, E.S., DeBerardina, T.M., Brooks, D.E., and Judson, K., *In vivo* comparison of a metal versus a biodegradable suture anchor, *Arthroscopy*, 20(5), 511, 2004.
108. Koh, J.L., Szomor, Z., Murrell, G.A., and Warren, R.F., Supplementation of rotator cuff repair with a bioresorbable scaffold, *Am. J. Sports Med.*, 30(3), 410, 2002.

Section C

Development in Preparative, Processing, and Evaluation Methods

7 Physicochemical Properties of Bioactive Polymeric Composites: Effects of Resin Matrix and the Type of Amorphous Calcium Phosphate Filler

J.M. Antonucci and D. Skrtic

CONTENTS

7.1 INTRODUCTION

For decades, polymeric composites have been used in several dental and orthopedic applications because of the ability to tailor-make these materials to meet specific requirements at different biological sites. The recognition that the bony tissues that these composites interface with are partly made of calcium phosphate–based materials led consistently to the use of these materials as fillers in a number of polymeric composites. The use of calcium phosphate–based fillers has been associated with excellent biocompatibility of several commercial and experimental dental and orthopedic composites. A key determinant for the success of the calcium phosphate–based fillers is their *in vivo* absorption profile and subsequent release of their biologically active ions. In most cases, the absorption profile of these inorganic materials is controlled not only by their chemical composition, but also by whether they are amorphous or crystalline as well as the surface-to-volume ratio of filler particles. Among the most useful calcium phosphate–based fillers is amorphous calcium phosphate (ACP), which offers a great deal of flexibility in terms of property modulation to meet demanding clinical requirements. This chapter focuses on the chemistry of ACP and its effective use in composites for dental applications.

7.2 AMORPHOUS CALCIUM PHOSPHATE (ACP): CHEMISTRY AND IMPORTANCE IN DENTISTRY

Calcium phosphates (CaPs) are of significant relevance to dentistry because of their involvement in both normal dentition (enamel and dentin formation) and pathological mineralization (dental calculus) and demineralization (dental caries). ACP is unique among the CaPs as the only noncrystalline compound within the group (see Table 7.1).

ACP forms instantaneously during the spontaneous precipitation from supersaturated basic Ca^{2+} and PO_4^{3-} aqueous solutions. Its structural, chemical, and thermodynamic properties are extensively discussed in a recent review article by Eanes. ACP is generally viewed as a precursor to hydroxyapatite (HAP) formation both *vitro* and *in vivo.*[1,2] HAP is a thermodynamically stable form of CaP in neutral and basic environments. The rate of ACP conversion to HAP depends primarily on the chemistry of the microenvironment. As a result of this conversion, the crystallinity of the solid and its Ca^{2+}/PO_4^{3-} ratio increase with time. The process can be affected by the presence of inorganic anions, cations, or organic molecules, which can adsorb on the ACP surface, incorporate into the ACP structure, and/or coprecipitate with ACP.

CaP-based dental restorative and sealant materials are primarily appealing because of their biocompatibility. ACP-based materials provide a virtually continuous

TABLE 7.1
Calcium Phosphate (CaP) Compounds of Biological Importance

CaP	Compositional Formula	Ca/PO$_4$ Molar Ratio	Acronym
Amorphous calcium phosphate	$Ca_3(PO_4)_2{\cdot}3H_2O$[b]	1.50	ACP
Monocalacium phosphate anhydrous	$Ca(H_2PO_4)_2$	0.50	MCPA
Dicalcium phosphate anhydrous	$CaHPO_4$	1.00	DCPA
Dicalcium phosphate dihydrate	$CaHPO_4{\cdot}2H_2O$	1.00	DCPD
Tricalcium phosphate (α- or β- form)	α-$Ca_3(PO_4)_2$; β-$Ca_3(PO_4)_2$	1.50	α-TCP; β-TCP
Tetracalcium phosphate	$Ca_4O(PO_4)_2$	2.00	TTCP
Octacalcium phosphate pentahydrate	$Ca_8H_2(PO_4)_6{\cdot}5H_2O$	1.33	OCP
Hydroxyapatite	$Ca_{10}(PO_4)_6(OH)_2$	1.67	HAP
Fluorapatite	$Ca_{10}(PO_4)_6F_2$	1.67	FAP

[a] Indicated acronyms will be used throughout this chapter.
[b] Approximate formula.

supply of Ca^{2+} and PO_4^{3-} ions needed to re-form damaged mineral structures and counteract recurrent decay, such as occurs near the surfaces of teeth in contact with conventional fillings (almost 50% of all dental fillings require replacement because of recurrent caries). These ACP materials fall into the category of bioactive dental materials. Such antidemineralizing–remineralizing composites may be particularly useful for patients that are susceptible to cavities as a result of radiation therapy, and diseases or medications that cause dry mouth. When embedded in polymerized methacrylate matrices and exposed to an aqueous environment, ACP releases sufficient levels of remineralizing ions in such a way as to promote redeposition of thermodynamically stable, apatitic tooth mineral.[3–6]

A problem with ACP based composites is their inability to resist cracking under masticatory stress because of their low strength and toughness. The uncontrolled aggregation of ACP particles was identified as one of the main reasons for a poor interfacial interaction with dental resin matrices, which leads to the mechanical inferiority of these materials when compared with glass-reinforced composites.[7] overcome this shortcoming, we have focused on developing strategies for improving the ACP filler–polymer matrix interfacial properties (and, in turn, composite properties) by better controlling the particle size distribution and surface properties of ACP fillers and/or by fine-tuning the chemical structures of the resin.[7–11] These issues were the main targets of our ACP studies to date.

From an application perspective, our goals were to formulate ACP base and lining materials, pit and fissure sealants, and adhesive cement capable of minimizing the demineralization that frequently occurs under orthodontic brackets. Extensive physicochemical studies are being performed in our group on various ACP polymeric composites.[3–11] The knowledge obtained through the combined ACP surface modification and resin matrix selection will serve as the basis for extending the utility of ACP composites to endodontic applications in near future. By employing innovative composite approaches, we will broaden ACP's clinical utility beyond already proposed topical gels, toothpastes, and/or mouthrinses[12] or as phosphopeptide-ACP nanoclusters in sugar-free chewing gums and glass ionomers.[13,14] In this chapter methodologies used for evaluating the effect(s) of the types of resin matrices and bioactive ACP fillers on the selected physicochemical properties of copolymers and composites are presented. Also discussed is a possible correlation(s) between some of the physicochemical parameters and the biocompatibility of ACP-based resin materials.

7.3 ACP BASED COMPOSITES: PHYSICOCHEMICAL AND BIOCOMPATIBILITY ASPECTS

Dental composites are made up of a polymer matrix phase (usually methacrylate based), a filler phase (commonly glass, quartz, or ceramic oxide particulates; in our case ACP), and a little understood interphase that results from interaction of the organic and inorganic phases. Coupling agents such as silanes are commonly used to improve the bonding at the filler–polymer matrix interface, typically when the filler is siliceous. It is important to review the chemistry of composites for an appreciation of the potential for interactions of monomer components of these materials and the oral environment. It is also important to consider the biodegradation of composite and adhesive chemistries at the interface with tooth structures. The susceptibility to degradation (inherent in the choice of chemistries selected for the formulation of dental composites) is promoted by salivary enzymes and related cofactors, generating defined chemical products.[15] The latter products may modulate the biological activity of cells and oral bacteria that interface with restorative material.

Typically dental resins contain a relatively viscous base monomer and a diluent comonomer. The base monomer in the resin serves to minimize the polymerization shrinkage by virtue of its relatively large molecular volume and to enhance the modulus of the cured polymer, while the diluent monomer provides good handling properties and improves copolymer conversion because of its greater flexibility and smaller molecular volume.[16] The list of the monomer acronyms to be used throughout this chapter is provided in Table 7.2. The most commonly utilized copolymers are

TABLE 7.2
Monomers and Components of the Photoinitiator Systems with their Commonly Used Acronyms

2,2-*bis*[p-(2'-Hydroxy-3_-methacryloxypropoxy)phenyl]propane	Bis-GMA
Tri(ethyleneglycol) dimethacrylate	TEGDMA
Ethoxylated bisphenol A dimethacrylate	EBPADMA
Urethane dimethacrylate	UDMA
2-Hydroxyethyl methacrylate	HEMA
Methacryloyloxyethyl phtalate	MEP
Camphorquinone and ethyl-4-*N,N*-dimethylaminobenzoate	CQ & 4EDMAB
bis(2,6-Dimethoxybenzoyl)-2,4,4-trimethylpentyl phosphine oxide and 1-hydroxycyclohexyl phenyl ketone	IRGACURE 1850

based on the base monomer Bis-GMA and the diluent monomer TEGDMA. The hydroxyl groups of Bis-GMA and the ethylene oxide segments of TEGDMA contribute to the relatively high water sorption of Bis-GMA/TEGDMA copolymers. High concentrations of the more rigid structure of Bis-GMA typically result in monomer systems with relatively low degrees of cure or conversion. Polymerization shrinkage, relatively low cure efficiency at ambient temperatures, and plasticization of Bis-GMA/TEGDMA copolymers by oral fluids affect the service life of these composites. Alternative base monomers and/or diluent monomers have been explored to overcome some of the known shortcomings of the Bis-GMA/TEGDMA copolymers. Dental polymers based on EBPADMA, a relatively hydrophobic analog of Bis-GMA with a more flexible structure and lower viscosity, show higher degrees of cure and lower polymerization shrinkages than Bis-GMA/TEGDMA mixtures.

The mechanical properties of polymeric composites crucially depend upon the condition of the interface between surfaces of the inorganic filler particles and the polymerized organic resin in which the filler particles are embedded.[19] The homogeneity of the filler–matrix interface may directly control the sorption of water and the subsequent release of potentially irritating organic moieties. To better resist the destructive environment that exists inside the human oral cavity, the filler in the polymer matrix must have a fairly uniform distribution, i.e., the uneven formation of filler-rich and filler-poor areas (voids, non-bonding spaces) must be minimized. Usually, the improved mechanical performance of composite is achieved with a high degree of conversion (DC) of methacrylate groups. However, the dilemma is that whatever enhances the DC can lead to the clinically unfavorable condition of enhanced polymerization shrinkage (PS) and to the development of internal stresses that can lead to adhesive or cohesive failures. PS can also cause microleakage (passage of fluids, bacteria, ions, molecules, etc., between a restorative material and the prepared tooth surface). This hostile microenvironment can yield to secondary caries and further diminish the biostability of the material.[20]

The ultimate goal of resin design and selection is to achieve matrices suitable for the uniform incorporation of particulate ACP fillers that yield high DC upon curing and improved adhesion of the composite to tooth structures without having adverse effects on PS. We hypothesize that through the enhanced interaction(s) with the ACP filler certain resin systems will also improve matrix–filler coherence. Our systematic studies are expected to provide information on the relationship(s) among the chemical structure, DC, and relative cross-link density of polymeric matrices and the thermodynamic stability and mechanical behavior of their ACP composites.

As mentioned previously, the main advantages of CaP-based biomaterials designed for dental and/or orthopedic bone tissue regeneration are their osteoconductivity and biocompatibility.[21–23] Both vary with the type of CaP utilized.[24–28] The biocompatibility arises from their chemical composition, which resembles that of the inorganic phase of natural mineralized tissues. HAP is the main inorganic constituent of hard tissues, and free calcium and phosphate ions can be used in metabolism.[23,29] Reportedly, the biocompatibility of various CaP cements is attributed to either the biocompatibility of their individual constituents (α- and β-TCP, DCPD, TTCP, and HAP) or the biocompatibility of the reaction product(s) (predominantly Ca-deficient

HAP, traces of DCPD).[30–34] CaPs with solubility above that of hydroxyapatite (HAP) are reactive and expected to contribute to bone formation by osteoblasts.[35]

Despite considerable research efforts, the mechanism by which the more soluble CaPs promote osteogenesis remains unclear.[31,35–37] We have found that copolymers derived from highly converted resins also yield polymeric ACP composites with high DC (i.e., the low leachability of unreacted monomeric species, which is taken as an indirect measure of high biocompatibility) and favorable ion (Ca^{2+} and PO_4 release profiles.[7,38] In our evaluations thus far we have consistently used the DC as an indirect indicator of the material's biocompatibility. More recently, to shed some light on the possible interactions between the ACP filler and/or ACP composites and osteoblastlike cells, we have performed an *in vitro* study of their cytotoxicity.[39]

It is important to mention that in preparing the fast-setting CaP cements described in the literature, no ions other than calcium, phosphate, sodium, and/or potassium are utilized. The ACP used in our experimental composite was synthesized in the presence of zirconyl chloride for the purpose of improving ACP's intracomposite stability upon exposure to aqueous milieu.[3] Such Zr-stabilized ACP usually contains a mass fraction of $(8.6 \pm 1.4)\%$ Zr.[6] Although the significance of Ca ions in bone mineralization is well established, the ability of extracellular calcium to regulate specific cell responses has been demonstrated only recently.[40,41] The ability of osteoblasts to transport PO_4^{3-} was also recognized as a prerequisite for bone mineralization.[42] Cellular receptors for both Ca^{2+} and PO_4^{3-} have been identified.[40,43] There is also evidence that Si plays an important role in bone metabolism, but a cellular receptor for Si has not been identified.[41,42] At this point no evidence on the potential role of Zr in hard tissue mineralization and its interaction(s) is available. It is, however, possible that the coprecipitation of Zr into the ACP solid could have some effect on mitochondrial dehydrogenase activity of cells cultured in the extract of Zr–ACP-filled resin matrices. A series of cell viability experiments using nonstabilized ACP (ACP synthesized without any hybridizing or tabilizing ion) would be necessary to test this possibility.

Polymerization of dental resin composites is usually less complete than that of the unfilled resin, and almost every component can be detected in the extracts of polymerized materials.[44,45] Some of the released, unpolymerized resin monomers may elicit various biological effects such as genetic mutations *in vitro*.[46] Among commonly used methacrylate monomers, TEGDMA has been reported as directly mutagenic in a mammalian cell gene mutation assay while no mutagenic effects were detected with UDMA and HEMA. No information was available for EBPADMA, a base monomer frequently used in our experimental copolymer and composite formulations. On the other hand, cytotoxicity of the resin components of composites and adhesives (expressed as a concentration that suppresses the mitochondrial activity by 50%, i.e., TC_{50} concentration) was ranked as follows UDMA > TEGDMA > HEMA after 72 h exposure to Balb/c 3T3 mouse fibroblasts.[47]

The chemical-structure property relations of the constituent monomers, compositional differences involving polymers and photoinitiator systems, and DC, especially as it relates to the potential presence of leachable monomers, are important contributing factors that control the cellular response. The total residual vinyl unsaturation from photopolymerization that is measured by FTIR consists of the pendent vinyl groups in the matrix phase plus residual monomeric species that arise from the polymerization process. The combined DC studies and leachability measurements should be correlated with the physicochemical evaluation of both copolymers and their composites as well as with cytotoxicity tests.

7.4 METHODS AND TECHNIQUES FOR PHYSICOCHEMICAL EVALUATION OF COPOLYMERS AND ACP COMPOSITES

The main objectives of the ongoing research on ACP based dental materials are: (1) to develop strategies that better control ACP's dispersion in the polymer matrix and (2) to investigate intracomposite and composite–tooth interactions to determine the mechanisms that govern mineral redeposition from the composites. The methodologies and techniques that are used to validate ACP fillers and physicochemically evaluate the unfilled resins (copolymers) and their ACP composites are summarized in Table 7.3. The indicated acronyms are used throughout this chapter.

7.4.1 X-Ray Diffraction (XRD), Fourier Transform Infrared (FTIR) Spectroscopy, and FTIR-Microspectroscopy (FTIR-M)

The amorphous state of ACP is verified by powder X-ray diffraction (XRD; Rigaku DMAX 2000 X-ray diffractometer, Rigaku/USA Inc., Danvers, MA) and Fourier-transform spectroscopy (FTIR; Nicolet Magna-IR FTIR 550 spectrophotometer,

TABLE 7.3
Methods and Techniques Utilized in Physicochemical Characterization of ACP Fillers, Monomers, Copolymers, and Composites

Method	Property
Fourier-transform infrared (FTIR) spectroscopy and microspectroscopy (FTIR-m)	Structure/composition of the monomers, ACP fillers and composites
	Degree of conversion (DC) of copolymers and composites
	Surface characterization of copolymers and composites
X-ray diffraction (XRD)	Long-range crystalline order of the fillers
Particle size analysis	Particle size distribution (PSD) of ACP fillers
Scanning electron microscopy (SEM)	Morphology and/or topology of ACP fillers
Thermogravimetry	Water content (structural vs. surface-bound) of ACP fillers
Ultraviolet/visible (UV/VIS) spectrophotometry	Compositional analysis of ACP fillers (Ca/PO_4 ratio)
	Kinetics of Ca^{2+} and PO_4^{3-} release from composites
Dilatometry	Polymerization shrinkage (PS) of composites
Mechanical testing	Biaxial flexure strength (BFS) of copolymers and composites
Gravimetry	Water sorption (WS) of copolymers and composites

Nicolet Instrumentations Inc., Madison, WI).[6,7] XRD patterns are recorded from 4 to 60° 2θ with CuKα radiation (λ = 0.154 nm) at 40 kV and 40 mA. ACP samples are step-scanned in intervals of 0.010° 2θ at a scanning speed of 1.000°/min. The FTIR spectra (4000–400 cm–[1]) of ACP specimens are recorded using a KBr pellet technique (0.8–1.0 mg solid/400 mg KBr). The FTIR spectra of the resins are obtained in transmission mode from thin films of the neat resins between KBr plates.

Mid-FTIR is also used to determine the degree of vinyl conversion (DC) of the unfilled resins (copolymers) and their ACP-filled composites by monitoring the reduction in the 1637 cm–[1] absorption band for the vinyl group against that of an unchanged aromatic peak.[11] FTIR spectra are usually acquired before photopolymerization, immediately after cure, as well as 24 h and 7 d postcure by collecting 64 scans at 2 wavenumber resolutions. Triplicate measurements are performed for each experimental group.

The FTIR spectrophotometer equipped with a video camera and a computerized motorized mapping stage (FTIR-m; Spectra-Tech Inc., Shelton, CT) is used to analyze intact copolymer and composite surfaces as well as cross-sections of copolymer and composite specimens in dry and wet states (after exposure to aqueous environment). The usefulness of FTIR-m in producing functional group maps representative of the organic matrix and the inorganic filler distributions is described in detail in Skritic et al.[7]

7.4.2 Particle Size Distribution (PSD)

The PSD of the ACP fillers is measured using a laser light scattering particle size analyzer (Ankersmid C100 computerized inspection system for particle size analysis and dynamic shape characterization, Metropolitan Computing Corporation, E. Hanover, NJ). ACP powder is dispersed in isopropanol and ultrasonicated for 10 min at room temperature prior to the analysis (triplicate runs for each experimental group). From the PSD(s), the median particle size diameter (d_m) of the sample is obtained. Changes in d_m are taken as a primary indicator of alterations in the aggregation of the ACP particulates (the higher the d_m value, the more aggregated the ACP).[8,48] In addition to PSD analysis, the ACP specimens are also routinely compared morphologically (SEM analysis).

7.4.3 Scanning Electron Microscopy (SEM)

Surface morphology and topology of ACP powders is conveniently determined by SEM (JSM-5400 instrument JEOL Inc., Peabody, MA). SEM is also used to examine: (a) composite disk surfaces before, during (disks may be cut perpendicular to their flat surfaces and the cut faces examined), and after immersion in the test solutions.[6,38] In composite–dentin bonding studies, argon ion etching techniques are used to observe the dentin-adhesive interphase.

7.4.4 Thermogravimetry

Thermal decomposition profiles of ACP fillers are determined by thermogravimetric analysis (TGA; Perkin Elmer 7 Series Thermal Analysis System, Perkin Elmer,

Norwalk, CT) by heating 5–10 mg of powdered ACP at the rate of 20°C/min (30–600°C temperature range) in air. The overall water content (mass fraction, %), relative ratio of the surface-bound to structural water, and the level of structurally incorporated organics is then determined from the TGA profiles.

7.4.5 Chemical Analysis

Calcium and phosphate ion concentrations of various ACPs are determined following the dissolution of fillers in HCl. For the spectrophotometric determination of Ca ion complexation with Arsenazo-III has been adopted. Phosphate ion is determined as a blue molybdato complex in an acidified ammonium molybdate solution. The absorbances are measured spectrophotometrically (UV/VIS Carey Model 219 spectrophotometer, Varian Analytical Instruments, Palo Alto, CA) at the wavelengths of 650 and 882 nm for Ca^{2+} and PO_4^{3-}, respectively. Detailed description of the analytical procedures are provided in references 4 and 6.

7.4.6 Polymerization Shrinkage (PS)

The PS of composite resin samples is measured by a computer-controlled mercury dilatometer (Paffenbarger Research Center, American Dental Association Foundation, Gaithersburg, MD). A schematic diagram of the dilatometer is given in Figure 7.1. Composite pastes are irradiated twice, initially for 60 s followed by a second irradiation of 30 s after 60 min. Data acquisition is for a total of 90 min. A minimum of triplicate runs are performed for each experimental group.[6] Volumetric shrinkage of a specimen corrected for temperature fluctuations during the measurement is plotted as a function of time. The overall shrinkage (volume fraction, %) is calculated

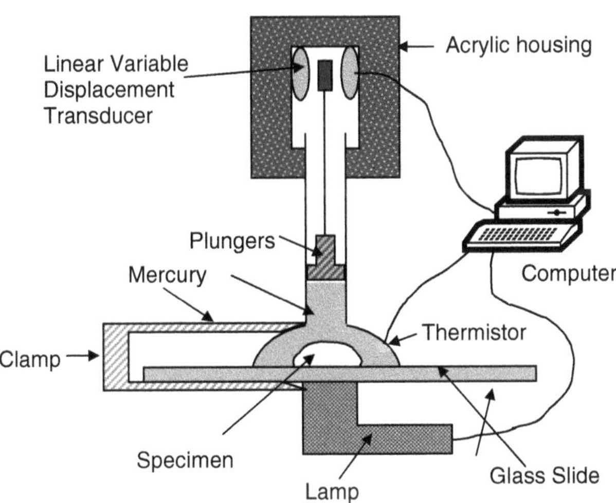

FIGURE 7.1 Schematic diagram of a computer-controlled mercury dilatometer utilized for polymerization shrinkage (PS) measurements.

based on the known mass of the sample (50–100 mg) and its density. The latter is conveniently determined by means of the Archimedean displacement principle using an attachment to a microbalance (Sartorius YDK01 Density Determination Kit; Sartorius AG, Goettingen, Germany).

7.4.7 Mechanical Strength

Biaxial flexure strength (BFS) testing (Figure 7.2) is systematically used to evaluate the mechanical strength of various bioactive ACP composites.[4,6,8–11,48] To determine the BFS of copolymers and composites, we utilize a piston-on-three-ball loading cell and a computer-controlled Universal Testing Machine (Instron 5500R, Instron Corp., Canton, MA) operated by Testworks 4 software. The BFS values are calculated according to the following equation[49]:

$$\mathrm{BFS} = AL/t^2$$

where $A = -[3/4\pi(X - Y)]$, $X = (1 + \nu)\ \ln\ (r_1/r_s)^2 + [(1 - \nu)/2](r_1/r_s)^2$, $Y = (1 + \nu)[1\ \ln(r_{sc}/r_s)^2]$, and where ν = Poisson's ratio, r_1 = radius of the piston applying the load at the surface of contact, r_{sc} = radius of the support circle, r_s = radius of disk specimen, L = applied load at failure, and t = thickness of disk specimen.

When required, the same testing machine and software are utilized for the diametral tensile strength (DTS), flexural strength (FS), and modulus (E) determinations.

7.4.8 Gravimetry and Water Sorption

Water sorption (WS) of composite specimens is determined as follows. A minimum of seven replicate disks in each experimental group is initially dried over CaSO

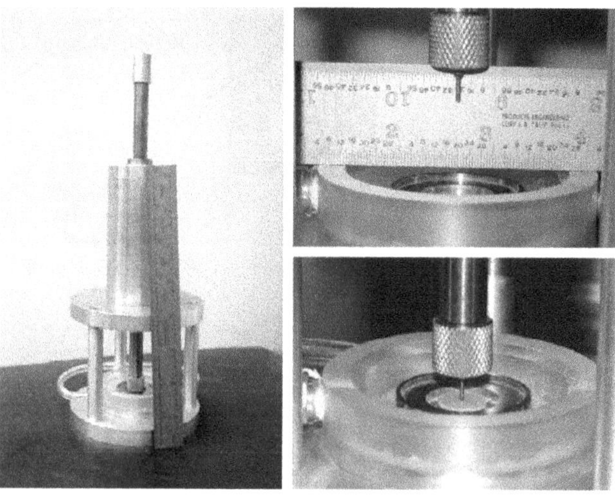

FIGURE 7.2 Biaxial flexure strength (BFS) testing jig (left side) and the close-up of the piston-on-three-ball loading arrangement (images on the right side).

until a constant mass is achieved (±0.1 mg).[8,9] Specimens are then exposed to an air atmosphere of 75% relative humidity (RH) at 37°C by keeping them suspended over a saturated aqueous NaCl slurry in closed systems. Gravimetric mass changes of dry-padded specimens are recorded at predetermined time intervals. The degree of WS of any individual specimen at a given time interval (t), expressed as a percent mass fraction, is calculated using a simple equation:

$$\mathrm{WS} = [(W_t - W_0)/W_0] \times 100$$

where W_t represents the sample mass at the time and W_0 is the initial mass of dry sample.

7.4.9 Ion Release

Mineral ion release from composite disk specimens is examined at 37°C, in a continuously stirred, HEPES-buffered saline (0.13 mol/L) solution. Kinetic changes in the Ca^{2+} and PO_4^{3-} levels are determined by utilizing spectroscopic methods described in Section 7.3.4. Ion release data are corrected for variations in the total area of the disk exposed to the immersion solution using the simple relation for a given surface area, A, wherein the normalized value x equals $500/A$. The ion release profiles are used to semiquantitatively compare the antidemineralizing–remineralizing capacity of differently formulated ACP composites.[4,6]

7.4.10 Cytotoxicity Testing

In vitro cytotoxicity of the copolymer matrix, ACP filler, and ACP composite is evaluated on specimens extracted in media overnight followed by culturing MC3T3-E1 osteoblastlike cells in extracts for 3 days.[50] Cytotoxicity is evaluated by phase contrast microscopy and an enzymatic assay for mitochondrial dehydrogenase activity (Wst-1, Dojindo, Gaithersburg, MD). Colorimetric measurements are performed with a plate reader (Wallac 1420 Victor², Perkin Elmer Life Sciences, Gaithersburg, MD). Detailed description of the cell culture maintenance, extract experiments, and Wst-1 viability measurements are provided in Simon et al.[51]

One standard deviation is identified in this paper for comparative purposes as the estimated standard uncertainty of the measurements. These values should not be compared with data obtained in other laboratories under different conditions.

7.5 PHYSICOCHEMICAL PROPERTIES OF ACP FILLERS, COPOLYMERS, AND COMPOSITES

7.5.1 ACP Fillers: Structure, Morphology, and Particle Size Distribution

The various types of ACPs employed in our studies are listed in Table 7.4. Syntheses of unmodified (u-ACP) and cation hybridized (Ag-, Al-, Fe(II)-, Fe(III)-, Si-, Zn-, and, Zr-ACP) ACPs were carried out according to a modified version of the preparation protocol proposed by Eanes et al.[52] Similarly, various surfactants and polymer

TABLE 7.4
Median Particle Diameter (d_m) and Water Content of Different Types of ACP Evaluated in Our Studies

ACP	Additive	Acronym	d_m (μm)	H_2O (mass %)
Unmodified	None	u-ACP		
Hybridized and/or surface-modified	AgCl	Ag-ACP	3.5 (1.9)	14.0 (2.2)
	$AlCl_3$	Al-ACP	2.2 (1.3)	16.8 (2.8)
	$FeCl_2$	Fe(II)-ACP	3.8 (1.9)	15.4 (1.2)
	$FeCl_3$	Fe(III)-ACP	2.1 (0.6)	14.1 (2.3)
	PEO[a]	PEO-ACP	14.3 (2.3)	13.7 (0.3)
	PAA[b]	PAA-ACP	9.2 (1.9)	15.8 (1.0)
	TEOS[c]	Si-ACP	8.9(1.8)	13.2(1.6)
	TEOS/APTMS[d]	Si/APTMS-ACP	nd	14.2(1.1)
	TEOS/APTES[e]	Si/APTES-ACP	nd	15.0(1.1)
	TEOS/ MPTMS[f]	Si/MPTMS-ACP	5.8(1.6)	13.8(1.2)
	Triton-100[g]	Triton-ACP	8.3 (1.4)	16.3 (1.2)
	Tween-80[h]	Tween-ACP	8.9 (2.1)	16.9 (0.9)
	$ZnCl_2$	Zn-ACP	1.4 (0.5)	16.6 (2.5)
	$ZrOCl_2$	Zr-ACP	7.4 (2.3)	16.1(2.0)
	$ZrOCl_2$/ZrDMA[i]	Zr/Zr-ACP	7.5(1.5)	15.9(1.7)
	ZONYL FSN[j]	FSN-ACP	6.5(1.2)	19.7(1.1)
	ZONYL FSP[k]	FSP-ACP	4.1(0.4)	17.6(2.1)
Milled	$ZrOCl_2$	Zr-ACP/m	0.9(0.2)	nd

All syntheses were performed with 2 mole% sodium pyrophosphate utilized as a stabilizer for ACP. Additives: [a]PEO, poly(ethylene oxide); [b]PAA, poly(acrylic acid), [c]TEOS, tetraethoxy silane; [d]APTMS; 3-aminopropyltrimethoxy silane; [e]APTES, 3-aminopropyltriethoxy silane; [f]MPTMS, methacryloxypropyltrimethoxy silane; [g]Triton, alkyl aryl polyether alcohol; [h]Tween, poly(oxyethylene) sorbitane monolaureate, [i]ZrDMA, zirconyl dimethacrylate; [j]ZONYL FSN, nonionic fluoro surfactant, [k]ZONYL FSP, anionic fluoro surfactant, nd,not determined.

modified ACPs were prepared by the same basic protocol. The names of the surfactants, polymers, and silane agents utilized as well as their acronyms are provided in Table 7.4. Cations were introduced *ab initio* at the relative molar ratio Ca:cation = 9:1, surfactants at the level of 0.1 mass % relative to Ca reactant, and polymers at 0.5 mass % total concentration. A mixture with mass fractions of 10% TEOS, 10% ethanol, 10% tartaric acid, and 70% water, proven to effectively prevent premature TEOS gelation, was used to introduce the silica elements during hybridization. Si-ACP was surface treated by introducing a mass fraction of 10% of various silane agents (APTMS, APTES, or MPTMS) relative to ACP from a cyclohexane–*n*-propyl amine solution. Zr-ACP was surface treated by introducing a mass fraction of 2% ZrDMA relative to ACP from a methylene chloride solution.

The amorphous state of the each filler was routinely verified by FTIR and XRD — typical patterns are presented in Figures 7.3a and 7.3b. The PSD of the typical, heterodispersed Zr-ACP is shown in Figure 7.4. The corresponding SEM image is

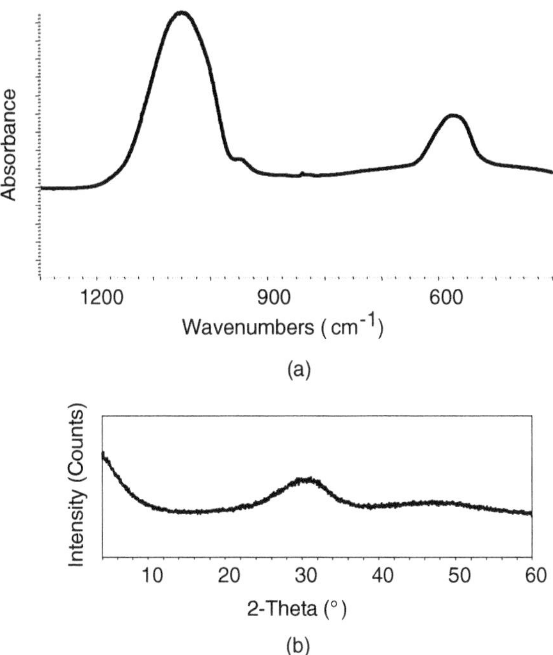

FIGURE 7.3 (a) Typical FTIR spectrum and (b)x-ray diffraction pattern of Zr-ACP filler.

provided in Figure 7.5. All ACP groups (u-, hybrid-, surfactant-, and polymer-ACP, as well as the surface modified solids) had heterogeneous PSD with particle diameters (expressed as the equivalent spherical diameter) ranging from 0.1 to 80 μ Apparent differences in the mean values of d_m between different groups (Table 7.4) could be explained by slight modifications in the different degree (extent) of ACP

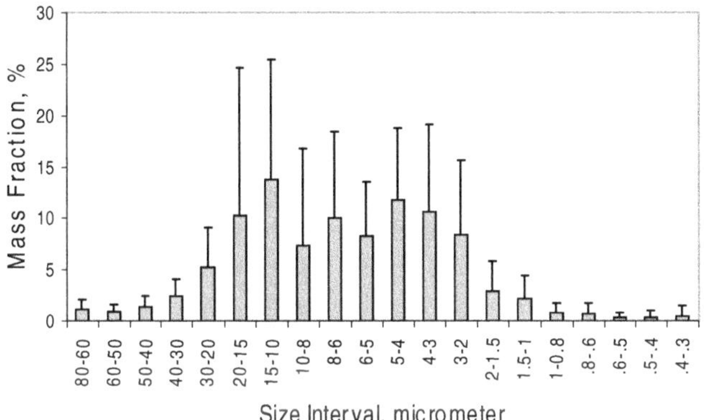

FIGURE 7.4 Particle size distribution of unmilled Zr-ACP after dispersion in isopropanol.

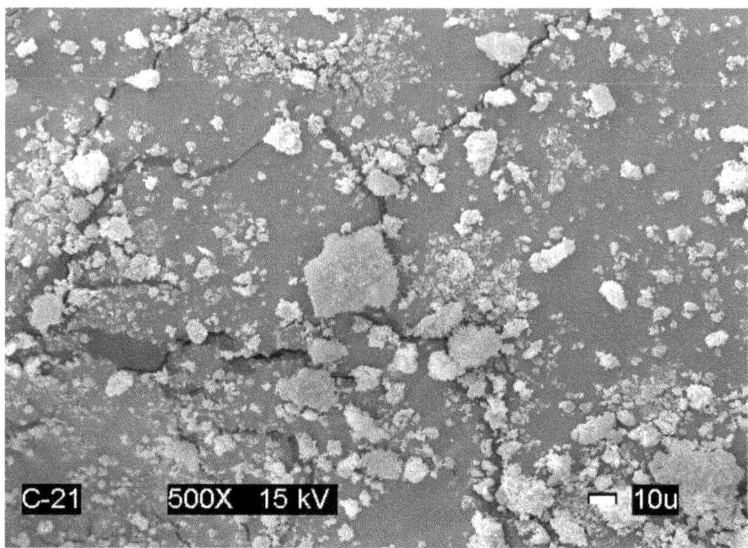

FIGURE 7.5 SEM image of the unmilled Zr-ACP.

agglomeration, which were more or less random and not related to the treatment method (hybridization vs. surface modification). Similarly, the total water content of the solids (TGA data; Table 7.4, far right column) was also independent of the type of the cocation or the surface-active agent added. The average value of approximately 16 mass % total water corresponds to the approximate compositional formula $Ca_3(PO_4)_2 \cdot 2.7H_2O$. It correlates very well with the values reported in literature[1] (18 mass %). Roughly 70% of water is surface bound (weight loss below 130°C) and the rest (weight loss in the temperature region (130–600°C) is structurally incorporated.

Additionally, ball milling of the ACP powder was evaluated as an alternative way to reduce the average size of ACP by breaking up large aggregates into smaller agglomerates that will more intimately interact with the resin and, therefore, more homogeneously disperse in the composite. Dry solid (as-synthesized Zr-ACP) was mixed with very high density zirconia oxide balls (2 mm in diameter) at the mass ratio 1:20 (25 g ACP/500 g zirconia oxide) and 150 mL isopropanol and sealed in the grinding jar. The milling was performed at 400 rpm for 2 h with rotation being reversed every 15 min. The ball mill and a close-up of the jar are shown in Figure 7.6. Milled ACP was separated from grinding balls by sieving, excess isopropanol was evaporated in a vacuum oven (Mo. 3608-5; Barnstead Lab-line, Melrose Park, IL) overnight at 70°C. Approximately 85–90 mass % of the initial ACP was retrieved after the process. The proposed milling protocol has consistently reduced the d_m up to 70–80%.[8] Dry, milled ACP (Zr-ACP/m) powder was, as were all the other types of ACP, stored under vacuum to avoid the exposure to humidity and possible conversion to HAP prior to its utilization in the composite preparation and evaluation. While having no apparent effect on the structure, composition, and/or morphology

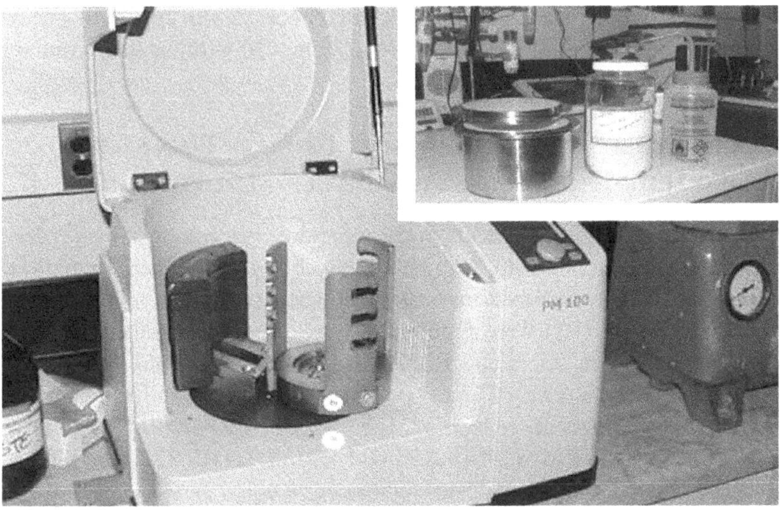

FIGURE 7.6 Planetary ball mill utilized for the grinding of Zr-ACP. Inlet: grinding jar (500 mL total volume) with the latching brackets.

or topology of the fillers, milling significantly reduced the average size of Zr-ACP/m particulates (median diameter, $d_m = 0.9 \pm 0.2$ μm) and the spread of their PSD (Figure 7.7). Better dispersion of Zr-ACP/m in the resin is expected to improve the BFS of the composites, especially after aqueous immersion. Results of the physicochemical comparison of the unmilled Zr-ACP and milled Zr-ACP/m are presented

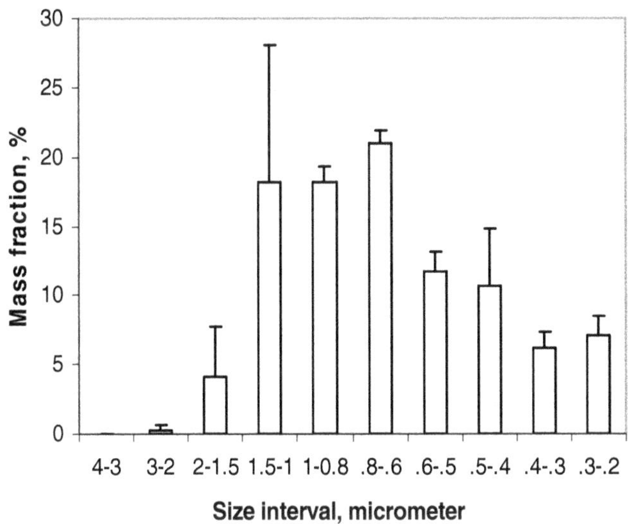

FIGURE 7.7 Particle size distribution of milled Zr-ACP (Zr-ACP/m) after dispersion in isopropanol.

in Section 7.5.2. Such an assessment is deemed necessary to ensure that improvement in mechanical strength of composite is achieved without compromising its antidemineralizing–remineralizing ability.

7.5.2 Copolymers and ACP Composites: Effects of Resin Matrix and Filler Type on Chemical and Mechanical Performance

The effect(s) of fine tuning the chemical structure and composition of the resin matrix on the antidemineralizing–remineralizing ability, mechanical strength (BFS), water sorption (WS), photopolymerization efficacy (degree of vinyl conversion, DVC), and shrinkage (PS) were preliminarily assessed in Antonucci and Skrtic. Zr-ACP and Zr-ACP/m fillers and EBPADMA-based resins were formulated into composites with two series of matrices. In the first series, the molar ratio of EBPADMA/TEGDMA decreased in the range (0.50–0.125) at a constant HEMA/MEP molar ratio of 4.28 (ETHM0.50, ETHM0.33, ETHM025, and ETHM0.13). The photoinitiator system consisted of equal parts by mass of *bis*(2,6-dimethoxybenzoyl)-2,4,4-trimethylpentyl phosphine oxide and 1-hydroxycyclohexyl phenyl ketone (IRGACURE 1850®). The second resin system had increasing EBPADMA/TEGDMA molar ratios in the range 0.50–1.35 and a constant HEMA/MEP molar ratio of (8.26 ± 0.33) (ETHM0.50*, ETHM0.85, and ETHM1.35). The photoinitiator system consisted of camphorquinone (CQ) and ethyl-4-*N*,*N*-dimethylamino benzoate (4EDMAB). The monomers and the components of photoinitiator systems employed are given in Table 7.2. The compositions of the ETHM resins are indicated in Table 7.5. The structures of the main components of ETHM resins are provided in Figure 7.8.

The results of the physicochemical and mechanical testing of ETHM-based composites are summarized in Table 7.6. Compositional variation of the resin matrix did not significantly affect the DC, WS, or the BFS of Zr-ACP/ETHM composites.

TABLE 7.5
Compositions of the Experimental EBPADMA/TEGDMAHEMA/MEP (ETHM) Resins (Mass %)

Monomer/Resin	ETHM 0.50	ETHM 0.33	ETHM 0.25	ETHM 0.13	ETHM 0.50*	ETHM 0.85	ETHM 0.35
EBPADMA	42.00	33.60	28.00	16.80	43.17	54.45	62.85
TEGDMA	42.00	50.40	56.00	67.20	43.24	31.94	23.22
HEMA	10.00	10.00	10.00	10.00	10.08	10.00	10.36
MEP	5.00	5.00	5.00	5.00	2.51	2.56	2.57
IRGACURE 1850	1.00	1.00	1.00	1.00	—	—	—
CQ	—	—	—	—	0.20	0.20	0.20
4EDMAB	—	—	—	—	0.80	0.80	0.80
EBPADMA/TEGDMA molar ratio	0.50	0.33	0.25	0.13	0.50	0.85	1.35

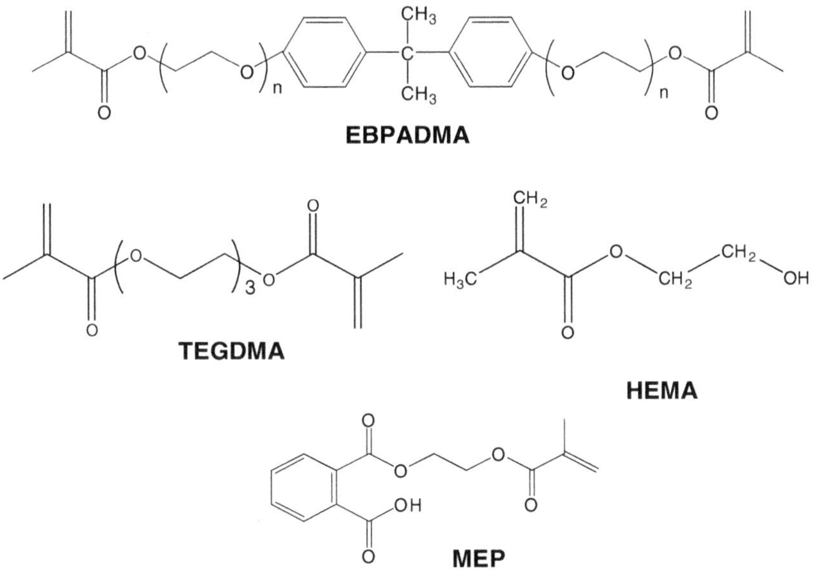

FIGURE 7.8 Chemical structure of monomers utilized to formulate EBPADMA/TEGDMA/HEMA/MEP (ETHM) resins.

The reduction in Ca^{2+} release, which was observed in formulations with the higher MEP levels, only marginally affected the overall remineralizing potential of composites. The attained supersaturations were consistently above the theoretical minimum necessary for remineralization ($\Delta G^0 < 0$). However, the chemical structure and resin matrix composition influenced the PS of the resin composites. The dominant factor controlling the PS of ETHM formulations seems to be the relative content of the high molecular mass EBPADMA; the PS increased when the EBPADMA/TEGDMA molar ratio in the resin matrix was lowered. Significant improvements in DC, WS, and BFS are achieved by replacing the coarse as-synthesized ACP filler with milled ACP in ETHM0.50*–ETHM0.85–ETHM1.35 series. The improved strength and lower WS of milled ACP composites is related to the improved dispersion of milled ACP (median diameter, $d_m = 0.9$ μm) filler throughout the composites compared with the unmilled, coarse ACP with $d_m = 5.7$ μm. Ultimately, milled ACP composites have fewer water sorption-prone voids or defects, which have been identified as the main reason for the poor mechanical stability of the unmilled ACP-based composites.

In addition, ETHM1.35 matrices were evaluated for the effects of the Zr-ACP filler's size on the biaxial and three-point flexural strength (FS), Young's modulus (E), and diametral tensile strength (DTS). The mechanical testing data were correlated with the water sorption of Zr-ACP and Zr-ACP/m composites. Results of mechanical testing are presented in Figure 7.9 a–d. WS results are shown in Figure 7.10. A marked improvement in BFS and a moderate improvement in FS upon aqueous exposure of Zr-ACP/m composites were again attributed to the more homogeneous

TABLE 7.6
Degree of Conversion (DC), Polymerization Shrinkage (PS), Water Sorption (WS), Biaxial Flexure Strength (BFS; Wet Specimens), and the Theoretical Supersturation (ΔG^0)[6] Corresponding to the Maximum Released Calcium and Phosphate from Unmilled (Zr-ACP), Milled (Zr-ACP/M) ETHM Composites with Different Resin Compositions

Monomer/ Resin	ETHM 0.50	ETHM 0.33	ETHM 0.25	ETHM 0.13	ETHM 0.50*	ETHM 0.85	ETHM 1.35
DC (%)							
Zr-ACP	85.8(5.3)	84.4(5.0)	82.2(6.5)	86.6(5.0)	76.9(3.5)	70.5(3.8)	69.1(4.2)
Zr-ACP/m	—	—	—	—	80.3(1.4)	74.8(3.9)	75.1(1.2)
PS (vol %)	6.1(0.5)	6.5(0.7)	7.2(0.4)	7.8(0.6)	—	—	—
WS (mass %)							
Zr-ACP	3.3(0.5)	3.6(0.5)	3.2(0.5)	3.3(0.5)	2.5(0.2)	2.3(0.2)	2.5(0.3)
Zr-ACP/m	—	—	—	—	2.1(0.2)	1.8(0.2)	1.6(0.1)
BFS_{wet} (MPa)							
Zr-ACP	43.6(7.8)	48.5(6.9)	45.9(4.2)	44.4(8.2)	36.3(4.9)	35.0(4.2)	36.4(6.7)
Zr-ACP/m	—	—	—	—	60.9(9.4)	52.9(8.9)	55.8(17.2)
$-\Delta G^0$ (kJ/mol)							
Zr-ACP	4.50(0.19)	4.61(0.13)	4.44(0.30)	5.07(0.31)	4.35(0.21)	4.65(0.22)	4.67(0.23)
Zr-ACP/m	—	—	—	—	3.42(0.39)	4.32(0.36)	4.79(0.20)

Source: Skrtic, D., Antonucci, J.M., and Eanes, E.D., *J. Res. Natl. Inst. Stands. Technol.*, 108(3), 167–182, 2003.

Indicated are mean values with SD in parentheses. Number of repetitive experiments in each group: DC, $n \geq 6$; PS, $n = 3$; WS, $n = 5$; BFS, $n = 5$;and ΔG^0,$n = 4$.

distribution of the finer ACP particles within the composite. The reduced WS of the milled composites is linked to fewer voids and defects existing throughout the body of composite disk specimens. However, the DTS and modulus appeared to be less affected by the filler's size in both dry and wet stage. Modifications in the milling protocol may be required to further improve the mechanical interlocking at the filler–matrix interface and in turn boost the mechanical performance of composites.

7.5.3 ACP Composites: *In Vitro* Cytotoxicity

Our hypothesis was that ACP, because of its compositional similarity to HAP, would show very little or no adverse effect on cell morphology and/or viability. To prove that hypothesis, we exposed an osteoblastic cell culture system MC3T3-E1 to extracts of the Zr-ACP/m filler, the experimental copolymers (mass ratio EBPADMA:UDMA:TEGDMA:HEMA = 1.7:1.7:1.5:1.0) and their ACP composites, and their effects were compared with commercially available orthodontic

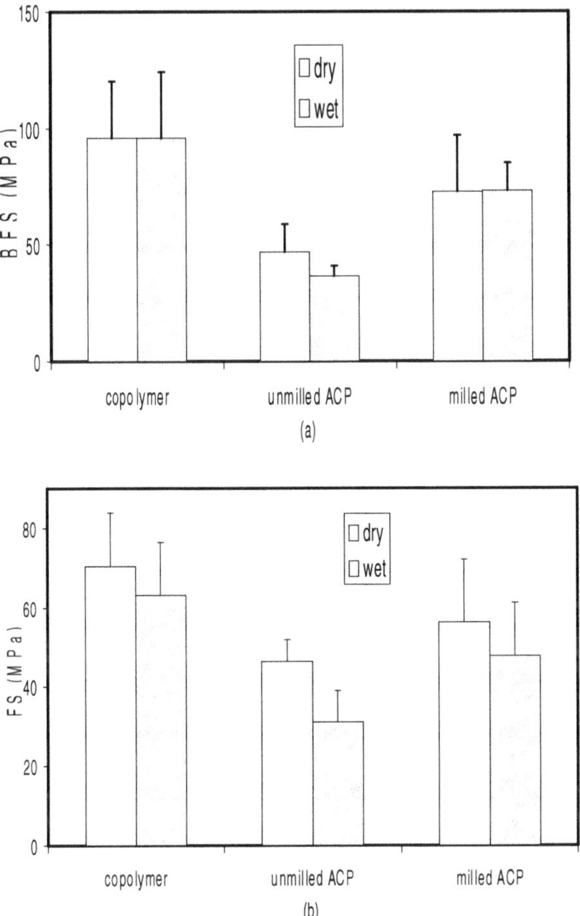

FIGURE 7.9 Mechanical properties of ETHM copolymers and their Zr-ACP and Zr-ACP/m composites containing a mass fraction of 40% filler: (a) BFS, (b) FS, (c) DTS, and (d) E. Values represent mean values and standard deviations (SD; indicated by bars). The SD is taken as a measure of the standard uncertainty. Number of runs in each experimental group: (a) $n \geq 7$, (b) $n \geq 7$, (c) $n \geq 5$, and (d) $n \geq 38$.

adhesive (COA) of similar matrix composition. Cytotoxicity data were correlated with DC and the kinetics of the release of the remineralizing Ca^{2+} and PO_4^{3-} ions from the composites. Phase contrast images of MC3T3-E1 cells cultured in extracts from ACP powder and different resin composites for 3 days (not shown here) showed a normal, spread, polygonal morphology. Only cell remnants were seen in positive control, detergent-containing samples, indicating that 0.1 mass % detergent in the medium was cytotoxic. Qualitatively, an approximately equivalent amount of cells was found in each experimental system, suggesting no adverse cellular response to

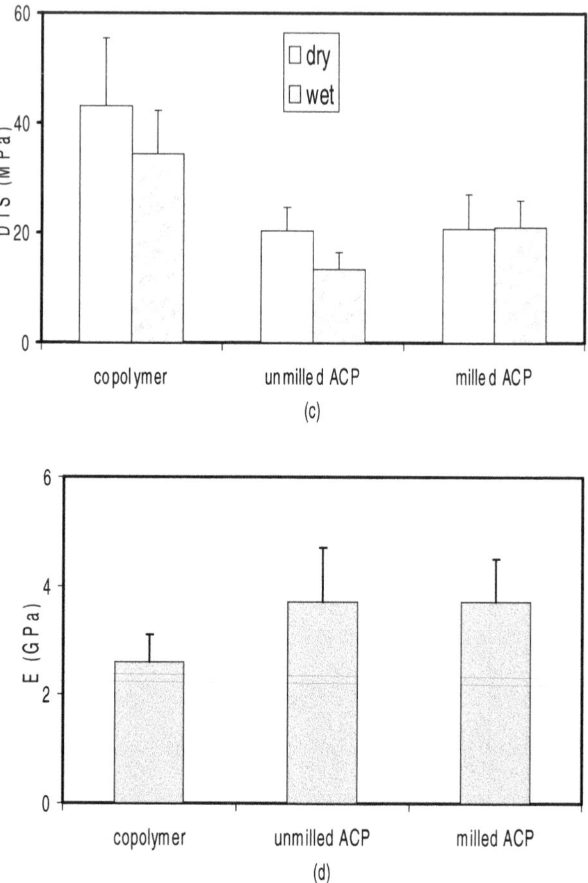

FIGURE 7.9 (Continued)

ACP powder, composite, copolymer, or COA. Based on a colorimetric assay of cellular dehydrogenase activity (Wst-1; Figure 7.11) the extracts from the resins caused a mild drop in the viability of cells compared with the negative control. This drop was found significant [ANOVA ($\alpha = 0.05$) and Tukey pairwise comparison (95% confidence interval)] for ACP powder, ACP composite, and commercial control, but it was not significant for copolymer (unfilled resin). However, there was no significant difference between ACP composite and the copolymer or COA. These results suggest that the experimental ACP is no more toxic than the commercial adhesive chosen as the control. The DC results (24 h postcure; Figure 7.12) show that the attained level of conversion in ACP composite was 24% higher than the DC of COA. Zr-ACP/m EBPADMA/UDMA/TEGDMA/HEMA composites steadily released calcium and phosphate ions into buffered

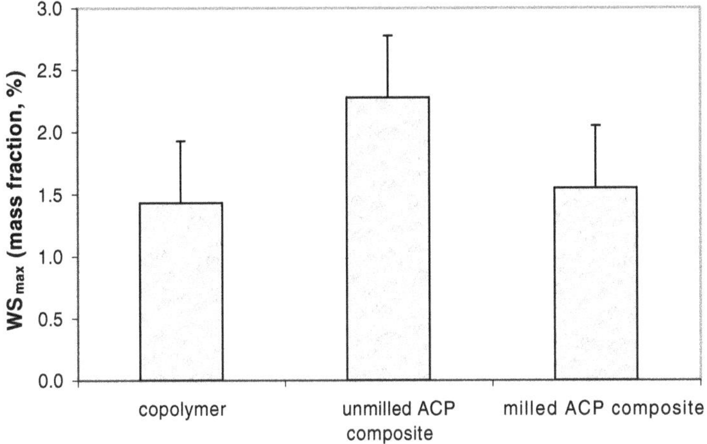

FIGURE 7.10 Maximum water sorption (WS_{max}) expressed as the mean value + SD of ETHM0.35 copolymer and the corresponding Zr-ACP and Zr-ACP/m composites. Number of specimens $n > 7$ in each experimental group.

saline solution (Figure 7.13). The levels of the mineralizing ions released were adequate for attaining the supersaturation required for the internal (intracomposite) reprecipitation of HAP.

Cytotoxicity is more likely to depend on leachable residual monomers and other leachable organic species in the composite. It is likely that the mild effects of the

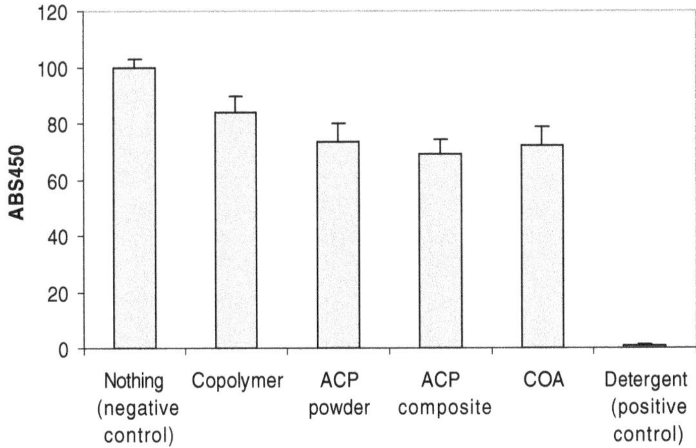

FIGURE 7.11 Cell viability for EBPADMA/UDMA/TEGDMA/HEMA copolymer, Zr-ACP/m powder, the corresponding composite and the commercial light-cured orthodontic adhesive (COA) compared with negative (nothing) and positive (detergent) controls. Indicated results represent the mean value + SD of the absorbance at 450 nm (ABS450 is proportional to the amount of dehydrogenase activity in the cell). Number of samples in each group $n =$

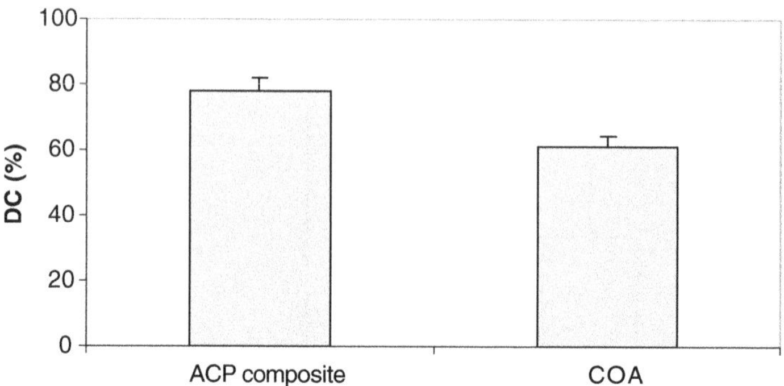

FIGURE 7.12 Degree of conversion (DC) attained 24 h after curing: the experimental Zr-ACP/m EBPADMA/UDMA/TEGDMA/HEMA composite compared with the commercial adhesive (COA). Indicated values represent mean value + SD of five measurements in each group.

resins on cell viability observed in our study are a result of the effects on cells of leachable monomeric species, initiator components, or their by-products. Therefore, for ACP composites, as for traditional dental composites, the correlation of cytotoxicity with the DC would require the assessment of leachable organic moieties as well as the total vinyl unsaturation in the composite. Nevertheless, favorable DC, sustainable release of mineral ions, and the satisfactory cellular response confirm the potential of bioactive ACP composites as a tool for hard tissue regeneration.

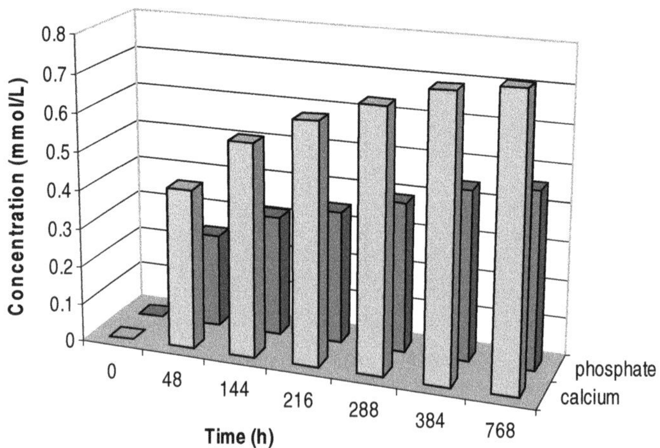

FIGURE 7.13 Kinetics of the release of calcium and phosphate ions from Zr-ACP/m EBPADMA/UDMA/TEGDMA/HEMA composites. Indicated values correspond to the mean values obtained from six repetitive specimens in each group. SDs of the reported values were <0.16 mmol/L and <0.06 mmol/L for calcium and phosphate, respectively.

7.6 CONCLUSION AND PERSPECTIVE ON THE FUTURE

Polymer matrix composition and particle size distribution of the ACP filler phase play a major role in shaping the physicochemical properties of these bioactive composites. Essentially no significant improvement in mechanical properties could be achieved via hybridization and or surface modification of the filler. However, significant improvement in composite's performance upon aqueous exposure is obtained with milled ACP. In addition, fine tuning of the resin matrix did not significantly affect the extent of vinyl conversion, the mechanical stability or the water sorption of the composites. However, chemical structural and resin matrix composition may play an important role in controlling the polymerization shrinkage of the composites. To optimize the composite's potential for apatite reprecipitation (remineralization), it is essential to maintain the level of surface active, bifunctional monomers such as methacryloxyethyl phthalate in the resin formulation at the lowest effective concentration and avoid excessive uptake of calcium ions released from the composite. This requires fine tuning the resin composition with respect to carboxylate content. It appears that the particle size distribution, and in particular the level of uncontrolled ACP agglomeration, are the key factors that determine the filler's ability to homogeneously distribute throughout the matrix without creating voids at the filler–matrix interface. The presence of such voids, frequently seen in composites based on coarse (unmilled) ACPs, hinders the interfacial filler–resin interactions and diminishes the mechanical strength of composites. No adverse response regarding morphology and viability of osteoblastlike cells with ACP composites was seen, whichconfirms their exceptional potential as antidemineralizing–remineralizing materials in dental applications.

REFERENCES

1. Eanes, E.D., Amorphous calcium phosphate: thermodynamic and kinetic considerations, in *Calcium Phosphates in Biological and Industrial Systems,* Amjad, Z., Ed., Kluwer, Dordrecht, 1998, pp. 21–39.
2. Boskey, A.L., Amorphous calcium phosphate. The contention of bone, *J. Dent. Res.,* 76, 1433–1436, 1997.
3. Skrtic, D., Antonucci, J.M., Eanes, E.D., and Brunworth, R.T., Silica- and zirconia-hybridized amorphous calcium phosphate. effect on transformation to hydroxyapatite, *J. Biomed. Mater. Res.,* 59(4), 597–604, 2002.
4. Skrtic, D., Antonucci, J.M., Eanes, E.D., Eichmiller, F.C., and Schumacher, G.E., Physicochemical evaluation of bioactive polymeric composites based on hybrid amorphous calcium phosphates, *J. Biomed. Mat. Res. (Appl. Biomater.),* 53, 381–391, 2000.
5. Skrtic, D., Antonucci, J.M., and Eanes, E.D., Improved properties of amorphous calcium phosphate fillers in remineralizing resin composites, *Dent. Mater.,* 12, 295–301, 1996.
6. Skrtic, D., Antonucci, J.M., and Eanes, E.D., Amorphous calcium phosphate-based bioactive polymeric composites for mineralized tissue regeneration, *J. Res. Natl. Inst. Stands. Technol.,* 108(3), 167–182, 2003.
7. Skrtic, D., Antonucci, J.M., Eanes, E.D., and Eidelman, N., Dental composites based on hybrid and surface-modified amorphous calcium phosphates — a FTIR microspectroscopic study, *Biomaterials,* 25, 1141–1150, 2004.

8. O'Donnell, J.N.R., Antonucci, J.M., and Skrtic, D., Amorphous calcium phosphate composites with improved mechanical properties, *J. Bioact. Compat. Polym.,* 21(3), 169–184, 2006.
9. Skrtic, D. and Antonucci, J.M., Effect of bifunctional co-monomers on mechanical strength and water sorption of amorphous calcium phosphate- and silanized glass-filled Bis-GMA-based composites, *Biomaterials*, 24, 2881–2888, 2003.
10. Antonucci, J.M., McDonough, W.G., Liu, D.W., and Skrtic, D., Effect of polymer matrices on methacrylate conversion and mechanical strength of bioactive composites based on amorphous calcium phosphate, *Polymer Preprints*, 43(2), 741–742, 2002.
11. Antonucci, J.M., McDonough, W.G., Liu, D.W., and Skrtic, D., Effect of acidic comonomers on methacrylate conversion and mechanical strength of bioactive composites based on amorphous calcium phosphate, *Polym. Mater.: Sci. Eng.*, 88, 50–51, 2003.
12. Tung, M.S. and Eichmiler, F.C., Dental applications of amorphous calcium phosphates, *J. Clinical Dent.*, 10, 1–6, 1999.
13. Reynolds, E.C., Cai, F., Shen, P., and Walker, G.D., Retention in plaque and remineralization of enamel lesions by various forms of calcium in a mouthrinse or sugar-free chewing gum, *J. Dent. Res.*, 82(3), 206–211, 2003.
14. Mazzaoui, S.A., Burrow, M.F., Tyas, M.J., Dashper, S.G., Eakins, D., and Reynolds, E.C., Incorporation of casein phosphopeptide-amorphous calcium phosphate into a glass-ionomer cement, *J. Dent. Res.*, 82(11), 914–918, 2003.
15. Santerre, J.P., Shajii, L., and Leung, B.W., Relation of dental composite formulations to their degradation and the release of hydrolyzed polymeric-resin-derived products, *Crit. Rev. Oral Biol. Med.*, 12(2), 136–151, 2001.
16. Stansbury, J.W. and Dickens, S.H., Network formation and compositional drift during photo-initiated copolymerization of dimethacrylate monomers, *Polymer*, 42, 6363–6369, 2001.
17. Antonucci, J.M. and Stansbury, J.W., Molecularly designed dental polymers, in *Desk Reference of Functional Polymers Syntheses and Applications,* Arshady, R., Ed., American Chemical Society, Washington DC, 1997, pp. 719–738.
18. Antonucci, J.M., Liu, D.W., and Stansbury, J.W., Synthesis of hydrophobic oligomeric polymers for dental applications, *J. Dent. Res.*, 72, 369, 1993.
19. Nihei, T., Kurata, S., Kondo, Y., Umemoto, K., Yoshino, N., and Teranaka, T., Enhanced hydrolytic stability of dental composites by use of fluoroalkyltrimethoxysilanes, *J. Dent. Res.*, 81(7), 482–486, 2002.
20. Kidd, E.A.M. and Beighton, D., Prediction of secondary caries around tooth-colored restoration: a clinical and microbiological study, *J. Dent. Res.*, 75, 1942–1946, 1996.
21. Hollinger, J.O., Brekke, J., Gruskin, E., and Lee D., Role of bone substitute, *Clin. Orthop.*, 324, 55–66, 1996.
22. Legeros, R.Z. and Legeros, J.P., Calcium phosphate biomaterials in medical application, *Bioceramics*, 9, 7–10, 1996.
23. Yuan, H., Li, Y., De Bruijn, J.D., De Groot, K., and Zhang, X., Tissue responses of calcium phosphate cement: a study in dogs, *Biomaterials*, 21, 1283–1290, 2000.
24. St. John, K.R., Zardiackas, L.D., Terry, R.C., Teadsall, R.D., and Cooke, S.E., Histological and electron microscopic analysis of tissue response to synthetic composite bone graft in the canine, *J. Appl. Biomater.*, 6, 89–97, 1995.
25. Oonishi, H., Kushitani, S., Iwaki, H., Saka, K., Ono, H., Tamura, A., Sugihara, T., Hench, L.L., Wilson, J., and Tsuji, E., Comparative bone formation in several kinds of bioceramic granules, *Bioceramics*, 8, 137–144, 1995.

26. Drissen, F.C.M., Boltong, M.G., Zapatero, M.I., Verbeeck, R.M. H., Bonfield, W., Bermudez, O., Fernandez, E., Ginebra, M.P., and Planell J.A., *In vivo* behavior of three calcium phosphate cements and a magnesium phosphate cement, *J. Mater. Sci.: Mater. Med.*, 6, 272–278, 1995.
27. Nakamura, T., Bioceramics in orthopedic surgery, *Bioceramics*, 9, 31–34, 1996.
28. Ten Huisen, K.S. and Brown, P.W., Variation in solution chemistry during calcium-deficient and stoichiometric hydroxyapatite formation from $CaHPO_4{\cdot}2H_2O$ and $Ca_4(PO_4)_2O$, *J. Biomed. Mater. Res.*, 36, 233–241, 1997.
29. Jarcho, M., Calcium phosphate ceramics as hard tissue prosthetics, *Clin. Orthop.* 157, 260–268, 1981.
30. Kurashina, K., Kurita, H., Hirano, M., De Blieck, J.M. A., Klein, C.P.A.T., and De Groot, K., Calcium phosphate cement: *in vitro* and *in vivo* studies of the α-tricalcium phosphate - dicalcium phosphate dibasic - tetracalcium phosphate monoxide system, *J. Mater. Sci.: Mater. Med.*, 6, 340–347, 1995.
31. Kurashina, K., Kurita, H., Kotani, A., Klein, C.P.A.T. and De Groot, K., *In vivo* study of calcium phosphate cements: implantation of an α-tricalcium phosphate/dicalcium phosphate dibasic/tetracalcium phosphate monoxide cement paste, *Biomaterials*, 18, 539–543, 1997.
32. Koshino, T., Kubota, W., and Morii, T., Bone formation as a reaction to hydraulic hydroxyapatite thermal decomposition product used as bone cement in rabbits, *Biomaterials*, 16, 125–128, 1996.
33. Miyamoto, Y., Ishikawa, K., Takeuchi, M., Yuasa, M., Kon, M., Nagayama, M., and Asaoka, K., Non-decay type fast-setting calcium phosphate cement: setting behavior in calf serum and its tissue response, *Biomaterials*, 17, 1429–1435, 1996.
34. Nishimura, N., Yamamura, T., Taguchi, Y., Ikenaga, M., Nakamura, T., Kokubo, T., and Yoshihara, S., A new bioactive bone cement: its histological and mechanical characterization, *J. Appl. Biomater.*, 2, 219–229, 1991.
35. Ehara, A., Ogata, K., Imazato, S., Ebisu, S., Nakano, T., and Umakoshi, Y., Effects of α-TCP and TetCP on MC3T3-E1 proliferation, differentiation and mineralization, *Biomaterials*, 24, 831–836, 2003.
36. Constantino, P.D., Friedman, C.D., Jones, K., Chow, L.C., and Sisson, G.A., Experimental hydroxyapatite cranioplasty, *Plast. Reconstr. Surg.*, 90, 174–191, 1992.
37. Wiltfang, J., Merten, H.A., Schlegel, K.A., Schiltze-Mosgau, S., Kloss, F.R., Rupprecht, S., and Kessler, P., Degradation characteristics of α and β tri-calcium phosphate in minipigs, *J. Biomed. Mater. Res.*, 63, 115–121, 2002.
38. Antonucci, J.M. and Skrtic, D., Matrix resin effects on selected physicochemical properties of amorphous calcium phosphate composites, *J. Bioact. Comp. Polym.*, 20, 29–49, 2005.
39. Simon, C.G., Jr., Antonucci, J.M., Liu, D.W., and Skrtic, D., *In vitro* cytotoxicity of amorphous calcium phosphate composites, *J. Bioact. Compat. Polym.*, 20(5), 279–295, 2005.
40. Yamaguchi, T., Chattopadhyay, N., Kifor, O., Butters, R.R., Jr., Sugimoto, T., and Brown, E.M., Mouse osteoblastic cell line (MC3T3-E1) expresses extracellular calcium (Ca^{2+})-sensing receptor and its antagonists stimulate chemotaxis and proliferation of M3CT3-E1 cells, *J. Bone Miner. Res.*, 13, 1530–1538, 1998.
41. Hynos, I., Edgar, A.J., Buttery, L.D.K., Hench, L.L., and Polak, J.M., Gene-expression profiling of human osteoblasts following treatment with the ionic products of Bioglass® 45S5 dissolution, *J. Biomed. Mater. Res.*, 55, 151–157, 2001.

42. Keeting, P.E., Oursler, M.J., Wiegand, K.E., Bonde, S.K., Spelsberg, T.C., and Riggs, B.L., Zeolite A increases proliferation, differentiation and transforming growth factor beta production in normal adult human osteoblast-like cells *in vitro, J. Bone Miner. Res.*, 7, 1281–1289, 1992.
43. Beck, G.R., Jr., Zerler, B., and Moran, E., Phosphate is a specific signal for induction of osteopontin gene expression, *Proc. Natl. Acad. Sci.*, 97, 8452–8357, 2000.
44. Spahl, W., Budzikiewicz, H., and Geurtsen, W., Determination of leachable components from four commercial dental composites by gas and liquid chromatography/mass spectrometry, *J. Dent.*, 26, 137–145, 1998.
45. Pelka, M., Distle, R.W., and Petshelt, A., Elution parameters and HPLC-detection of single components from resin composite, *Clin. Oral Invest.*, 3, 194–200, 1999.
46. Schweikl, H., Schmalz, G., and Spruss, T., The induction of micronuclei *in vitro* unpolymerized resin monomers, *J. Dent. Res.*, 80(7), 1615–1620, 2001.
47. Ratanasathien, S., Wataha, J.C., Hanks, C.T., and Denison, J.B., Cytotoxic interactive effects of dentin bonding components on mouse fibroblasts, *J. Dent. Res.*, 74, 1602–1606, 1995.
48. Lee, S.Y., Regnault, W.F., Antonucci, J.M., and Skrtic, D., Effect of particle size of an amorphous calcium phosphate filler on the mechanical strength and ion release of polymeric composites, *J. Biomed. Mater. Res.*, in press, 2005.
49. ASTM F394–78, Standard test method for biaxial strength (modulus of rapture) of ceramic substrates, reapproved 1991.
50. Sudo, H., Kodama, H.A., Magai, Y., Yamamoto, S., and Kasai, S., *In vitro* differentiation and calcification in a new clonal osteogenic cell line derived from newborn mouse calvaria, *J. Cell Biol.*, 96, 191–198, 1983.
51. Simon, C.G., Jr., Khatri, C.A., Wight, S.A., and Wang, F.W., Preliminary report on the biocompatibility of a moldable, resorbable, composite bone graft consisting of calcium phosphate cement and poly(lactide-co-glycolide) micospheres, *J. Orthopaed. Res.*, 20, 473–482, 2002.
52. Eanes, E.D., Gillessen, I.H., and Posner, A.S., Intermediate states in the precipitation of hydroxyapatite, *Nature*, 208, 365–367, 1965.

8 New Approaches to Improved Polymer Implant Toughness and Modulus

Meng Deng and Shalaby W. Shalaby

CONTENTS

8.1 INTRODUCTION

The properties of polymers span a very broad range, from viscous fluids, to rubber, and to hard solids. In the field of biomaterials, polymers as implants or medical devices have found wide application in treating patients with tissue loss and organ failure. Yet one of the major drawbacks of polymeric biomaterials is that their mechanical properties may not be sufficient for high load-bearing applications, such as in orthopedics, if these materials are compared with metallic implants, which have a very high stiffness and strength. However, when implants made of metals are used in the body, it may lead to a phenomenon called the stress-shielding effect because of the mismatch between the modulus of the implants and the surrounding tissues. Furthermore, metal alloys may be subject to corrosion in the biological environment. As a result, there have been tremendous efforts in the past few decades to improve the stiffness and toughness of polymers so that their properties match those of hard tissue. One practical way to do so is to introduce into a polymer matrix a reinforcing phase of high strength and modulus to produce a composite material. Compared with metals and ceramics, the polymer-based composite materials are less stiff, have high fatigue strength, and their properties and structures can be easily tailored to meet specific requirements.

If used for hard tissue replacement, polymer composite materials have a number of potential advantages over metal alloys because it is possible to modulate their strength and stiffness to achieve better mechanical compatibility with bone and other tissues while maintaining durability. For example, composite materials in orthopedics may provide the opportunity of reinforcing bone cement and load-bearing materials to improve their durability, incorporating bioactive agents to improve the performance of internal fixation implants, and using resorbable phases that help incorporation of the material into the bone. Practically, many bone cements containing fillers that can be classified as particulate reinforced composites. However, because of the need to design composite materials and components to achieve certain desired mechanical and biological properties, their design and manufacturing are far more complex than those of conventional monolithic materials. This is because of the large number of additional design and processing variables that must be considered and controlled. In composite technology, the dispersion of reinforcement phase and the interfacial bonding between components play important roles in achieving the desired mechanical properties.

Other methods used in improving the performance of polymeric biomaterials include cross-linking and solid-state orientation. For example, high energy radiation-induced cross-linking is used to modify ultrahigh molecular weight polyethylene (UHMWPE), a widely used orthopedic load-bearing material. Cross-linking and annealing lead to an increase in surface hardness and modulus, and a significantly improved wear resistance of UHMWPE. Forced orientation of polymer chains and chain segments by solid-state deformation results in a polymeric biomaterial of the same chemical composition with significantly enhanced mechanical properties. This solid-state orientation technology has been applied to UHMWPE, polyether ether ketone (PEEK), and degradable polymers.

8.2 NEW APPROACHES TO POLYMER IMPLANTS OF IMPROVED TOUGHNESS AND MODULUS

8.2.1 Composite Technology

8.2.1.1 Fiber Reinforcement

Composites offer more design flexibility than monoliths. In recent years, there has been a great deal of research activity in the development of biomaterials based on polymer composites. By selecting and controlling the fraction and distribution of the different combinations of matrices and reinforcements for improving the interfacial bonding in the composites, one can tailor the properties of these composites to meet the mechanical and physiological requirements for implants. The experimental and analytical studies of the mechanical behaviors of fiber-reinforced composites of high performance polymers such as PEEK suggest that these composites can potentially be used in load-bearing orthopedic dental applications, for example, crowns and bridges. PEEK is a rigid semicrystalline, high-temperature melting polymer with excellent mechanical properties and high resistance to various chemicals and types of radiation, which makes it suitable for use as a load-bearing biomaterial. There have been quite a few studies on this polymer for biomedical uses. However, the modulus of PEEK is still lower than that of cortical bone. Therefore, to further increase the mechanical properties of PEEK for potential load-bearing applications, glass fibers and carbon fibers have been used to reinforce this polymer.[1,2] The results indicate that the fibers cause an increased stiffness of PEEK. Knitted carbon–PEEK composites were investigated for orthopedic bone plates. Compared with braided carbon–PEEK composites, the knitted carbon–PEEK composites were shown to have relatively lower stiffness and bending moment, but higher deformability.[4]

The modulus of polylactic acid (PLA)-based materials is relatively low (~4 GPa) compared with that of cortical bone (~15 GPa). Efforts have been made to prepare osteoconductive composites consisting of PLA or its copolymers and calcium phosphate–based reinforcing agents such as hydroxyapatite (HA) or β-tricalcium phosphate (TCP). When an HA having a high aspect ratio is introduced into PLA, its modulus increases significantly. Accordingly, HA short fibers were prepared and used to reinforce poly-L-lactide (PLLA).[5] The respective testing results show that the bending modulus of the composites was increased significantly with increasing fiber content as shown in Figure 8.1. However, the bending strength and breaking elongation tended to decrease with the increasing fiber fraction at high fiber content, where

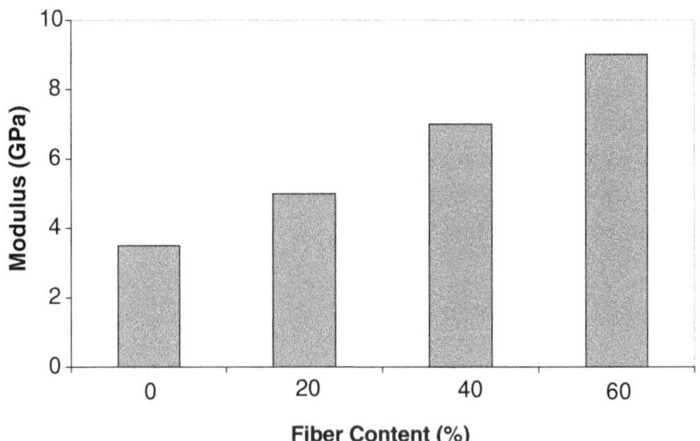

FIGURE 8.1 Change of modulus with fiber content for HA–PLA composites.

the interfacial bonding strength may start to decrease. Such results indicate that there is still a need to improve the mechanical properties of these types of composites.

Chopped and networked glass fibers were used to reinforce dental resins.[6,7] Heat-curing and postcure heat treatment may be used during the manufacturing process to further enhance the strength and toughness of these composites. However, the relatively high brittleness and low fracture resistance of current dental composites still limit their use in high load-bearing applications. In a unique approach, Xu et al. developed a ceramic whisker filler system for dental composites.[8,9]

The whiskers, with much smaller diameter than chopped glass fibers, possess high strength and toughness. To increase the interaction between resin matrix and the fillers, Xu et al. thermally fused silica glass particles onto the surfaces of the whiskers to facilitate silanization and to roughen the whisker surfaces for improved interfacial bonding of their composites. This approach led to a twofold increase in composite flexural strength compared with currently available dental resin composites. The whisker-to-silica ratio was shown to be a key microstructural parameter that controlled the strength of composites. However, the effects of whisker-to-silica ratio on modulus and hardness were not well investigated in that study. In a recent report, the effect of whisker-to-silica ratio on the performance of silica-fused whisker composites was studied,[10] and it was found that the fracture toughness increased when the whisker-to-silica ratio was increased from 0:1 to 2:1. Then the toughness plateaued. With increasing whisker-to-silica ratio, the elastic modulus of the composites increased significantly, but the brittleness of whisker composites steadily decreased. During composite cracking, whiskers and fibers in the composite were observed to pin and deflect the crack propagation, thus significantly increasing the roughness of fracture surfaces by creating steps and tortuous topographies. At high whisker-to-silica ratios, the possibility of whisker entanglement and agglomeration increases, leading to a plateaued toughness. However, the composite hardness was less sensitive to this ratio. The toughening mechanisms consisted of crack deflection and bridging by, and frictional pullout of, the silica-fused whiskers in the composites.

UHMWPE fibers have been used to reinforce poly(methyl methacrylate) (PMMA) and epoxy resins. Realizing the important role that interfacial bonding plays in the performance of reinforced composites, Shalaby and coworkers developed a phosphonylation process that could be used to render UHMWPE fiber surfaces less hydrophobic and more compatible, chemically, with common polymeric matrices.[11,12] And these phosphonylated fibers were incorporated as reinforcing fillers for PMMA matrices.[13,14] The experimental results indicated that phosphonylation was an effective approach to improving the bending strength and modulus of UHMWPE fiber- and fabric-reinforced composites.

8.2.1.2 Particulate Reinforcement

Inorganic phosphate-based particulates with good mechanical properties are well-suited for use as reinforcement in polymer composites. Hydroxyapatite (HA) and tricalcium phosphate (TCP) particles with a calcium-to-phosphorus ratio close to that of natural bone's inorganic component are also bioactive. Additionally, they can be processed to have high mechanical strength and modulus. Therefore, it is a logical consequence to use HA or TCP as a reinforcing phase for polymeric biomaterial composites. The first use of bioactive HA particles to reinforce polymers in an implant was in the early 1980s. A few studies have been published on the use of HA to reinforce high density polyethylene (HDPE) and UHMWPE for bone substitutes.[15–18] Particulate HA–HDPE composites were developed as an analog material for bone replacement and used successfully in clinical practice.[15,19] The close modulus matching of HA–HDPE composite to bone shows promise in solving the problem of bone resorption that has been associated with the use of implants made up of conventional high modulus materials such as metals and ceramics, which are less compliant than human cortical bone. It was found that an optimum combination of mechanical and biological performance was achieved with 40% HA for HA–HDPE composites. However, composites with only HA and HDPE achieve their integrity through mechanical interlocking or coupling, and their performance improvement over pure HDPE is limited. This is particularly the case for load-bearing applications because of the lack of strong interfacial bonding between HA and HDPE. In a more recent study, Juhasz et al. used a bioactive glass-ceramic, apatite-wollastonite (A-W) to reinforce HDPE.[20] Compared with HA–HDPE, which is used in maxillofacial applications, the new composites have higher modulus, which makes their use in orthopedic applications possible. Silanation of HA and acrylic acid grafting of polyethylene (PE) were employed to improve the filler-matrix interfacial bonding in HA–HDPE composites.[21] The introduction of silane-coupled HA and acrylic acid grafted PE has resulted in new HA–HDPE composites with improved ductility and tensile strength. An increase in the HA content led to increases in both Young's modulus and strength, but with a corresponding decrease in fracture elongation. Improved bonding between the ceramic particles and the polymer, which is achieved by both chemical adhesion and tight mechanical coupling, resulted in the improved mechanical properties of new HA–HDPE composites. The study further showed that particulate size and morphology of HA had significant effects on the performance of the HA–PE composites.[22] HA particles of large median sizes reduced the strength and modulus but increased the ductility of the composites.

For UHMWPE, HA was used as a reinforcement to improve its mechanical properties.[23] The HA–UHMWPE composites were prepared by wet ball-mill compounding and swelling in a nontoxic solvent. The composites had about 100% increase in both yield strength and modulus as compared with bulk UHMWPE because (1) ball milling in ethanol reduced the HA particle size and improved the dispersion of HA in the matrix, and (2) swelling enhanced the polymer chain mobility leading to the formation of an interpenetrating network. Xie et al. incorporated quartz powders into UHMWPE, and the composites were further cross-linked in the presence of organosiloxane.[24] Their results indicated that the organosiloxane acted as a cross-linking agent for UHMWPE as well as a coupling aid between the quartz particles and the UHMWPE matrix. At low organosiloxane content, the mechanical properties (tensile strength, modulus, impact resistance, and wear resistance) were substantially improved. This was attributed to the improved interfacial adhesion and the cross-linking of the matrix. However, excess cross-linking led to a deterioration of the properties because of the increase in material brittleness. Anderson et al. incorporated Al–Cu–Fe quasi-crystals in UHMWPE, and the mechanical properties of the resulting composites were evaluated.[25] While there was no statistical difference in wear performance between the composite and control samples, the Al-Cu-Fe/UHMWPE composites showed significantly higher moduli than pure UHMWPE.

The mechanical and osteoinductive properties of PEEK were modified with HA. The experimental results showed that the Young's modulus of injection-molded HA–PEEK composites can be as high as 10 GPa, which is in the range known for cortical bone, thus making them potential candidates for use in load-bearing applications. HA–PEEK composites may also improve the bone-implant bonding over pure PEEK, because of the osteoinductive property of HA particles.[27] Abu Bakar et al. investigated the tensile and tension-tension fatigue properties of HA-reinforced PEEK composites for orthopedic applications.[28] It was found that for the HA volume fraction of 0 to 40%, Young's modulus and the fatigue residual modulus increased with the increase in the HA percentage. These composites had a modulus within the low to middle range of natural bone modulus. However, the increases in modulus were achieved at the expense of tensile strength — at 40% HA, the tensile strength drop was about 30–40% compared with pure PEEK. These composites showed both ductile and brittle behavior, depending on the amount of HA incorporated into the polymer matrix. Such results might suggest that interfacial bonding plays a very important role in HA–PEEK composites.

HA particles were also used to reinforce biodegradable polymers. Advantages with this type of composites are that HA may become part of adjacent tissues after the matrix is degraded. The composites made of HA particles and PLLA are very stiff, totally bioresorbable, and osteologically bioactive — they may find applications in the areas of oral-maxillocraniofacial, plastic, and reconstructive surgeries.[29] A thin composite plate made of HA and PLLA shows an elastic modulus of 9 GPa compared with a pure PLLA with a modulus of 6 GPa. Devices made of PGA and PLLA copolymers, enantiomeric PDLLA, and reinforced lactide copolymers and their mixture usually were reported to have lower strength than reinforced PLLA.[30] Kikuchi et al. prepared powder calcium phosphate–copoly-L-lactide composites.[30] Their testing data showed that the Young's modulus of the composites was significantly higher than those of the individual component materials.

It has long been realized that distribution of fillers in the matrix is important to the performance of composites. For PMMA or bone cement, a nonuniform dispersion (i.e., agglomerates) of the radiopacifier has been reported to decrease tensile strength, fatigue life, and fracture toughness of the implants because of the stress concentrations caused by these agglomerates. In an attempt to solve this problem, Shalaby and Demian developed a microencapsulated radiopacifier enabling a uniform dispersion of the radiopacifier in the matrix of the cured bone cement.[31] The specially formulated radiopacifier–PMMA composite was shown to have an improved *in vitro* fatigue behavior over commercial orthopedic acrylic bone cements.

In other areas, HA has been used as a filler for poly(methyl methacrylate) (PMMA) to improve its mechanical properties.[18] Various bioactive ceramics, such as HA and tricalcium phosphate (TCP), have also been used to reinforce polysulfone and polyhydroxybutyrate to produce bone substitutes.[32,33]

8.2.1.3 Nanocomposites

Application of nanotechnology in biomaterials has become a very active research area. This was reflected in the consistently increasing number of publications dealing with nanobiomaterials in recent years.[34–39] One of the important areas has been the incorporation of nanofillers into degradable matrices. If a homogenous dispersion of the nanofillers can be achieved at the microscopic and/or nano levels, the mechanical properties of the composites would be significantly improved. In concert with this, Deng et al. studied the effect of incorporating Ca-deficient hydroxyapatite (d-HAP) nanocrystals on the properties of the resulting composite of poly(D,L-lactide) (PDLLA).[34] The composite was prepared by the solvent-cast technique. The tensile testing results showed that the modulus of the composites increased with the increase in the d-HAP fraction. At 10.5% d-HAP content, the modulus of the composite was 2.47 GPa as compared with 1.66GPa for the pure PDLLA. Results of the study indicated that incorporating d-HAP nanocrystals into the PDLLA polymer matrix could significantly improve the rigidity of the materials without compromising strength. This preservation of strength for PDLLA–d-HAP nanocomposites may be attributed to the homogeneous dispersion of d-HAP nanocrystals in the PDLLA matrix as well as to good interfacial bonding. Similarly, nanoparticles of calcium carbonate (vaterite) were incorporated into the PLLA matrix to form particle-reinforced nanocomposites.[35] This is a new type of ceramic-polymer biomaterial that may have excellent apatite-forming ability. At 30% content of the reinforcing phase, the modulus of the composites is twice as high as pure PLLA. The composites had a relatively high bending strength of ~50 MPa with no brittle fracture behavior, compared with pure PLA with a bending strength of ~35 MPa. However, the mechanical properties of the composite started to decrease after the vaterite content reached 50%. An *in vitro* study showed that the composite formed a thin layer of bonelike apatite on its surface after soaking in simulated body fluid at 37°C for 1–3 days. In a similar study, nanohydroxyapatite (NHA) particles were used to form PLLA composite scaffolds with high porosity and different pore structures for bone tissue engineering using a thermally induced phase separation technique.[36] The study showed that the compressive modulus of the scaffolds increased with increasing NHA content. The modulus almost doubled at 50% NHA. It was found that processing conditions had a large effect on the final properties of the scaffolds.

Ruan et al. used multiwalled carbon nanotubes (MWCNT) to reinforce UHMWPE. Their results indicate that even at 1% MWCNT content, the composites showed remarkable increases in tensile strength and modulus for nondrawn samples. For the samples with high draw ratios, the materials showed an increase in strain energy density of up to 150% and an increase of ductility up to 140%. It was observed that there existed a good load transfer at the interfaces between the matrix and reinforcement. Liu et al. reported mechanical properties of nano-HA–polymer composites. The polymer was a block copolymer of poly(butylenes terephthalate) and poly(ethylene glycol). The composites were prepared by hot-press compression molding. The tensile test indicated that compared with pure polymer the composite had a significantly higher modulus, but a slightly lower strength. In other areas, effects of resin formulation and nanofiller surface treatment on the properties of experimental hybrid resin composites were investigated.[39] The results indicated that the addition of a nonbonded nanofiller does not negatively affect the initial or long-term properties of hybrid dental composites, but the polymerization contraction stress was significantly reduced.

8.2.2 Self-Reinforced Composites

Self-reinforced composites consist of a polymer matrix filled with oriented high strength and modulus polymer fibers of the same chemical composition. Because of the chemical similarity and therefore, the compatibility between fiber and matrix, the formation of an intimate, interfacial bonding in the composite becomes feasible. The advantage of a self-reinforced material entails producing a composite having improved properties over the single-component system without introducing a second phase of different chemical composition. The lower entropy state (oriented polymer chains) can be associated with several strengthening and toughening mechanisms that may result in significant improvements in the mechanical performance of the composite. If the preparation of a self-reinforced composite is through thermal processing, the process temperature should be carefully controlled because the reinforcement phase and matrix phase will have very close melting temperatures. Representative examples of self-reinforced composites include UHMWPE, PMMA, and degradable polymers.

8.2.2.1 UHMWPE

UHMWPE is currently the choice of materials for load-bearing components articulating with metal- or ceramic-counterpart surfaces, as in the majority of joint endoprostheses. However, UHMWPE bulk material has its inherent weakness, such as low modulus and yield strength, as compared with much stiffer metal stem and cortical bone. As a result, the polymer shows wear and creep as an implant. Composite technology has been used in the past to improve its performance, as in the case of carbon-fiber reinforced UHMWPE composites. Although carbon fiber reinforcement brought about high modulus (stiffness), the inherent nature of brittleness of the carbon fiber led to a decreased wear resistance in the carbon fiber–UHMWPE composite as compared with bulk UHMWPE. On the other hand, reinforcement of UHMWPE has also been explored with other fillers, such as ceramics, quartz, and metal. But, the disadvantages of these reinforcements are their incompatibility with the matrix, not to mention the extremely high melt viscosity of UHMWPE, which makes it very difficult to mix fibers with matrix during melt processing. In a novel approach, Shalaby and Deng successfully incorporated high strength and modulus UHMWPE fibers into a UHMWPE matrix by a thermal-compression molding process.[40,41] The mechanical properties of the resulting self-reinforced UHMWPE composites showed significant improvement over bulk UHMWPE. Even for UHMWPE composites with a 5% fiber fraction, substantial increases in tensile strength and modulus were achieved. The composites exhibited significant reduction in creep over bulk UHMWPE deformation, as shown in Figure 8.2. At the same time, the wear performance of the materials did not show any significant change after the incorporation of UHMWPE fibers. Additionally, the composites showed an increase in impact

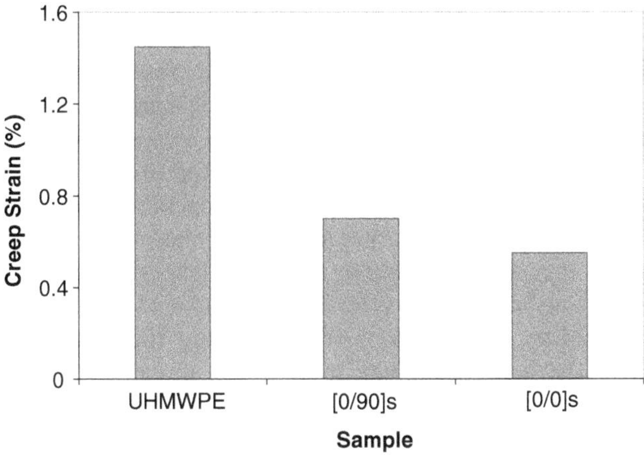

FIGURE 8.2 Comparison of tensile creep deformation between bulk UHMWPE and self-reinforced composites-cross-ply [0/90]s and unidirectional [0/0]s at 5 MPa and room temperature.

strength in notched specimens because of the toughness of polyethylene fiber and the energy dispersion occurring along the laminate interfaces. The thermal properties of the fiber were not affected significantly by the compression-molding process at the elevated temperature.

8.2.2.2 PMMA

Poly(methyl methacrylate) (PMMA) or bone cement is widely used in a variety of orthopedic and dental applications. PMMA is a glassy, amorphous, thermoplastic material with relatively low strength if used in load-bearing applications. The polymer also exhibits brittle, less than optimal properties at body temperature because of its high glass transition. Because of these weaknesses, PMMA displays poor fatigue performance. The presence of the porosity and other stress concentrating factors introduced during application further contributes to the weakness of the polymer. The fatigue fracturing has been found to be one of the main causes for loosening and cement fragmentation during the long-term survival of this material. Although a few techniques have been used to address the problems associated with the PMMA, long-term cement fatigue failure still exists.

To improve the mechanical properties of PMMA, researchers have explored composite technology. For example, fibers of carbon, steel, Kevlar, polyethylene, and titanium have been incorporated into PMMA matrix with the idea that these materials would improve the mechanical properties of the polymer. Although these composites did show some improvement in mechanical properties such as fracture toughness and fatigue resistance, the incompatibility between fibers and matrix posted possible weak interfacial bonding. To overcome the problems with the traditional composites, investigators developed a new composite technology that uses PMMA fiber as a reinforcement to produce the self-reinforced PMMA composites. While commercial PMMA in bulk form has a strength of about 50 MPa and a breaking elongation of about 5%, PMMA fibers having a strength of 220 MPa, modulus of 8 GPa, and a breaking elongation of 25% were successfully prepared by melt extrusion and drawing.[42] Such fibers are highly oriented. Because of the increased elongation at break, the PMMA fiber exhibited significant improvement in ductility compared with bulk polymer. Using PMMA fibers, Gilbert et al. prepared self-reinforced PMMA composites with a 60% fiber fraction and tested their mechanical properties.[43] The results indicated that although the modulus of composites showed a limited increase in comparison to pure PMMA, the elongation at breaking achieved significant increases as shown in Figure 8.3, suggesting high toughness for the self-reinforced PMMA composites. The single edge notched tests showed an increase of almost 100% in fracture toughness for composites. The study of failure mechanisms revealed that the composites absorbed much energy before fracture. Fatigue experimental results showed that the composites had significant fatigue strength improvement over that of bulk PMMA. It was claimed that the fiber-matrix bond in self-reinforced PMMA composites is uniform and continuous through the composite.

8.2.2.3 Biodegradable Polymers

Tormala and coworkers pioneered development of biodegradable, self-reinforced composites based on polylactide (PLA), polyglycolide (PGA), and their copolymers (PLGA) in the middle of 1980s. Their work led to the clinical application of these materials as bone screws and plates.[44–47] The initial objective of their studies was to develop biodegradable biomaterials of high strength and modulus for load-bearing applications such as internal bone fixation devices. The first absorbable rods investigated in early clinical studies were made of self-reinforced glycolide–lactide materials. This was followed by the introduction of a group of similar composites.

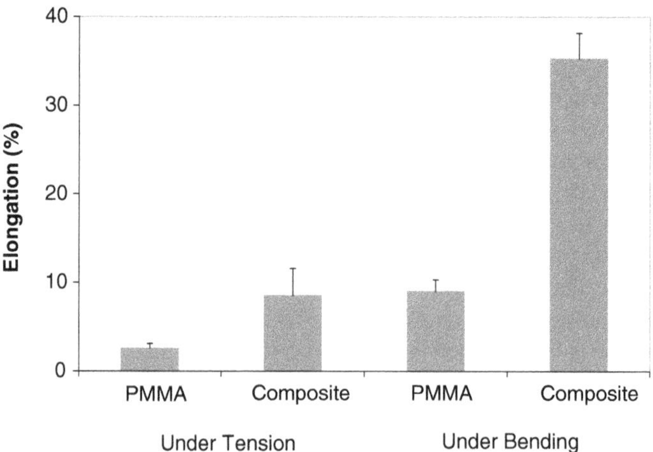

FIGURE 8.3 Comparison of tensile and flexural elongation between bulk PMMA and self-reinforced composites.

These composites consist of degradable fibers imbedded in the same degradable polymer matrix. For example, one such composite was to incorporate degradable sutures of high strength into a matrix of the same polymer by sintering at high temperature and pressure, resulting in the consolidation of the fiber and polymer into a composite structure. The processing temperature was usually maintained above the glass transition temperature but below the melting temperature. The careful control of processing temperature is important because it may result in the partial melting and/or loss of orientation of the reinforcement phase, leading to the reduction in its reinforcing efficiency. Self-reinforced PGA–PLA rods have fairly good initial flexural strength (250 MPa), and they lose most of their mechanical strength *in vitro* in 4 weeks.[48] Meanwhile, the self-reinforced PGA composites have a much higher initial strength (~370 MPa).[44] These composites were shown to have a strength reduction of ~14% at 1 week and it takes more than 5 weeks for them to lose most of their strength when they were immersed in the distilled water at 37°C. It was also reported in the same study that gamma-irradiation with 25 kGy decreased the strength by ~20%. However, after the first week, the irradiated PGA and the nonirradiated PGA composites displayed very similar degradation profiles. The self-reinforced PGA composites have been used clinically to treat certain types of cancellous bone fractures. One additional advantage with self-reinforced PGA and PGA–PLA composites is that they show a ductile fracture behavior compared with the pure PGA and PGA–PLA rods, which undergo brittle fracture. Such properties may allow the composites to exhibit a delayed fracture, which offers a warning that a fracture is taking place. To further illustrate effects of self-reinforcement on mechanical properties of PLL and PGA, the data from Tormala's study is replotted in Figure 8.4 and Figure 8.5.[46] These figures clearly indicate that incorporating PGA fibers into a PGA polymer matrix significantly increased the bending modulus of the polymer. In the meantime, the bending strength has also shown improvement over both bulk PGA and PLL polymers. The overall results suggest that the initial strength and modulus values of self-reinforced composites would be significantly higher than

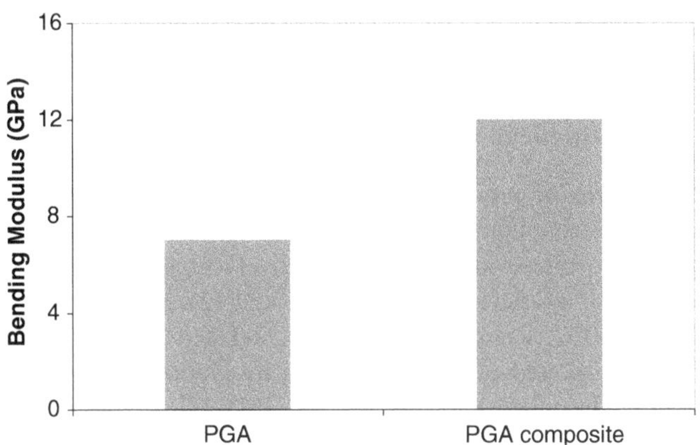

FIGURE 8.4 Effects of self-reinforcement on bending modulus of PGA.

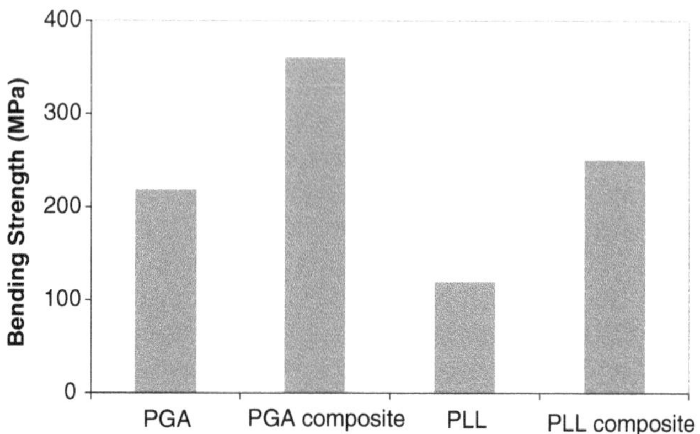

FIGURE 8.5 Effects of self-reinforcement on bending strength of PGA and PLL.

the corresponding values of injection molded bulk materials. It was also reported that the use of self-reinforced PGA rods and screws in fixation of cancellous bone fractures is comparable with the results associated with metallic device fixation. Still, an obvious advantage with absorbable implants is that they do not need a removal operation as the metallic ones may. In a recent study, a third phase (bioceramic) was added to the self-reinforced PLLA composites.[49] However, the testing results indicate that addition of the bioceramic to self-reinforced composites does not improve the mechanical properties of these composites.

8.2.3 Cross-Linking

Two types of cross-linking methods have been used in cross-linking polymeric biomaterials for the improved mechanical properties. They are radiation-induced cross-linking and chemical-induced cross-linking. The radiation-induced cross-linking entails subjecting the polymer to high energy ionizing radiation. The chemical-induced cross-linking is based on the use of a suitable free radical-generating chemical or cross-linking agent.

8.2.3.1 Radiation-Induced Cross-Linking

This type of cross-linking process is currently used to improve the performance of UHMWPE orthopedic implants. The processes include normally two steps: (1) cross-linking by gamma or electron beam at a relatively high dose (e.g., 150 kGy) at ambient condition or at elevated temperature and (2) annealing at temperatures between 130 and 150°C. The purpose of the second step is to stabilize the polymer by neutralizing the free radicals formed during irradiation. Although cross-linking is mainly used to reduce the wear particles of UHMWPE, the mechanical properties of the polymer are improved. Muratoglu et al. and Mckellop et al. used gamma and electron beams to cross-link UHMWPE in an effort to improve its wear resistance, which is critical for the long-term successful application of the polymer for use in orthopedic implants.[50,51] A controlled cross-linking and postprocessing (such as in annealing and remelting) led to a reduction in the formation of wear particles. Free radicals formed during irradiation were eliminated to prevent a continuous change in the properties. The mechanism of improving the wear resistance through increasing cross-link density is based mainly on decreasing the conformational chain segmental mobility in cross-linked polymers. Hence, this leads to a significant reduction in surface deformation and orientation, which are the primary causes of wear particle generation. However, over–cross-linking may affect other mechanical properties (such as toughness) to varying degrees. Cross-linking will reduce creep deformation, and the irradiation environment and postirradiation treatments will affect the final outcome.[52,53] Limiting cross-linking to the polymer surface may have benefits to the wear property without affecting other properties significantly.[54]

8.2.3.2 Chemical-Induced Cross-Linking

One type of chemical-induced cross-linking process involves mixing a free-radical–generating chemical with the polymer resin powder and then consolidating the mixture at elevated temperature. This process generates free radicals, leading to the cross-linking of the polymer. Another type of chemical-induced cross-linking process is the grafting of a silane compound onto the polymer chain. Both of these processes could result in a significant increase in the mechanical properties of polymeric biomaterials. The study also showed that chemical crosslinking of UHMWPE–quartz composites by organosiloxane significantly improved the mechanical performance of the materials.[24]

8.2.4 Solid-State Orientation

When the polymer microstructure is oriented in the preferable directions, mechanical strength, modulus, and toughness of the polymer may increase significantly in those directions. An effective way to create an oriented structure in a polymeric material is mechanical deformation. The deformation process is normally carried out at a temperature higher than glass transition temperature but lower than the melting temperature. Unidirectional orientation is a widely used solid-state deformation process to produce oriented, high performance polymeric material. By definition, this technique is a process resulting in mainly a one-direction orientation, which leads to dramatic increase in the mechanical properties in that direction. This method can be applied to most semicrystalline polymeric biomaterials. Tormala investigated the solid-state orientation of poly(L-lactide) (PLL) and PGA by free-drawing or die-drawing.[46] Their data are replotted in Figure 8.6 and Figure 8.7. For PGA rods, free-drawn samples (PG-O1 and PG-O2) showed significant increase in modulus compared with injection-molded samples (PG-IM), about an 86 to 160% increase was achieved. The bending strength improvement was ~50 to 90%. For PLL rods, die-drawn samples (PL-O) displayed significant increase in modulus compared with injection-molded samples (PL-IM), about 230%, and the bending strength improvement was about 150%. For both polymers, the shear strength showed significant improvement following the drawing process. Despite a slightly weaker initial mechanical strength compared with drawn PGA pins, the strength of the drawn PLL

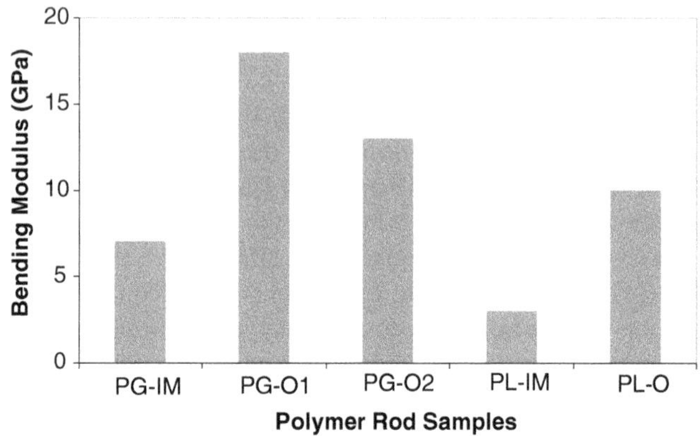

FIGURE 8.6 Effects of unidirectional orientation on bending modulus of PGA and PLL.

is maintained at a high level for a longer time compared with PGA pins. This technique was also extended to other biodegradable polymers and their composites such as poly(DTE carbonate) and poly(DTE carbonate) bioglass.[55]

In a novel approach, Shalaby et al. developed an orthogonal solid-state orientation (OSSO) process for polymeric biomaterials.[56] In this process, a uniaxial orientation is achieved by applying a perpendicular, high compressive force at a temperature lower than the melting temperature, which forces the orientation of polymer microstructures, such as chains, in one direction. The process was successfully applied to UHMWPE and PEEK. The results for UHMWPE are shown in Figure 8.8. Clearly, the modulus of the polymer was significantly increased following orientation, and the tensile strength was also significantly increased.

The OSSO technique was also applied successfully to three types of crystalline absorbable copolymers for suitable use in orthopedic devices.[57] The three types of

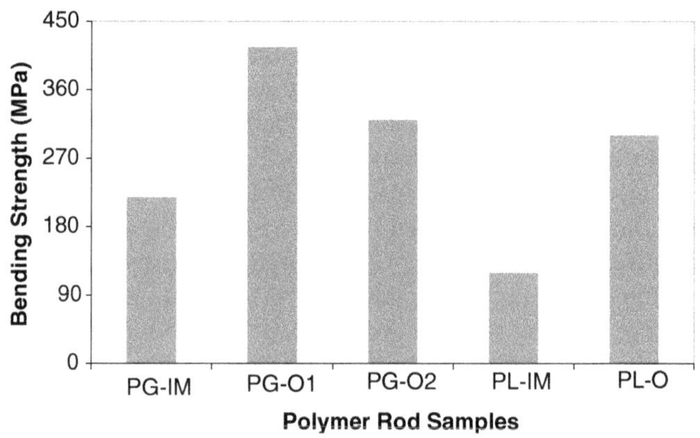

FIGURE 8.7 Effects of unidirectional orientation on bending strength of PGA and PLL.

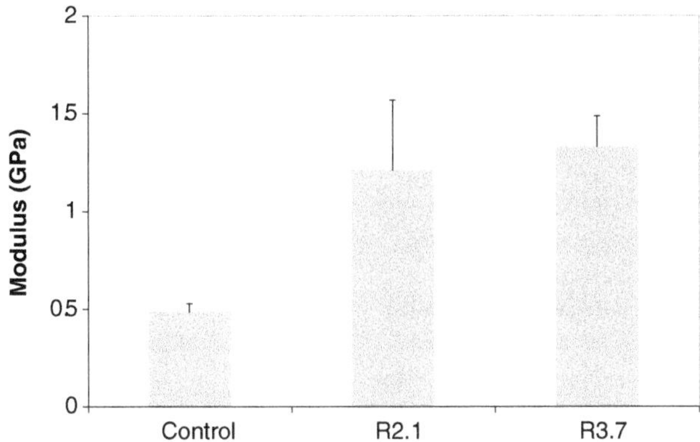

FIGURE 8.8 Effect of unidirectional orientation on tensile modulus of UHMWPE (processing temperature 125°C; R2.1 and R3.7 = compression ratios of 2.1 and 3.7, respectively).

copolymers were in turn made from three different combinations of monomers to provide different chain microstructures: random 95/5 poly(glycolide-co-*l*-lactide), segmented 70/30 poly(*l*-lactide-co-*d,l*-lactide), and segmented 88/12 poly(*l*-lactide-co-trimethylene carbonate). The heat of fusion (ΔH_f) of each polymer was determined using differential scanning calorimetry. Both molding and orthogonal solid-state orientation were performed using a Carver hydraulic press. The 95/5 samples were molded by pressing at 220°C and 0.8 MPa for 10 min. The 70/30 and 88/12 samples were pressed at 173 and 206°C, respectively, for 10 min at 4.3 MPa. Prior to solid-state orientation, samples were annealed to induce crystallization. The 70/30 samples were annealed at 120°C in air for 3 h, whereas, the 88/12 samples were heated (1) at 120°C in air for 5 h, or (2) at 100°C in nitrogen for 4 h. The OSSO was achieved by pressing samples sized ~5 × 19 × 19 mm in a 19 × 38 mm heated steel chamber. The 95/5, 70/30, and 88/12 samples were oriented for 10 min at 85°C, 93 MPa; 120°C, 12 MPa; and 165°C, 12 MPa, respectively. The changes in crystallinity were determined in terms of respective changes in ΔH_f due to annealing and orientation; this is represented as $\Delta H_f/\Delta H_{f,0}$ where $\Delta H_{f,0}$ and $\Delta H_{f,}$ are the heat of fusion of polymer before molding and following orientation, respectively. Samples tested under three-point bending were ~3 × 4 × 38 mm (30-mm span).

The heats of fusion of 95/5, 70/30, and 88/12 samples before molding were 53.0, 44.4, and 59.8 J/g, respectively. The effect of orthogonal solid state orientation on the tangent modulus and strength of 95/5, 70/30 and 88/12 samples is shown in Table 8.1. The most pronounced modulus increases were observed for the 95/5 and 88/12 samples. Each of the oriented strength values was in the range of that for cortical bone (100–200 MPa). Orientation increased the strength of the 88/12 sample by 44% to 121 MPa, and the modulus by 80.0% to 3.9 GPa. Furthermore, the strength and modulus of sample 88/12 were dependent on crystallinity level (measured in terms of $\Delta H_f/\Delta H_{f,0}$) (Figure 8.9). Annealing the molded 88/12 sample in air for 5 h at 120 increased ΔH_f from 21.5 to 43.9 J/g. The level of crystallinity, strength, and modulus of samples heated under nitrogen at 100°C for 4 h were 67%, 110 MPa, and 3.4 GPa, respectively.[57]

TABLE 8.1
Effect of Orthogonal Solid-State Orientation on Tangent Modulus and Strength

Composition, State	Strength (MPa)	Modulus (GPa)
95/5 poly(glycolide-co-*l*-lactide), unoriented	49 ± 16	1.3 ± 0.3
95/5 poly(glycolide-co-*l*-lactide), oriented	122 ± 11	4.8 ± 1.1
70/30 poly(*l*-lactide-co-*d,l*-lactide), unoriented	104 ± 6	3.5 ± 0.0
70/30 poly(*l*-lactide-co-*d,l*-lactide), oriented	122 ± 2	3.6 ± 0.1
88/12 poly(*l*-lactide-co-trimethylene carbonate), unoriented	84 ± 12	2.2 ± 0.3
88/12 poly(*l*-lactide-co-trimethylene carbonate), oriented	121 ± 8	3.9 ± 0.4

These results led to the conclusion that orthogonal solid-state orientation can be used to increase the strength and tangent modulus of three types of absorbable polymer systems: random 95/5 poly(glycolide-co-*l*-lactide), segmented 70/30 poly (*l*-lactide-co-*d,l*-lactide), and segmented 88/12 poly(*l*-lactide-co-trimethylene carbonate). Variation in crystallinity prior to orientation has a pronounced effect on the oriented absorbable polymer strength and modulus.[57]

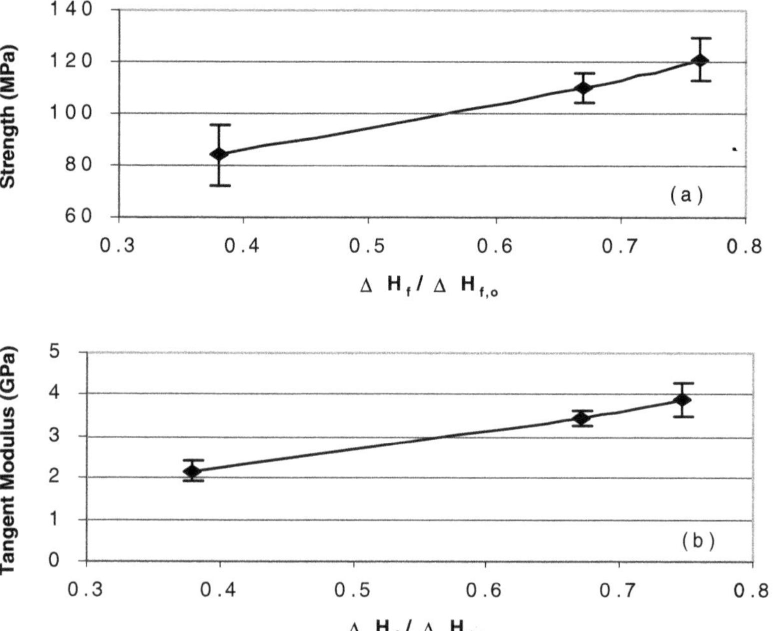

FIGURE 8.9 Level of crystallinity (in terms of $\Delta H_f/\Delta H_{f,0}$) versus one three-point bend strength, and tangent modulus of 88/12 poly(*l*-lactide-co-trimethylene carbonate).

8.3 CONCLUSION AND PERSPECTIVE ON THE FUTURE

Great progress has been made in the past two decades in the area of polymeric biomaterials to improve their toughness and modulus. The composite technology, cross-linking, and solid-state orientation are effective means to improving the mechanical and biological properties of biomaterials. One way to further enhance the mechanical property of the polymer-based composites is to improve interfacial bonding through silane coupling, polymer grafting, and introduction of an interphase layer between the reinforcement and the matrix.[58–60] In general, such an interphase layer promotes the adhesion between the reinforcement and the matrix and hence improves mechanical properties of composites. And the function of the interphase layer in composite materials needs further investigation because it may have significant effects on end performance of the composites.[60] New processing methods are needed to promote uniform distribution of reinforcing components because clustering of particles or fibers in composites may become a crack initiation site under excess loading. Development of UHMWPE processing in conjunction with interfacial bonding and new processing techniques of high viscosity melts and dispersion of reinforcement are also needed. Application of the orthogonal solid-state orientation to both absorbable and nonabsorbable polymers for orthopedic and dental devices is likely to receive considerable future attention. One will continue to see the increased efforts in biodegradable polymers and nano-biomaterials in coming years.

REFERENCES

1. Yildiz, H., Ha, H.K., and Chang, F.K., Composite hip prostheses design I. Analysis, *J. Biomed. Mater. Res.*, 39, 91, 1998.
2. Yildiz, H. and Chang, F.K., Composite hip prostheses design I. Simulation, *J. Biomed. Mater. Res.*, 39, 102, 1998.
3. Fujihara, K., Huang, Z.M., Ramakrishna, S., Satknanantham, K., and Hamada, H., Feasibility of knitted carbon/PEEK composites for orthopedic bone plates, *Biomaterials*, 25, 3877, 2004.
4. Fujihara, K., Huang, Z.M., Ramakrishna, S., Satknanantham, K., and Hamada, H., Performance study of braided carbon/PEEK composite compression plates, *Biomaterials*, 24, 2661, 2003.
5. Kasuga, T., Ota, Y., Nogami, M., and Abe, Y., Preparation and mechanical properties of polylactic acid composites containing hydroxyapatite fibers, *Biomaterials*, 22, 19, 2001.
6. Krause, W.R., Park, S.H., and Straup, R.A., Mechanical properties of Bis-GMA resin short glass fiber composites, *J. Biomed. Mater. Res.*, 23, 1195, 1989.
7. Bayne, S.C. and Thompson, J.Y., Mechanical property analysis of two admixed PRIMM-modified commercial dental composites, *Acad. Dent. Mater. Trans.*, 9, 238, 1996.
8. Xu, J.H.K., Martin, T.A., Antonucci, J.M., and Eichmiller, F.C., Ceramic whisker reinforcement of dental resin composites, *J. Dent. Res.*, 78, 706, 1999.
9. Xu, H.H.K. and Eichmiller, F.C., Reinforcement of Dental and Other Composite Materials, U.S. Patent No. 5,861,445, 1999.
10. Xu, H.H.K., Quinna, J.B., Smith, D.T., Antonuccic, J.M., Schumachera, G.E., and Eichmillera, F.C., Dental resin composites containing silica-fused whiskers — effects of whisker-to-silica ratio on fracture toughness and indentation properties, *Biomaterials*, 23, 735, 2002.

11. Shalaby, S.W. and Rogers, K.R., Polymeric Prosthesis Having a Phosphonylated Surface, U.S. Patent (to Clemson University) 5,558,517, 1996.
12. Shalaby, S.W. and McCaig, S., Surface Phosphonylation of Polymers, U.S. Patent (to Clemson University) 5,491,198, 1996.
13. Allan, J.M., Biggers, L., Duncan, M., Atkins, T., and Shalaby, S.W., New approach to development of fiber-reinforced bone cement, *Trans. Soc. Biomater.*, 21, 285, 1998.
14. Deng, M., Allan, J.M., Lake, R.A., Gerdes, G.A., and Shalaby, S.W., Effects of phosphonylation on UHMWPE fabrics reinforced composites, *Trans. Soc. Biomater* 22, 470, 1999.
15. Bonfield, W., Grynpas, M.D., Tully, A.E., Bowman, J., and Abram, J., Hydroxyapatite reinforced polyethylene — a mechanically compatible implant material for bone replacement, *Biomaterials*, 2, 185, 1981.
16. Reis, R.L., Granja, P.L., and Cunha, A.M., Impact behavior of UHMWPE/HA composites for orthopedic prostheses, in *Frontiers in Biomedical Polymer Applications* Ottenbrite, R.M., Ed., Technomic Publishing, Lancaster, PA, 1998, pp. 252.
17. Knets, I.V., Bunina, L.O., and Filipenkov, V.V., Ultrahigh-molecular weight polyethylene and hydroxylapatite-based materials for replacement of bone tissue, *Mech. Compos. Mater.*, 1993, 29, 181, 1993.
18. Cunha, A.M., Reis, R.L., Ferreira, F.G., and Granja, P.L., The influence of processing conditions on the mechanical behavior of UHMWPE/HA and PMMA/HA composites, in *Advances in Materials Science and Implant Orthopedic Surgery*, Kossowsky R. and Kossowsky N, Eds. (NATO Science Series E: Vol. 294, June 19–July 2), Academic Publishers, Netherlands, 1994, pp. 163–176.
19. Evans, G.P., Behiri, J.C., Currey, J.D., and Bonfield, W., Microhardness and Young's modulus in cortical bone exhibiting a wide range of mineral volume fractions and in a bone analogue, *J. Mater. Sci. Mater. Med.*, 1, 38, 1990.
20. Juhasz, J.A., Best, S.M., Brooks, R., Kawashita, M., Miyata, N., Kokubo, T., Nakamura, T., and Bonfield, W., Mechanical properties of glass-ceramic A-W-polyethylene composites: effect of filler content and particle size, *Biomaterials*, 25, 949, 2004.
21. Wang, M. and Bonfield, W., Chemically coupled hydroxyapatite-polyethylene composites: structure and properties, *Biomaterials*, 22, 1311, 2001.
22. Wang, M., Joseph, R., and Bonfield, W., Hydroxyapatite-polyethylene composites for bone substitution: effects of ceramic particle size and morphology, *Biomaterials*, 19, 2357, 1998.
23. Fang, L., Leng. Y., and Gao, P., Processing of hydroxyapatite reinforced ultrahigh molecular weight polyethylene for biomedical applications, *Biomaterials*, 26, 3471, 2004.
24. Xie, X.X., Tang, C.Y., Chan, K.Y.Y., Wu, X.C., Tsui, C.P., and Cheung, C.Y., Wear performance of ultrahigh molecular weight polyethylene/quartz composites, *Biomaterials*, 24, 1889, 2003.
25. Anderson, B.C., Bloom, P.D., Baikerikar, K.G., Sheares, V.V., and Mallapragada, S.K., Al–Cu–Fe quasicrystal/ultra-high molecular weight polyethylene composites as biomaterials for acetabular cup prosthetics, *Biomaterials*, 23, 1761, 2002.
26. Abu Bakar, M.S., Cheang, P., and Khor, K.A., Mechanical properties of injection molded hydroxyapatite-polyetheretherketone biocomposites, *Composites Sci. Tech.* 63, 421, 2003.
27. Yu, S., Hariram, K.P., Kumar, R., Cheang, P., and Aik, K.K., *In vitro* apatite formation and its growth kinetics on hydroxyapatite/polyetheretherketone biocomposites, *Biomaterials*, 26, 2343, 2005,

28. Abu Bakar, M.S., Cheng, M.H.W., Tan, S.M., Yu, S.C., Liao, K., Tan, C.T., Khor K.A., and Cheang, P., Tensile properties, tension-tension fatigue and biological response of polyetheretherketone-hydroxyapatite composites for load-bearing orthopedic implants, *Biomaterials*, 24, 2245, 2003.
29. Shikiami, Y. and Okuno, M., Bioresorbable devices made of forged composites of hydroxyapatite (HA) particles and poly L-lactide (PLLA). Part II: Practical properties of miniscrews and miniplates, *Biomaterials,* 22, 3197, 2001.
30. Kikuchi, M., Suetsugu, Y., Tanaka, J., and Akao, M., Preparation and mechanical properties of calcium phosphate/copoly- L -lactide composites, *J. Mater. Sci. Mater. Med.*, 8, 361, 1997.
31. Demian, H.W. and Shalaby, S.W., Bone Cement Composition Containing Micro-Encapsulated Radiopacifier and Methods of Making Same, U.S. Patent (to Clemson University) 5,795,922, 1998.
32. Wang, M., Wang, J., and Ni, J., Developing tricalcium phosphate/polyhydroxybutyrate composite as a new biodegradable material for clinical applications, *Biomechanics*, 192-1, 741, 2000.
33. Wang, M., Yue, C.Y., and Chua, B., Production and evaluation of hydroxyapatite reinforced polysulfone for tissue replacement, *J. Mater. Sci. Mater. Med.*, 9, 821, 2001.
34. Deng, X., Hao, J., and Wang, C., Preparation and mechanical properties of nanocomposites of poly(D,L-lactide) with Ca-deficient hydroxyapatite nanocrystals, *Biomaterials*, 22, 2867, 2001.
35. Kasuga, T., Maeda, H., Kato, K., Nogami, M., Hata, K., and Ueda, M., Preparation of poly(lactic acid) composites containing calcium carbonate (vaterite), *Biomaterials* 24, 3247, 2003.
36. Wei, G., and Ma, P.X., Structure and properties of nano-hydroxyapatite/polymer composite scaffolds for bone tissue engineering, *Biomaterials*, 25, 4749, 2004.
37. Ruan, S.L., Gao, P., Yang, X.G., and Yu, T.X., Toughening high performance ultrahigh molecular weight polyethylene using multiwalled carbon nanotubes, *Polymer*, 44, 5643, 2003.
38. Liu, Q., de Wijn, J.R., and van Blitterswijk, C.A., Nano-apatite/polymer composites: mechanical and physicochemical characteristics, *Biomaterials*, 18, 1263, 1997.
39. Musanje, L. and Ferracane, J.L., Effects of resin formulation and nanofiller surface treatment on the properties of experimental hybrid resin composite, *Biomaterials*, 25, 4065, 2004.
40. Shalaby, S.W. and Deng, M., Self-Reinforced Ultra-High Molecular Weight Polyethylene Composite Medical Implants, U.S. Patent (to Poly-Med, Inc.) 5,834,113, 1998.
41. Deng, M. and Shalaby, S.W., Properties of self-reinforced ultra-high-molecular-weight polyethylene composites, *Biomaterials*, 18, 645, 1997.
42. Buckley, C.A., Gilbert, J.L., and Lautenschlager, E.P., Thermomechanical processing of PMMA into high strength fibers, *J. Appl. Polym. Sci.*, 44, 1321, 1992.
43. Gilbert, J.L., Ney, D.S., and Lautenschlager, E.P., Self-reinforced composite poly(methyl methacrylate): static and fatigue properties, *Biomaterials*, 16, 1043, 1995.
44. Vainionpaa, S., Kilpikari, J., Laiho, J., Helevirta, P., Rokkanen, P., and Tormala, P., Strength and strength retention in vitro, of absorbable, self-reinforced polyglycolide (PGA) rods for fracture fixation, *Biomaterials*, 8, 46, 1987.
45. Tormala, P., Vasenius, J., and Vainionpaa, S., Ultra-high strength absorbable self-reinforced polyglycolide (SR-PGA) composite rods for internal fixation of bone fractures: in-vitro and in-vivo study, *J. Biomed. Mater. Res.*, 25, 1, 1991.

46. Tormala, P., Ultra-high strength, self-reinforced absorbable polymeric composites for applications in different disciplines of surgery, *Clinic. Mater.*, 13, 35, 1993.
47. Tiainen, J., Soini, Y., Tormala, P., Waris, T., and Ashammakhi, N., Self-reinforced polylactide/polyglycolide 80/20 screws take more than 1.5 years to resorb in rabbit cranial bone, *J. Biomed. Mater. Res.*, 70B, 49, 2004.
48. Tormala, P., Vainionpaa, S., Kilpikari, J., and Rokkanen, P., The effects of fiber reinforcement and gold plating on the flexural and tensile strength of PGA/PLA copolymer materials in vitro, *Biomaterials*, 8, 42, 1987.
49. Bleach, N.C., Nazhat, S.N., Tanner, K.E., Kellomaki, M., and Tormala, P. Effect of filler content on mechanical properties of particulate biphasic calcium phosphate-polylactide composites, *Biomaterials*, 23, 1579, 2002.
50. Muratoglu, O.K., Bragdon, C.R., O'Connor, D.O., Jasty, M., and Harris, W.H., A novel method of crosslinking UHMWPE to improve wear, reduce oxidation and retain mechanical properties, *J. Arthroplasty*, 2001;16, 1, 2001.
51. McKellop, H., Shen, F-W., Lu, B., Campbell, P., and Salovey, R., Development of an extremely wear resistant ultra-high molecular weight polyethylene for total hip replacements. *J. Orthop. Res.*, 17, 157, 1999.
52. Deng, M. and Shalaby, S.W., Effects of gamma irradiation, gas environments and postirradiation aging on ultrahigh molecular weight polyethylene, *J. Appl. Polym. Sci.*, 58, 2111, 1995.
53. Deng, M. and Shalaby, S.W., Long-term gamma irradiation effects on ultrahigh molecular weight polyethylene, *J. Biomed. Mater. Res.*, 54, 428, 2001.
54. Muratoglu, O.K., O'Connor, D.O., Bragdon, C.R., Delaney, J., Jasty, M., Harris, W.H., Merrill, E., and Venugopalan, P., Gradient crosslinking of UHMWPE using irradiation in molten state for total joint arthroplasty, *Biomaterials*, 23, 717, 2002.
55. Pyhalto, T., Lapinsuo, M., Patiala, H., Pelto, M., Tormala, P., and Rokkanen, P., Fixation of distal femoral osteotomies with self-reinforced polymer/bioactive glass rods: an experimental study on rabbits, *Biomaterials*, 26, 645, 2005.
56. Shalaby, S.W., Johnson, R.A., and Deng, M., Process of Making a Bone Healing Device, U.S. Patent (to Clemson University) 5,529,736, 1996.
57. Cluper, D.C., Carpenter, K.A., Anneaux, B.L., and Shalaby, S.W., Orthogonal solid-state orientation of absorbable polymers for orthopedic devices, 7th World Biomaterial Congress, *Trans. Soc. Biomater.*, 27, 458, 2004.
58. Wang, M., Deb, S., and Bonfield, W., Chemically coupled hydroxyapatite-polyethylene composites: processing and characterization, *Mater. Let.*, 44, 119, 2000.
59. Fu, Q. and Wang, G., Polyethylene toughened by ridge inorganic particles, *Polym. Eng. Sci.*, 32, 94, 1992.
60. Fan, J.P., Tsui, C.P., Tang, C.Y., and Chow, C.L. Influence of interphase layer on the overall elasto-plastic behaviors of HA/PEEK biocomposite, *Biomaterials*, 25, 5363, 2004.

9 Physicochemical Modification of Polymers for Bone-Implant Osseointegration

Shalaby W. Shalaby and Bruce L. Anneaux

CONTENTS

9.1 INTRODUCTION

Traditionally, most biomaterials are developed or selected to meet biological requirements based on their (1) initial mechanical properties and their retention profiles in the biologic environment, (2) mechanical biocompatibility, such as having practically smooth surface morphology, and (3) chemical biocompatibility, i.e., being free of toxic leachables and inert with no tendency for biological interaction. In fact, inertness was the primary criterion early investigators used for material selection; a biocompatible material was denoted as one that does not elicit toxic, carcinogenic, or significant local inflammatory reactions.[1] An ideal biomaterial for use in long-term or permanent (nontransient) implants was typically described by a list of negative adjectives: nontoxic, noncarcinogenic, and nonallergenic.[2] Because our understanding of implantable biomaterials and the biological reactions at the implant–tissue interface have increased significantly over the past two decades, the definition of biocompatible materials has evolved beyond being simply bioinert, and the significance of positive interaction of a biomaterial implant with the surrounding biological environment has been widely acknowledged.[3] Contemporary biomaterial scientists and engineers are calling for the development of a new generation of implants having chemically and/or physically tailored and/or modified surfaces to provide positive interaction with the biological environment and capable of directing pertinent biological events to meet specific functional requirements of such implants. This ideology was the driving force for pursuing most of the studies reported in this chapter, which deal with the introduction of functional groups capable of positive interaction with osteoblasts to encourage osseointegration. A second aspect of these studies deals specifically with dental and orthopedic implants, which need to meet certain strength and modulus requirements. Accordingly, a segment of the studies reported in this chapter describe a new process for enhancing the bulk properties of the pertinent material. A third aspect of the reported studies pertains to the advantage of having microtextured surfaces that support interlocking with bony tissues. And a novel process for surface microtexturing is discussed in the text of the chapter.

9.2 TECHNOLOGY EVOLUTION OF PHYSICOCHEMICAL SURFACE MODIFICATION AND BULK ORIENTATION

Since the beginning of interest in polymers as implantable dental and orthopedic biomaterials, most investigators focused on exploring means to increase the polymer modulus to match or approach those of pertinent bony tissues for optimum biomechanical compatibility. Until recently, most of the studies dealt with solid-state orientation in the tensile mode.[5–7] With the introduction of orthogonal solid-state orientation by Shalaby and coworkers, the application of exceptionally high forces to achieve maximum orientation became possible.[8] However, with the exception of random efforts to modify polymeric surfaces through cold plasma oxidation radiation grafting of unsaturated monomers and introduction of bioactive molecules of hydrophilic polymers, early efforts on physicochemical surface modification of polymeric implants to optimize their biomechanical and biochemical compatibility were limited.[9–14] More specifically, earlier approaches to the chemical modification of polymeric implant surfaces dealt mostly with blood-contacting surfaces. These and related modifications were addressed by a number of authors and dealt primarily with increasing the surface hydrophilicity of hydrophobic polymeric substrates and entailed (1) surface oxidation using gas plasma, (2) grafting of hydrophilic monomers, and (3) covalently immobilizing hydrophilic or water-soluble polymers on the specific surface.[11–14] In spite of recent emphasis on the implant–tissue interfaces and their key relevance to optimal performance of dental and orthopedic implants, efforts of contemporary investigators in this area were minimal. This led Shalaby and coworkers to pursue part of the studies described in this chapter on the physicochemical surface modification of model polymers, such as polyethylene and polypropylene, as well as high modulus implantable materials, such as polyether ether ketone and its carbon fiber–reinforced composites.[15,16]

9.2.1 Surface Sulfonation of Model Polyolefins

Since it early use in polymer science and technology, polyethylene (PE) has been used as a model polymer to investigate new approaches to surface and bulk modification of other polymers because low density polyethylene (LDPE) has the simplest possible chemical structure of all known polymers. Furthermore, the ultrahigh molecular version of PE, that is UHMW-PE, is a key biomaterial used in artificial joints; surface modification is an important aspect as is seen in Chapter 10. On the other hand, polypropylene (PP), which is still a simple polymer, is more reactive than LDPE and can be used as another model polymer for those having methyl side groups. In addition, isotactic polypropylene (*i*-PP) is currently used in several biomedical implants and most notably in surgical sutures.

LDPE and *i*-PP as model polymers for studying surface modification; however, these polymers are hydrophobic. Many investigators have attempted to introduce polar moieties, such as carboxylic and sulfonic groups, on the polymer surface to determine their effect on the surface hydrophilicity and the ability to modulate their interaction with the surrounding tissue as part of an implant. For this, introduction of selected types of carboxylic groups is being investigated at Poly-Med, Inc. (Anderson, SC), while efforts at introducing more polar groups, such as sulfonic and phosphonic, are addressed in this chapter.

A sulfonation protocol employing fuming sulfuric acid developed at Poly-Med, Inc. (Anderson, South Carolina) was used to surface sulfonate thin films of LDPE and *i*-PP to render their surfaces more hydrophilic and capable of displaying a negative charge.[17] This study was designed to assess the effect of sulfonation on blood compatibility of LDPE and *i*-PP as model surfaces.[17,18] More specifically, the study was designed to determine how changes in surface chemistry of a model implant influence the degree of conformational change of adsorbing proteins and to investigate the correlation between this change and platelet response. Results of the first segment of the study showed that both LDPE and *i*-PP became more wettable with water in terms of dynamic contact angle measurements — the contact angle of LDPE and *i*-PP changed from about 88° to 47° and from about 82° to about 52°, respectively.[17] In the study, sulfonated film (LDPE and *i*-PP) surfaces were treated with poly-D-lysine (PDL) to achieve a positively charged surface resulting from ionically immobilized PDL. To determine the effect of surface modification on the conformation of adsorbed proteins, we used porcine serum albumin and porcine fibrinogen as model proteins. In effect, thin films of LDPE and *i*-PP were surface modified using sulfonation and immobilized (or preadsorbed) PDL to create a range of surface chemistries. Circular dichroism (CD) studies were then conducted to assess how each surface influenced the secondary structure of adsorbed albumin and fibrinogen as a measure of adsorption-induced conformational changes, and platelet adhesion studies were conducted to investigate how the degree of structural change in the adsorbed proteins influenced the platelet response. From the results of these studies, it was concluded that platelet adhesion to surfaces with a preadsorbed layer of either albumin or fibrinogen is directly related to the degree of adsorption-induced structural change to the protein. It was further concluded that the ability of albumin to serve as a passivation layer to resist platelet adhesion is not a universal property of albumin, but rather is related to albumin's inherent resistance to adsorption-induced structural changes Although controversial, it was suggested that for the same degree of conformational change, nonactivated platelets will adhere to adsorbed albumin as readily as to adsorbed fibrinogen. And collectively, it was concluded that surface treatment of LDPE and *i*-PP by sulfonation and preadsorption of PDL is an effective means of reducing the degree of surface-induced conformational change of adsorbed albumin and fibrinogen and subsequently to reduce albumin and fibrinogen-mediated platelet adhesion.

The results of this study also suggest that the use of surface chemistry to influence protein adsorption in a manner that minimizes the degree of adsorption-induced structural change may be one of the most important principles for the design of blood-compatible biomaterials to minimize platelet adhesion, subsequent platelet activation, and thrombus formation on biomaterial surfaces.

9.2.2 Surface Phosphonylation of Model Polyolefins and Polyether-ether Ketone (PEEK)

Treatment of saturated hydrocarbon with phosphorous trichloride in the presence of oxygen was shown to yield alkyl phosphonyl chloride, which can be hydrolyzed to produce the corresponding alkyl phosphonic acid according to the following reaction scheme:

$$R\text{–}H + 2PCl_3 + O_2 \longrightarrow R\text{–}POCl_2 + POCl_3 + HCl$$

Alkyl phosphonyl chloride

$$R\text{–}POCl_2 + 2H_2O \longrightarrow R\text{–}PO(OH)_2 + 2HCl$$

Alkyl phosphonic acid

The general reaction scheme was later adopted by Shalaby and coworkers to develop new methods for surface activation of preformed polymeric articles, including those made of LDPE, *i*-PP, and on PEEK.[15,16] The surface treatment scheme was devised as a liquid phase reaction in which a thermoplastic polymer was suspended in a phosphorus trichloride solution in an inert solvent with a continuous flow of oxygen through the system.[16] A gas phase process was also developed in which polymers were suspended directly over a reservoir of phosphorus trichloride in a static oxygen environment.[15] Both schemes led to the introduction of phosphonyl chloride groups, which were subsequently hydrolyzed to phosphonic acid groups at the LDPE, *i*-PP, and PEEK surfaces, without imparting discernable changes in the bulk properties of these polymers. The phosphonic acid–bearing surfaces were then reacted with calcium ion–containing solutions to produce calcium phosphonate moieties at the polymeric surfaces.[16–20] Such surfaces approximate bioglass and hydroxyapatite, which were recognized earlier for their bone-binding properties.[21,22] Formation of calcium phosphonate as bound moieties PEEK and other polymers of orthopedic significance created the interesting possibility of direct fixation of orthopedic devices to bone without the need for an intermediate grouting material.

Recognizing the simplicity of the gas phase surface phosphonylation of the thermoplastics led to the pursuit of a new study on a modified version.[2,3] In this particular study, surface phosphonylation of LDPE was conducted, and the phosphonylation process was modified using a two-chamber reactor and a dynamic oxygen flow in an effort to secure greater control of the gas phase reaction.[23] Using such a reaction scheme, the study was designed to determine the effect of the physicochemical properties of LDPE surface, as a model for orthopedic materials on bone binding and apposition to phosphonylated surfaces. And, to determine the effect of phosphonylation time and temperature on the surface properties, low-density polyethylene films were phosphonylated at both ambient and elevated temperatures for periods ranging from 15 to 60 min. After hydrolyzing the phosphonyl chloride groups, the films were analyzed by scanning electron microscope (SEM), electron dispersive X-ray (EDX) analysis, horizontal ATR-FTIR, surface roughness, and dynamic contact angle measurements. The experimental numerical data are summarized in Table 9.1.

Horizontal ATR-FTIR (using a Paragon 1000 spectrophotometer) spectra of representative control and films phosphonylated for 15 min were identical and provided no evidence of phosphonylation. For all other groups, the spectra indicated surface

TABLE 9.1
Surface Analysis Data of Phosphonylated LDPE

Reaction		Elemental Analysis[a]		Roughness[b]		Contact Angle (in.)	
Time (min)	Temp (°C)	%P	%Cl	R_q (nm)	R_z (μm)	Water	CH_2I_2
0	—	0.20	0.04	75.59	1.40	96.81	69.32
15	25	0.26	0.04	78.02	1.23	93.49	78.45
30	25	9.59	0.22	127.19	1.90	52.19	67.15
60	25	6.13	0.27	130.43	1.81	56.36	66.47
60	45	13.65	0.35	201.42	2.81	50.70	64.02

[a] Using JEOL JSM-1c 848 electron microscope (JEOL, Peabody, Massachusetts) equipped for electron dispersive X-ray (EDX) analysis.
[b] Using WYKO NT 2000 Profilometer (Veeco Corp., Tuscon, Arizona).

modification with the same characteristic group frequencies present in samples treated at 25°C for 30 and 60 min, or 45°C for 60 min. The P–O–H group exhibited four characteristic frequencies at 2525– 2725, 2080–2350, 1600–1740, and 917–1040 cm The first of these frequencies appeared as a slight shoulder on the spectra, while the last three were readily apparent. Coupled with the identification of phosphorus at the surface, these spectra provided conclusive evidence that phosphonic acid moieties exist on the surfaces of films phosphonylated for more than 15 min.

EDX spectra of the control and treated surfaces indicated the absence of phosphorus and chlorine on the control and 15-min treatment groups, while it was present on all other surfaces. More revealing than the EDX spectra is the semiquantitative analysis computed from five such spectra for each treatment group as shown in Table 9.1. For all cases, the amount of chlorine present is quite low — only a fraction of a percentage — indicating that samples were adequately hydrolyzed following phosphonylation.

After 15 min of phosphonylation time, the surface does not show phosphorus above the amount detected in the control film, again an indication that the LDPE film does not phosphonylate to a detectable degree in this period. After a 30-min treatment, the film surface is composed of approximately 10% phosphorus. Polyphosphonic acids obtained after hydrolysis are highly hydrophilic, and previous research has shown that these moieties dissolve in water at phosphorus contents in excess of 10%. Therefore, it is no surprise that after a 60-min treatment time the phosphorus content decreases to 6%; isolated surface hydrocarbon chains are excessively phosphonylated and pulled from the bulk during hydrolysis. Solubilization of overphosphonylated surface molecules upon hydrolysis is consistent with pitting of this film group seen using SEM. Finally, the highest phosphorus incorporation, i.e., 13%, is achieved after 60 min phosphonylation at 45°C, indicating that the material is phosphonylated well below the surface without the concomitant solubilization of overphosphonylated surface molecules.

Surface roughness measurements data are summarized in Table 9.1. The film treated for 15 min shows essentially the same degree of roughness as the control, reflecting that practically no phosphonylation has taken place. For the 30- and 60-min phosphonylation at room temperature, the surface roughness values were similar to each other and notably rougher than the control. Phosphonylation did appear to cause a physical change in the polymer surface, as also noted from the SEMs in addition to the known chemical modification. Also, while excessively phosphonylated molecules of the 60-min treatment group delaminate from the surface, the overall surface roughness did not change substantially because of this process. Finally, for 60 min treatment at 45°C, both the average roughness and peak-to-valley height were substantially greater than those of other treatment groups. This is consistent with the thesis that the treatment affects the subsurface and is not limited to the surface.

Dynamic contact angle measurements were considered in conjunction with the physicochemical differences of the surfaces described; the contact angles values are summarized in Table 9.1. As expected, water proved to be a superior probe liquid for discriminating between differences in the treated and untreated surfaces, while methylene iodide (CH_2I_2) was none too revealing. This is because phosphonylation renders the polymer surface hydrophilic, and water, a polar liquid, is quite responsive to this change, while methylene iodide, a nonpolar liquid, is not. Therefore, treatments are discussed in terms of their advancing dynamic contact angle in water.

Results of the Allan et al. study led to the conclusion that using a two-chamber dynamic flow system, phosphonylation of LDPE can be regulated to control the extent and uniformity of surface modification.[23] Under the prevailing reaction conditions, LDPE films do not phosphonylate to a detectable degree at 15 min. Within 30 min, the surface undergoes phosphonylation, and at 60 min, the surface becomes overphosphonylated at localized sites with concomitant surface pitting being observed. Phosphonylation at 45°C results in phosphonylation at the surface as well as the subsurface. Overall, gas phase phosphonylation of LDPE was noted as being best regulated at 25°C, with reaction times greater than 15 min but less than 60 min providing the most uniform surface treatment.[23]

For preparing surface phosphonylated *i*-PP films, a protocol similar to the one described for LDPE was used, but the reaction time was limited to 15 and 60 min periods at 45°C. The hydrolysis of the phosphonyl chloride groups of the phosphonylated surface was achieved by sonicating the films in distilled water for 30 min using a Branson Model 3210 Ultrasonic Cleaner (Branson Ultrasonic Corp., Danbury, CT). The films were characterized for surface composition, surface roughness, and contact angle as described previously for LDPE films. Although most of the results were generally similar to those of LDPE, the *i*-PP films revealed (1) measurable phosphonylation for the 15-min reaction time, (2) a slightly higher level of surface phosphonylation, (3) a slightly more noticeable decrease in contact angle, and (4) a slightly more pronounced surface roughness or microtexturing.[23]

Attempts to surface phosphonylate PEEK or carbon fiber-reinforced (CFR) PEEK were first made using the protocols applied successfully to LDPE and *i*-PP. However, it was observed that the aromatic PEEK-based surfaces are far less reactive than their aliphatic counterparts, especially in the case of the gas phase method. Accordingly, a study on the surface phosphonylation of PEEK and CFR-PEEK was conducted on practically unoriented thin films, using the liquid phase method and carbon tetrachloride (CCl_4) as a medium to maximize the effectiveness of the phosphonylation reaction. The phosphonyl chloride groups of the phosphonylated films were hydrolyzed. The films were dried and subjected to the same analytical methods employed for LDPE and *i*-PP counterparts with the exception of using electron spectroscopy for chemical analysis (ESCA) in addition to EDX for surface elemental analysis. Analytical data obtained using the different methods indicated that phosphonylation occurs mostly at the uppermost layers of the PEEK-based films, while in the polyolefin films, the reaction proceeds well below the surface. This was associated with the finding that the surfaces of PEEK-based films have much lower phosphorus contents than their polyolefin-based counterparts. When EDX was used, it showed comparable and sometimes lower phosphorus concentrations than when the less penetrating ESCA was used. Accordingly, phosphonylation of PEEK-based films appears to be affected by their lower chemical reactivity and high glass transition temperature (T_g) as aromatic substrates.

9.2.3 Surface Microtexturing of Model Polyolefins and PEEK-Based Substrates

The term surface microtexturing was initially used relative to improving tissue regeneration and short- and long-term mechanical stability of the soft tissue implants. On the other hand, for high modulus dental and orthopedic implants, the term microroughness or microroughening was used as the equivalent of the term surface microtexture, or microtexturing. Contemporary orthopedic and dental investigators, while acknowledging the importance of an implant's chemical inertness, emphasize the importance of bioactivity and surface roughness of such an implant relative to its short- and long-term mechanical stability at a bony site.[24,25] Meanwhile, practically all efforts to impart the required surface microroughness or higher level of roughness focused on ceramic and metallic implants to improve their osseointegration with surrounding bony tissue.[25,26] And numerous surface modification schemes have been developed and are currently used to enhance clinical performance of ceramic and metallic implants. Such modifications dealt primarily with blasted, acid-etched, porous sintered, oxidized, plasma-sprayed, and hydroxyapatite-coated surfaces.[26] However, until Shalaby and coworkers developed a process denoted as crystallization-induced microphase separation (CIMS) to produce microporous foam with a continuous cellular structure and an extension thereof, surface microtexturing of crystalline thermoplastic polymers was virtually unknown for dental and orthopedic implants.[27,28] The CIMS process entails

1. Dissolving the crystalline polymer in the melt of a crystalline, low-melting organic compound or diluent to form a one-phase liquid system of the polymer and diluent
2. Quick-quenching the polymer–diluent system to form two bicontinuous crystalline microphases of the polymer and diluent
3. Removing the diluent from the two-phase system by sublimation below the melting temperature of the polymer or extracting the diluent with a solvent that does not dissolve the polymer phase

This process results in a microporous foam with continuous cell structure. The average size of the pores can be modulated primarily by controlling the polymer-diluent ratio, wherein larger pores can be achieved by decreasing this ratio. The CIMS process has been applied successfully for the production of PE and *i*-PP microporous foams.[29] On the other hand, limiting the CIMS process to the surface of a crystalline polymer results in the formation of a microporous surface that is, in effect, a microtextured surface.[27,28] Application of the CIMS process for surface microtexturing of a preformed implant made of crystalline thermoplastic polymer entails

1. Heating the selected diluent to liquefy and acquire a temperature below the polymer melting temperature (T_m)
2. Dipping the preformed polymeric article or implant in the molten diluent for a specific period to attain a transient, high viscosity, one-phase solution of the polymer with the diluent at the surface
3. Removing the treated implant and quick-quenching it to form a thin, bicontinuous solid coating that is molecularly intermixed with the surface
4. Extracting or subliming the diluent as described for the production of microporous foam

Forming such a coating on the implant surface that yields mostly a microtextured surface that may have a microporous subsurface can be achieved by controlling the (1) type of diluent in which the polymer exhibits limited solubility, (2) temperature of the molten diluent, and (3) contact time of the polymer with the diluent.

Early attempts in the study of microtexturing dealt with the preparation of microtextured films of *i*-PP and LDPE using molten naphthalene as a diluent.[27,28] Removal of the naphthalene microphase from the bicontinuous system was achieved by sublimation. Further purification of the microtextured films can be accomplished by extracting residual naphthalene by a solvent such as hexane or methylene chloride. However, surface microtexturing of thin films of PEEK and CFR-PEEK using the CIMS process proved to be more demanding, and the conditions applied successfully for microtexturing polyolefin films were modified substantially in terms of the type of diluent used, reaction temperature, polymer–diluent contact time, and the cooling rate of the treated films. More specifically, the modified CIMS process required the use of (1) high melting diluents for application at temperatures near the T_g of PEEK and (2) more polar diluent than naphthalene with higher solubilizing effect relative to PEEK. Specific conditions for microtexturing LDPE, *i*-PP, PEEK, and CFR-PEEK as implantable devices are outlined in Section 9.4 in conjunction with the preparation and evaluation of surface-phosphonylated rods.

9.2.4 Orthogonal Solid-State Orientation of Crystalline Thermoplastic Polymers

The concept of orthogonal solid-state orientation (OSSO) of crystalline thermoplastic polymers was first disclosed by Shalaby and coworkers.[30] One aspect of the OSSO process deals with the following steps.[30,31]

1. Placing a sheet or block of practically unoriented crystalline polymer in a U-shaped mold with an adjustable frame to allow precise contact of the polymer in the three sides of the mold
2. Heating the polymer above its T_g but below its T_m to allow for controlled deformation under pressure
3. Applying a compressive force perpendicular to the top surface through a movable plate that fits precisely within the horizontal space of the U-shaped mold
4. Allowing the polymer to deform uniaxially to exit through the open end of the U-shaped mold. The OSSO process was used successfully to produce a number of oriented forms of thermoplastic polymers, such as UHMW-PE and PEEK

Most relevant to the subject of this chapter is the study of tailoring the mechanical properties of PEEK implants using the OSSO process.[31,32] In this study, PEEK samples were subjected to the OSSO process at different temperatures. Properties of oriented PEEK were compared with those of unoriented PEEK and carbon fiber–reinforced PEEK (CFR-PEEK). For processing and testing PEEK, dried, molding grade resin (PEEK 450PF, Victrex USA, Inc.) was melt processed into 76 × 76 32 mm blocks using a Carver hot press (Model 3895) at 370°C and 9100 kg with a load bearing area of 152 × 152 mm. The blocks were cut into six bars measuring 76 × 12.7 × 32 mm for orientation. For surgical implants, a solid-state orientation was accomplished at 315°C and 13,600 kg with a final load bearing area of 152 × 152 mm in a custom designed mold used to achieve uniaxial orientation by applying a compressive force at 90° to the sample surface. The thickness of the oriented material was 10 mm, for a final compression ratio of approximately 3 to 1. Samples of molded and oriented PEEK, prepared as described above, were machined into rods with a diameter of 5 mm and a length of 10 mm using a JET-1240PD lathe. For comparison purposes, two similar sets of rods were prepared using molded PEEK and CFR-PEEK without implementing the OSSO process. Both sets of rods were used for implantation studies and evaluation of compressive properties. For evaluation of flexural properties, three-point bend samples were prepared as rectangular specimens measuring approximately 28 × 6 × 1 mm. All mechanical testing was accomplished using an MTS 858 MiniBionix universal testing apparatus. Compression tests were conducted at a displacement rate of 1 mm/min. Three-point bend tests were conducted at a rate of 0.54 mm/min with a span of 18 mm. For each test method, force versus displacement curves were captured, and the yield stress and modulus of the materials were calculated.

Results of oriented PEEK, unoriented PEEK, and CFR-PEEK specimens tested for flexible strength and modulus are depicted in Figure 9.1 and Figure 9.2, respectively, and Table 9.2. PEEK's yield strength and modulus, as determined by compression and three-point bend, were improved by solid state orientation. Table 9.2 shows compression test results of oriented PEEK and CFR-PEEK rods prepared according to the scheme just described. Values are presented as averages with corresponding standard deviations. PEEK orientation at 315°C and a compression ratio of 3 to 1 resulted in an increase in yield strength and modulus of 15 and 24%,

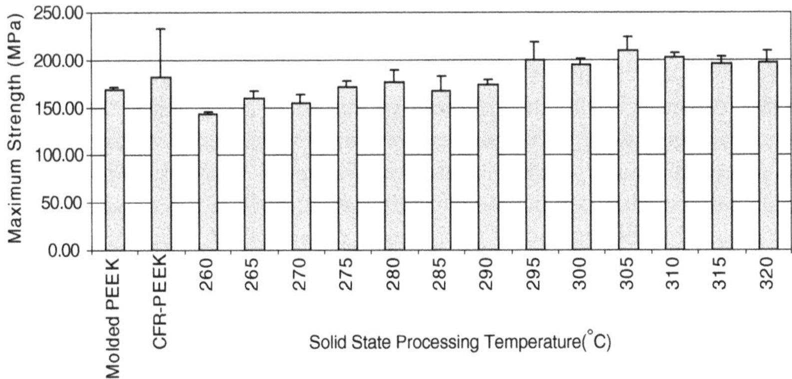

FIGURE 9.1 Maximum strength of oriented PEEK compared to molded and CFR-PEEK using three-point bend.

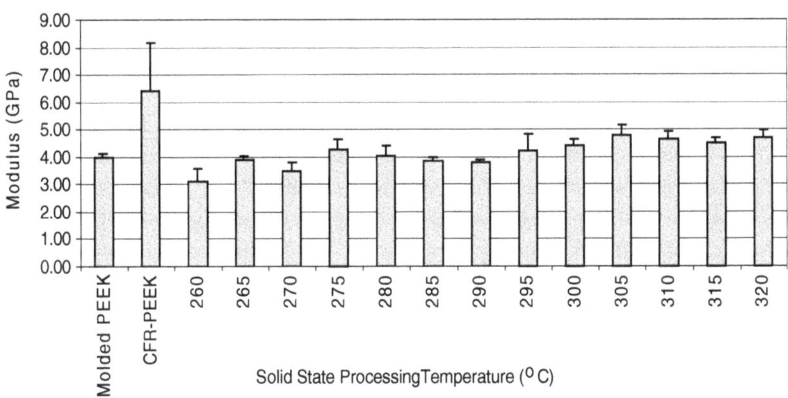

FIGURE 9.2 Modulus of oriented PEEK compared to molded and CFR-PEEK using three-point bend.

TABLE 9.2
Compressive Properties of Typical PEEK-Based Rods

Sample	Compressive Properties	
	Yield Strength (MPa)	Modulus (GPa)
Unoriented PEEK	114.2 ± 9.82	2.24 ± 0.16
Oriented PEEK	128.0 ± 4.21	2.77 ± 0.18
Unoriented CFR-PEEK	124.4 ± 21.2	3.20 ± 0.61

respectively, over the molded control. Further, the yield strength of the oriented PEEK was approximately equal to that of CFR-PEEK.

Figure 9.1 and Figure 9.2 show results of three-point bend studies conducted on PEEK oriented over a range of temperatures and a compression ratio of 5 to 1. Values on the graphs are shown as averages with corresponding standard deviations. Solid-state orientation of PEEK between 295 and 320°C resulted in increased strength and modulus over the molded PEEK control. Over this range, the strength of the oriented PEEK was equal to or greater than the CFR-PEEK.

The effect of the OSSO process on PEEK T_m as determined by DSC was an increase of 4°C. The results, summarized in Table 9.2 and Figure 9.1 and Figure 9.2, led to the conclusion that solid state orientation of PEEK results in an increase in the strength and modulus of the material over the unoriented PEEK control. The strength of oriented PEEK is approximately equal to that of CFR-PEEK; however, the modulus is less than that of CFR-PEEK

9.3 INTERACTION OF CELLS WITH CHEMICALLY MODIFIED SURFACES

Interactions of biomaterial surfaces with different types of cells in the biological environment determine, to a great extent, the successful short- and long-term use of polymeric implants. The long-term use of polymeric biomaterials in blood is limited by surface-induced thrombosis and biomaterial-associated infections.[14,33–35] Meanwhile, positive interactions and attachment of osteoblasts to biomaterial surfaces are key to the successful application of various dental and orthopedic implants and their osseointegration with surrounding bony tissues.[35–37] In this section, however, discussion of cell interactions with biomaterial surfaces are limited to those related to infection and osseointegration.

9.3.1 Interaction of Bacteria

Biomaterial-associated infection is known to occur as a result of adhesion of bacteria onto the surface.[38] And it is well acknowledged that the biomaterial surface provides a site for bacterial attachment and proliferation.[14] Adherent bacteria can be covered with a biofilm that supports bacterial growth and provides protection against phagocytes and antibiotics.[14,39] Acknowledging the relationship between bacterial cell attachment and device-induced infection, Gerdes and coworkers evoked the strategy of reducing or eliminating the cell attachment as an effective means of reducing the incidence of bacterial infections.[40] To this end, these investigators (1) adopted the findings of an earlier study where polymers with negatively charged surfaces allowed lower bacterial adherence as compared with chargeless controls and (2) applied the technology of gas phase phosphonylation discussed in Section 9.2 to impart negatively charged functional groups on LDPE as a model implant material.[40,41] It was also suggested that (1) in addition to the effect of the negative charge, the phosphonylated surface is more hydrophilic than the LDPE control, which rendered the surface unfavorable for bacterial colonization, and (2) phosphonylation-induced microtexturing may increase the charge density and decrease cell adherence further.

TABLE 9.3
Data from EDX and Contact Angle Analysis

Sample Treatment	C/P Ratio from EDX	Contact Angle
LDPE	—	84.46 ± 1.04
LDPE + HD	—	89.88 ± 1.57
LDPE + 30 m P	11.92	49.58 ± 3.48
LDPE + 45 m P	10.21	45.75 ± 3.24
LDPE + 60 m P	4.21	19.83 ± 2.37

In this study, LDPE films were phosphonylated to different degrees in the gas phase by treating the LDPE for 30, 45, and 60 min. Following phosphonylation the samples were sonicated in distilled water for a minimum of 1 h and dried under reduced pressure. SEM and electron EDX analysis confirmed the presence of phosphorus as well as its relative amounts attached to the surface. Contact angle measurements reconfirmed surface changes with varying intensities of the treatment. Controls included untreated and amine-bearing LDPE. For the latter, the amine-bearing surface was created by phosphonylation of LDPE followed by a 5-h incubation in a 5% solution of hexane diamine; the final surface exhibited a positive charge. LDPE was treated using the CIMS method at 92°C at intervals from 25 to 300 s. Following the CIMS treatment, samples were quenched in ice water for a minimum of 2 min. After air drying, the samples were sonicated in toluene for 30 min. Samples were dried under reduced pressure. SEM and noncontacting profilometry was conducted to analyze these surfaces.

Staphylococcus epidermidis, the most common pathogen in device-induced infections, was used as a model bacterium for studying cell attachment and was first characterized for growth. A growth curve was created in tryptic soy broth (TSB) at 37°C. Antibiotic resistance was evaluated to help facilitate the use of the organism in the planned testing.

Results of the study are summarized in Table 9.3 and Table 9.4. SEM and EDX confirmed the presence of phosphorus on the treated surfaces. The presence of

TABLE 9.4
Data from Profilometry Analysis

Sample	Roughness Average (nm)
LDPE	105.90 ± 7.40
LDPE + 25 s CIMS	161.65 ± 32.71
LDPE + 50 s CIMS	163.30 ± 43.60
LDPE + 160 s CIMS	5688.71 ± 682.32
LDPE + 30 m P	204.49 ± 68.06
LDPE + 45 m P	219.26 ± 9.53
LDPE + 60 m P	297.73 ± 31.27

hydrophilic phosphonate groups was verified by contact angle measurements. The gas phase phosphonylation process imparted microtexturing on the surface bearing the functional groups. EDX also showed relative decreases in the carbon to phosphorus ratio (C/P) with increases in treatment time. The contact angle data of the phosphonylated surface confirmed increases in hydrophilicity. However, the amine-bearing surfaces displayed a slight increase in surface hydrophobicity as compared with the control surface. The examined CIMS samples exhibited microtexture for all periods (25, 50, and 160 s) used for the treatment. Noncontacting profilometry showed an increase in the roughness average with an increase in CIMS treatment time and phosphonylation reaction time. During the course of this study, the need for reliable methods to assess and quantitate the level of cell attachment was evident. In a subsequent report, the different methods were critically evaluated for their effectiveness in studying the attachment of *S. epidermides* on surface activated LDPE, which may be also applicable to similar systems.[42] The methods used and critically assessed were colony count analysis, SEM analysis, dye-elution technique, total DNA isolation, and total protein quantification. Comparative assessment of these methods led to the conclusion that colony counts and SEM are useful methods of monitoring cell attachment under the conditions used in this study, colony counting being the most effective. Colony counts gave repeatable results and enabled the study to be quantitative. The SEM qualitative analysis was helpful and may have been more informative as an extensive study. The dye-elution technique, total DNA, and surface protein methods of quantitating bacterial cells were ineffective in monitoring cell attachment under the conditions used in this study. Because of the active surfaces, both cationogenic and anionogenic, dyeing the cells without binding the dye to the surface was not possible. Total DNA was an ineffective method because of the difficulty in lysing Gram positive species. Although newer protocols claiming to be capable of penetrating the cell wall were used, no DNA was isolated.[42] The study to quantitate proteins on the cells' surfaces was not sensitive enough to distinguish between 10-fold changes in cell numbers. This was found to be an unacceptable method of quantitating cell numbers.

9.3.2 Interaction of Osteoblasts

It has been shown by Shalaby and coworkers that surface phosphonylated surfaces of LDPE, *i*-PP, and PEEK-based bone implants do encourage bone ingrowth, resulting in osseointegration with surrounding bony tissues, as discussed in more detail in Section 9.4.[43–50] This led to the postulate that surfaces capable of immobilizing and chelating calcium ions, as in the case of phosphonylate-bearing surfaces, provide a preferred active substrate for the attachment and proliferation of osteoblasts.[46,47] In an effort to test this hypothesis and demonstrate the relevance of previously noted osseointegration of different implants to osteoblast attachment, a study was conducted on osteoblast attachment to phosphonylated *i*-PP film as a model substrate for typical orthopedic and dental polymeric substrates.[51] In this study, attachment, proliferation, and differentiation of osteoblast to phosphonate-bearing *i*-PP film, pretreated with calcium hydroxide to immobilize Ca^{2+}, was explored. The attachment of osteoblasts and their presence on the activated surface was verified using alkaline phosphatase activity assays and alizarin red staining. Results showed clearly that phosphonylated surfaces do encourage osteoblast attachment, thus providing a preliminary verification of the aforementioned hypothesis. This may also have impact on the growing interest in the *in situ* tissue engineering, where bioactive scaffolds are placed in defective biological sites to recruit pertinent cells to initiate tissue regeneration within and about the scaffolds. In an extension of this study on phosphonylated *i*-PP, a novel form of surface activated *i*-PP and PEEK-based films were examined for osteoblast attachment.[52] More specifically, the surface activation entailed the carboxylation of these films to produce a special form of carboxylic moieties on the surface, which are capable of binding and/or chelating calcium.[52–54] Osteoblast attachment to these surfaces was measured in terms of cell viability. For conducting the study, human fetal osteoblasts (ATCC, Manassas, VA) were maintained under recommended culture conditions in a 33.5°C, humidified, 5% CO_2–95% air environment in a 1:1 mixture of Dulbecco's modified Eagle's medium and Ham's nutrient mixture F12 supplemented with 10% fetal bovine serum (ATCC), 15 mm HEPES, and 0.3 mg/mL G418 (Invitrogen, Carlsbad, CA). Polypropylene and CFR-PEEK films of less than 1 mm thickness were prepared using a heated, automatic hydraulic press (Carver, Wabash, IN) and then surface carboxylated to introduce a special form of carboxylic acid side groups or left untreated. The individual films were cut into 1 cm^2 pieces and sterilized by ultraviolet irradiation for 20 min. Prior to cell seeding, films were fixed to the bottom of tissue-culture wells with a small amount of sterile silicone grease and soaked in media for 2 h. The osteoblasts were seeded onto films at a density of 1.3×10^4 cells/cm^2. After 7 days of culture, films were transferred to a new tissue-culture plate and visualized with propidium iodide or alizarin red staining. As part of the preliminary outcome of this study, direct microscopic examination of alizarin red–stained specimens are illustrated in Figure 9.3 and Figure 9.4. Compared to untreated polypropylene controls (Figure 9.3), there was enhanced osteoblast attachment and proliferation on carboxylated polypropylene films (Figure 9.4). Specimens stained with propidium iodide and viewed with fluorescence microscopy revealed that there was osteoblast adhesion on both control and carboxylated CFR-PEEK films (Figure 9.5 and Figure 9.6), but adhesion was hardly enhanced on carboxylated films. Available results of this preliminary study

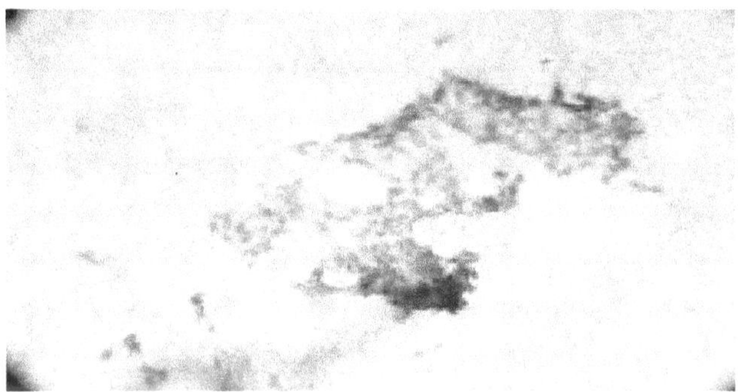

FIGURE 9.3 Control polypropylene.

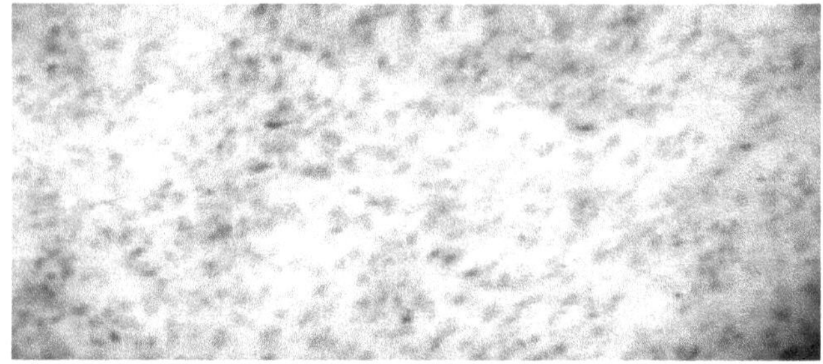

FIGURE 9.4 Carboxylated polypropylene.

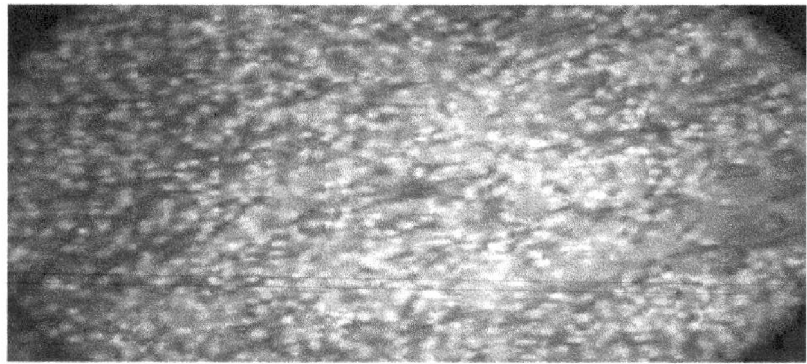

FIGURE 9.5 Control CFR-PEEK.

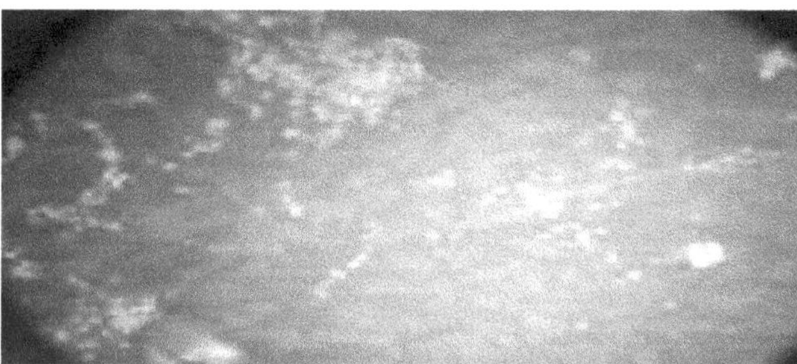

FIGURE 9.6 Carboxylated CFR-PEEK.

suggest that specially carboxylated surfaces, at least for *i*-PP films, encourage the attachment and proliferation of osteoblasts.

9.4 OSSEOINTEGRATION OF PHOSPHONYLATED POLYOLEFINS AND PEEK RODS AS TIBIAL IMPLANTS

Discussion in the previous sections dealt with demonstrating

1. The viability of LDPE and *i*-PP as model substrates for achieving phosphonylation
2. The successful extension of the phosphonylation technology to PEEK and CFR-PEEK
3. The ability to increase the modulus of crystalline polymers of interest in dental and orthopedic applications using the OSSO process so as to approach the moduli of typical bony tissues
4. The ability to achieve microtexturing of key polymers

A logical follow-up, this section deals with the use of simple implants, such as rods, to study their osseointegration in simple animal models, such as the rabbit and goat tibial models.

9.4.1 Osseointegration of Chemically and Physicochemically Modified Polyethylene and Propylene Rods as Goat Tibial Implants

In general, the sterilized implants were prepared by (1) melt extrusion of LDPE and *i*-PP into rods, (2) surface activation with or without surface microtexturing, and (3) sterilization.[43] More specifically, for the test implants, *i*-PP and LDPE were extruded using a Randcastle Microtruder laboratory extruder. Extruded polymers were subjected to the types of treatments outlined in Table 9.5. Implants were phosphonylated

TABLE 9.5
Types of Treatment of LDPE and *i*-PP Implants

Material	Group	Treatment
i-PP	I-A	Control, no treatment.
i-PP	I-B	Phosphonylated.
i-PP	I-C	Microtextured.
i-PP	I-D	Microtextured and phosphonylated.
i-PP	I-E	Phosphonylated and calcium treated.
LDPE	II-A	Control, no treatment.
LDPE	II-B	Phosphonylated and calcium treated.
LDPE	II-C	Microtextured.
LDPE	II-D	Microtextured, phosphonylated, calcium treated.

in the gas phase and hydrolyzed by sonicating in distilled water for 30 min. Random sets were selected and treated with calcium hydroxide. Rods with microtextured surfaces were produced by immersion into a molten diluent at a temperature between their melting and glass transition temperatures. The *i*-PP implants were sterilized using a General Purpose Model 2120 autoclave; the LDPE implants were sterilized via ethylene oxide gas at 25°C for 24 h. Sterilized implants were characterized using SEM, EDX, and surface roughness measurements.

Bone apposition and binding to the implant surface were evaluated using a transcortical plug model in the goat.[43,55] Four rods were implanted through the medial cortex of both tibias in nine goats to give a total of eight implants per surface treatment. The tibial positioning of implants in each group was randomized. *i*- and LDPE implants were harvested at 6 and 8 weeks postimplantation, respectively. Six implants per treatment group were used for mechanical tests, and the remaining two were used for histological evaluation. Mechanical push out tests were accomplished using an MTS 858 MiniBionix universal testing apparatus at a displacement rate of 1 mm/min. Samples for histological evaluation were prepared using standard hard tissue techniques and stained with basic fuschin and methylene blue.

In general, results of this study show that *i*-PP and LDPE rods were successfully extruded and surface treated. The EDX spectra of the materials indicated the presence of phosphorus and calcium on all phosphonylated and calcium hydroxide treated implants, respectively. Microtexturing of *i*-PP and LDPE produced the expected irregular surface topography with porosities on the order of 10 to 100 μm. Microtextured implants exhibited greater surface roughness values than smooth implants. Results of mechanical tests are shown in Figure 9.7 and Figure 9.8. Histological evaluation indicated no significant differences in bone apposition among groups. The biomechanical testing results and histological evaluation data led to the conclusion that formation of a calcium phosphonate surface on thermoplastic polymers through phosphonylation and subsequent treatment with calcium hydroxide resulted in an increased propensity for bone binding in both the *i*-PP and LDPE sets of implants.

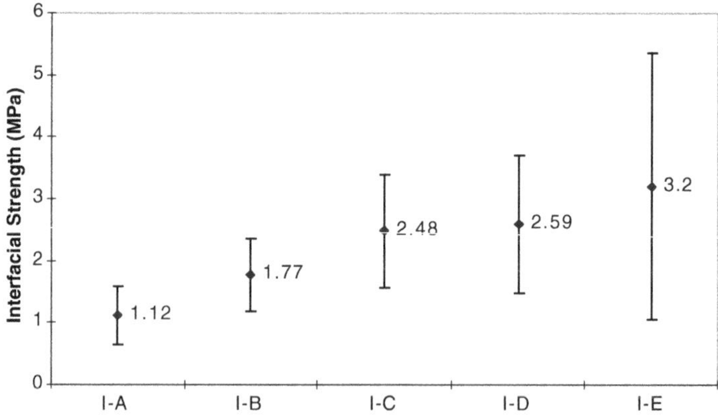

FIGURE 9.7 Strength of the *i*-PP implant–bone interface.

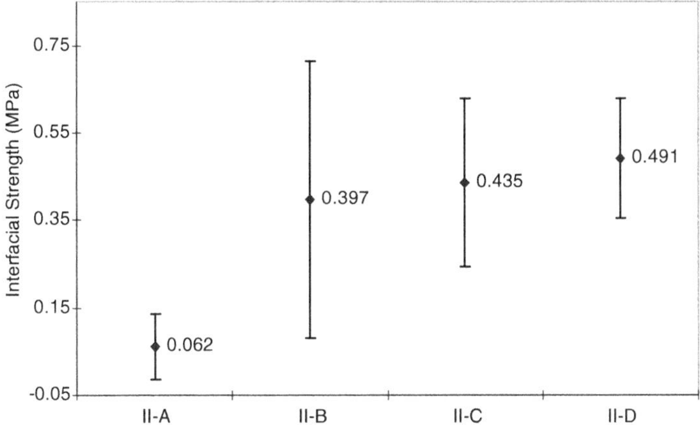

FIGURE 9.8 Strength of the LDPE implant–bone interface.

9.4.2 Osseointegration of Phosphonylated PEEK Rods as Rabbit Tibial Implants

Successful results of the study on the osseointegration of phosphonylated LDPE and *i*-PP rods using a goat tibial model prompted the pursuit of a limited study on the osseointegration of phosphonylated PEEK rods as rabbit tibial implants.[47] The selection of PEEK as a potential substitute for metallic dental and orthopedic implants was justified following the successful use of the OSSO process for increasing the modulus of the polymer to approach those of typical bony tissues.[31] For preparing and evaluating the test implants, PEEK pellets were compression molded into 32 mm thick blocks using a 30-ton Carver hydraulic press. The blocks were subsequently oriented using the OSSO process.[31] Once oriented, the blocks were machined into rods 3.00 mm in diameter and approximately 5 mm in length.

PEEK rods were divided into two groups, untreated controls and calcium phosphonate bearing surfaces. Control rods were cleaned after machining by sonication, first in acetone and then in water. Rods in the surface treated group were phosphonylated in the liquid phase and then incubated in a saturated solution of calcium hydroxide. The rods were evaluated using EDX analysis to confirm the presence of phosphorus and calcium on the surface of the treated rods and their absence on the control. SEM was used to visualize the material surfaces. Rods were individually packaged in sterilization bags and autoclaved prior to surgery. Sterilized rods were reexamined by EDX and SEM.

Bone apposition and binding to the implant surface were evaluated using a transcortical plug model in the rabbit. Rabbits were premedicated and then anesthetized via 2% isofluorane inhalation. The right leg was shaved and scrubbed, and an incision was made along the medial tibia from the tibial crest to the fibula insert. Three holes were drilled into the medial tibia using a 7/64-in. drill bit with an approximate spacing of three diameters between holes. Positioning of the rods in the tibias was randomized. Four rabbits were implanted with three rods each to give a total of six implants per treatment group.

Twelve weeks postimplantation, the rabbits were euthanized, and the implants were harvested with the surrounding bone. The strength of the bone–implant interface was measured via a push out test, which was accomplished using an MTS 858 MiniBionix universal testing apparatus at a displacement rate of 1 mm/min. Explanted rods were stained with a blue marking dye and then examined under a microscope to detect adhering bone fragments.

Results of the push out test are shown in the Figure 9.6. The PEEK rods bearing calcium phosphonate surfaces imparted by phosphonylation with calcium hydroxide posttreatment exhibited an interfacial strength with bone that was twice that of the untreated controls. The two groups were compared using a two-tailed, pairwise comparison t-test and were found to be different at a probability level of 99.3%. Observation of explanted rods indicated areas of adhered bone on the calcium phosphonate surfaces. Little to no bone was detected on the control implants. The results of this study led to the conclusion that phosphonylation and calcium hydroxide posttreatment is effective in enhancing the propensity for bone binding and apposition to PEEK tibial implants.

9.5 OSSEOINTEGRATION OF CHEMICALLY AND PHYSICOCHEMICALLY MODIFIED PEEK-BASED RODS AS GOAT MANDIBULAR IMPLANTS

Successful results of the study on the osseointegration of phosphonylated PEEK implants as rabbit tibial implants (Section 9.4.2) prompted a more detailed study of similar implants in the goat mandible.[32,56]

9.5.1 Preparation of Implantable Sterilized Rods

The PEEK rods were processed by melt extrusion and oriented using the OSSO protocol as described earlier in Section 9.4.2. On the other hand, CFR-PEEK pellets (RTP 2285LF series, RTP Co.) were melt processed into 76 × 76 ×32 mm blocks using a Carver hot press at 370°C and 9100 kg with a load bearing area of 152 × 152 mm. The blocks were then cut into 8 mm wide strips for further processing.

For chemical treatment, solid-state oriented PEEK and practically unoriented CFR-PEEK rods were fabricated as described previously with a diameter of 5 mm and a length of 10 mm. Subsequently, the rod surfaces were chemically and morphologically modified as described in Table 9.6.

To impart the desired surface microtexture and to develop surface microporosity, we treated a fraction of the PEEK and CFR-PEEK cylinders with molten phenylsulfone, rapid cooled them, and then extracted following the general procedure described in Section 9.2.3. Thus, the PEEK and CFR-PEEK rods were immersed in phenyl sulfone at 267°C for 2 min and 305°C for 45 s, respectively. The rods were then quenched in ice water for 3 min, and extracted (to remove the phenylsulfone phase) by sonicating in toluene for 30 min at room temperature.

To maximize the effectiveness of the phosphonylation process, Allan and coworkers acylated the PEEK and CFR-PEEK with an aliphatic anhydride having a long paraffin chain.[56] This is because the early finding showed that surface

TABLE 9.6
PEEK and CFR-PEEK Implants Treatment Schemes

Oriented PEEK		CFR-PEEK Composite	
Group	**Surface Treatment**	**Group**	**Surface Treatment**
1	Control, no treatment	5	Control, no treatment
2	Acylated, phosphonylated, calcium post-treatment	6	Acylated, phosphonylated, calcium post-treatment
3	Microtextured using CIMS	7	Microtextured using CIMS
4	Microtextured, acylated, phosphonylated, calcium posttreatment	8	Microtextured, acylated, phosphonylated, calcium posttreatment

phosphonylation of the aliphatic polyolefin was much more effective than in the case of PEEK (Section 9.2.2). Accordingly, to promote phosphonylation of the PEEK and CFR-PEEK surfaces (both smooth and microtextured), rods marked for phosphonylation were first acylated by immersion in phenyl sulfone in the presence of a catalytic amount of aluminum chloride at 120°C for 2 h. The samples were then rinsed in a series of steps using distilled water, chloroform, and acetone. Samples were dried under reduced pressure at room temperature for at least 12 h before further treatment. Surface phosphonylation was then accomplished as per the liquid-phase method (Section 9.2.2). The rods were rinsed in toluene, and the surface P–Cl groups were hydrolyzed to P–OH groups by sonicating in distilled water. To immobilize calcium ions by surface P–OH groups, the rods were allowed to bind Ca through immersion in a saturated solution of calcium oxide in water as described by Campbell.[20] Samples were removed from the solution and dried under reduced pressure at room temperature.

Prior to conducting the *in vivo* evaluation, all implants were sterilized and random samples of were characterized. Accordingly, after all sample preparations and drying were completed, rods were packaged in Chex-all® II Instant Sealing sterilization pouches. Rods were autoclaved prior to surgery. Sterilized implants were characterized using SEM and EDX. Representative sterile rods, which have been surface treated according to the different schemes shown in Table 9.6, were analyzed by EDX. The EDX data showed the presence of phosphorus and calcium on the surface of these implants.

9.5.2 *In Vivo* Study of Sterilized Rod Implants Using Goat Mandibles

9.5.2.1 Animal Model and Surgical Protocol

Bone apposition and binding to the implant surface were evaluated using a recently developed dental implantation model in goats.[45] Sixteen Nubian goats weighing 25–30 kg were procured for use in this study. Prior to surgery, animals were premedicated with glycopyrrolate (0.005–0.01 mg/kg) and buprenex (0.005 mg/kg) via subcutaneous injection. Anesthesia was induced with a mixture of ketamine (3 mg/kg) and xylazine (0.03 mg/kg) intravenously and maintained via inhalation of isofluorane (1.5–3%) in oxygen. A ventral approach was made to the hemimandible, bilaterally just caudal to the last incisor. The subcutaneous tissue and platysma muscle were incised, and the ventral aspect of each hemimandible was isolated. The soft tissues were retracted laterally to expose the mandible caudal to the incisors. On each hemimandible, two holes were drilled in the lateral aspect, avoiding the mental foramen and associated neurovascular bundle. With the gingiva reflected, a 1.9 mm diameter hole was drilled using a 13/64-in. drill bit to a depth of 10 mm. The 5.0 mm diameter cylindrical implants were gently tapped into the prepared holes, and the fascia, subcutaneous, and subcuticular layers were closed using simple interrupted sutures. Eight implants per treatment group were implanted. Buprenex (0.005–0.01 mg/kg) and flunixin meglumine (1.1 mg/kg) were administered via subcutaneous injection every 4–8 h. and 24–48 h, respectively, until there were no clinical or behavioral signs of pain.

9.5.2.2 Harvesting of Implants in Bone and Their Biomechanical Testing

After 12 weeks healing time, the animals were euthanized via intravenous injection of ketamine (3 mg/kg), xylazine (0.03 mg/kg), and Beuthanasia (1 m/10 lbs. to effect). The implants were harvested along with the surrounding bone. One specimen per goat was immersed in 10% neutral buffered formalin for histological evaluation. The remaining three implants were stored in cups with saline-soaked paper towels for mechanical push out tests. For the biomechanical testing, samples marked for push out tests were prepared by milling the bone on one side to ensure a level support face for testing. Tests were conducted on an MTS 858 MiniBionix universal testing apparatus. Implanted rods were pushed from the bone using the smooth end of a 9/16-in. drill bit at a displacement rate of 0.43 mm/s. Force versus displacement curves were recorded, and the contact area of the implant and bone was measured. The interfacial strength was calculated as the force required to dislodge the rod from the bone divided by the bone–implant contact area.

9.5.2.3 Histological Evaluation

Samples for histological evaluation were fixed in 10% neutral buffered formalin for 1 week and processed using a standard dehydration cycle of alcohols of increasing concentration in a Tissue-Tek VIP. The samples were infiltrated with a proprietary Poly-Med, Inc. methacrylate resin for 1 week under reduced pressure, and then embedded in the resin[56] by curing for 2.0 h under white light and 6.0 h under blue light in a Histolux.[56] Embedded samples were sectioned using an Isomet 2000 precision saw and then ground and polished to a thickness of 50 μm using an EXAKT. Finished slides were stained with basic fuschin and methylene blue. Histological slides were evaluated qualitatively and quantitatively to ascertain bone apposition and ingrowth. Images of the histology slides were taken using a Dage-MTI, Inc. 3 CCD camera connected to an Olympus BH-2 microscope at an objective magnification of 2×. The presence of inflammatory cells, fibrous tissue, bone resorption, new bone growth, and other pertinent features of the interface were noted. Image-Pro Plus version 3.0.01.00 for Windows 95/NT was used to measure the length of the implant embedded in bone and the length of bone in direct apposition with the implant. These measurements were expressed as a ratio of implant in contact with bone to the total length of the implant.

9.5.2.4 Outcome of the *In Vivo* Study

Implantation surgeries required approximately 30 min for each animal. Within 1 h of surgery, all goats recovered from anesthesia. All animals healed without significant signs of pain and no incidence of infection. At 12 weeks, the animals were sacrificed and implants were harvested. The interfacial strength data of the implants are shown in Table 9.7 and Figures 9.9 and 9.10. Values are presented as averages with corresponding standard deviations. The scatter in the data is attributed to many factors, including straightness of bore upon implantation, variability in healing and bone remodeling rates from animal too animal, and positioning of the specimen in the test grips to ensure central loading of the implant. While care was taken to manage and minimize the variability of each of these and other factors, some deviation occurred. This variability notwithstanding, the trends in mechanical test data are decidedly clear. Groups 2, 6, 7, and 8 showed increases in interfacial strength over their corresponding, untreated controls. Phosphonylation followed by calcium ion immobilization posttreatment resulted in a stronger bond with bone than both PEEK and CFR-PEEK. Further, microtexturing CFR-PEEK also resulted in a stronger interfacial bond. Microtexturing PEEK did not result in an increase in strength, which may be attributed to the difficulty in actually achieving a microtextured surface on the material.

Statistical analysis of the interfacial strength data from the push out test for PEEK and CFR-PEEK dental implants was conducted and results are presented in

TABLE 9.7
Mechanical and Histological Evaluation Data of Rod Implants

Implant Group	Interfacial Strength (MPa)	% Implant in Contact with Bone
1	0.80 ± 0.70	46.1 ± 14.8
2	2.18 ± 2.07	44.7 ± 16.6
3	0.80 ± 1.24	43.1 ± 17.8
4	0.99 ± 1.23	40.3 ± 4.8
5	0.92 ± 1.23	45.2 ± 8.5
6	4.05 ± 2.71	54.2 ± 18.4
7	7.56 ± 5.59	46.7 ± 21.5
8	7.26 ± 5.67	65.4 ± 24.9

Note: Implant surfaces of groups 2, 4, 6, and 8 contain Ca^{2+} immobilized by the phosphonate functionalities as noted in Table 9.6.

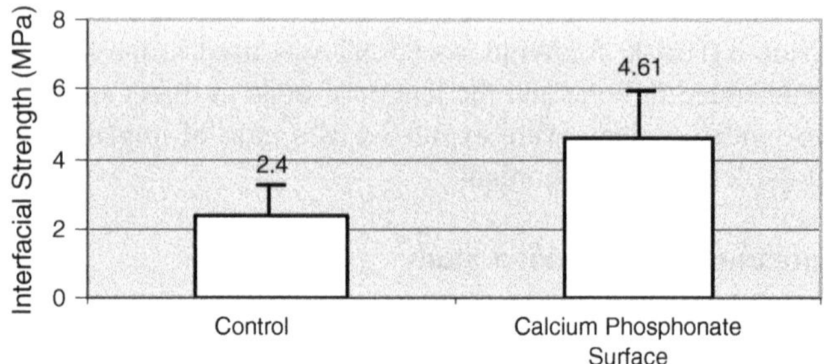

FIGURE 9.9 Interfacial strength comparison of untreated PEEK and calcium phosphonate–bearing PEEK tibial implants.

Table 9.8. Overall, the phosphonylated PEEK with calcium posttreatment had an interfacial strength greater than that of the untreated control at a probability level of 80% Figure 9.9. All treatment groups of CFR-PEEK showed improvements in interfacial strength over the untreated control at a probability level of 95%.

In the study of bone apposition through histological analysis and interfacial strength measurement, limited correspondence between the two evaluations is common.[57,58] This is due in part to fundamental differences in the methodology of each test. Mechanical evaluation of the bone–implant interface via a push out test assays the entire implant surface as a whole. Conversely, histological analysis provides an image of a singular plane of the interface. In addition, tissue processing and grinding to produce slides for microscopic evaluation can result in implant displacement with respect to the bone, resulting in difficult to interpret or misleading observations regarding tissue interaction with the implanted material. Recognizing this, we selected interfacial strength as determined by mechanical testing as the primary measure of bone ingrowth and apposition in this study. Histology was pursued on a limited basis to explore possible relevance to the mechanical test results. Values obtained from this analysis for fraction of bone in contact with the implant are presented in Table 9.8 and Figure 9.11. Representative histology slides revealed

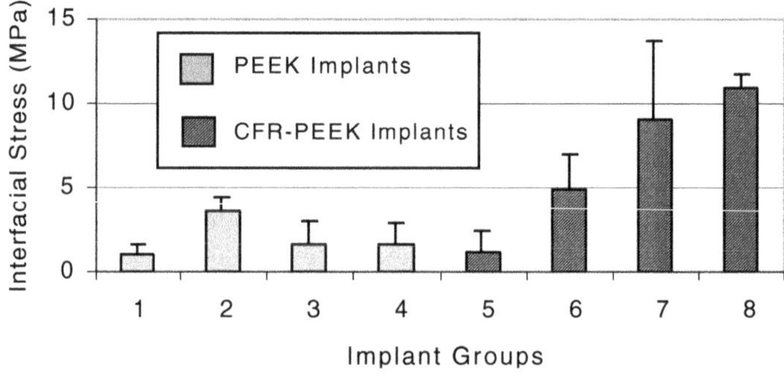

FIGURE 9.10 Implant–bone interfacial strength: the implant surface of groups 2, 4, 6, and 8 contain immobilized Ca^{2+}.

TABLE 9.8
Statistical Analysis of Push-Out Data

Sample Group	Average (MPa)	St. Dev. (MPa)	95% Confidence Interval (MPa)	t-Test Probability (%)
1	0.80	0.70	0.62	—
2	2.18	2.07	1.82	19.6
3	0.80	1.24	0.99	99.6
4	0.99	1.23	1.12	78.9
5	0.92	1.23	0.98	—
6	4.05	2.71	2.17	2.8
7	7.56	5.59	4.47	1.8
8	7.26	5.67	4.53	2.3

extensive remodeling of the cortex and bone adjacent to the implant. PEEK control slides, group 1, indicated fibrous tissue growth adjacent to the implant. While group 2, phosphonylated and calcium treated PEEK, also showed extensive remodeling at the bone–implant interface, new bone growth was observed in apposition to isolated portions of the implant surface. CFR-PEEK control implants, group 5, showed a mixed response with both fibrous tissue and new bone growth found at the interface. While groups 6, 7, and 8 of the treated CFR-PEEK materials also exhibited extensive remodeling at the implant–bone interface, new bone was observed in apposition to the implant. In spite of the limited histological findings, there is a correlation between the push out data and bone apposition for groups 6, 7, and 8. Additionally, there is practically no fibrous tissue formation about the surface of the implants corresponding to those groups.

Collectively, the results of the study of PEEK-based implants in the goat mandible led to the conclusion that solid-state orientation of PEEK (using the OSSO process) results in an increase in the strength and modulus of the material over the unoriented PEEK control. The strength of oriented PEEK is approximately equal to that of CFR-PEEK; however, the modulus is less than CFR-PEEK. Phosphonylation

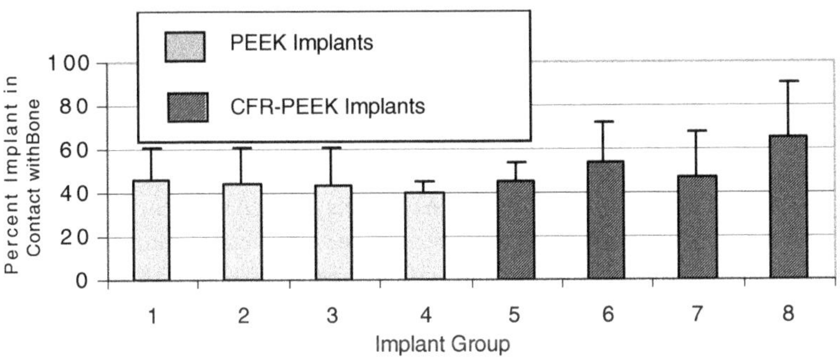

FIGURE 9.11 Histological evaluation of PEEK-based implants.

and calcium posttreatment of PEEK and CFR-PEEK surfaces led to a stronger interfacial strength over untreated controls as measured by the push out test. Micro-texturing CFR-PEEK resulted in an increase of the joint strength at the bone–implant interface. Image analysis of histology slides to assess bone apposition to implants was of limited value in verifying bone ingrowth and providing a strong correlation with the push-out results.

9.6 OSSEOINTEGRATION OF PHOSPHONYLATED PEEK AND CFR-PEEK ENDOSTEAL DENTAL IMPLANTS

In a review by Lemon on dental implants, the author noted that modern dental implants began with metallic endosteal systems, such as blades, root forms, endodontic stabilizers, plates, and screws.[59] Most pertinent to the subject of this section are the endosteal screws. An endosteal screw is the major component of a typical prosthesis used to replace a natural tooth. In such a prosthesis, the endosteal screw represents the implant body anchored in the bony tissue of the jaws. To the screw is attached an abutment connector, and the artificial crown is affixed to this connector. Endosteal implants, including those in the form of screws, are usually based on alloys, such as Ti-Al-V and Co-Cr-Mo types. Concerns about the use of metallic implants in bony tissues and associated stress-shielding and subsequent bone resorption directed the attention of contemporary investigators, as discussed earlier in this book, to explore the use of high modulus polymeric alternatives to currently used metallic implants, including those used in dental applications. This provided an incentive to pursue the subject discussed in this section; a second incentive pertains to the limited success associated with the ability of metallic implants to osseointegrate with the surrounding dental bony tissues and attain long-term mechanical stability therein. Among the many early attempts and associated studies to stabilize dental implants through design and surface treatment, those noted below are most pertinent to the subject of this section. Langer and coworkers noted that a 5.0 mm diameter self-tapping metallic dental implant was used successfully for patients who have inadequate bone height, poor bone quality, and who need immediate replacement of nonintegrated or fractured implants.[60] This was followed by a study by Kaito and coworkers that showed that the pull-out force for large diameter implants (4.5 mm diameter) was 16% higher than that of the small diameter (3.25 mm diameter) implants.[61] In a study by Mukherjee and coworkers on the fatigue of hydroxyapatite-coated dental metal implants, it was concluded that microcracks widened in some if the samples were fatigued; the surface composition in terms of Ca/P did not change significantly; some P, but not Ca, was released from the samples into the immersion solution during fatigue testing.[62] In a study to determine the effect of surface roughness on TiO_2-coated titanium implant screws, Wennerberg and Albrektsson arrived at the following conclusion: Implants with a surface structure that had no dominating pattern, an average surface roughness of 1.4 μm, an average wavelength of 11.1 μm, and a developed area ratio of 1.5 provide the firmest bone fixation.[63]

Contents of this section are designed to take into account the (1) aforementioned discussion pertaining to the growing interest in polymeric alternatives to presently used metallic dental implants while featuring a new design and unique surface physicochemical properties, and (2) discussion in Section 9.5 outlining the promising properties of phosphonylated materials as dental implants capable of osseointegration. The first segment of this section deals with the development of a new design of a typical endosteal dental implant (EDI) in the form of a screw for evaluation in beagles. This is followed by the development of a suitable animal model and its use in evaluating osseointegration, both histomorphometrically and biomechanically.

9.6.1 Development of a New Endosteal Dental Implant Design for Evaluation in Beagles

Toward the development of a PEEK-based EDI and its coronal components for evaluation in beagles, a number of requirements were recognized and addressed accordingly in terms of having the following features[64,65]:

1. An EDI with a threaded neck for screwing a metallic abutment connector to which a metallic or ceramic crown is affixed to transfer the load during mastication
2. A screw that can be mechanically placed in the mandibular bone without being distorted
3. A thread design coupled with radially positioned creators and vertical grooves to prevent axial and radial micromotions, respectively, following implantation and during the sought after early EDI bone osseointegration

An illustration of the screw design is depicted in Figure 9.12.

In preparation for the animal study using PEEK-based implants and a titanium alloy control for implantation in beagle mandibles, bars of oriented PEEK, unoriented CFR-PEEK, and Ti alloy were formed and micromachined into the design depicted in Figure 9.12. More specifically, PEEK and CFR-PEEK pellets were molded into blocks of desired dimensions using a Carver press after which they were cut into bar stock. The PEEK bars were subjected to OSSO using high

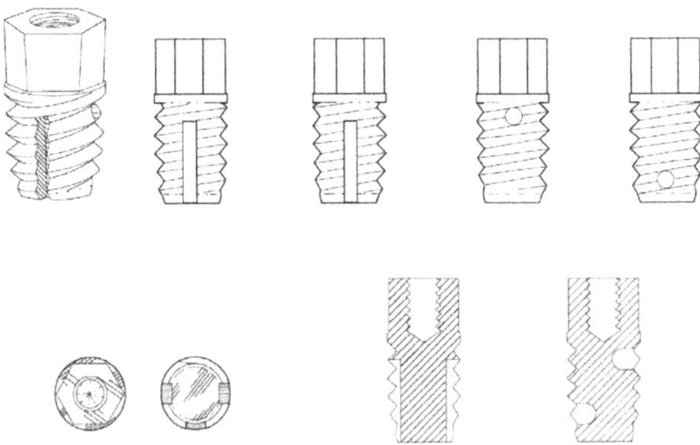

FIGURE 9.12 Optimized endosteal implant design.

compressive forces. The oriented PEEK and CFR-PEEK bars were micromachined into the implant forms using a Benchman XT machining center. The machined implants were scoured by sonication in isopropyl alcohol. The implants were surface phosphonylated and processed to immobilize calcium ions on their activated surfaces to allow for osseointegration as discussed earlier. Implants made of Ti alloy (Ti6-6Al-4V) were micromachined and scoured as noted for the PEEK-based implants.

9.6.2 Development of a Beagle Animal Model and Pilot Study of the EDI

During the initial stage of development, a series of EDIs made of PEEK, CFR-PEEK, and Ti alloy having the same preliminary design that was slightly different from the later-optimized design shown in Figure 9.12. In the first segment of the pilot study, the three types of EDIs were used. Conventional wisdom was to compare the implants under two modes of placement, immediate and delayed. In the immediate placement scheme, implants were to be placed in the mandibular bone following extraction of the selected premolars in the canine model. Conversely, the delayed placement scheme was to extract the appropriate premolars, reapproximate the gingiva, and allow a 12-week healing period prior to the placement of the implants in the mandibular bone. However, it was found that the immediate placement presented certain challenges that could not be overcome, at least early on in this study. Namely, the condition of the implant bed following extraction of healthy, multirooted teeth was less than ideal. Given the narrow dimensions of the furcation bone remaining after extraction, immediate placement caused a collapse of the adjacent, empty root cavity. Additionally, success of the immediate placement method is highly dependant on no load being applied to the implant in the early healing period. This led to the focus on delayed placement using an optimized implant design of the EDI in the second segment of the pilot study. More details of the protocol and outcomes of the pilot study are described below.

9.6.2.1 Beagle Mandibular Model and Placement Protocols

In preparation of the pilot study, female beagles of approximately 18 months of age and weighing 15–25 lb were purchased from Harlan (Indianapolis, IN) and held in quarantine for acclimation and observation for not less than 2 weeks. The animals were evaluated for skeletal maturity by radiographic confirmation of closure of the distal femoral and proximal tibial epiphyses. Tooth extraction was performed under anesthesia with the assistance of a certified veterinary surgeon and a registered dental veterinary technician. Complete extraction was verified radiographically. In the immediate placement group, one root cavity was chosen from each of the extracted teeth to receive an implant. This root cavity was prepared to receive an implant by first drilling with a 1/8-in. hole using sterile saline irrigation. The hole was then threaded using a tap custom made to the same thread form as that on the implants. The tapped hole was then irrigated to remove any debris and the implant inserted to a depth that brought the head to the same level as the surrounding gingival tissue followed by gingival closure. In the delayed placement group, the teeth were extracted in the same fashion and the implant bed allowed to heal for a period of 12 weeks. Following the healing period, radiographs were taken to ensure good bone formation and proper healing. The sites for implantation were then selected and the sites drilled and tapped as before. Implants were then placed and the gingiva closed.

9.6.2.2 Pilot Study of the EDIs

To assess the efficacy of the immediate placement approach, we placed EDIs of the original design into two animals on the left side of their mandible in the P2, P3, and P4 (P = premolar) positions. After 2 weeks, several implants were lost and an oral exam revealed that the remaining EDIs were loose. Radiographs were taken and revealed two distinct problems. The first was that the adjacent empty root cavity had collapsed, which eliminated the anchoring of the EDI on one side. This loss of anchoring not only compromised the security of the EDI but also allowed for movement, which prevented any healing at the bone–implant interface. The second source of problems was due to incomplete tooth root extraction. Careful examination of early radiographs showed evidence of root fragments remaining. In subsequent surgeries, radiographic procedures have been modified to improve the quality of the films and aid in the detection of root fragments during the extraction procedure and eliminate this as a source of error. However, the stability issues associated with empty root cavities and thin furcation bone segments have led to suspending the use of the immediate placement approach. After implementing revised extraction techniques and improving the design of the EDIs, a second series of 5 animals have been implanted with a total of 22 EDIs using the delayed placement method. Of these 22 implants, 21 remain intact with good bone remodeling and implant security as evidenced by radiographic and oral examination. The one implant that was lost was due to incomplete insertion secondary to a sheared head during implantation.

Results of the pilot study led to the conclusion that a refined beagle model, using delayed implant placement, can be used for evaluation of optimally designed surface phosphonylated PEEK-based endosteal dental implants to demonstrate their ability to osseointegrate with mandibular bone tissue.

9.6.3 Biomechanical Evaluation of Osseointegration of Metallic and PEEK-based EDIs

Results of the *in vivo* study discussed in Section 9.6.2 on the preliminary evaluation of the EDI design of phosphonylated PEEK-based EDIs reflected the increased propensity of these implants to osseointegrate with mandibular bone following a delayed placement protocol.[48,64] This prompted the pursuit of a more comprehensive study, subject of this section, dealing with the effect of the implantation period on the extent of osseointegration measured in terms of the biomechanical properties of EDI–bone interface.[49] Experimentally, this study was pursued by following the processing protocols described earlier (Section 9.6.2) for preparing ready-to-implant EDIs, multiple-member sets were made using solid-state oriented PEEK (by the OSSO process), CFR-PEEK, and titanium alloy.[48,49,64] The number of implants in each set was sufficient to ensure having at least four test specimens per segment of the study and, hence, statistically viable test results. For the animal study, female beagles of approximately 18 months of age and weighing 15–25 lb were used. The study was pursued following the delayed placement protocol and associated preoperative, surgical, and postoperative procedures as discussed earlier.[48] At the conclusion of each study period for different EDIs, animals were euthanized and mandibles removed. Using a band saw, the mandible was cut into proper size blocks (or test specimens) with bone tissue adequately surrounding the test implant to allow conducting reproducible torsional measurements. These were conducted following a protocol similar to one described recently for titanium dental implants.[66] The test specimens were placed immediately in saline and tested within 2 h of removal. The peak torque (or maximum removal torque, MRT) required to disengage the EDI from surrounding bone tissue was measured using a Multitorque Analyzing System. For this, the individual test specimen was affixed in a metallic holder and rotated at a rate of 16 radians per minute until failure.[49]

Collectively, the study included:

1. Optimization of the direct surface phosphonylation of the PEEK-based EDIs to ensure reproducibility and formation of highly functionalized substrates for immobilizing the calcium ion without compromising the mechanical integrity of the thread.
2. Modification of the EDI head to a hexagonal geometry that is compatible with a specially designed hexagonal applicator to facilitate its insertion without deformation (this was particularly useful for OSSO-PEEK and led to elimination of the notches in the preliminary head design).
3. Use of an acrylic model of the premolar crown to revise the micromachining program to produce the optimum stem design as shown in Figure 9.12. The design program modification was implemented directly on the preliminary design program in a stepwise manner following several *in vitro* attempts to simulate the device assembling steps and to determine the design requirements for facile insertion of the stem into the dog mandible.
4. Combining the crown-holding post (or abutment connector) and the crown into one component that can be securely attached into the thread receptacle of the EDI head using a commercial dental resin cement (Calibra™). This was pursued to avoid mechanical instability of the post–crown joint and shearing-off of the ceramic- or acrylic-based crown shortly after implant assembling at the mandibular site
5. Use of direct phosphonylation of the EDIs as the method of choice as per the comparative ESCA data of specimens made using the indirect method (i.e., surface acylation following by phosphonylation).
6. Use of heat, radiochemical, or radiation sterilization for preparing sterile EDIs for implantation, depending on the time constraints and coordination with the ESCA verification of surface functionality and testing for implant sterility (see Table 9.9 for typical ESCA data of randomly selected EDIs from three evaluated sets); standard method for sterility testing employing liquid culture media was used.

TABLE 9.9
Typical ESCA[a] Data of Phosphonylated EDIs, with and without Immobilized Calcium Ion

	EDI Type					
	OSSO-PEEK Specimen No.			CFR-PEEK Specimen No.		
Treatment	1	2	3	1	2	3
After phosphonylation						
Atomic phosphorous, %	2.34	2.42	2.46	3.07	3.17	3.61
After phosphonylation and Ca^{2+} immobilization						
Atomic phosphorous, %	1.04	1.40	2.07	1.82	1.86	1.81
Atomic calcium, %	0.50	0.46	0.56	0.41	0.42	0.47

[a] ESCA = electron spectroscopy for chemical analysis.

7. Use of delayed placement of the EDIs as the only viable protocol for conducting the balance of the studies. This decision was made as a result of many unsuccessful attempts based on immediate placement, which led to loss of time and animals.
8. A brief study on the effect of loading on the biomechanical properties. The results showed that under the prevailing conditions, loading the implant has practically no effect or can lead to minimum improvement in the biomechanical properties in the case of the metallic and OSSO-PEEK or CFR-PEEK EDIs, respectively (Table 9.10).
9. Completion of three sets of studies on the effect of postloading healing period (namely, 10, 15, and 20 weeks following complete assembling of the EDI stem–crown components) on biomechanical stability (Table 9.11 and Figure 9.13).

TABLE 9.10
Effect of Loading on the Biomechanical Properties of Representative EDI Implants

	Maximum Removal Torque (N-cm)		
Loading Period (weeks)	Titanium Alloy EDI	Oriented PEEK EDI	CFR-PEEK EDI
0	77.2	96.3	93.2
10	73.6	—	—
20	—	95.4	117.1

Titanium EDIs were implanted for 20 cumulative weeks posthealing following the tooth extraction (loaded + unloaded) while PEEK and CFR-PEEK EDIs were implanted for 30 cumulative weeks posthealing following the tooth extraction.

TABLE 9.11
Effect of Post-Loading Period and Composition on Biomechanical Properties of Representative EDI Implants

	Maximum Removal Torque (N-cm)		
Loading Period (weeks)	Titanium Alloy EDI	Oriented PEEK EDI	CFR-PEEK EDI
10	73.6 ± 4.6	81.0 ± 7.1	98.8 ± 3.7
15	83.4 ± 9.1	91.7 ± 6.5	107.3 ± 8.5
20	77.6 ± 8.9	95.4	117.1 ± 8.6

Measured in terms of maximum torque (N-cm) to disengage the EDI from the mandible.

It is important to note that the data in Table 9.11 and Figure 9.13 dealing with the effect of loading time (namely 10, 15, and 20 weeks following complete assembly of the EDI stem and crown components) on osseointegration–bone apposition, measured in terms of MRT, indicate that

1. At any of the three periods, extent of bone apposition and osseointegration is lowest for titanium alloy and highest for CFR-PEEK EDIs, respectively, with the OSSO-PEEK EDI displaying intermediate values.

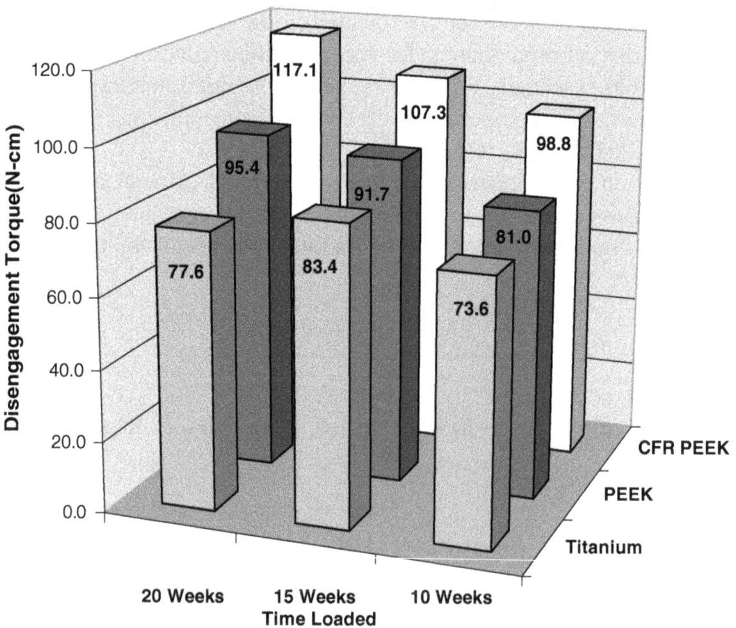

FIGURE 9.13 Effect of postloading period and EDI composition on maximum torque required for disengagement.

2. For both PEEK-based EDIs, the bone apposition–osseointegration values increase progressively with time, thus supporting the postulate that the relatively moderate modulus of the polymeric EDI, as compared with the Ti alloy and surface phosphonylation do support osseointegration and bone formation.
3. For the Ti alloy EDIs, osseointegration and bone apposition or bone formation reached a maximum at 15 weeks, then decreased at 20 weeks, thus supporting the thesis that metallic implants can cause bone resorption upon prolonged presence at implant site.
4. The MRT values for the Ti alloy EDI exceeded those reported by Cho et al. on commercial titanium alloy EDIs with or without surface texturing, thus suggesting that the newly patented proprietary design of the endosteal implant, shown in Figure 9.12, contributes positively to the biomechanical properties of the Ti alloy EDI.[65,66]

Results of the study on the biomechanical properties of EDI–bone interface led to the conclusion that surface phosphonylated PEEK-based EDIs and particularly those made of CFR-PEEK, having surface-immobilized calcium ions, should be viewed as clinically preferred alternatives to those made of Ti alloys.

9.6.4 Histomorphometric Evaluation of Osseointegration of Metallic and PEEK-Based EDIs

Extension of the studies described in the preceding sections of the chapter on maximizing the effectiveness and clinical relevance of surface phosphonylated implants with hydroxyapatite-like surfaces capable of osseointegration with bone tissue has led to the following

1. The development of an optimized endosteal dental implant (EDI) that minimizes or prevents axial and radial micromotion at the implant site
2. The identification of the delayed placement protocol as the choice approach for introducing mandibular implants after tooth extraction
3. The demonstration that osseointegration, as measured in terms of mechanical properties, of an endosteal implant is time dependent, particularly for PEEK implants
4. The conclusion that both the surface morphology and bulk properties do affect the biomechanical properties, which may be related to the extent of osseointegration[48]

The latter observation provided the incentive to conduct the study, subject of this section, to determine the relevance of the time-dependent mechanical properties of PEEK-based and metallic implants to osseointegration as measured in terms of bone apposition.[48,50,64]

In preparation for conducting the histomorphometric evaluation of osseointegration of the different EDIs, multiple-member sets of ready-to-implant EDIs were prepared as per the processing protocols described earlier, and test specimens made from OSSO, CFR, and titanium alloy were prepared.[48,50,64] The number of implants in each set was sufficient to provide at least two implants per specimen for individual histological evaluation. For the animal study, female beagles of approximately 18 months of age and weighing 15–25 lb were used. The study was pursued following the delayed placement protocol and associated preoperative, surgical, and postoperative procedures. At the conclusion of each study period, the animals were euthanized and the mandibles were removed and placed in 10% neutral buffered formalin (NBF) for at least 48 h. Using a band saw, the mandible was cut into properly sized blocks with bone tissue adequately surrounding the test implant. The blocks were then transferred individually to 70% ethanol and stored for histological evaluation. With the exception of a few specimens, histology and histomorphometric evaluations were conducted at SkeleTech (Bothell, WA). The samples were scanned by a SkyScan 1076 micro-CT system for a quick turnaround on the three dimensional visualization of bone ingrowth to the implant materials within 2 weeks. The samples were then processed, undecalcified, and embedded in PMMA (polymethyl methacrylate) for sectioning by using the EXAKT system to obtain two vertical and two horizontal sections of the implants and surrounding bone tissue. Sections were stained with toluidine blue. Microscopic evaluation for histopathology and histomorphometry was focused on cell–tissue reaction and percentage bone ingrowth within and surrounding the implant. The bone ingrowth to the grooves of the implanted EDIs was estimated by the groove surface that is in contact with the ingrown bone. Histomorphometric measurements were performed by using the point-counting method for obtaining percent bone ingrowth within and surrounding the implant and by using the OsteoMeasure™ software adjunct to a Nikon Camera Lucida Imaging hardware. Typical histomorphometry data are summarized in Table 9.12 and illustrate the effect of postloading period and EDI type and composition on percent bone–implant contact.

Histology specimens were subjected to histomorphometric evaluation. No significant differences in the histopathology of the three types of EDIs could be observed.[50,64] In general the results of the study indicated, specifically, that

TABLE 9.12
Effect of Postloading Period and Composition on Percentage Bone–Implant Contact for Different EDIs: Typical Data

Post-loading Period	Titanium Alloy EDI	OSSO-PEEK EDI	CFR-PEEK EDI
10 weeks	36	35	33
20 weeks	57	56	72

This represents the ratio of implant surface in contact with bone tissue divided by the total surface.

1. The osseointegration, or mechanical stability, of the titanium alloy EDI exceeded that reported earlier, which may be attributed to the new design of the EDI depicted in Figure 9.12.
2. The OSSO-PEEK functional performance is slightly better in comparison to the Ti-based control in terms of biomechanical stability and osseointegration.
3. CFR-PEEK-based EDI functional performance is superior to both the Ti- and OSSO-PEEK-based EDIs.

A representation of a typical histology photomicrograph depicting osseointegration at the EDI–bone interface is shown in Figure 9.14. The photomicrograph shows the extent of osseointegration for a CFR-PEEK EDI implanted for a 20-week (10 weeks unloaded and 10 weeks loaded) posthealing period.

Analysis of the histomorphometric data summarized in Table 9.12 in terms of percentage of bone in contact with different EDIs, which are relevant to the extent of bone apposition and osseointegration at the bone–implant interface, does reflect significant differences among these implants. More specifically, Table 9.12 outlines the percentage of bone in contact with the surface of different EDIs, which reflects primarily the extent of bone apposition and osseointegration, and can be related to the overall tendency for bone formation at the implant site. Taking this into account, the data in Table 9.12 and Figure 9.14 indicate that

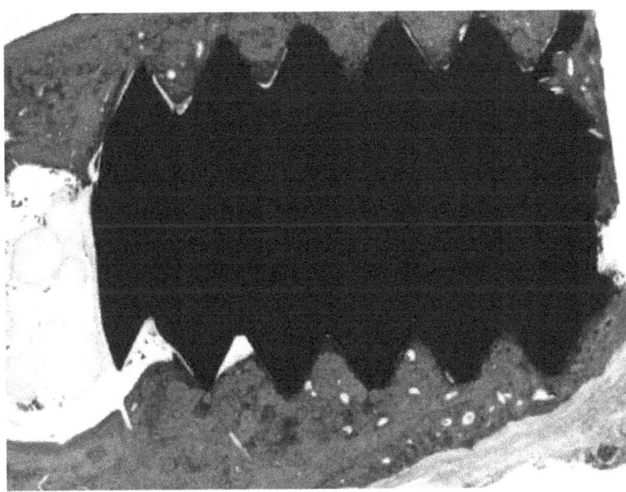

FIGURE 9.14 Histological photomicrograph of a typical longitudinal section of a CFR-PEEK EDI implanted for 20 weeks (10 weeks unloaded and 10 weeks loaded) posthealing period.

1. At a postloading period of 10 weeks, limited increase in bone apposition and osseointegration takes place for all types of implants, with the EDIs made of CFR-PEEK showing minimum values.
2. At a postloading period of 20 weeks, when sufficient bone formation was allowed to take place, a maximum bone apposition and/or osseointegration was associated with CFR-PEEK EDIs.
3. There is no significant difference between percentage of bone in contact with the titanium and with OSSO-PEEK EDIs.
4. A 30-week posthealing period, including a 20-week loading period, is associated with extensive osseointegration for the CFR-PEEK EDI.

Collective analysis of the results of biomechanical and histomorphometric data of Sections 9.6.3 and 9.6.4, respectively, led to the conclusion that

1. The osseointegration and mechanical stability of the Ti alloy EDI exceeded that reported earlier by Cho and Jung,[66] which may be attributed to the newly patented design of the EDI depicted in Figure 9.12.
2. The OSSO-PEEK functional performance is slightly better in comparison to the Ti-based control in terms of biomechanical stability and osseointegration.
3. CFR-PEEK-based EDI functional performance is superior to both the Ti- and OSSO-PEEK-based EDIs.

9.7 CONCLUSION AND PERSPECTIVE ON THE FUTURE

Results of the studies discussed in this chapter led to the conclusions that:

1. Solid-state orientation of PEEK, among other thermoplastic crystalline polymers, can be used to increase the compression-molded polymer modulus and allow its micromachining to yield useful bone implants, including endosteal dental implants with different designs.
2. Direct surface phosphonylation is well-suited as a practical and economical method to create a hydroxyapatite-like surface after the immobilization of calcium ions thereon.
3. Surface microtexturing and/or phosphonylation of high modulus crystalline polymeric bone implants, such as those based on PEEK, can result in their osseointegration and hence, mechanical stability in the bony tissue.
4. CFR-PEEK is the most suitable form of PEEK-based constructs for the production of EDIs. Micromachining is a well-suited method for the production of metallic and PEEK-based EDIs.
5. Using the beagle mandibular model, 10–12 weeks is a sufficient period to allow adequate bone formation following extraction and make available the mandibular site for drilling and preparing the mandibular bone for delayed placement of the EDI.
6. Following the delayed placement of the EDI, most bone formation and osseointegration takes place within a 10-week period followed by variable

degrees of bone remodeling and densification after an additional 10, 15, and 20 weeks. The remodeling and densification were minimal in the case of the titanium-based and OSSO-PEEK-based EDIs, but quite discernable in the case of the CFR-PEEK-based EDIs. Under these conditions, the loading of the EDI did not appear to have a significant effect on the amount of bone formation or its quality.

7. Biomechanical properties measured in terms of the torsional force required for disengaging the implant from the surrounding bone is most effective in evaluating the EDI biomechanical stability and the overall extent of osseointegration.

Based on the technical outcome of the studies noted in this chapter, the surface-activated CFR-PEEK system is recommended for further use in the production of not only screw-type, but also other forms of endosteal implants. Additionally, it is recommended that (1) surface activated OSSO-PEEK be explored for use in maxillofacial applications, (2) surface carboxylation be explored as a facile means of producing substrates capable for osseointegration, and (3) the technological achievement associated with the development of dental implants be explored for suitable applications in the orthopedic area.

REFERENCES

1. von Recum, A.F., Ed., *Handbook of Biomaterials Evaluation*, Macmillan, New York, 1986, p. vii.
2. Williams, D., *Concise Encyclopedia of Medical and Dental Materials*, MIT Press, Cambridge, MA, 1990, p. 52.
3. Williams, D.G., *Definitions in Biomaterials: Proceedings of a Consensus Conference of the European Society for Biomaterials*, Chester, England, Elsevier, Amsterdam, March 3–5, 1989.
4. Ratner, B.D., New ideas in biomaterials science — a path to engineered biomaterials, *J. Biomed. Mat. Res.*, 27, 837, 1993.
5. Tunc, D, Absorbable Bone Fixation Devices, U.S. Patent 4,539,981, 1985.
6. Tunc, D., Absorbable Bone Fixation Devices, U.S. Patent 4,550,449, 1985.
7. Zachariades, A.E., Process for Producing a New Class of Ultra-High Molecular Weight Polyethylene Orthopedic Prostheses with Enhanced Mechanical Properties, U.S. Patent 5,030,402, 1991.
8. Shalaby, S.W., Johnson, R.A., and Deng, M., Process of Making a Bone Healing Device, U.S. Patent 5,529,736, 1996.
9. Kim, S.W. and Feijen, J., Surface modification of polymers for improved blood compatibility, *CRC Crit. Revs. Biocomp.*, 1, 229, 1980.
10. Lelah, M.D., Jordan, C.A., Pariso, M.E., Lambarecht, L.K., Albrecht, R.M., and Cooper, S.L., Blood compatibility of polyethylene and oxidized polyethylene in canine A-V shunt: Relationship to surface properties, in *Polymers as Biomaterials,* Shalaby, S.W., Hoffman, A.S., Ratner, B.D., and Horbett, T.A., Eds., Plenum Press, New York, 1984, p. 257.
11. Hoffman, A.S., Modification of material surfaces to affect how they interact with blood, *Ann. N.Y. Acad. Sci.*, 516, 96, 1987.

12. Ikada, Y., Blood compatible surfaces, *Adv. Polymer Sci.*, 57, 103, 1984.
13. Nagaoka, S., Mori, Y., Tanzawa, T., Kikuchi, Y., Inagaki, F., Yokota, Y., and Nioshiki, Y., Hydrated dynamic surfaces, *Trans. Am. Soc. Artific. Intern. Organs* 33, 76, 1987.
14. Amiji, M. and Park, K., Surface modification of polymeric biomaterials with polyethylene oxide, in *Polymers of Biological and Biomedical Significance,* vol. 54, Shalaby, S.W., Ikada, Y., Langer, R., and Williams J., Eds., ACS Symposium Series, Amer. Chem. Soc., Washington, D.C., 1992, chap. 11.
15. Shalaby, S.W. and McCaig, M.S., Process for Phosphonylating the Surface of Polymeric Preforms, U.S. Patent 5,491,198, 1996.
16. Shalaby, S.W. and Rogers, K.R., Polymeric Prothesis Having a Phosphonylated Surface, U.S. Patent 5,558,517, 1996.
17. Hylton, D.M., The Effect of Sulfonation of Polyethylene and Polypropylene on Blood Compatibility, M.S. thesis, Department of Bioengineering, Clemson University, Clemson, SC, 2002.
18. Hylton, D.M., Shalaby, S.W., and Latour, R.A., Jr., Direct correlation between adsorption-induced changes in protein structure and platelet adhesion, *J. Biomed. Mater. Res.*, 73, 349, 2005.
19. Clayton, J.O. and Jensen, W.L., Reaction of paraffin hydrocarbons with phosphorus trichloride and oxygen to produce alkanephosphonyl chlorides, *J. Am. Chem. Soc.* 70, 3880, 1948.
20. Campbell, C.E., Surface-Phosphonylated Polyethylene and Its Binding Capacity, Doctoral dissertation, Department of Bioengineering, Clemson University, Clemson, SC, 1996.
21. Hench, L.L. and Paschal, H.W., Histochemical responses at a biomaterial's interface, *J. Biomed. Mater. Res.*, 4, 25, 1973.
22. Holmes, R.E. and Hagler, H.K., Porous hydroxyapatite as a bone graft substitute in mandibular augmentation: a histometric study, *J. Oral Maxillofac. Surg.*, 45, 421, 1987.
23. Allan, J.M., Dooley, R.L., and Shalaby, S.W., Surface phosphonylation of low-density polyethylene, *J. Appl. Polymer Sci.*, 76, 1870, 2000.
24. Williams, D.E., The inert-bioactivity conundrum, in *Bio-Implant Interface* Ellingsen, J.E. and Lyngstadaas, S.P., Eds., CRC Press, Boca Raton, FL, 2003, chap. 23.
25. Szmukler-Moncler, S., Zeggel, P., Perrin, D., Bernard, J-P., and Neuman, H.G., From micro-roughness to resorbable bioactive coating, in *Bio-Implant Interface*, Ellingsen, J.E. and Lyngstadaas, S.P., Eds., CRC Press, Boca Raton, FL, 2003, chap. 5.
26. Esposito, M., Worthington, H.V., Coulthard, P., Wennerberg, A., and Thomsen, P., Role of implant surface properties on the clinical outcome of osseointegrated oral therapy: an evidence-based approach, in *Bio-Implant Interface*, Ellingsen, J.E. and Lyngstadaas, S.P., Eds., CRC Press, Boca Raton, FL, 2003, chap. 1.
27. Shalaby, S.W. and Roweton, S.L., Continuous Open Cell Polymeric Foam Containing Living Cells, U.S. Patent 5,677,355, 1997.
28. Shalaby, S.W. and Roweton, S.L., Microporous Polymeric Foams and Microtextured Surfaces, U.S. Patent 5,847,012, 1998.
29. Roweton, S.L. and Shalaby, S.W., Microcellular foams, in *Polymers of Biological and Biomedical Significance,* Vol. 520, Shalaby, S.W. Ikada, Y., Langer, R., and Williams, J., Eds., A.C.S. Symp. Series, American Chemical Society, Washington, DC, 1993.
30. Shalaby, S.W., Johnson, R.A., and Deng, M., Process of Making a Bone Healing Device, U.S. Patent 5,529,736, 1996.

31. Deng, M., Wrana, J., Allan, J.M., and Shalaby, S.W., Tailoring mechanical properties of polyether-ether ketone for implants using solid-state orientation, *Trans. Cos. Biomater.*, 22, 477, 1999.
32. Shalaby, S.W., Highly Oriented PEEK/PEEK Composites for Dental Implants, Phase I Report, NIH-supported SBIR, Grant No. R43 DE12558-01, March 8, 1999.
33. Andrade, J.D., Nagaoka, S., Cooper, S.L., Okeno, F., and Kim, S.W., Surfaces and blood compatibility, current hypothesis, *Trans. Am. Soc. Artif. Intern. Organs*, 33, 75, 1987.
34. Hanker, J.S. and Giammara, B.L., Biomaterials and biomedical devices, *Science*, 242, 885, 1988.
35. Tengvall, P., How surfaces interact with the biological environment, in *Bio-implant Interface,* Ellingsen, J.E. and Lyngstadaas, S.P., Eds., CRC Press, Boca Raton, FL, 2003, chap. 16.
36. Jansen, J.A., ter Brugge, P.J., van der Wal, E., Vredenberg, A.M., and Wolke, J.G.C., Osteocapacities of calcium phosphate ceramics, in *Bio-implant Interface,* Ellingsen, J.E. and Lyngstadaas, S.P., Eds., CRC Press, Boca Raton, FL, 2003 chap. 17.
37. Paine, M.L. and Wong, J.C., Osteoblast response to pure titanium and titanium alloy, in *Bio-implant Interface,* Ellingsen, J.E. and Lyngstadaas, S.P., Eds., CRC Press, Boca Raton, FL, 2003, chap. 7.
38. Gristina, A.G., Biomaterial-centered infection: microbial adhesion versus tissue integration. *Science*, 237, 1588, 1987.
39. Costerton, J.W., Marrie, T.J., and Change, K.J., Phenomena of bacterial adhesion in bacterial adhesion mechanism and physiological significance (Sawage, D.C. and Fletcher, M., Eds), Plenum Press, New York, 1985, p. 3.
40. Gerdes, G.A., LaBerge, M.L., Barefoot, S.E., Dooley, R.L., and Shalaby, S.W., Surface phosphonylated substrate for studying bacterial cell attachment, *Trans Soc. Biomater.*, 23, 1535, 2000.
41. Jansen, B. and Kohnen, W., Prevention of biofilm formation by polymer modification, *J. Ind. Microbiol.*, 15, 391, 1995.
42. Atkins, G.G., Barefoot, S.G., LaBerge, M.L., Dooley, R.E., and Shalaby, S.W., Critical evaluation of methodologies for studying bacterial cell attachment to polymeric material, *Trans Soc. Biomater.*, 24, 353, 2001.
43. Allan, J.M., Wrana, J.S., Dooley, R.L., Budsberg, S., and Shalaby, S.W., Bone ingrowth into surface phosphonylated polyethylene and polypropylene, *Trans Soc. Biomater.*, 22, 468, 1999.
44. Allan, J.M., Wrana, J.S., Budsberg, S.C., Farris, H.M., Dooley, R.L., Powers, D.L., and Shalaby, S.W., Surface modified polyolefins for improved adhesion to bone, *Proc. 22nd Ann. Meeting,* Adhesion Soc., 1999, Virginia Tech., Blacksburg, VA. p. 106.
45. Wrana, J.S., Allan, J.M., Budsberg, S.C., Powers, D.L., Dooley, R.L., and Shalaby, S.W., Dental implants with modified surfaces for improved bioadhesion, *Proc. 22nd Ann. Meeting*, Adhesion Soc., 1999, p. 111.
46. Allan, J.M., Wrana, J.S., Linden, D.E., Farris, H., Budsberg, S., Dooley, R.L., and Shalaby, S.W., Bone formation into surface phosphonylated polymeric implants, *Crit. Rev. Biomed. Eng.*, 28, 377, 2000.
47. Allan, J.M., Wrana, J.S., Kline, J.D., Gerdes, G.A., Anneaux, B.L., Budsberg, S.C., Farris, H.E., and Shalaby, S.W., Bone ingrowth into phosphonylated PEEK rabbit tibial implants, *Sixth World Biomaterials Congress, Trans. Soc. Biomat.*, 23, 631, 2000.
48. Anneaux, B.L., Hollinger, J.O., Budsburg, S.C., Fulton, L.K., and Shalaby, S.W., Surface activated PEEK-based endosteal implants, *7th World Biomaterials Congress, Trans. Soc. Biomater.,* 27, 967, 2004.

49. Anneaux, B.L., Taylor, M.S., Johnston, S.A., and Shalaby, S.W., Biomechanical properties of osseointegrated PEEK-based and metallic endosteal implants, *Trans. Soc. Biomater.,* 28, 129, 2005.
50. Anneaux, B.L., Taylor, M.S., Shih, M., Fulton, L.K., and Shalaby, S.W., Histomorphometric evaluation of osseointegration of metallic and PEEK-based endosteal dental implants, *Trans. Soc. Biomater.*, 28, 431, 2005.
51. Tate, P.L., Taylor, M.S., Perry, D.M., and Shalaby, S.W., Attachment of osteoblasts to surface activated biomaterials, Abstract of Second Annual Southeastern Tissue Engineering and Biomaterial Conference, Birmingham, Alabama, February 11, 2005.
52. Tate, P.L., Hucks, M.A., Nagatomi, S., Vaughn, M.A., Shalaby, M., and Shalaby, S.W., Attachment of osteoblasts to surface modified substrates — a preliminary report, *Trans. Soc. Biomater.*, 29 (2), 611, 2006.
53. Shalaby, S.W., Surface Functionalized Absorbable Medical Devices, U.S. Patent Application, 2005.
54. Shalaby, S.W., Surface Electroconductive Biostable Polymeric Articles, U.S. Patent Application, 2005.
55. Tencer, A.F., Holmes, R.E., and Johnson, K.D., *Handbook of Biomaterials Evaluation* von Recum, A.F., Ed., Macmillan Publishing Co., New York, 1986, p. 324.
56. Allan, J.M., Wrana, J.S., Linden, D.E., Dooley, R.L., Farris, H., Budsberg, S., and Shalaby, S.W., Osseointegration of morphologically and chemically modified polymeric dental implants, *Trans. Soc. Biomater.*, 22, 37, 1999.
57. Maxian, S.H., Zawadsky, J.P., and Dunn, M.G., Effect of Ca/P coating resorption and surgical fit on bone/implant interface, *J. Biomed. Mater. Res.*, 28, 1311, 1994.
58. Wei, H., Hero, H., Solheim, T., Kleven, E., Rorvik, A.M., and Haanaes, H.R., Bonding capacity in bone of HIP-processed HA-coated titanium: mechanical and histological investigations, *J. Biomed. Mater. Res.*, 29, 1443, 1995.
59. Lemon, J.E., Dental implants, in *Biomaterials Science*, Ratner, B.D., Hoffman, A.S., Schoen, F.J., and Lemons, J.E., Eds., Academic Press, New York, 1996, chap. 7.
60. Langer, B., Langer, L., Hermann, I., and Jorneus, L., The wide fixture: a solution for special bone situations and a rescue for the compromised implant. Part 1, *Int. J. Oral Maxillofac. Impl.*, 8, 400, 1993.
61. Kato, K., Eika, Y., and Ikada, Y., Depositon of a hydroxyapatite thin layer onto a polymer surface carrying grafted phosphate polymer chains, *J. Biomed. Mater. Res* 32, 687, 1996.
62. Mukherjee, D.R., Wittenberg, J.M., Rober, S.H., Kruse, R N., and Albright, J.A., A fatigue study of hydroxyapatite dental implants, *Trans. Soc. Biomater.*, 28, 283, 1995.
63. Wennerberg, A. and Albrektsson, T., The influence of surface roughness on implant take, *Trans. Fifth World Biomater. Congr.*, 2, 459, 1996.
64. Shalaby, S.W., Highly Oriented PEEK/PEEK Composites for Dental Implants, Phase II Report, NIH-supported SBIR, Grant No. 2R 44 DE 012558-02A2, August 18, 2004.
65. Shalaby, S.W., Anneaux, B.L., and Taylor, M.S., Endosteal Dental Implant, U.S. Patent D 503,803, 2005.
66. Cho, S-A. and Jung, S-K., A removal of torque of the laser-treated titanium implants in rabbit tibia, *Biomaterials*, 24, 4859, 2003.

10 Surface Modification of Articulating Surfaces and Tribological Evaluation

Sunita P. Ho, Rebecca A. Caldwell, and Martine LaBerge

CONTENTS

10.1 INTRODUCTION

Polymeric materials have been used extensively for many engineering applications as bulk materials, coatings, adhesives, composites, and electronic devices at macrometer and nanometer scales.[1] A polymeric material that has gained utmost prominence, especially for high impact and high and low load bearing applications is ultra high molecular weight polyethylene (UHMWPE).[2,3] This chapter emphasizes the influence of UHMWPE microstructure on nanofriction and nanowear. It takes into account the surface topography and chemistry of the cobalt chromium (CoCr) femoral component articulating against a semicrystalline UHMWPE tibial plateau of a total knee replacement prostheses, using an atomic force microscope (AFM) as a test bed (Figure 10.1).

10.2 TOTAL JOINT REPLACEMENT (TJR) PROSTHESES — UHMWPE AND COCR ALLOY COMPONENTS

Total joint replacement (TJR) prostheses have allowed thousands of patients to regain painless motion in diseased (osteo and rheumatoid arthritis) and injured diarthroidal joints over the past five decades. In 1996, approximately 400,000 total hip and knee replacements were performed within the United States. By 2030, it is anticipated that this number may increase to over 700,000 annually.[4] Although the life expectancy of a TJR prosthesis is suitable for older and less active patients, it often necessitates revision operations in younger patients because of excessive wear and/or total failure of the joint.[5] During the late 1980s and early 1990s, the life expectancy of an artificial hip joint was limited to a few surviving beyond 25 years. With an increased number of prostheses being implanted into younger patients, the need to understand the failure mechanisms and to develop TJR prostheses with extended life expectancy have become major issues within the orthopedic community.[6] Hence, the long-term performance of the articulating system and materials in the design of artificial joints are very important, particularly for younger, heavier, and more active patients.

A typical total joint replacement consists of a smooth hard metal or ceramic counterface, articulating on a softer UHMWPE component (Figure 10.1). UHMWPE is the principal material used to replace damaged cartilage in joint arthroplasties. The first application of this material was in 1962 by Sir Charnley in the acetabular cup component of total hip joint prostheses.[2] UHMWPE has been the material of choice for high load bearing applications in TJR prostheses including hip, knee, ankle, shoulder, and prosthetic cruciate ligament.[7] UHMWPE is the sole polymeric bearing material currently being used as a liner for the acetabular cup in total hip arthroplasties, the tibial insert, and patellar component in total knee arthroplasties.

10.2.1 CoCr Femoral Component

CoCr alloy femoral components are used in TJR prosthesis because of their excellent wear resistance (Figure 10.1). The alloys currently being used in the manufacture

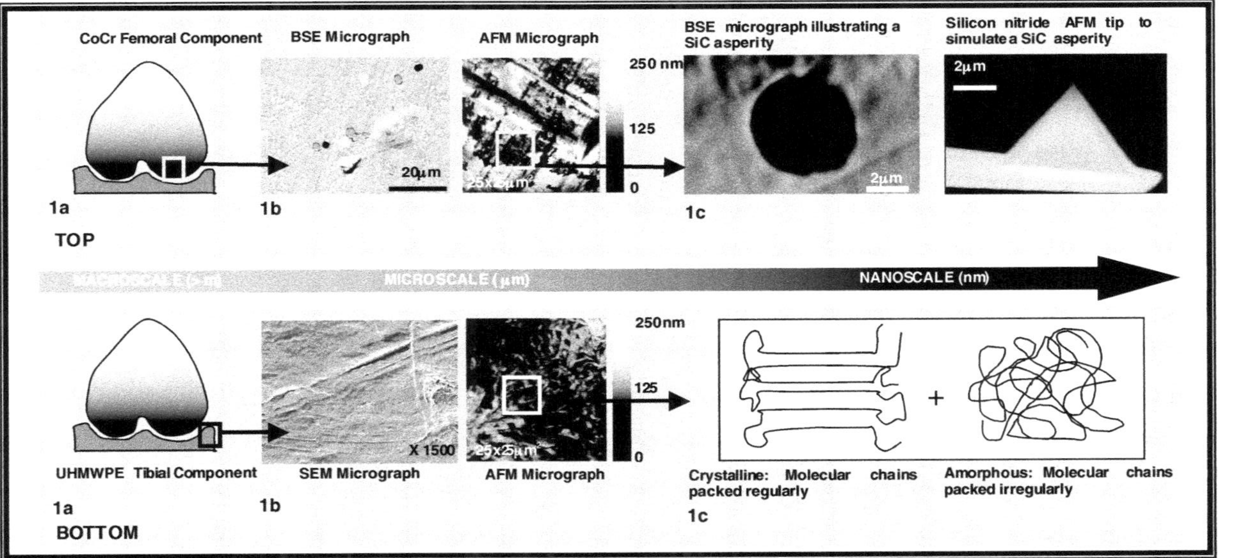

FIGURE 10.1 Schematic representation of transition from macroscale (device) to nanoscale substructures of CoCr and UHMWPE. (a) Macroscale: top, femoral and bottom, tibial components of a total knee replacement prosthesis device. (b) Microscale: top, BSE micrograph illustrating scratches and pits forming a rough metallic articulating surface. The black spots determined using BSE and EDXA illustrate SiC particles embedded within CoCr component, a remnant of SiC particles used during polishing of CoCr components, and a representative AFM micrograph illustrating scratches and pits. Bottom, SEM micrograph illustrating molding imperfections of a virgin compression molded UHMWPE and a representative AFM micrograph illustrating lamellar structure of UHMWPE. (c) Top, A SiC asperity equivalent to a Si_3N_4 AFM tip of nanometer radius of curvature. Bottom: A schematic representation of the semicrystalline molecular structure of UHMWPE — the basic structural units that define the long-term longevity of UHMWPE tibial component. *Note*: CoCr, cobalt chromium; UHMWPE, ultra high molecular weight polyethylene; BSE, back scattered electron; EDXA, energy dispersive X-ray

of these components are alloys that meet the requirements of the ASTM specification for Wrought Cobalt-28 Chromium-6 Molybdenum Alloy for surgical implants (F 1537).[9] It has been suggested that alloys with higher carbon composition may be superior in wear resistance because of the size and distribution of the carbides within the alloy, and particularly at the polished bearing surface.[9] The choice of the two bearing materials, cast CoCr alloy and UHMWPE for TJR prostheses, stems from their superior mechanical properties, including high toughness, low friction coefficient, and good biocompatibility.[2,3]

10.2.2 Ultra High Molecular Weight Polyethylene (UHMWPE) Tibial Component

Polyethylene in general is called ultra high molecular weight (UHMW) when its molecular weight exceeds 1×10^6 g/mole. The molecular weight of UHMWPE is the number of ethylene groups (C_2H_4) that make up one molecule of polyethylene polymer, multiplied by the molecular weight of ethylene (Figure 10.2). The highly linear homopolymer of ethylene namely, UHMWPE (molecular weight, $M_w \sim 2 \times$ to 6×10^6 g/mole, density, $\rho \sim 0.930$–0.945 g/cm^3) formed by Ziegler-Natta catalysis, belongs to a family of polyethylenes, including high-density polyethylene (HDPE) and low density polyethylene (LDPE) (M_w~0.05–0.2×10^6 g/mole, $\rho \sim 0.952$–0.965 g/ cm^3) (Figure 10.2).[2,8,10]

UHMWPE is distinctly different from HDPE, in microstructure, molecular weight, density, and impact strength, eventually leading to a relatively high wear-resistant material (Figure 10.3).[8] In addition, UHMWPE has several advantageous properties over other polymeric materials, which include high abrasion wear resistance, low friction, high impact strength, excellent toughness, low density, ease of fabrication, biocompatibility, and biostability. These positive attributes define UHMWPE to be the sole polymeric biomaterial for high load bearing applications such as in TJR prostheses.[2,8,10]

The arrangement of molecular chains of the polyethylene material is a function of molecular weight and thermal history, which in turn is governed by primary fabrication parameters, namely, temperature, pressure, and virgin polyethylene resin. The evolved microstructure defines the physical properties and the structural integrity of the material thus elucidating the response of the material to the applied stress in load bearing applications.[2,3,8]

At a nanometer scale, the UHMWPE is a two-phase viscoplastic semicrystalline composite solidlike material defining both a crystalline domain and the amorphous

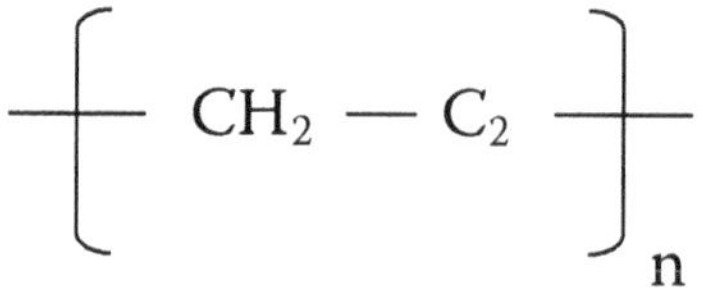

$$\left[CH_2 - C_2 \right]_n$$

FIGURE 10.2 General structure of polyethylene.

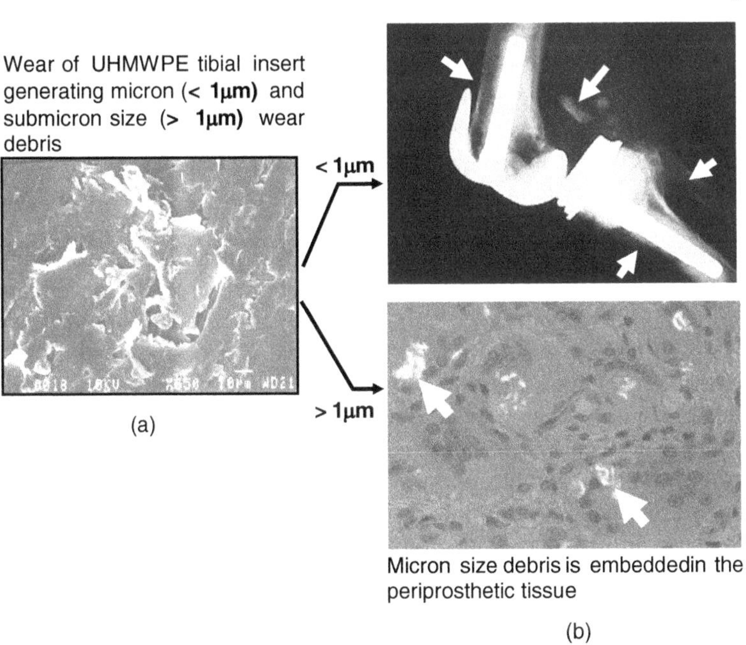

FIGURE 10.3 Clinical relevance of UHMWPE micron (≥1 μm) and submicron (<1 μ wear debris.

(noncrystalline) matrix that contains it. The long chains of UHMWPE, contrary to the short chains in HDPE and LDPE, prevent the molecules from ordering themselves into crystalline arrays, thus limiting the percentage of the crystalline material. The surrounding amorphous phase consists of randomly oriented and entangled polymer chains transversed by tie molecules with interconnected lamellae, which provide resistance to mechanical deformation.[2,3] The resulting structure consists of long molecular chains folded into dispersed crystalline lamellae connected by tie molecules within an amorphous matrix, thus defining a compositelike structure. The crystalline arrays of UHMWPE are composed of groups of orthorhombic unit cells with four carbon atoms and eight hydrogen atoms forming several lamellae.[11–13] The lamellae formed are 10– 50 nm thick and 10–50 μm long.[3] As long as these microconstituents within the amorphous matrix retain their specific arrangement, UHMWPE provides excellent toughness and mechanical integrity unmatched by most homopolymers.[14] In addition, owing to the high molecular weight of UHMWPE, the long molecular chain structures give rise to extensive mechanical entanglements of the molecular chains, imparting relative high abrasion resistance over the family of polyethylenes and other polymeric bearing materials used in TJR prostheses.[15]

10.3 WEAR OF UHMWPE COMPONENT IN TJR PROSTHESIS

Despite the many added advantages of UHMWPE over the other biomaterials for high load bearing applications, it was found that the weak link in the design of both total knee and hip replacements is the wear of the UHMWPE component.[8] In TJR prosthesis, several types of wear mechanisms have been found to occur in UHMWPE when articulating against its metallic counterpart. The primary types of wear that have been observed in both *in vivo* and *in vitro* studies are abrasive, adhesive, and fatigue wear.[14]

Wear of the UHMWPE insert in TJR prosthesis is identified by performing *vitro* (laboratory simulation) and *in vivo* (clinical retrieval) studies following revisions.[15–19] In general, abrasive wear in any tribosystem occurs when an intimate contact between the two surfaces of the tribosystem is developed with the harder surface asperities abrading against the softer polymeric bearing surface, which develops scratches. Abrasive wear in TJR prosthesis is due to trapping of a third particle (such as bone cement) or the penetration of hard CoCr alloy asperities into the soft polymeric UHMWPE material, resulting in the plowing of the surface, eventually developing a deep scratch and forming wedges around the scratch.[20] For polymers, abrasive wear is further subclassified into plowing and wedge formation, primarily within the softer surface of the two contacting bodies.[21]

Adhesive wear in lubricated systems could be due to the breakdown of the boundary lubricant, which causes an intimate contact between the two articulating surfaces, releasing loose wear particles or causing transfer of material from softer to the harder surface. In nonlubricated systems, adhesive wear is primarily due to the intimate contact of the two sliding surfaces. Surface fatigue wear occurs at a microscopic level because of repeated loading of the large number of asperity to asperity contacts between the hard and the soft components of two articulating components.[15–18] This surface fatigue could eventually lead to subsurface fatigue wear due to initiation and propagation of cracks leading to excessive pitting and delamination of UHMWPE tibial components.[19] In a UHMWPE tibial insert, a single individual wear mechanism occurs very rarely; the total wear debris produced is thus a combination of the various types of wear mechanisms. The contribution of wear debris from an individual wear mechanism could vary as a function of alignment of the prosthesis, the patient's activity, method of fixation, prosthesis design and fabrication, and surgical skills. For example, total hip replacement prostheses are more conforming and are defined predominantly by the occurrence of abrasive and adhesive wear mechanisms. On the other hand, considering the least conforming type of total joint replacement prosthesis, namely the knee implant, pitting and delamination seem to be the predominant type of wear mechanism despite the frequent abrasive and adhesive wear mechanisms observed.

10.3.1 Clinical Relevance of UHMWPE Wear Debris

Wear debris in TJR prostheses has been of primary concern for the past four decades. The clinical implication of wear debris is adverse. Based on retrieval studies, size of the UHMWPE wear debris particles that are generated are categorized into micron (≥1 μ and submicron (<1 μm) (Figure 10.3). The micrometer and submicrometer size

UHMWPE wear debris particles generated at the articulating surfaces accumulate in tissues surrounding the prostheses, causing inflammation, bone resorption, and joint loosening (Figure 10.3).[22,23] The physiological tissue and cellular response to the wear debris is not only a function of the shape but also size, number, and morphology of the particles.[17,24,25] TJR prostheses most often fail because of aseptic loosening. A certain degree of wear causes the fixation of joint into the bone to become loose, necessitating revision surgery. In the absence of infection, aseptic loosening may occur as a result of the biological response of the bone to stress shielding; micromotion at the bone cement, cement–prosthesis, or bone–prosthesis interface; or biological loosening due to osteolysis caused by adverse cellular reactions to debris generated by wear (Figure 10.3). Poor alignment, poor fixation leading to micromotion, and fluid pressure have been identified as important factors in late aseptic loosening, and the lack of initial stability of an implant is a strong predictor of later symptomatic loosening.[6,25–27] It is currently believed that UHMWPE wear debris generated at the articulating surfaces enters the periprosthetic tissue where it is phagocytosed by macrophages. The macrophages then release proinflammatory cytokines that include interleukin-1 (IL-1), interleukin-3 (IL-3), interleukin-6 (IL-6), tumor necrosis factor α (TNF-α), granulocyte-macrophage colony stimulating factor (GM-CSF), macrophage colony stimulating factor (M-CSF), stem cell factor (SCF), and platelet-derived growth factor (PDGF). Activated macrophages may also secrete matrix metalloproteinases (enzymes which degrade collagens) and prostagladin E2 (PGE2). It has been suggested that a rise in endogenous PGE2 may stimulate osteoblasts to produce an osteoclast activating factor.[6,28] The osteoclast activating factor stimulates bone resorption, leading to osteolysis and eventual loosening of the prosthesis. This cascade of events defines the need for revision surgery, leading to an increase in health care costs.

10.3.2 Factors Related to UHMWPE Wear Debris Generation

Over the past four decades, pharmacological and nonpharmacological methods have been considered when addressing the question of "How to increase the efficacy of TJR prosthesis?" Understanding the generation of UHMWPE wear debris by the articulating surfaces in TJR prostheses and evaluating wear debris dimensions play a primary role in defining the pathway for the origination of these wear particles. Based on the scope of this book, in the following pages only some of the current nonpharmacological methods are addressed.

The influential wear related factors could be classified into two categories: exogenous and endogenous. The factors that are related to virgin or fabricated UHMWPE material alone are termed endogenous while those that are not material related are termed exogenous. The endogenous factors include physical properties, composition of UHMWPE resin powder, fabrication parameters of the UHMWPE component, sterilization methods, packaging, and aging conditions. The exogenous factors include geometry of bearing components and entire total joint prosthesis; bearing surface characteristics; surgical alignment; and age, weight, and exercise condition of subject.[8,29–31] In this chapter, some of the endogenous factors are considered to explain the cause of submicron wear debris generation.

Thus far, the causes of generation of wear debris have been addressed and studied at different modeling scales, namely, macro-, micro- and nanoscales, taking into account both exogenous and endogenous factors. At a macroscale, various joint simulation studies, finite element modeling, and numerical modeling studies have been performed to date in an attempt to understand the cause of submicron wear debris generation by evaluating the cause of failure of the TJR prosthesis.[32,33]

Over the past four decades, the school of thought for the submicron wear debris generation was divided primarily into two major sources, when considering only the endogenous factors: (1) classical adhesive, abrasive, and third-body wear processes occurring *in vivo* and (2) release of particles that already exist in UHMWPE's microstructure. The first source of submicron wear debris generation was studied from purely a mechanistic approach. The combined effort of *in vitro* joint simulation, finite element modeling, and numerical modeling studies elucidate the cause of different wear mechanisms in UHMWPE at a macroscopic scale, defining the failure of the UHMWPE insert in the TJR prosthesis. In these studies, the bulk material properties of the two contacting surfaces and the macroscopic loading and boundary conditions were taken into account. The *in vitro* and macroscale experimental and numerical models attempted to define the cause of submicron wear debris by addressing the accumulation of large amounts of plastic strain. It was suggested that large scale deformations, texture evolution, fracture, and surface rupture within the surface region of UHMWPE components over repeated cyclic motion between the two components of the TJR prosthesis could cause macroscopic failure in the material, eventually leading to total failure of the TJR prosthesis.[14] However, while these studies attempt to connect the total failure of the insert observed to the generation of submicron wear debris particles, they do not explain the initiating cause of the submicron wear debris generation that occurs before the familiar wear processes such as delamination, pitting, and scratches are observed in TKR prostheses, leading to total failure of the UHMWPE insert.

The second source of submicron wear debris generation was studied from purely a materials approach. A microscopic examination of the morphology of retrieved UHMWPE wear debris nanostructure was compared with the morphology of virgin UHMWPE resin nanostructure and the morphology of sectioned samples fabricated from virgin UHMWPE resin. Although the evidence supporting this second source of particles is circumstantial, mostly based on qualitative analysis, it is worthy of further investigation.[2,14,24,34] Despite the many possible sources of submicron wear debris considered, these studies in their entirety do not bridge the gap between the cause of origination of the wear debris particles and total failure of the polymeric UHMWPE softer component of TJR prosthesis.[2,14,24,34]

10.4 FRICTION AND WEAR OF UHMWPE AT A NANOSCALE

One of the primary tribological parameters, friction or frictional work, is loss of energy that leads to deformation and dissipation within the contacting elements and under some circumstances mechanical or chemical damage of the interface zones. This leads to significant chemical, morphological, mechanical, and topographical modification of the interface zone, which could eventually lead to a third body particle formation as well as production of significant amounts of heat at the interface.[36] This damage produces debris, which when displaced from the interfacial zone is observed as wear debris.[35–37]

The influence of mechanical loading on UHMWPE bearing surfaces could be amplified when the inhomogeneity of the polymer is taken into account. UHMWPE is inhomogeneous either because of machining marks, poor consolidation of the material, or local changes in mechanical properties resulting from processing or sterilization.[2,8,38–41] In addition, the intrinsic compositelike semicrystalline nature of the polymer could cause variability in mechanical properties, leading to variability in mechanical response upon multiaxial loading (normal and shear loading). The variable mechanical response could cause a differential in shear resistance of the material, leading to variable friction at the interface of the two contacting surfaces of a TJR prosthesis.[42,43] Subsequently, the differential coefficient of friction at the tribocontact can cause a stress concentration within the polymeric material, eventually leading to submicron wear debris generation.[43]

10.4.1 Nanotribology of CoCr-UHMWPE TJR Prosthesis Using Atomic Force Microscopy

Over the past four decades, it has been thought that the generation of submicron wear debris was the result of two material related factors: (1) classical adhesive, abrasive, and third-body wear processes occurring *in vivo* and (2) release of particles that are inherent to the microstructure of UHMWPE. The first source of submicron wear debris generation was studied from a purely mechanistic approach. The combined effort of *in vitro* joint simulation, finite element modeling, and numerical modeling studies elucidated the cause of different wear mechanisms in UHMWPE at a macroscopic scale, defining the failure of the UHMWPE insert in the TJR prosthesis. These studies attempted to define the cause of submicron wear debris by addressing the accumulation of large amounts of plastic strain. It was suggested that large scale deformations, texture evolution, fracture, and surface rupture within the surface region of UHMWPE components over repeated cyclic motion could cause macroscopic failure in the material, eventually leading to total failure of the implant. However, as stated above, while these studies attempt to connect the failure of the insert to the generation of submicron wear debris particles, they do not explain the initiating cause of the generation of submicron wear debris.

The second source of submicron wear debris generation was studied from a purely materials approach. A microscopic examination of the morphology of the retrieved UHMWPE wear debris nanostructure was compared with the morphology of virgin UHMWPE powder nanostructure and with sectioned samples fabricated from virgin UHMWPE powder. Despite the many possible sources of submicron wear debris considered in these studies, the initiating origination of UHMWPE wear debris particles in TJR prostheses was not discussed.[44] At the present time there is a strong transition from continuum macroscale to asperity-to-asperity discrete nanoscale contact (Figure 10.1) that may give new insight into basic problems of tribology. For tribomechanical studies, mechanical properties of contact materials should be taken into account at any scale. However, depending on the scale, such parameters as modulus and hardness can differ not only in magnitude but also in their physical interpretation.[36] In simulating real contact, mechanical properties along with conventional factors such as temperatures, velocity, loading, to name a few, should be properly taken into account.[36] The mechanical properties of the compositelike structure of polyethylene (PE) could play a pivotal role in defining the frictional response of the material when an asperity-to-asperity contact of a TJR prosthesis is established.

Multiple asperity contact, adhesion-induced deformation, and plowing of the surfaces by wear particles or hard asperities on the countersurface could occur at the solid–solid interface during sliding of articulating surfaces of TJR prostheses or any other tribosystem. The real area of contact between the two surfaces is then equal to the sum of all the individual areas of contact established between the asperities of the two contacting surfaces. As stated earlier by several researchers, the dependence of material response upon load is a result of complex interface phenomena at each one of these nanoscale asperity-to-asperity contacts.[45–48]

Nanometer-scale single asperity contacts are essential elements in microscopic models of macroscopic contacts as formulated by Bowden and Tabor (Figure 10.1).[47,48] Their sizes are comparable to mechanical contacts in MEMS devices, and they are widely used as models of AFM contacts.[49–51] In each of these areas, it is essential to understand the frictional response of these contacts, particularly under combined normal and resulting shear loading at the interface of the various tribosystems.

Prior to the early 1980s, the fundamental explanation for not being able to define nanoscale tribological phenomena at the buried interface between various contacting surfaces was due to the lack of tribosystems that can access the complexity within the interfacial zone of two contacting surfaces. The invention of atomic force microscopy (AFM) in 1986 by Bening and Quate has made it possible to understand the macroscopic failure in a tribological contact of TJR prostheses by evaluating the nanotribological properties at the contact.[37] Before a tribological parameter can be measured, the primary objective is to define if the sharp atomic force microscope tip sliding on a surface could simulate just one such nano asperity contact.[43] The idea is to define the nanofrictional response as a function of nanomechanical properties resulting from their intrinsic physical properties for a given range of load at the contact of a TJR prosthesis.[43]

10.4.2 Effects of Sample Preparation Temperature on Nanostructure of UHMWPE

For macroscale and nanoscale tribological applications, determining whether the principal cause of failure is deformation or reorientation of UHMWPE lamellae is of practical importance to many technological processes such as manufacture of fiber, film, and TJR prostheses.[52] At a nanometer scale, when mechanical loading is placed on a polymer above its glass transition temperature, T_g, orientation of the material could occur because of the movement of polymeric chains. The resulting arrangement of the polymer molecular chains can redefine the mechanical response of the nanostructure of the polymer. On the other hand, the movement or rearrangement of polymeric chains is much more restricted when the material is loaded at an operating temperature below the T_g of the polymer.[52–54] Hence, the T_g of the polymer

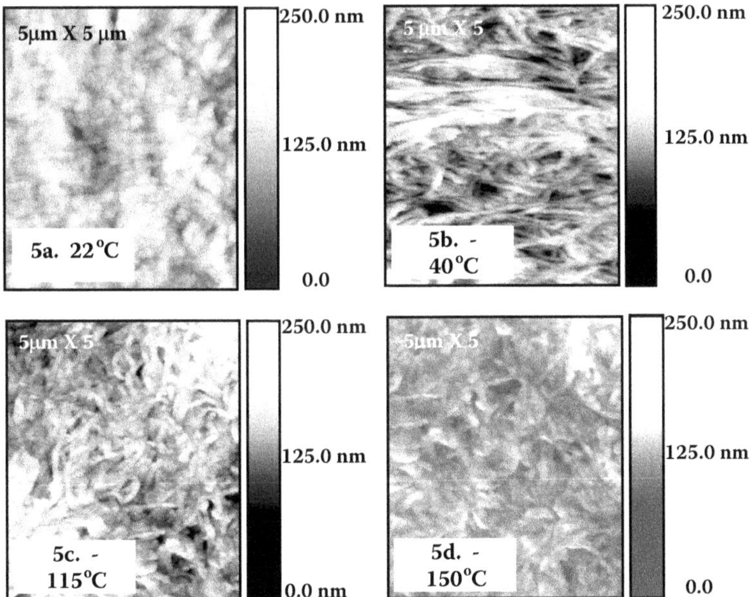

FIGURE 10.4 Ultramicrotomed surfaces of surgical grade direct compression molded UHMWPE at (a) 2°C; (b) 40°C (notice the preferential orientation of the UHMWPE fibers); (c) 115°C (notice there is no preferential orientation of UHMWPE fibers); (d) 150°C (notice there is no preferential orientation of UHMWPE fibers).

plays a pivotal role during preparation of samples to study the polymer nanostructure. This phenomenon is illustrated in Figure 10.4 using a cryoultramicrotome, a diamond knife, and an AFM.[55]

10.4.3 Nanomechanical Properties of Compression Molded UHMWPE

In a compositelike system such as UHMWPE, nanoscale mechanical properties that control various aspects of material performance can be different from bulk properties. Previous works focused on determining the average mechanical properties, assuming isotropy within the material. While this approach is suitable for macroscale study, it does not hold true at a nanometer scale. Scaling from macro to nano (Figure 10.1) can be related to transition from bulk properties of material to surface layer properties, local modulus, and nanoindentation data.[36]

At a nanoscale, the mechanical and subsequently frictional response of the individual nanoconstituents defines the overall behavior of the nanometer scale interface contact between an asperity of CoCr and UHMWPE (Figure 10.1). While there are several factors that can influence the mechanical failure of a material, one of these factors is primarily the frictional response of the nanostructure of the UHMWPE insert in the TJR prosthesis. To study the mechanical response of the

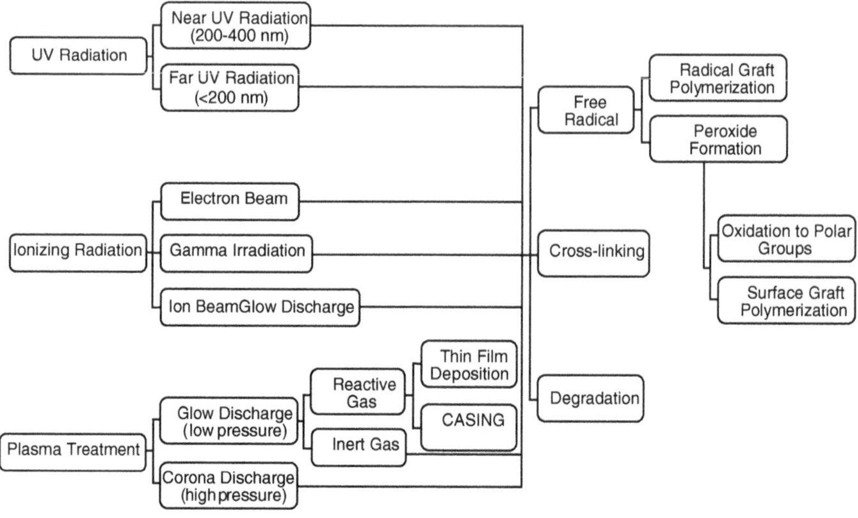

FIGURE 10.5 Common physical methods used for surface modification of polymers (adapted from Ikada, Y. and Uyama Y., *Lubricating Polymer Surfaces*, Technomic, Lancaster, England, 1993).[63]

nanostructure, we need a proper sample preparation method that calls for knowledge of sectioning techniques and the T_g of the polymer material.

Over the past decade, the damage threshold for materials such as mica, alkali halides, and low and high density polyethylene was defined using an AFM by measuring lateral force as a function of normal load.[35,56,57] AFM was used to model several plowing wear mechanisms of UHMWPE and subsequently the generation of nanoscale wear debris particles in the TJR prosthesis.[58,59] Although these studies explain the failure of the material, they do not explain the damage threshold of the UHMWPE insert, else defined as onset of plastic deformation in the TJR prosthesis. Plastic strain accumulation and the underlying assumptions of onset of plasticity have yet to be explicitly explored for UHMWPE in the context of total joint replacement wear simulation.[43,60]

Nanoindentation techniques can be employed to evaluate nanohardness and nanomodulus of the nanoscale basic building blocks that are responsible for the macroscale build-up of UHMWPE, which can then be related to resistance to local deformation.[20,61] Additionally, the mechanical properties of the nanostructure govern the evolution of the nanoscale morphology caused by plastic strain. These nanomechanical properties of the basic building blocks would therefore be essential to the understanding of the mechanisms of fracture and wear in polymers, subsequently defining the macroscale tribological performance and failure of TJR prosthesis at a macroscopic scale.[20]

On a nanoscale, UHMWPE has a compositelike semicrystalline structure consisting of more highly ordered crystalline constituents (lamellae) distributed within an amorphous (noncrystalline) matrix (Figure 10.1). The lamellae formed are typically

10–50 nm thick and 10– 50 μm long.[62] Considering the asperity-to-asperity contact or nanocontact of a TJR prosthesis, it is possible that either amorphous or crystalline regions will lead to results exhibiting the individual mechanical differences of the respective regions, such as amorphous and crystalline within UHMWPE. The combination of these significant mechanical differences at a nanoscale between the regions and their distribution could affect the frictional forces at the nanocontact.[43] This could lead to a change in surface mechanical behavior of UHMWPE on a nanoscale and subsequently the tribological characteristics of the TJR prosthesis.[42,43]

In an attempt to improve the surface quality and minimize the subsurface long-term plastic strain phenomenon, many surface treatments for polymers have been developed.[43] These modifications range from chemical to physical treatments that generate a multitude of altered PE properties. Thus, by modifying the surface of UHMWPE it may be possible to improve the friction and lubrication properties, and increase the wear resistance of the material. The following sections illustrate in detail the various existing surface modification techniques for various forms of PE.

10.5 SURFACE MODIFICATION OF POLYMERS

Surface modification of polymers is performed to provide the material with properties not inherent to the bulk material such as wettability, adhesiveness, biocompatibility, or lubricity. However, these surface modifications should not change the physical properties of the bulk material when applied. Altering the surface energy by making the polymer either hydrophilic or hydrophobic can enhance the surface properties and increase the longevity of an implant. For example, wettability can be increased by making the surface of the polymer more hydrophilic, whereas surface lubricity can be improved by making the surface more hydrophobic, which decreases the attractive forces between the opposing materials. However, a hydrated surface with large amounts of water-soluble polymers immobilized at the surface, which produces a hydrophilic surface, also interacts less with the opposing surface, improving the lubricity of the modified surface.[63]

10.5.1 Thickness of Surface Modification

An optimum thickness of surface modifications must be attained to prevent excessive delamination of thick coatings, surface reversal, and mechanical erosion of thin coatings. Delamination can be hindered by covalently bonding the surface layer to the substrate. However, thin-surface modifications are often desirable because modified surface layers that are too thick can change the mechanical and chemical properties of the material. Ideally, the treatment should alter only the outermost molecular layers (3–10 Å). Nevertheless, the surface modification should be applied at a thickness that achieves uniformity, durability, and functionality, but no thicker.

10.5.2 Surface Rearrangement

Even after a successful surface modification, surface rearrangement may occur. The surface structures and chemistries may change because of diffusion or translation of the atoms or molecules as the material interacts with the environment. Thus, to retain the desired surface properties, this surface reversal should be prevented or inhibited by such means as cross-linking, sterically blocking the ability of surface structures to move, and incorporating rigid, impermeable layers between the surface modification and the substrate.[64]

10.6 CLASSIFICATION OF SURFACE MODIFICATIONS

The most common surface modifications involve either coating the polymers with materials that have different chemical and physical properties, or the altering of the surface by forming or removing functional groups. Normally, the techniques that impart these altered surfaces can be divided into five general categories: chemical modifications, physical modifications, surface grafting, biologically functional modifications, and physical coatings. These surface modifications are discussed in the following sections with emphasis placed on the applicability to PE usage.

10.6.1 Chemical Modification

Chemical modifications of polymers are imparted by reagents that react with atoms or molecules at the surface but do not coat the surface atoms or molecules with a new layer. There are many chemical reactions that can be employed to modify the surfaces of polymers, and these techniques are typically more reliable and simpler than other methods allowing for the treatments to be performed on an industrial scale.[64] All of the chemical modifications have the following in common: (1) the chemicals used are highly reactive with the polymers being treated, (2) the treatment usually causes the oxidation of the surface, and (3) the modified surface that is formed is different in composition, structure, or functionality from the bulk material after oxidation of the surface.[65] Likewise these chemical modifications can be classified as either nonspecific or specific. Nonspecific reactions leave a distribution of different functional groups at the surface. An example of a nonspecific reaction is chromic acid oxidation of PE. On the other hand, specific chemical reactions change only one functional group into another with a high yield and few side reactions.

The most simple and rudimentary chemical modifications are those induced by acidic and alkaline treatments and flame exposure that produce hydrophilic polymer surfaces by introducing oxidized hydrophilic polar groups onto the surface of the polymer.[63] Another chemical treatment is direct chemical modification of a polymer surface, which is characterized by reactive groups with the capability of chemically interacting with other components. This direct chemical modification often takes place in water-soluble polymers such as polyethylene glycol binding to cellulose.[63] Both methods produce a modified top layer, which is chemically different than the bulk material.

Many different methods of chemical modifications exist for PE. Table 10.1 lists a few of the more commonly used chemical ones. These chemical treatments typically alter the PE surfaces both chemically and morphologically through the introduction of polar groups and etching of the surface, respectively. The resulting chemically modified surfaces exhibit enhanced surfaces with a wide variety of properties including increased wettability, improved adhesion, and decreased coefficient of friction.

TABLE 10.1
Chemical Surface Modifications of Polyethylene

Chemical Modification	Materials	Observations	Ref.
Chlorosulfonic acid treatment	LDPE HDPE	Produces surface modifications with depths of <14 μm and as the treatment time increases, the depth increases.	102
Chromic acid treatment	LDPE	Increased ionic content, surface roughness, hydrophilicity.	103,104
Decalin treatment (solvent immersion)	UHMWPE	Increases metal–polymer adhesion.	105
	UHMWPE	Removes short chains of PE at or near the surface and causes swelling and toughening of subsurface thereby reducing wear rate and coefficient of friction.	106
Flame treatment	LDPE	Increases the surface energy and improves peel strength; however, causes weight loss and an increase in surface roughness.	107
	LDPE	Formation of C—O, C—O, and C(—O)—O groups; carbonyl groups detected, thereby, increasing adhesion with epoxy; causing cohesive failure within PE	108
Fluorination	PE	200–400 Å fluorocarbon surface layer, providing good barrier to diffusion of solvents.	109
	PE	Depth of penetration is a diffusion-limited reaction providing effective permeation protection against solvents.	
Permanganate treatment	LDPE HDPE	Oxidized deposits are highly adherent to the surface resisting mild abrasion; causes surface corrosion.	110
	LDPE	Adsorption increases with relative concentrations of oxygen-containing groups. Increases adhesion strength to aluminum.	111
	LDPE HDPE	Increases average peeling force with epoxy. Produces corroded (surface roughened) PE with greater wettability.	112
	LDPE	Increases polar contributions, surface energies and adhesion strength. Peel force and thermodynamic work of adhesion increased.	113
Nitric acid treatment	PE	Removes the surface layer.	114
	LDPE LLDPE	Formation of polar groups including –COOH, >C–O, $-NO_2$, and –NO providing better adhesion with epoxy.	115
Ozone treatment	PE	Surface oxidation decreased degradation and bulk oxidation temperature due to chain scission, ablation, and loss of crystallinity.	116
Sulfuric acid treatment (sulfonation)	Linear PE, LDPE, HDPE	Surface hardness, conductivity, microindentation hardness, critical surface tension; Preferential hardening of lamellae.	61

Another important chemical modification of PE is phosphonylation. This modification involves the creation of phosphonate groups at the surface of the polymers. Phosphonylation can be produced by two different methods: liquid-phase and gas-phase. The liquid-phase process involves the immersion of PE in a solution of phosphoryl tricloride in carbon tetrachloride with oxygen bubbled through the solution. The samples are then rinsed in carbon tetrachloride, acetone, or water. The gas-phase process attaches phosphoryl chloride groups to the surface of the UHMWPE by exposing the material to phosphorus trichloride and oxygen gases followed by immersion in water. The groups created by this chemical modification are highly reactive and can be converted to different functionalities for molecular binding. This chemical modification has shown to attach —$P(O)Cl_2$, —P(O)(OH) —$P(OR)_2$ or —$P(NR)_2$ groups onto the surface, decrease the contact angle (increase surface energy), and allow binding of calcium ions, hydroxyapatite crystals, and phospholipids.[66–71]

10.6.2 Physical Modification — Ultraviolet Radiation

Physical modifications alter the surface properties of polymers without the use of a wet chemical reagent, but through the use of multiple types of high energy sources. Figure 10.6 outlines the commonly used physical methods of surface modifications.

Ultraviolet (UV) radiation is a form of ionizing radiation that promotes cross-linking and produces thin film deposits on the surface of polymers.[63,72] In UV lamps, mercury plasma is formed that emits UV, visible, and infrared wavelengths. It is possible to control the wavelengths emitted by doping the lamps with other elements or fluorescent materials that allow very specific wavelengths (typically between 200 and 300 nm) to reach the polymer surfaces. UV exposure of polymers in the presence of oxygen generally exhibits enhanced wettability and adhesion. However, the main disadvantage of the use of UV radiation is that it is difficult to employ UV light on irregularly shaped objects because the UV intensity is reduced by the square of the distance from the UV source and may cause an uneven distribution on the surface.[72]

Often UV modifications are coupled with chemical treatments such as ozone. The resulting physiochemical modification method, which employs the use of an ultraviolet light irradiation apparatus with the introduction of ozone, has been termed ultraviolet light–ozone (UVO) treatment. The surface of the PE became oxidized as detected by the oxygen-containing functional groups such as carbonyl, carboxyl, and ether groups. The hydrophilicity, adhesion to epoxy resin, and dyeability are shown to improve with UVO treatment.[73] In addition, this treatment causes material erosion and preferential etching in the amorphous regions with the UV light principally responsible for the chain scission.[74] A study compared the effects of pure ozonation with photooxidation (UV and an oxygen atmosphere) on PE surfaces. Photooxidation was shown to oxidize the surface more extensively than the ozone treatment with both treatments producing carboxyl and C—O groups.[75]

10.6.3 Physical Modification — Electron Beam Radiation

Electron beam (e-beam) radiation is similar to UV radiation in that it induces a chain reaction at the surface of the material. When performed under vacuum, e-beam radiation produces radicals on the polymer surface, which subsequently react with oxygen in air to form surface functionality. E-beams are produced with an electron accelerator, which bombards the surface of the polymer with a narrow beam of electrons.[72]

The use of e-beams with PE has not been extensively investigated as a surface modification method. However, e-beam irradiation of UHMWPE in air has induced the formation of hydroperoxide groups into the polymer without the formation of any other oxygen-containing groups. The hydroperoxides could be decomposed by subsequent heat treatments to produce cross-linking at the surface of the material, resulting in an increased surface hardness.[76]

10.6.4 Physical Modification — Gamma Irradiation

Gamma irradiation is produced from a radiation source (a radioactive isotope) that emits two monochromatic gamma rays with energy outputs. The common radiation source is ^{60}Co, which is housed *in vacuo*, and produces gamma rays that are directed out of the vacuum chamber onto the substrate. Gamma irradiation treatments performed in air produce radicals on the surface that can react with oxygen to yield functional groups.[72]

Gamma irradiation, which is a commonly used sterilization method for PE, has been extensively examined for its modification abilities. Research has shown that sterilization by gamma irradiation improves the wear resistance of the material by producing cross-linking and increasing the density of the polymer.[77–81] However, the combination of oxidation and cross-linking increases the rate of crack propagation, and reduces ultimate tensile strength, fatigue strength, and elongation.[81–83] Because of the free radicals in the material, either oxidation or cross-linking can occur. Because oxidation degrades whereas cross-linking tends to improve at least the wear resistance of PE, it is desirable to promote the cross-linking.[84,85] Therefore, a low oxygen or an inert environment, often either nitrogen or vacuum conditions, can be used, which reduces the amount of oxidation and increases cross-linking, and ultimately lowers the wear rate of the material.[85–87] Although irradiation in an inert environment produces cross-linking by a free radical recombination process, some primary free radicals remain in the core of the material, which promotes oxidation over time.[88,89]

Oxidation of gamma irradiated PE in an oxygen environment decreases the molecular weight due to chain scission and increases the density due to crystallization.[62,90] In fact, a maximum level of oxidation and crystallinity occurs on the UHMWPE surface immediately after irradiation. Large concentrations of secondary alkyl radicals are formed from C—H bond scission and primary alkyl radicals are produced by main chain scission. These alkyl radicals are rapidly converted to peroxy radicals, which generate carbonyls such as ketone.[90] This process of oxidation is initiated at the surface of the material and progresses inward.[91]

As the irradiated UHMWPE ages, the crystallinity increases as a result of oxidative chain scission. However, the concentration of carbonyls and the degree of crystallinity are limited to the reduced concentrations of oxygen present. Also, the subsurface oxidation tends to increase faster than that if the surface over long periods after irradiation.[90] Studies have shown that oxidation does not occur for about 5 or more years after sterilization in air when shelf aged (and even longer when implanted), but after this time the cross-linking decreases and promotes oxidation.[92,93] Because the benefits of gamma sterilization due to cross-linking are lost over time as a result of oxidation, Sanford et al. propose the use of nonirradiating methods such as gas plasma, which provide better long term wear performance.

10.6.5 Physical Modification — Ion Beam Implantation

Ion beam implantation involves accelerating ions with energies ranging from 10 to 10 electron volts onto the surface of the polymer.[64] Ion beams can be divided into two energy categories, low-ion beam and high-ion beam. Low-ion beam methods only interact with the first few layers of the material being treated, whereas the high-ion beam methods can penetrate several micrometers into the substrate. Presently, these techniques are mainly used in polymer adhesion applications.[65] When performed under vacuum, ion beam implantation produces radicals at the polymer surface, which can react with oxygen to produce surface functionality.[72]

Ion beam implantation of PE has been performed with various ions including argon, fluorine, nitrogen, and xenon. The concentration of the radicals formed in the polymer by ion bombardment is a decreasing function of the ion energy.[95] addition, ion implantation tends to increase the roughness, wettability, and hardness of PE. However, degradation of the polymer is also promoted by this modification method. Table 10.2 highlights some of the observed behaviors of PE treated with ion implantation.

10.6.6 Physical Modification — Plasma

Plasma modifications provide another type of physical modifications to polymer surfaces. "Plasma" is a mixed state of ionized gases that consists of electrons, positive ions, negative ions, free radicals, photons gas atoms, and molecules in their ground or excited state.[63,64] Different types of wave frequencies are used to produce the plasma, including radio waves, microwaves, or acoustic energy.[64,72] Plasma exposure tends to make a hydrophobic surface more hydrophilic, although this tendency normally disappears with time.[63] Also, plasma treatment increases the cross-linking at the surface, which can result in increased hardness of the polymer.[96]

The formation of polymeric materials in this plasma environment is known as plasma polymerization. Typically, a thin layer of the polymer is deposited on the substrate by the plasma polymerization of the monomer, which tends to become highly cross-linked and branched, but the treatment is not commonly employed to make the substrate more hydrophilic.[63] In addition, these plasma treatments can be employed to ablate or etch the polymer surfaces, which can substantially change the substrate both chemically and morphologically. Etching is characterized by the

TABLE 10.2
Ion Implantation of Polyethylene

Ion Implantation Materials	Ions	Observations	Ref.
LDPE HDPE UHMWPE PE Oriented PE	Argon (Ar^+)	Layered structure: the outermost carbon layer (75% C and 25% O) and the subsurface layer with O—H and C—O groups as well as ester and double bonds. Free radicals and conjugate double bonds formed. Leads to oxidation of surface layer. Concentration of incorporated water (mostly in the form of isolated molecules) increases with ion fluence until a maximum is attained from carbonization and cross-linking. Decreases surface resistivity. Increases bulk conductivity with increasing dose. Improves wear resistance and increases subsurface hardness. Decreases contact angle. Increases surface roughness with higher ion fluences.	95,117–122
PE	Fluorine (F^+)	Splits molecular bonds and creates conjugate unsaturated bonds and oxidized structures (carbonyl groups) producing degradation and etching of the polymer surface Produces homogeneous oxidation Increases electrical conductivity	123
LDPE UHMWPE	Nitrogen (N^+)	Layered structure: upper layer containing various products of oxidation and the lower layer containing products of decomposition (condensed aromatic structures) Increases content of the nitrogen and oxygen at surface Increases wettability with water Decreases surface resistivity Increases bulk conductivity with increasing dose	117,118,125
Oriented PE	Xenon (Xe^+)	Causes degradation (free radicals and conjugate double bonds formed) that is greater than Ar^+ because of the heavier ions, but surface morphology is altered less than Ar^+ because of the stronger compaction of the surface layer and a reduction of free volume Increases surface roughness with higher ion fluences	120

removal of surface material in the form of volatile products.[72] In fact, a competition between the deposition and ablation exists, and when ablation is more rapid than deposition, no deposition will occur.[64]

Plasma induces surface reactions between the species in the gas plasma and the polymer surface, or between the surface species alone. These surface reactions form functional groups or cross-linking at the surface and enhance interactions between the coating and substrate. Typical gases that are used to produce these surface reactions are argon, ammonia, carbon monoxide, carbon dioxide, fluorine, hydrogen, helium, nitrogen, nitrogen dioxide, oxygen, air, and water vapor. Oxygen, nitrogen, ammonia, argon, and helium gases tend to decrease the contact angle with water (increase surface energy), whereas carbon tetrafluoride and sulfur hexafluoride tend to increase the water contact angle (decrease surface energy).[97] In addition, oxygen- and fluorine-containing plasmas tend to induce etching of the surface, resulting in enhanced wettability and spreading of the coating over the substrate. Important parameters that can be controlled in plasma treatments to optimize these surface modifications include gas flow rate, power input, and reactor pressure. In addition, as the temperature of the substrate in the plasma reactor is increased, the degree of interaction between the plasma and polymer is increased.[72]

Even though the advantages are numerous, several disadvantages do exist. First, the chemistry produced on the surface is not well defined. For example, if tetrafluoroethylene gas is introduced into the plasma reactor, tetrafluoroethylene will not be deposited, but a complex, branched fluorocarbon polymer will be produced. Also, a uniform reaction is difficult to achieve in long, narrow crevices, and contamination or extraneous gases and pump oils may cause problems. Lastly, the plasma apparatus is rather costly.

The surface modification by plasma treatment typically extends less than 1 μm into the surface of polymer. Surface rearrangement begins immediately after the removal of the material from the plasma reactor as a result of its thermodynamic response to reduce its overall surface energy. The ultimate longevity of a plasma treated surface in air is usually less than 1 week because the nonpolar groups migrate to the surface and the reactive groups formed migrate inward toward the bulk. This aging phenomenon is dependent on the storage temperature: with elevated temperatures, the rate of aging increases.[72]

Plasma treatments can be categorized into either glow or corona discharge. Glow discharge occurs when the high electric energy is produced at reduced pressure, whereas corona discharge is produced at atmospheric pressures.[63,97] Thus, corona discharge plasma treatments may be simpler because evacuation of the system is not required, but they are less effective, less consistent, and less uniform.[63,72] However, glow discharge treatments allow not only the normal plasma treatments of surfaces but also direct deposit of organic layers onto the surfaces by introducing various gases into the reduced pressure atmosphere.

10.6.7 Physical Modification — Glow Discharge

In general, oxygen-containing plasmas induces surface reactions, etching, and degradation of the PE at the surface depending on the parameters of the treatment.

The common functional groups are formed with the oxygen containing plasmas include C—O, C=O, O—C=O, C—O—O, and CO_3. The formation of these moieties can be optimized using short cycle times and lowering the gas pressure and the power input.[72]

Wettability, bondability, and biocompatibility can be enhanced with nitrogen-containing plasmas, which form nitriles such as –C—N, –C—N, and –C=N. If ammonia is introduced into the plasma reactor, amino compounds are formed including –NH and –NH_2. In addition, the oxygen-containing functional groups described previously will also be incorporated into the PE surface. This is because the free radicals formed in the oxygen-free plasma react with ambient oxygen when the surface is removed from the reaction chamber. Also, plasmas containing fluorine will produce the oxygen-containing functionalities and fluorinated moieties such as —CF, —CF_2, and —CF_3.[72] These and other glow discharge plasma treatments are presented in Table 10.3.

10.7 BIOLOGICALLY FUNCTIONAL MODIFICATIONS OF POLYETHYLENE

Generally after a polymer surface is brought into contact with a biological system, proteins are adsorbed onto the surface followed by cell attachment. The protein adsorption and cell attachment to the surface of the polymer initiates a complex series of biological reactions toward the material. Thus regulating adsorption and attachments can control these biological reactions. Surfaces with water-soluble polymer chains minimize protein adsorption and cell adhesion.[63]

Active biomolecules, such as heparin and albumin, have been immobilized on the surfaces of synthetic polymers to create physiologically active surfaces.[63] Functional groups such as hydroxyl, carboxyl, and amino groups must be present on the surface of the polymer to induce biomolecule immobilization.[63] Many different functional molecules can either be chemically or physically immobilized on both solid or soluble polymer matrices. Therefore, immobilization can refer to temporary or permanent biomolecular attachment depending on the type of attachment.[98]

Immobilization can also be produced by physical adsorption to the surface or physical entrapment within the polymer. Physical adsorption can occur through van der Waal forces, electrostatic forces, affinity of the surface to the biomolecule, or absorption and cross-linking of the molecule to the polymer surface, whereas barrier systems, hydrogels, and dispersed (matrix) systems produce physical entrapment. To covalently bind a biomolecule to an inert solid polymer surface, it must first be chemically modified to provide reactive groups, such as hydroxyl, carboxyl, and amino groups, for subsequent immobilization. If the surface does not contain these moieties, surface modifications must be employed including photochemical grafting, plasma treatment, ionizing radiation graft polymerization, and chemical modification.[98]

Several of the aforementioned modifications, especially grafting techniques, can be employed to immobilize biomolecules on the surface of PE. Table 10.4 provides an overview of biologically functional modifications of PE.

TABLE 10.3
Glow Discharge Treatments of Polyethylene

Glow Discharge Materials	Atmosphere	Observations	Ref.
LDPE LLDPE HDPE Oriented PE	Air	Formation of hydroxyl, carbonyl, and carboxyl groups, which increases with increasing O/C ratio Increases surface roughness and surface energy Provides increased depth of cross-linking with increasing treatment time and power	125–129
LDPE HDPE Oriented PE UHSPE	Ammonia	Formation of amine and other nitrogen- and oxygen-containing groups on the surface Increases surface energy No change in surface morphology Decreases tensile strength Improves strength and durability of adhesive bonding in hot and humid conditions by covalent bonding of amine groups to cyanoacrylate adhesive	127,130–132
LDPE HDPE UHMWPE	Argon	Formation of radicals (midchain radicals, allylic radicals, and dangling bond sites), which subsequently induces cross-linking Methyl groups and double bonds on surface Increases shear strength Improves wear resistance and microhardness because of cross-linking of surface region Increases surface energy Provides increased depth of cross-linking with increasing treatment time and power	96,126,133–135
LDPE	Carbon dioxide	Produces oxidization of the surface by the introduction of oxygen functionalities including carboxylic acid, ketone/aldehyde, and hydroxyl/epoxide Increases surface roughness Increases surface energy, which is decreased when stored in air	136
LDPE HDPE PE	Fluorination by CF_4, CF_3H, CF_3Cl, CF_3Br, F_2	Formation of CHF—CH_2, CHF—CHF, and CF_2 groups Cross-linking occurs at surface Increases crystallinity Increases surface roughness with increasing treatment time More fluorinated surfaces, decreases the wettability of the surface	137–144
PE	Iodine	Chemically bound iodine atoms on surface that increases with increasing treatment time and plasma voltage	145

TABLE 10.4
Biologically Functional Modifications of Polyethylene

Material	Observations	Ref.
	Adherence	
LDPE	Sulfur containing functionalities were incorporated into the surface.	146
	Treatment increases surface hydrophilicity, but decreases with time.	
	Allyl phenyl sulphone plasma-treated LDPE is less platelet-activating in terms of platelet adhesion and spreading and is independent of plasma excitation energies.	
LDPE	Increases wettability.	147
	Cells adhere best to surface grafted with amine groups because its positive charge.	
PE	Free surface energy is not a decisive factor affecting the non–self-recognition of the grafted PE by macrophages.	119
LDPE	Increases surface wettability.	148
	Provides nonfouling surface (protein an platelet resistant).	
LDPE	Heparin is covalently bound in the coating.	149
	Acid solution increases surface wettability to provide good adhesion between the substrate and the coating.	
	Prolonged partial thromboplastin times occurred on coated samples without significant heparin release.	
	Heparin Coatings	
LDPE	HA-heparin is immobilized to surface-modified PE by reductive amination.	150
	Highest anticoagulant activity observed for HA-heparin immobilized to PE modified by NVP with a PEO spacer.	
LDPE	Heparinlike surfaces containing carboxylate and sulfate groups were formed.	151
	Thickness of layer = 55 Å.	
	The ratio of carboxylate to sulfate groups can be controlled by changing the composition of the coated surfactant layer.	
PE	^{125}I-labeled antibodies covalently attached to the amino groups via glutaraldehyde.	152
	Surface morphology remained essentially unaffected.	
	Immobilization of BiologicallyDerived Molecules	
LDPE	Protamine immobilized on surface.	153
	Protamine characteristic nitrogen traces were present.	
HDPE	Collagen immobilization reduces the tumorigenic potential of PE.	154
	Collagen immobilized surfaces increase gap-junction intercellular communication of cells, whereas RGDS peptide, RGES peptide, or bovine serum albumin did not reduce the activity.	

10.8 MISCELLANEOUS SURFACE MODIFICATIONS

Other surface modifications have been employed for polymers. Surface modifications relating to PE are the use of magnetic fields, sonochemical modifications, and laser irradiation. The introduction of a magnetic field to LDPE or HDPE has been shown to decrease the polymer's microhardness.[99] In addition, CO_2 laser radiation at low radiation intensity has reduced HDPE permeability to unleaded gasoline because of an increase in surface crystallinity.[100] Lastly, oxidation of LDPE with mild oxidizing agents, such as hydrogen peroxide and persulfate salts, can be enhanced with the use of ultrasound (sonochemical modification).[101]

10.9 CONCERNS OF SURFACE MODIFICATION

When a modification is applied to a polymer, two important surface characteristics should be considered: the thickness of the modification and the possible surface rearrangement. An optimum thickness of surface modifications must be attained to prevent excessive delamination of thick coatings and surface reversal and mechanical erosion of thin coatings. Delamination can be hindered by covalently bonding the surface layer to the substrate. However, thin surface modifications are often desirable because modified surface layers that are too thick can change the mechanical and chemical properties of the material. Ideally, the treatment should alter only the outermost molecular layers (3–10 Å). Nevertheless, the thickness of the surface modification should be such that it achieves uniformity, durability, and functionality, but no thicker.

Even after a successful surface modification, surface rearrangement may occur. The surface structures and chemistries may change because of diffusion or translation of the atoms or molecules as the material interacts with the environment. Thus, to retain the desired surface properties, this surface reversal should be prevented or inhibited by such means as cross-linking, sterically blocking the ability of surface structures to move, and incorporating rigid, impermeable layers between the surface modification and the substrate.[63]

10.10 CONCLUSION AND PERSPECTIVE ON THE FUTURE

Surface modification has clearly been shown to improve the frictional behavior of biomaterials for many clinical applications including endovascular surgery, general surgery, ophthalmology, and orthopedic surgery to name a few. Distinct advantages of surface modification are related to physicochemical properties of the surface where hydrophilicity, profilometry, and surface charges can be tailored to accommodate specific needs. As mentioned, numerous techniques have been proposed to modify surfaces with the goal of reducing the frictional properties of materials. Major advances have been made toward obtaining a better understanding of the effect of surface modification of the tribological properties of materials on the nano- and macroscale. For total joint replacements, surface modification of polymeric bearing materials is challenged by their impact on mechanical properties and consequently on wear properties. Wear of bearing materials remains one of the leading causes of clinical failure of total joint replacements. Therefore, better *in vitro* characterization methods to predict clinical wear are needed. Implant wear can be predicted *in vitro* by coupling nanoscale and macroscale device testing. The former allows the prediction of nanoscale wear debris generation while the latter focuses on the effects of macroscale wear simulation kinematics on wear and the quantifying of wear volumes. Multi-interdisciplinary research initiatives focused on understanding the nanomechanics of clinical wear from a tribological perspective, and on improving simulation methods as predictive tools for the clinical wear performance of devices and alternative bearing materials are essential to fully assess the potential of new surface modification methods.

REFERENCES

1. Van Landingham, M.R., McKnight, S.H., Palmese, G.R., Elings, J.R., Huang, X., Bogetti, T.A., Eduljee, R.F., and Gillespie, J.W., Nanoscale indentation of polymer systems using the atomic force microscope, *J. Adhesion*, 64, 31, 1997.
2. Li, S. and Burstein, A.H., Current concepts review or ultra-high molecular weight polyethylene, *J. Bone Joint Surg.*, 76-A(7), 1080, 1994.
3. Kurtz, S.M., Muratoglu, O.K., Evans, M., and Edidin, A.A., Advances in the processing, sterilization, and crosslinking of UHMWPE for total joint arthroplasty, *Biomaterials*, 20, 1659, 1999.
4. National Institutes of Health, Strategic Research Plan to Reduce and Ultimately Eliminate Health Disparities, U.S. Department of Health and Human Services, Fiscal Years 2002–2006.
5. Klapperich, C., Komvopoulos, K., and Pruitt, L., Tribological properties and microstructure evolution of ultra-high molecular weight polyethylene, *J. Tribol.* 121(2), 394, April 1999.
6. Ingham, E. and Fisher, J., Biological reactions to wear debris in total joint replacement, *Proc. Inst. Mech. Eng. Part H—J. Eng. Med.*, 214-H, 21, 2000.
7. Deng, M., Latour, R.A., Ogale, A.A., and Shalaby, S.W., Study of creep behavior of ultra-high-molecular-weight-polyethylene systems, *J. Biomed. Mater. Res.*, 40, 214, 1998.
8. Lewis, G., Polyethylene wear in total hip and knee arthroplasties, *J. Biomed. Mater. Res. (Appl. Biomater.)*, 38, 55, 1997.
9. St. John, K.R., Poggie, R.A., Zardiackas, L.D., and Afflitt, R.M., Comparison of two cobalt-based alloys for use in metal-on-metal hip prostheses: evaluation of the wear properties, in *Simulator, Cobalt-Base Alloys for Biomedical Applications,* Disegi, J.A., Kennedy, R.L., and Pilliar, R., Eds., American Society for Testing and Materials, West Conshohocken, PA, 1999, pp. 1365.
10. Coughlan, J.J. and Hug, D.P., Ultra high molecular weight polyethylene, in *Encyclopaedia of Polymer Science and Engineering*, Mark, H.F., Bikalls, N.M., Overberger, C.G., Menges, G., and Kroschurtz, J., Eds., Wiley, New York, 1986. p. 490.
11. Bunn, C.W., The crystal structure of long-chain normal paraffin hydrocarbons. The "shape" of the <CH_2 group,, *Trans Faraday Soc.*, 35, 482, 1939.
12. Teare, P.E. The crystal structure of orthorhombic hexatriacontane, $D_{36}H_{74}$, *Acta Crystal.*, 12, 294, 1959.
13. Odajima, T.M., Calculation of the elastic constants and the lattice energy of the polyethylene crystal, *J. Polym. Sci.*, Part C, 15, 55, 1966.
14. Wang, A., Edwards, B., Yau, S., Polineni, V.K., Essner, A., Klein, R., Sun, D.C., Stark, C., and Dumbleton, J.H., Orientation softening as a mechanism of UHMWPE wear in artificial hip and knee joints, in *Characterization and Properties of UHMWPE* Gsell, R.A., Stein, H.L., and Ploskonlea, J.J., Eds., ASTM STP, ASTM, Washington, DC 1998, p.56.
15. Nusbaum, H.J., Rose, R.M., Paul, I., Crognola, A.M., and Radin, E.L., Wear mechanisms for ultrahigh molecular weight polyethylene in the total hip prostheses, *J. Appl. Polym. Sci.*, 23, 777, 1979.

16. McKellop, H.A., Campbell, P., Park, S.H., Schamalzried, T., Grigoris, P., Amstutuz, H.C., and Sarmiento, A., The origin of submicron polyethylene wear debris in total hip arthroplasty, *Clin. Orthopaed. Related Res.*, 311, 3, 1995.
17. Cooper, J.R., Dowson, D., and Fisher, J., The mechanisms of the generation of wear particles of ultra high-molecular-weight polyethylene, *Proceedings, Leeds/Lyon Tribology Conference,* Elsevier, Amsterdam, 1992, p. 29.
18. Wang, A., Stark, C., and Dumbleton, J.H., Role of cyclic plastic deformation in the wear of UHMWPE acetabular cups, *J. Biomed. Mater. Res.*, 29, 619, 1995.
19. Hood, R.W., Wright, T.M., and Burstein, A.H., Retrieval analysis of total knee prostheses: a method and its application to 48 total condylar prostheses, *J. Biomed. Mater. Res.*, 17, 829, 1983.
20. Ho, S.P., Riester, L., Drews, M., Boland, T., and LaBerge, M., Nanoindentation properties of compression-molded ultra-high molecular weight polyethylene, *Proc. Inst. Mech. Eng. Part H—J. Eng. Med.*, 217(H5), 357, 2003
21. Bhushan, B., *Handbook on Macro and Micro/Nanotribology*, CRC Press, Boca Raton, FL, 1995.
22. Revel, P.A., Al Safar, N., and Kobayashi, A., Biological reaction to debris in relation to joint prostheses. *Proc. Inst. Mech. Eng. Part H—J. Eng. Med.*, 211(H2), 187, 1997.
23. Fisher, J., Bell, J., Barbour, P.S.M., Tipper, J.L., Matthews, J.B., Besong, A.A., Stone, M.H., and Ingham, E., A novel method for the prediction of functional biological activity of polyethylene wear debris, *Proc. Inst. Mech. Eng. Part H—J. Eng. Med.* 215, 127, 2001.
24. Pienkowski, D., Jacob, R.J., Hoglin, D.P., Saum, K.A., Kaufer, H., and Nicholls, P.J., Low voltage scanning electron microscopic examination of ultra high molecular weight polyethylene powder, *J. Biomed. Mater. Res.*, 29, 1167, 1995.
25. Asperberg, P. and Herbertsson, P., Periprosthetic bone resorption: particles versus movement, *J. Bone Joint Surg.*, 78B, 641, 1996.
26. Wroblewski, B.M., Wear of the high-density polyethylene socket in total hip arthroplasty and its role in endosteal cavitation, *Proc. Inst. Mech. Eng. Part H—J. Eng. Med.*, 211(H1), 109, 1997.
27. Ryd, L., Albrektsson, B.E.J., and Carlsson, L., Roentgen stereophotogrammetric analysis as a predictor of mechanical loosening of knee prostheses, *J. Bone Joint Surg.*, 77B, 377, 1995
28. Tashjian, A. and Levine, L., Epidermal growth factor stimulates prostagladin production and bone resorption in cultured mouse calvariae, *Biochem. Biophys. Res. Comm.* 85, 966, 1978.
29. Olley, R.H., Hosier, I.L., Bassett, D.C., and Smith, N.G., On morphology of consolidated UHMWPE resin in hip cups, *Biomaterials*, 20, 2037, 1999.
30. Mintz, L., Tsao, A.K., McCrea, C.R., Stulberg, S.D., and Wright, T., The arthroscopic evaluation and characteristics of severe polyethylene wear in total knee arthroplasty, *Clin. Orthopaed. Related Res.*, 273, 215, 1991.
31, Premnath, V., Harris, W.H., Jasty, M., and Merrill, E.W., Gamma sterilization of UHMWPE articular implants: an analysis of the oxidation problem, *Biomaterials* 17(18), 1741, 1996.
32. Burgess, I.C., Kolar, M., Cunnigham, J.L., and Unsworth, A., Development of a six station knee wear simulator and preliminary wear results, *Proc. Inst. Mech. Eng.* 211, 37, 1997.
33. Currier, J.H., Duda, J.L., Sperling, D.K., Collier, J.P., Currier, B.H., and Kennedy, F.E., *In vitro* simulation of contact fatigue damage found in ultra-high molecular weight polyethylene components of knee prostheses, *Proc. Inst. Mech. Eng.*, 212, 294, 1998.

34. Pienkowski, D., Hoglin, D.P., Jacob, R.J., Saum, K.A., Nicholls, P.J., and Kaufer, H., Shape and size of virgin UHMWPE GUR 4150HP polyethylene powder, *J. Biomed. Mater. Res.* (*Appl. Biomater.*), 33, 65, 1996.
35. Carpick, R., The Study of Contact, Adhesion and Friction at the Atomic Scale by Atomic Force Microscopy, Ph.D. thesis, University of California at Berkeley, CA, 1997.
36. Myshkin, N.K., Petrokovets, M.I., and Chizhuk, S.A., Simulation of real contact in tribology, *Tribol. Int.*, 31, 79, 1998.
37. Bhushan, B., *Principles and Applications of Tribology*, Wiley. New York, 1999.
38. Halldin, G.W. and Kamel, I.L., Powder processing of ultra-high-molecular weight polyethylene. I. Powder characterization and compaction, *Polym.Eng. Sci.*, 17, 21, 1977.
39. Pruitt, L. and Bailey, L., Factors affecting the near-threshold fatigue behavior of surgical grade ultra high molecular weight polyethylene, *Polymer*, 39, 1545, 1998.
40. King, R., Devanathan, D., Gsell, R., Lin, S., and Rohr, W., Processing defects in UHMWPE, *Trans. 41st Orthoped. Res. Soc.*, 20, 759, 1995.
41. Devanathan, D., Bhambri, D., Nazre, A., Lin, S., Characterization of compression molded UHMWPE, *Trans. Soc. Biomater.*, 18, 113, 1995.
42. Joseph, P.F., Flood, L.M., Pullela-Ho, S., and LaBerge, M., Contact modeling of variable friction with application to bearing against polymeric surfaces, *Trans Soc. Biomater.*, 22, 130, 1999.
43. Ho, S.P., Joseph, P.F., Drews, M.J., Boland, T., and LaBerge, M., Experimental and numerical modeling of variable friction between nanoregions in conventional and crosslinked UHMWPE, *J. Biol. Eng.*, 126(1), 111, 2004.
44. Jacob, R.J., Penkowski, D., Hoglin, D.P., Saum, K.A., Kaufer, H., and Nicholls, P.J., *J. Biomed. Mater. Res.*, 37(4), 489, 1997.
45. Suh, N.P., *Tribophysics*, Prentice-Hall, Englewood Cliffs, NJ, 1986.
46. Rabinowicz, E., *Friction and Wear of Materials*, 2nd Ed., Wiley, New York, 1995.
47. Bowden, F.P. and Tabor, D., *Friction and Lubrication*, Wiley, New York, 1956.
48. Bowden, F.P. and Tabor, D., *Friction: an Introduction to Tribology*, Anchor Press, Garden City, NY, 1973.
49. Landman, U., Luedtke, W.D., Burham, N.A., and Colton, R.J., Atomistic mechanisms and dynamics of adhesion, nanoindentation, and fracture, *Science,* 248, 454, 1990.
50. Johnson, K.L., Adhesion and friction between a smooth elastic spherical asperity and a plane surface, *Procs R. Soc. London*, A453, 163, 1997.
51. Burham, N.A. and Colton, R.J., Force microscopy, in *Scanning Tunneling Microscopy and Spectroscopy*, Bonnell, D.A., Ed., VCH Publishers, New York, 1993, p. 191.
52. Wunderlich, B., *Macromolecular Physics Volume 1, Crystal Structure, Morphology, Defects,* Academic Press, New York, 1973, p. 489.
53. Lee, W.A. and Rutherford, R.A., The glass transition temperatures of polymers, in *Polymer Handbook*, Brandrup, J. and Immergut, E.H., Eds., Wiley, New York, 1975, p. III-140.
54. O'Reilly, J.M. and Karasz, F.E., Specific heat studies of transition and relaxation behavior in polymers, *J. Polymer. Sci.*, Part C, 14, 49, 1966.
55. Ho, S.P., Carpick, R.W., Boland, T., and LaBerge, M., Nanotribology of CoCr-UHMWPE TJR prosthesis using atomic force microscopy, *Wear*, 253(11–12), 1145, 2002.
56. Hu, J., Xiao, D.X, Ogletree F.D., and Salmeron, M., Atomic scale friction and wear of mica, *Surface Sci.*, 327, 358, 1995.
57. Niederberger, S., Gracias, D.H., Komvopoulos, K., and Somorjai, G.A., Transitions from nanoscale to microscale dynamic friction mechanisms on polyethylene and silicon surfaces, *J. Appl. Phys.*, 87(6), 3143, 2000.

58. Hampel, H., Hector, L.G., Nuhfer, N.T., and Piehler, H.R., Evolution of UHMWPE wear debris during single asperity plowing, *44th Annual Meeting, Orthopaedic Research Society*, Chicago, IL, March 16–19, 1998, p. 365.
59. Schmid, S.R., Hector, L.G., Elings, J., Hampel, H., and Piehler, H., Single asperity plowing of metallic and polymeric surfaces in an atomic force microscope: an overview of recent developments, *Mater. Res. Soc. Symp. Proc.*, 522, 391, 1998.
60. Ho, S.P., Riester, L., Drews, M., Boland T., and LaBerge, M., Effects of the sample preparation temperature on the nanostructure of compression molded ultra high molecular weight polyethylene, *Proc. Inst. Mech. Eng. Part H—J. Eng. Med.* 216(H2), 123, 2002.
61. Calleja, F.J.B., Fonseca, C., Perena, J.M., and J.G. Fatuo, Surface hardening of polyethylene through sulphuric acid exposure, *J. Mater. Sci. Letters*, 3, 509, 1984.
62. Kurtz, J.M., Rimnac, C.M., and Bartel, D.L., Degradation rate of ultra-high molecular weight polyethylene, *J. Ortho. Res.*, 15, 57, 1997.
63. Ikada, Y. and Y. Uyama, *Lubricating Polymer Surfaces*, Technomic, Lancaster, England, 1993.
64. Ratner, B.D. and Hoffman, A.S., Thin films, grafts, and coatings, in *Biomaterials Science: An Introduction to Materials in Medicine,* Ratner, B.D., Hoffman, A.S., Schoen, F.J., and Lemons, J.E., Eds., Academic Press, San Diego, 1996, p. 103.
65. Chou, N.J. and C. Chang, Surface modification of polymers, in *Characterization of Polymers* Chou, N.J., Kowalczyk, S.P., Saraf, R., and Tong, H., Eds., Butterworth-Heinemann, Boston, 1994, p. 169.
66. Rogers, K.R., The Formation and Reactivity of Surface Phosphonylated Thermoplastic Polymers, M.S. thesis, Department of Bioengineering, Clemson University, Clemson, SC, 1992.
67. Allan, J.M., The Molecular Binding of Inherently Conductive Polymers to Thermoplastic Substrate, M.S. thesis, Department of Bioengineering, Clemson University, Clemson, SC, 1994.
68. McCaig, M.S., Gas Phase Phosphonylation of Thermoplastic Polymer, M.S. thesis, Department of Bioengineering, Clemson University, Clemson, SC, 1994, p. 138.
69. Campbell, C.E., Surface-Phosphonylated Polyethylene and Its Ion-Binding Capacity, M.S. thesis, Department of Bioengineering, Clemson University, Clemson, SC, 1996.
70. Shalaby, S.W. and McCaig, M.S, Process for Phosphonylating the Surface of an Organic Polymeric Perform, U.S. Patent 5,491,198 (to Clemson University), 1996.
71. Caldwell, R.A., Allan, J.M., Shalaby, S.W., Powell, G.L., and LaBerge, M., Phospholipid attraction to phosphonylated low density polyethylene, *Trans Soc. Biomater* 21, 531, 1998.
72. LaPorte, R.J., *Hydrophilic Polymer Coatings for Medical Devices: Structure/Properties, Development, Manufacture and Applications*, Technomic, Lancaster, PA, 1997.
73. Gongjian, B., Yunxuan, W., and Xingzhou, H., Surface modification of polyolefins by UV light/ozone treatment, *J. Appl. Polym. Sci.*, 60, 2397, 1996.
74. Herbert, S., Shinozaki, D.M., and Collacott, R.J., Fine-scale morphology of ultraviolet ozone etched polyethylene, *J. Mater. Sci.*, 31(17), 4655, 1996.
75. Peeling, J. and Clark, D.T., Surface ozonation and photooxidation of polyethylene film, *J. Polym. Sci., Part A, Polym. Chem.*, 21, 2047, 1983.
76. Tretinnikov, O.N., Ogata, S., and Ikada, Y., Surface crosslinking of polyethylene by electron beam irradiation in air, *Polymer*, 39(24), 6115, 1998.
77. Clarke, I.C., Good, V., Williams, P., Oparaugo, P., Oonishi, H., and Fulisawa, A., Simulator wear study of high-dose gamma-irradiated UHMWPE cups, *Trans. Soc. Biomater.*, 20, 71, 1997.

78. Muratoglu, O.K., Biggs, S.A., Bragdon, C.R., O'Connor, D.O., Merrill, E.W., Premnath, V., Jasty, M., and Harris, W.H., Long term stability of radiation and peroxide cross-linked UHMWPE, *Trans. Soc. Biomater.*, 20, 49, 1997.
79. Polineni, V.K., Essner, A., Wang, A., Stark, C., and Dumbleton, J.H., Effect of sterilization methods on the wear behavior of UHMWPE acetabular cups, *Trans, 43rd Annu. Meeting Orthopaed. Res. Soc.* (San Francisco), 22, 779, 1997.
80. Sun, D.C., Schmidig, G., Yau, S.S., Jeanty, M., Wang A., and Stark, C., Correlations between oxidation, crosslinking, and wear performance of UHMWPE, *Transactions, 43rd Annu. Meeting Orthopaed. Res. Soc.* (San Francisco), 22, 783, 1997.
81. Goldman, M. and Pruitt, L., Comparison of the effects of gamma radiation and low temperature hydrogen peroxide gas plasma sterilization on the molecular structure, fatigue resistance, and wear behavior of UHMWPE, *J. Bone Mineral Res. (JBMR)* 40, 378, 1998.
82. Sauer, W.L., Weaver, K.D., and Beals, N.B., Fatigue performance of ultra-high-molecular-weight polyethylene: effect of gamma radiation sterilization, *Biomaterials* 17(20),1929, 1996.
83. Bell, C.J., Simmons, King, P., Walker, P.S., and Blunn, G.W., Is oxidation of ultra high molecular weight polyethylene the main cause of delamination wear in total knee replacement? *Trans. 43rd Annu. Meeting Orthopaed. Res. Soc.* (San Francisco), 22, 1997.
84. McKellop, H., Shen, F.W., Ota, T., Lu, B., Wiser, H., and Yu, E., Wear of UHMWPE acetabular cups after gamma steriliation in nitrogen, thermal stabilization and artificial aging, *Trans. Biomater. Soc.*, 20, 45, 1997.
85. McKellop, H.A., Shen, F.W., Yu, Y.J., Lu, B., and Salovey, R., Effect of sterilization method on the wear rate of UHMW polyethylene acetabular cups in a hip simulator, *Trans. 43rd Annu. Meeting Orthopaed. Res. Soc.* (San Francisco), 22, 1997.
86. Bapst, J.M., Valentine, R.H., and Vasquez, R., Wear simulation testing of direct compression molded UHMWPE irradiated in oxygenless packaging, *Trans. Soc. Biomater.*, 20, 72, 1997.
87. Wang, A., Polineni, V.K., Essner, A., Sun, D.C., Stark, C., and H. Dumbleton, H., Effect of radiation dosage on the wear of stabilized UHMWPE evaluated by hip and knee joint simulators, *Trans. Soc. Biomater.*, 20, 394, 1997.
88. King, R., Taylor, G., Devanathan, D., Lin, S., and Rohr, W., Gamma radiation effect on crosslinking of ultra-high molecular-weight polyethylene, *Trans. Soc. Biomater.* 20, 217, 1997.
89. Trieu, H.H., Haggard, W.O., Parr, J.E., Thomas, D.E., and Jahan, M.S., A study of long-lived free radicals in irradiated UHMWPE materials, *Trans. Soc. Biomater.*, 20, 47, 1997.
90. Yeom, B., Yu, Y.-J., McKellop, H.A., and Salovey, R., Profile of oxidation in irradiated polyethylene, *J. Polym. Sci., Part A: Polym. Chem.*, 36, 329,1998.
91. St. John, K.R., Takeuchi, M.J., and Poggie, R.A., Effects of radiation dose and packaging condition on the oxidation of UHMWPE, *Trans. Soc. Biomater.*, 20, 46, 1997.
92. Furman, B.D., Ritter, M.A., Perone, J.B., Furman, G.L., and Li, S., Effect of resin type and manufacturing method on UHMWPE oxidation and quality at long aging and implant times, *Trans. 43rd Annu. Meeting Orthopaed. Res. Soc.* (San Francisco), 22, 92, 1997.
93. Patel, A., Lee, K.-Y., Hamiliton, D.M., Higgins, J., Schroeder, D.W., and Pienkowski, D., Shelf-life effects on crosslinking of UHMWPE, *Trans. 43rd Annu. Meeting Orthopaed. Res. Soc.* (San Francisco), 22, 93, 1997.

94. Sanford, W.M., Moore, W.C., McNulty, D., Frisinger, C., and Schalzried, T.P., Hip simulator study of the effect of sterilization and oxidation on UHMWPE wear, *Trans. 43rd Annu. Meeting Orthopaed. Res. Soc.* (San Francisco), 22, 95, 1997.
95. Svorcik, V., Rybka, V., Stibor, I., Hnatowicz, V., Vacik, J., and Stopka, P., Synthesis of grafted polyethylene by ion beam modification, *Polym Degradation Stability*, 58, 143, 1997.
96. Farrar, D., Surface Treatment, International Patent WO 95/21212, 1995.
97. Fourche, G., An overview of the basic aspects of polymer adhesion. Part II: Application to surface treatments, *Polym. Eng. Sci.*, 35(12), 968, 1995.
98. Hoffman, A.S., Biologically functional materials, biomaterials science, in *An Introduction to Materials in Medicine*, Ratner, B.D. Hoffman, A.S. Schoen, F.J., and Lemons, J.E, Eds., Academic Press, San Diego, 1996, p. 124.
99. Zhorin, V.A., Mukhina, L.L., and Razumovskaya, I.V., The effect of magnetic treatment of microhardness of polyethylene and polypropylene, *Polym. Sci., Series B* 40(7–8), 233, 1998.
100. Duley, W.W., Ogmen, M., Steel, T., and Mihailov, S., Laser surfacing of high density polyethylene for reduction in fuel permeability, *J. Laser Appl.*, 4(1), 22, 1992,
101. Price, G.J., F. Keen, F., and A.A. Clifton, A.A., Sonochemically-assisted modification of polyethylene surfaces, *Macromolecules*, 29, 5664, 1996.
102. Kalnins, M.M., Brana, M.T.C., and Gedde, U.W., Treatment of polyethylene and polypropylene with chlorosulphonic acid to study the surface morphology, *Polym, Testing*, 11(2), 139, 1992.
103. Brack, H.-P. and Risen, W.M., Fourier transform mid- and far-infrared specular reflectance studies of the polarizability of ion-containing polymers and oxidized polyethylene and its application to adhesion, *J. Mater. Chem.*, 7(12), 2355, 1997.
104. Schonherr, H. and Vancso, G.J., Surface properties of oxidized LDPE by scanning force microscopy with chemically modified probes, *J. Polym. Sci., Part B: Polym. Phys.*, 36, 2483, 1998.
105. Gao, P. and Mackley, M.R., Surface treatment of ultra high molecular weight polyethylene to enhance adhesion and conductivity properties, *Polymer*, 33(19), 4075, 1992.
106. Dearnaley, G. and Lankford, J., Treatments to Reduce Frictional Wear between Components Made of Ultra-High Molecular Weight Polyethylene and Metal Alloys, International Patent WO 95/26169, 1995.
107. Piiroja, E.K. and Lippmaa, H.V., Intensification of low-temperature oxidation of low-density polyethylene by gas flame, *Acta Polym.*, 35(11), 669, 1984.
108. Sheng, E., Sutherland, I., Brewis, D.M., Heath, R.J., and Bradley, R.H., Surface studies of polyethylene modified by flame treatment, *J. Mater. Chem.*, 4(3), 487, 1994.
109. Volkmann, T. and Widdecke, H., Oxifluorination of polyethylene, *Kunststoffe German Plastics,* 79(8), 51, 1989.
110. Rubira, A.F., Costa, A.C.D., Galembeck, F., Escobar, N.F.L., Silva, E.C.D., and Vargas, H., Polyethylene and polypropylene surface modification by impregnation with manganese (IV) oxide, *Colliods Surfaces*, 15, 63, 1985.
111. Golander, C.-G. and Sultan, B.-A., Surface modification of polyethylene to improve its adhesion to aluminum, *J. Adhesion Sci. Technol.*, 2(2), 125, 1988.
112. Costa, R.A.D., Goncalves, M.D.C., Oliveira, M.G.D., Rubira, A.F., and Galembeck, F., Polyethylene adhesion: pretreatment with potassium permanganate, *J. Appl. Polym. Sci.*, 37, 3105, 1989.
113. Konar, J. and Ghosh, R., Studies on adhesion of polyethylene. Part I. Influence of functionality and phase transfer catalyst, *J. Adhesion Sci. Technol.*, 3(8), 609, 1989.

114. Ania, F., F. Calleja, F.J.B., and Cagiao. M.E., Diamagnetism and structure of nitric acid-treated bulk polyethylene, *Polym. Bull.*, 7, 317, 1982.
115. Bag, D.S., Ghosh, S.N., and Maiti, S., Surface modification and evaluation of polyethylene film, *Europ. Polym. J.*, 34(5/6), 855, 1998.
116. Chtourou, H., Riedl, R., and Kokta, B.W., Surface modification of polyethylene pulp fiber by ozone treatment. An analytical and thermal characterization, *Polym. Degradation Stability,* 43(1), 149, 1994.
117. Kuniyoshi, S., Kudo, K., and Tanaka, K., Surface modification of low density polyethylene by N^+, Ar^+ ion implantation for space charge devices, *Appl. Surface Sci.*, 43, 447, 1989.
118. Pichat, A., Rabbe, L.-M., Rieu, J., Rambert, A., Chabrol, C., and Robelet, M., Effect of ion implantation on titanium alloy/polyethylene and 316L stainless steel/polyethylene friction couples running in joint prostheses, *Surface Coatings Technol.*, 45, 15, 1991.
119. Svorcik, V., Rybka, W., Hnatowicz, V., and Smetana, K., Structure and biocompatibility of ion beam modified polyethylene, *J. Mater. Sci.: Mater. Med.,* 8(7), 435, 1997.
120. Svorcik, V., Arenholz, E., Hnatowicz, V., Rybka, V., Ochsner, R., and Ryssel, H., AFM surface investigation of polyethylene modified by ion bombardment, *Nucl. Instrum. Methods Phys. Res. B*, 142, 349, 1998.
121. Svorcik, V., Proskova, K., Rybka, V., and Hnatowicz, V., Water diffusion in polyethylene modified by ion irradiation, *Polym. Degradation Stability,* 60(2–3), 431, 1998.
122. Tretinnikov, O.N. and Ikada, Y., Surface characterization of ion-implanted polyethylene, *J. Polym. Sci., Part B: Polym. Phys.*, 36, 715, 1998.
123. Svorcik, V., Rybka, V., Endrst, R., Hnatowicz, V., Kvitek, J., and Seidl, P., Surface modification of polyethylene and polypropylene by ion implantation, *J. Appl. Polym. Sci.*, 49, 1939, 1993.
124. Gavrilov, N., Yakusheva, D., and Kondyurin, A., Structure of polyethylene after pulse ion beam treatment, *J. Appl. Polym. Sci.,* 69, 1071, 1998.
125. Foerch, R., Kill, G., and Walzak, M.J., Plasma surface modification of polyethylene: short-term vs. long-term plasma treatment, *J. Adhesion Sci. Technol.*, 7(10), 1077, 1993.
126. Yao, Y., Liu, X., and Zhu, Y., Surface modification of high-density polyethylene by plasma treatment, *J. Adhesion Sci. Technol.*, 7(1), 63, 1993.
127. Mercx, F.P.M., Improved adhesion properties of high-modulus polyethylene structures: 3. Air- and ammonia-plasma treatment, *Polymer*, 35(10), 2098, 1994.
128. O'Kell, S., Henshaw, T., Farrow, G., Aindow, M., and Jones, C., Effects of low-power plasma treatment on polyethylene surfaces, *Surface Interface,* .23(5), 319, 1995.
129. Kuzuya, M., Kondo, S.-I., Sugito, M., and Yamashiro, Y., Peroxy radical formation from plasma-induced surface radicals of polyethylene as studied by electron spin resonance, *Macromolecules*, 31, 3230, 1998.
130. Holmes, S. and Schwartz, P., Amination of ultra-high strength polyethylene using ammonia plasma, *Composites Sci. Technol.*, 38, 1, 1990.
131. Favia, P., Stendardo, M.V., and d'Agostino, R., Plasma-treatment of polyethylene in NH_3-H_2 RF glow discharges, *Polym. Preprints*, 36(1), 93, 1995.
132. Wu, D.Y., Gutowski, W.S., Li, S., and Griesser, H.J., Ammonia plasma treatment of polyolefins for adhesive bonding with a cyanoacrylate adhesive, *J. Adhesion Sci. Technol.*, 9(4), 501, 1995.
133. Ashida, M., Ikada, Y., Ueda, Y., and Aizawa, H., Properties of low-molecular-weight polyethylene treated with gas plasma, *J. Polym. Sci., Part A., Polym. Chem.*, 20, 3107, 1982.

134. Rossi, A., Incarnato, L., Tagliaferri, V., and Acierno, D., Modification of barrier properties of polymeric films of LDPE and HDPE by cold plasma treatment, *J. Polym. Eng.*,14(2–3), 191, 1995.
135. Kuzuya, M., Yamashiro, T., Kondo, S.-I. Sugito. M and Mouri, M., Plasma-induced surface radicals of low-density polyethylene studied by electron spin resonance, *Macromolecules*, 31, 3225, 1998.
136. Terlingen, J.G., Gerritsen, H.F.C., Hoffman, A.S., and Feijen, J., (1995). Introduction of functional groups on polyethylene surfaces by a carbon dioxide plasma treatment, *J. Appl. Polym. Sci.*, 57, 969, 1995.
137. Anand, M., Cohen, R.E., and Baddour, R.F., Conditions affecting surface fluorination of low density polyethylene in a fluoride glow discharge, *Polym. Preprints*, 21(1), 139, 1980.
138. Anand, M., Cohen, R.E., and Baddour, R.F., Fluorination of polyethylene surfaces using various plasma treatment methods, *Polym. Preprints*, 21(2), 182, 1980.
139. Anand, M., Cohen, R.E., and Baddour, R.F., Surface modification of low density polyethylene in a fluorine gas plasma, *Polymer*, 22, 361, 1981.
140. Yagi, T., Pavlath, A.E., and Pittman, A.G., Grafting fluorocarbons to polyethylene in glow discharge, *J. Appl. Polym. Sci.*, 27, 4019, 1982.
141. Inagaki, N., Tasaka, S., and Ishii, K., Surface modification of polyethylene and magnetite powders by combination of fluidization and plasma polymerization, *J. Appl. Polym. Sci.*, 48, 1433, 1993.
142. Khairallah, Y., Arefi, F., Amouroux, J., Leonard D., and Bertrand, P., Surface fluorination of polyethylene films by different glow discharges. Effects of frequency and electrode configuration, *J. Adhesion Sci. Technol.*, 8(4), 363, 1994.
143. Serpe, G., Huiban, Y., Lynch, J., Dole-Robbe, J.P., and Legeay, G., Polyethylene plasma fluorination and permeability relationships to methanol-gasoline mixtures, *J. Appl. Polym. Sci.*, 61, 1707, 1996.
144. Park, S.H. and Kim, S.D., Plasma surface treatment of HDPE powders by CF_4 plasma in a fluidized bed reactor, *Polym. Bull.*, 41, 479, 1998.
145. Fujishima, M., Kawabata, D., Funakoshi, C., Yoshida, Y., Yamashita, T., Kashiwagi, K., and Higashikata, K., Effect of I_2 plasma on the properties of polyethylene, *Polym. J.*, 27(6), 575, 1995.
146. Ko, T.-M., Lin, J.-C., and Cooper, S.L., Surface characterization and platelet adhesion studies of plasma-sulphonated polyethylene, *Biomaterials*, 14(9), 657, 1993.
147. Lee, J.H., Jung, Y.W., Kang, I.-K., and Lee, H.B., Cell behaviour on polymer surfaces with different functional groups, *Biomaterials*, 15(9), 705, 1994.
148. Sheu, M.-S., Hoffman, A.S., Ratner, B.D., Feijen, J., and Harris, J.M., Immobilization of polyethylene oxide surfactants for non-fouling biomaterial surfaces using an argon glow discharge treatment, *J. Adhesion Sci. Technol.*, 7(10), 1065, 1993.
149. Evangelista, R.A. and Sefton, M.V., Coating of two polyether-polyurethanes and polethylene with a heparin-poly(vinyl alcohol) hydrogel, *Biomaterials*, 7, 206, 1986.
150. Yuan, S., Szakalas-Gratzl, G., Ziats, N.P., Jacobsen, D.W., Kottke-Marchant, K., and Marchant, R.E., Immobilization of high-affinity heparin oligosaccharides to radiofrequency plasma-modified polyethylene, *J. Biomed. Mater. Res.*, 27, 811, 1993.
151. Lens, J.P., Terlingen, J.G.A., Engbers, G.H.M., and Feijen, J., Preparation of heparin-like surfaces by introducing sulfate and carboxylate groups on poly(ethylene) using an argon plasma treatment, *J. Biomat. Sci., Polym. Ed.*, 9(4), 357, 1998.
152. Hayat, U., Tinsley, A.M., Calder, M.R., and Clarke, D.J., ESCA investigation of low-temperature ammonia plasma-treated polyethylene substrate for immobilization of protein, *Biomaterials*, 13(11), 801, 1992.

153. Bai, G., Hu, X., and Yan, Q., Surface modification of polyethylene film by liquid phase photograft polymerization, *Polym. Bull.*, 36, 503, 1996.
154. Nakaoka, R., Tsuchiya, T., Kato, K., Ikada, Y., and Nakamura, A., Studies on tumor-promoting activity of polyethylene: Inhibitory activity of metabolic cooperation on polyethylene surfaces is markedly decreased by surface modification with collagen but not with RGDS peptide, *J. Biomed. Mater. Res.*, 35, 391, 1997.

11 Histopathological Evaluation of Hard Tissue Implant Performance

Mei-Shu Shih

CONTENTS

11.1 INTRODUCTION

The synthetic biomaterials for orthopedic and dental devices include polymer, metallic, and ceramic material constructs.[1] Refinements of synthesis of absorbable polymers for medical use have revolved mainly around reduction of host tissue reactions and promotion of functional integration. The fabrication of a device from polymers requires deciphering the key combinations of chemical characteristics and physical properties of the base materials, surface textures, and porosity of the end product, and general anatomical and physiological conditions of the target tissues and organs for optimal reparative actions. The shapes and sizes of the devices are often designed to press-fit when in direct contact with the target tissues, e.g., bone, cartilage, dentin, and to be held in position by physiological and functional loading from the local host anatomy. The surfaces of the devices are made to provide attachment and tissue ingrowths. The degradation rate of the base material decides the patency of the fabricated pores and channels, and the biomechanical plasticity of the repairing tissues and organs. These factors have been shown to directly influence the clinical longevity of the devices because the hard tissue modeling and remodeling adjacent to these designs are very different.[2,3] For example, resistance to load at the bone–polymer interface is one of the most important factor in deciding the success of the implant. Devices based on the new polymer technology avoid the excessive or unbalanced loads on titanium-based implant devices that often produce zones of high mechanical stress and cause bone resorption and implant loosening.[4] Around the implant region, cortical bone provides the most appropriate resistance to load for stabilizing the implant device.[5] On the other hand, trabecular bone provides cushion for elasticity, shear, and compression.

11.2 GENERAL PATHOLOGY

The intent of implantation is to restore the functionality of a defunct or malfunctioning unit of a tissue or organ. Debridement is always a prerequisite during the initial clinical steps to remove a volume of tissues slightly larger than the affected portion. The surgical procedures for implanting polymer based biomaterials in a targeted hard tissue site will elicit sequential events concerned with tissue healing. Besides the common elements of cell and tissues responses that occur during wound healing, the polymers used will certainly serve affect the healing processes, depending on the degree to which the implant is recognized as a foreign body. The common indicator of the foreign body reaction is the appearance of multinucleated giant cells.

The general stages of wound healing include clot formation, neutrophil and macrophage inflammatory reaction, neovascularization, fibroblast proliferation, devascularization, egress of inflammatory cells, fibroblast regression, and collagenous scar tissue.[6] The major additions to these stages at a bone implant site are the development of osteogenic repair tissue, apposition and ingrowths of osseous tissues into the implant, degradation of the polymers, and the remodeling of the osseous tissue during the stages of neovascularization and fibroblast proliferation. Dentin repair, although rarely successful, follows a similar route through the formation of tightly organized dentinal tubules. In contrast, at a cartilaginous defect implanted with a combinational device (biomaterial carrier plus biological agents), the additions to the wound healing stages are repopulation of chondrogenic cells, integration of newly formed cartilaginous matrix across the defect walls, and remodeling of the new cartilage from mostly fibrous to hyaline cartilage. Although all these stages may exhibit highs and lows, they often coexist throughout the repair period. The main determinants of their proportions in the healing processes are the antigenicity of the polymer, the capability of the biological agents to induce targeted tissue repair, the degradation rate of the polymer, and the stability of the integration between the polymer and the target tissues. Antigenicity drives the level and intensity of inflammatory responses against the polymer. It also sets the length of time for the continuation of inflammatory responses. The persistence of inflammatory responses shifts the repair toward potential tissue necrosis and/or fibroblastic scarring. For example, it is known that the fibrous sheet formed between the implant and the bone shortens the interval needed for a clinical revisit. When present at efficacious concentrations, biological agents, e.g., bone morphogenetic proteins, turn on differentiation of mesenchymal cells to osteogenic and chondrogenic precursors and subsequent bone formation on the surfaces of the polymers. The manner and rate of bone formation induced by biological agents may reduce the exposure period and the surface areas of polymer to the host immune system. Direct bone apposition under this circumstance also provides initial biomechanical support beyond the natural material properties of the polymer itself, which establishes the mode of integration with the adjacent existing bone and cartilage. Timely bone formation induced by biological agents likely uses the porous polymer as the building modules to form a framework of trabecular bone for the integration. The balance between the rate of polymer degradation and the tempo of bone formation decides the biomechanical stability and the final outcome of the repair. Therefore, an ideal combinational polymer device should possess low antigenicity, quick targeted tissue formation on its surfaces and ingrowths through its porous channels, tandem degradation of the polymer, and integration with the targeted tissues, and eventually a complete replacement of the defect area by host tissues. Histopathological evaluation in this regard facilitates grading how well the combinational device performs.[7]

11.3 HISTOPATHOLOGICAL EVALUATION

11.3.1 Hard Tissue Histological Preparation

It is a common practice that hard tissues, e.g., bone, cartilage, dentin, etc., be examined microscopically through the process of decalcification and embedding in polymethyl methacrylate media. The optimal preservation of cellular profiles, minimal shrinkage of tissues of various densities and compactness, and retention of integrity between the hard tissue and the polymer implant allow the evaluation to be done on histological sections that are relatively artifact-free. Details of the procedures for preparing hard tissue sections have been readily available in the literature since 1980s and are beyond the scope of this chapter.[8] However, the texture and the porosity of the implanted polymer may require a longer period of media infiltration and a lower temperature, 4°C or 20°C, for thorough penetration of the media and replacement of chemical reagents from the prior step. Similarly, polymerization of a hard tissue block is best done at a slow and steady rate to avoid excessive heat generation and explosion during methacrylate cross-linkage. Although a sledge microtome may be useful for producing 5 to 8 μm thin sections of hard tissues containing implanted polymer, ground sections between 25 and 50 μm in thickness are often the choice because they yield the best section quality. A variety of common staining methods for hard tissues is also suitable for histopathological evaluation of implanted polymer devices and depends on the researcher's personal preference. These stains include, but are not limited to, toluidine blue, von Kossa, Goldner's, or Masson trichrome, and Hematoxylin & Eosion. In addition, Safranin-O staining is commonly used to demonstrate the content of glycoaminoglycan in cartilage. The use of these stains can assist in the differentiation of newly formed matrix versus the preexisting one by the intensity and shades of colors.

11.3.2 Histopathological Evaluation of Hard Tissue Integration with Polymer Implant Device

Comparisons between the test and control implants regarding the amount of tissue reaction should focus on the thickness of the scar, presence of inflammatory or other cell types, presence of wear debris or particulates, and adverse interaction of tissue and material. The suggested criteria for evaluation from American Society for Testing and Materials International are listed in Table 11.1.

11.3.2.1 Histopathological Evaluation of Articular Cartilage Repair

The pathogenesis of articular cartilage degeneration that leads to osteoarthritis is not fully understood. However, the sequence of the degeneration follows the path of superficial layer fibrillation, fissures that reach and invade tidemarks, and erosion and loss of cartilage layers. The self-repair by chondrocytes in degenerating articular cartilage is slow and limited, although the remaining chondrocytes may have increased proliferative and synthetic activity via cloning. Therapeutic regimens

TABLE 11.1
Suggested Evaluation Format and Scoring Range

Animal number					
Duration of implant (weeks)					
Sample description					
Gross response					
Histopath-number					
Score					
Necrosis					
Degeneration					
Inflammation	0	0.5	1	2	3
Polymorphonuclear leukocytes					
Lymphocytes					
Eosinophils					
Plasma cells					
Macrophages					
Fibrosis					
Giant cells					
Foreign body debris					
Fatty infiltration					
Relative size of involved area in mm					
Histopathologic toxicity rating					

intended to restore the integrity of the lost cartilage often encounter the challenges of biomechanical loading and friction between the implanted device and preexisting cartilaginous tissue. These challenges impede the full restoration of hyaline cartilage. Therefore, the first goal in cartilage repair is to provide functional articular surfaces during locomotion. The success of a polymer-based therapeutic regimen is assessed by the reversibility of the abnormalities found in the structure, cells, and matrix of articular cartilage. The successful implant provides initial support to withstand physiological mechanical loading and is replaced in a timely fashion by host reparative osteochondral tissues. The criteria and scoring schemes in the literature for histopathological evaluation are largely similar to each other, although there are small variations.[9–16] It is crucial that the reparative cartilage in the defect region becomes level with the preexisting cartilage. Insufficient filling of the defect causes the collapse of defect walls from the adjacent cartilage. Overfilling of the defect mechanically affects the opposite articular surface and changes the local milieu of load distribution. The initial bonding and organization of the collagen fibers between the reparative cartilage and the preexisting cartilage decides the fate of the reparative process to continue toward functional restoration or toward deterioration that requires arthroplasty. The normalization in density of chondrocytes in the reparative and adjacent cartilage from hypocellularity and hypercellularity is indicative of a sound repair. The staining intensity by Safranin-O on glycoaminoglycan content indirectly shows the degree of normality of the matrix. Subchondral bone is interactive in the articular cartilage repair process. Sclerotic changes and microfractures are often found in mechanically weak repairs. Reestablished tidemarks are important indicators that the repair produces proper anatomical layers of tissues similar to their original form.

The criteria published in the literature each served an individual purpose in detailing the separations of conceptually better repair for the selected treatment regimens.[9–16] Universal histopathological evaluation criteria have recently been refined by a group of world renowned scientists and are provided by the International Cartilage Repair Society (www.cartilage.org); they are listed in Table 11.2.

11.3.2.2 Histopathology Evaluation of Bone Void Repair

Assessment of bone void repair can be both qualitative and quantitative. Bone formation at the initial healing stage goes at a fast pace and has a woven texture. Although the woven matrix produced in bulk may be sufficient to meet the requirement for biomechanical stability, it will be gradually replaced by a compact and lamellar type matrix. The organization of the bone matrix can be readily revealed under polarization microscopy. With the natural transition of woven to lamellar in the bone matrix, it is possible to determine the polymer–bone integration throughout the repair process. The material properties of the polymer interplay with the focal biomechanical environment and contribute to the modulation of surrounding preexisting bone structure. The orientations of the bone matrix lamella and of the trabecular spicules often indicate the biomechanical loading direction, which parallels the direction of the loading force. Bone matrix laid down in lamellar format along the surface contours of the implanted polymer reflects the biomechanical harmony

TABLE 11.2
Cartilage Repair Assessment

Criteria	Points		
	Degree of defect repair		
Protocol A[a]	In level with surrounding cartilage		
	75% repair of defect depth		
	50% repair of defect depth		
	25% repair of defect depth		
	0% repair of defect depth		
Protocol B[b]	100% survival of initially grafted surface		
	75% survival of initially grafted surface		
	50% survival of initially grafted surface		
	25% survival of initially grafted surface		
	0% (plug are lost or broken)		
Integration to border zone	Complete integration with surrounding cartilage		
	Demarcating border <1 mm		
	$^3/_4$ of graft integrated, $^1/_4$ with a notable border > 1 mm width		
	$^1/_2$ of graft integrated with surrounding cartilage, $^1/_2$ with a notable border > 1 mm		
	From noncontact to π of graft integrated with surrounding cartilage		
Macroscopic appearance	Intact smooth surface		
	Fibrillated surface		
	Small, scattered fissures or cracks		
	Several, small or few but large fissures		
	Total degeneration of grafted area		
Overall repair assessment	Grade I	Normal	12 P
	Grade II	Nearly normal	11–8 P
	Grade III	Abnormal	7– 4 P
	Grade IV	Severely abnormal	3–1 P

[a] Protocol A: Autologous chondrocyte implantation; periosteal or perichondrial transplantation; subchondral drilling; microfracturing; carbon fiber implants; others.
[b] Protocol B: Mosaicplasty; osteochondral allografts; others.

between the two types of texture. On the other hand, the bone matrix laid down perpendicular to the implanted polymer surface implies a changed load distribution in and around the implanted area. Bone responds to tensile force by adding more matrices, and to compression force by removing matrix. Therefore, a sclerotic reaction of the bone suggests excess tensile force exerted from the implanted polymer device, and an osteopenic reaction demonstrates excess compression force translated from the polymer implant. The summation of bone lamellar orientation within the proximity of polymer devices can serve as an indicator of directional changes in loading forces that resulted from implant degradation and bone adaptation.

In addition, the cement lines that appear in the bone matrix denote the end of resorbing activity by osteoclasts and the beginning of bone formation by osteoblasts can help distinguish newly formed bone from preexisting old matrix. However, the demarcations between new and preexisting matrices are often blurred by the substantial bone realignment with time. This is particularly true in a time course experiment where the interfaces between the two are being moved centrally in the later time points as the consequences of polymer degradation and the replacement of lamellar bone by woven bone. For the sake of safety, regulatory agencies are likely to require information regarding the degradation rate of an implanted polymer device in relationship to the original size of the defect that accommodated the device. The blurring effect of bone realignment poses a tall order for a post-hoc selected region on a histological section using the original defect diameter as a guide to the true region of the defect. Although fluorescent bone matrix mineralization markers may assist in identifying the preexisting bones if given prior to and after implantation, they are not specific enough to distinguish newly formed lamellar bone within the defect from those outside the defect.[17] In addition, the original outlines of the defect may not move in tandem when the direction of bone realignment is susceptible to the changes in the local biomechanical milieu. The assessment of the residual amount of implanted materials in a time course experiment can probably be done by histomorphometric measurements of the areas occupied by the implanted material and expressing those areas as a percent of the implant device area obtained immediately after the surgery.

Histomorphometry is a methodology using stereology principles to gauge structural relationships in three dimensions (3D) from two dimensional (2D) histological sections.[18] It translates the qualitative histopathological observations to quantitative manifestations. The most commonly applied parameters from the 2D measurements are area or region of interest, perimeter and interface, distance and width, and number of specific cells.[19] The inherent variations among levels of section planes on measured absolute values of any parameters may reflect the true 3D anisotropy of the anatomy. Therefore, it is a common practice to express the data in a relative manner, particularly for area and perimeter. The derived data facilitates the comparisons between samples. For example, a tangential histological section plane may make one specimen appear to have larger absolute values for the region of interest and for the bone ingrowths, but the percentage bone ingrown area within the region of interest may be comparable with another specimen from a horizontal section plane. It is crucial to include the absolute values of the common denominators in data presentation, e.g., total area (mm^2), total length of perimeter (mm), etc., in addition to the derived values, i.e., percent of the total. This provides reference to and allows unbiased comparisons on the derived values among treatment groups.

11.4 RECENT ADVANCES IN EVALUATING HARD TISSUES

The histopathological evaluations and histomorphometric assessments of hard tissue repair are 2D views of the dynamic healing processes, which relies on the unbiased section plane and the representation of the whole in this plane. In addition, histopathological evaluation requires long sample preparation, which makes it difficult to quickly reveal treatment effects and to refine subsequent treatment regimens. It is desirable to have tools that can display efficacy when the adverse effects manifested in general pathology are minimized by reduced antigenicity following favorable developments in polymer synthesis and fabrication. Although radiogrammetry, magnetic resonance imaging (MRI), computer-assisted tomography, and ultrasound imaging are useful tools in clinical settings to detect progression of healing and early signs of prosthesis loosening, their resolution is too coarse and time of exposure too long to allow similar assessments in animal species that are smaller than humans. The following sections describe current advances in methodologies to evaluate hard tissues repairs beyond histopathological assessments.

11.4.1 Cartilage Repair

The structural elements of the articular cartilage are not readily viewable by noninvasive imaging systems without histological preparation because their thickness is typically less than 2 to 3 mm and the homogeneity of the matrix shows little contrast. Several new methodologies are being developed along the lines of refinement of radiography, MRI, and ultrasound. Commercialization of these methodologies is imminent.

11.4.1.1 Diffraction Enhanced Imaging (DEI)

Instead of radioabsorption of X-rays, DEI collects refracted monochromatic light that differentiates structures in soft and hard tissues such as articular cartilage and subchondral bone.[20] Because the X-ray detector receives diffracted beams, articular cartilage can be visualized. The images can distinguish the articular region from its superficial zone, tidemark, subchondral bone, and structural defect within cartilage at a resolution of 0.5 mm and an exposure time of approximately 30 sec.

11.4.1.2 Quantitative Magnetic Resonance Imaging (qMRI)

The qMRI is a noninvasive means of revealing the structure, composition, and pathology of articular cartilage.[21] Delayed gadolinium-enhanced MRI of cartilage (dGEMRIC) can quantitatively detect the macromolecular structure and mechanical properties of articular cartilage topographically. The methodology uses the contrast agent gadolinium diethylenetriamine pentaacetic acid (Gd-DTPA). The enhanced T1 imaging is sensitive to cartilage proteoglycan content, while T2 relaxation time mapping is indicative of the integrity and arrangement of the collagen network. The higher the proteoglycan content in the cartilage, the longer the wave of T1, approximately 500 msec, as opposed to 240 msec in the depleted one.[22] As cartilage degeneration progressed, T2 increases in the superficial zone.

11.4.1.3 Optical Coherence Tomographic Imaging (OCT)

Microstructure of tissue viewed in cross-sectional images can be achieved with OCT at a high resolution of approximately 4 to 15 μm.[23] The methodology is based on fiber optic systems. The diameter of imaging catheters is constructed to have less than 150 μm, and OCT can identify articular cartilage surface fibrillation, cartilage thinning, and new bone growth. Coupled with the polarization state of the incident light, the OCT can define the collagen organization. Normal cartilage shown by the polarization sensitive OCT is uniform in intensity and has a banding pattern of collagen organization. An altered collagen organization in hypocellular cartilage loses the banding pattern on the OCT images.

11.4.2 Bone Void Repair

This section provides brief descriptions of noninvasive methods suitable for evaluating the effectiveness of the repair of bone voids or defects.

11.4.2.1 Peripheral Quantitative Computed Tomography (pQCT)

Peripheral quantitative computed tomography offers a noninvasive procedure for assessment of bone material quality and architectural indicators by means of 3D projections of X-ray images of both cortical and cancellous bone.[24] This technology compiles slices of bone images at 165 μm to 1.04 mm in thickness to form a 3D composite of the scanned tissue volume.[25,26] The calibrated pQCT to a known weight and volume density of calcium-phosphate phantom can automatically detect and evaluate bone mineral density and segregate bone tissues from nonbone tissues, provide an architectural pattern of bone distribution, and estimate biomechanical strength.[24]

11.4.2.2 Microcomputed Tomography (micro-CT)

Refinement of the X-ray emission and detection systems from pQCT allows the development of micro-CT that has a resolution of 2 to 56 μm.[26,27] Micro-CT images of the bone-implant specimen can reveal a clear distinction between the implant and the bone. The implant surface in direct contact with the implant can be clearly seen. The accuracy of the micro-CT on bone structural indices, i.e., bone volume fraction, bone surface density, trabecular thickness, trabecular separation, and trabecular number, is high ($r^2 > 0.90$) in relationship to 2D histomorphometry.[28] This is particularly useful for assessing the amount of bone ingrowth to the entire implanted device because the progression of ingrowth starts from the periphery toward the center of the device. Furthermore, because of the availability of complete digital data on the bone structure around the implant, it is possible to produce 2D slices in any chosen angle or plane for viewing the bone–implant interfaces.[29] The digitized data may be used to create finite-element models of the bone-implant system so that mechanical stress transfer at the interface can be realized and modeled to refine future implant devices for better bone–implant integration and stability.

11.5 CONCLUSION AND PERSPECTIVE ON THE FUTURE

Nanotechnology advances the fabrication of biomaterials, e.g., polymers, to a new era. Biomimetic devices being made for bone and cartilage commonly are composed of a core mass that is supposed to provide initial biomechanical support and a surface coating that provides a favorable ground for cell attachment and extracellular matrix adhesion, and consequently increases the rate of integration. A more sophisticated design may have multiple layers of various biomaterials to mimic the material property and structural characteristics of the natural tissue. Combination devices are engineered by incorporating biological factors and/or mesenchymal stem cells to further the rapid integration with the surrounding host tissues. The concerted gene expressions and cytokine secretions may shorten the repair period and quicken the normalization of tissue and organ functions.

The challenges for evaluation of enhanced repair rely on advances in the ability to detect in a timely way the healing progression, perhaps, down to the cellular and even molecular levels. Molecular imaging of musculoskeletal repair can be the next generation of noninvasive *in vivo* monitoring system.[30] Osteocalcin (OC) is expressed conspicuously in odontoblasts, hypertrophic chondrocytes, mature osteoblasts, and osteocytes. It is associated with matrix mineralization and accumulates in extracellular matrix. The luciferase gene from the firefly and green fluorescent protein are commonly used for monitoring gene expression because of their ability to generate light that can be captured by a cooled charged coupled device camera. Using a combination of these known techniques, hard tissue repair can be quantitatively evaluated and revealed with the spatial, temporal, and intensity of OC expression patterns.

Advancements in imaging soft tissues by MRI using a short tau inversion recovery (STIR) sequence that allows the differentiation of joint capsule, subchondral bone, bone marrow, ligament entheses, and ligaments.[31] It also can detect inflammation, including edema and foreign body reaction associated with intervertebral disc herniation.[32] It is conceivable that the methodology can be useful for monitoring the progression of tissue reactions to implant devices in a noninvasive manner.

When molecular imaging of the skeleton and STIR of soft tissue reaction is coupled, it is possible to realize the integration of the implant device with the host tissues in a timely fashion, particularly since the evaluations are noninvasive. Consequentially, improvements through biomimetic nanotechnology will quicken the development of host tissue friendly implant devices.

REFERENCES

1. *Medical Devices: Emergency Medical Services*, Annual Book of American Society for Testing and Material Standards, Standards, Philadelphia, Vol. 13, No.1, 1997.
2. Morrey, B.F., Ed., *Biological, Material, and Mechanical Considerations of Joint Replacement*, Bristol-Myers Squibb/Zimmer Orthopaedic Symposium Series, Raven, New York, 1993.
3. Pedersen, D.R., Brown, T.D., Hillis, S.L., and Callaghan, J.J., Prediction of long-term polyethylene wear in total hip arthroplasty, based on early wear measurements made using digital image analysis, *J. Orthop Res.*, 16(5), 557, 1988.
4. Vaccaro, A.R. and Madigan, L., Spinal application of bioabsorbable implants, *Neurosurg. Spine*, 97(4), 407, 2002.
5. Chacon, G.E., Ellis, J.P., Kalmar J.R., and McGlumphy E.A., Using restorable screws for fixation of cortical onlay grafts: an in vivo study in rabbits, *J. Oral Maxillofac. Surg.*, 62(11), 1396, 2004.
6. Slauson, D.O. and Cooper, B.J., Eds., Mechanisms of disease, in *A Textbook of Comparative General Pathology*, Williams & Wilkins, Baltimore, 1982.

7. Standard Practice for Assessment of Compatibility of Biomaterials for Surgical Implants with Respect to Effect of Materials on Muscle and Bone, ASTM, F-981-04, 2006.
8. Baron, R., Vignery, A., Neff, L., Silverglate A., and Santa Maria, A., Processing of undecalcified bone specimens for bone histomorphometry, in *Bone Histomorphometry: Techniques and Interpretation*, Recker, R., Ed., CRC Press, Boca Raton, FL, 1983, pp. 13–36.
9. Mankin, H.J., Dorfman, H., Lippiello, L., and Zarins, A., Biochemical and metabolic abnormalities in articular cartilage from osteo-arthritic human hips, *J. Bone Joint Surg.*, 53A(3), 523, 1971.
10. Kim, H.K.W., Moran, M.E., and Salter, R.B., The potential for regeneration of articular cartilage in defects created by chondral shaving and subchondral abrasion, *J. Bone Joint Surg.*, 73A(9), 1301, 1991.
11. Pineda, S., Pollack, A., Stevenson, S., Goldberg, V., and Caplan, A., A semiquantitative scale for histologic grading of articular cartilage repair, *Acta Anat.*, 143, 335, 1992.
12. Frenkel, S., Saadeh, P.B., Mehrara, B.J., Chin, G.S., Steinbrech, D.S., Brent, B., Gittes, G.K., and Longaker, M.T., Transforming growth factor beta superfamily members: Role in cartilage modeling, *Plast. Reconstr. Surg.*, 105, 980, 2000.
13. Solchaga, L.A., Yoo, J.U., Lundberg, M., Dennis, J.E., Huibregtse, B.A., Goldberg, V.M., and Caplan, A.I., Hyaluronan-based polymers in the treatment of osteochondral defects, *J. Orthop. Res.*, 18(5), 773, 2000.
14. Im, G-I., Kim, D-Y., Shin, J-H., Hyun, C-W., and Cho, W-H., Repair of cartilage defect in the rabbit with cultured mesenchymal stem cells from bone marrow, *J. Bone Joint. Surg.*, 83B(2), 289, 2001.
15. O'Driscoll, S.W., Marx, R.G., Beaton, D.E., Miura, Y., Gallay, S.H., and Fitzsimmons, J.S., Validation of a simple histological-histochemical cartilage scoring system, *Tissue Eng.*, 7(3), 313, 2001.
16. Solchaga, L.A., Gao, J-Z., Dennis, J.E., Awadallah, A., Lundberg, M., Caplan, A.I., and Goldberg, V.M., Treatment of osteochondral defects with autologous bone marrow in a hyaluronan-based delivery vehicle, *Tissue Eng.*, 8(2), 333, 2002.
17. Frost, H.M., Bone histomorphometry: choice of marking agent and labeling schedule, in *Bone Histomorphometry: Techniques and Interpretation*, Recker, R., Ed., CRC Press, Boca Raton, FL, 1983, pp. 37–52.
18. Parfitt, A.M., Stereolgic basis of bone histomorphometry: theory of quantitative microscopy and reconstruction of the third dimension, in *Bone Histomorphometry: Techniques and Interpretation*, Recker, R., Ed., CRC Press, Boca Raton, FL, 1983, pp. 53–88.
19. Kimmel, D.B. and Jee, W.S.S., Measurements of area, perimeter, and distance: details of data collection in bone histomorphometry, in *Bone Histomorphometry: Techniques and Interpretation*, Recker, R., Ed., CRC Press, Boca Raton, FL, 1983, pp. 89–108.
20. Mollenhauer. J., Aurich, M.E., Zhong, Z., Muehleman, C., Cole, A.A., Hasnah, M., Oltulu, O., Kuettner, K.E., Margulis, A., and Chapman, L.D., Diffraction-enhanced X-ray imaging of articular cartilage, *Osteoarthritis Cartilage*, 10(3), 163, 2002.
21. Nieminen, M.T., Toyras, J., Laasanen, M.S., Silvennoinen, J., Helminen, H.J., and Jurvelin, J.S., Prediction of biomechanical properties of articular cartilage with quantitative magnetic resonance imaging, *J. Biomech.*, 37(3), 321, 2004.
22. Williams, A., Gillis, A., McKenzie, C., Po, B., Sharma, L., Micheli, L., McKeon, B., and Burstein, D., Glycosaminoglycan distribution in cartilage as determined by delayed gadolinium-enhanced MRI of cartilage (dGEMRIC): potential clinical applications, *Am. J. Roentgen.*, 182(1), 167, 2004.

23. Li, X., Martin, S., Pitris, C., Ghanta, R., Stamper, D.L., Harman, M., Fujimoto, J.G., and Brezinski, M.E., High-resolution optical coherence tomographic imaging of osteoarthritic cartilage during opening knee surgery, *Arthritis Res. Therap.*, 7(2), R318, 2003.
24. Ferretti, J.L., Perspectives of pQCT technology associated to biomechanical studies in skeletal research employing rat models, *Bone*, 17(4 Suppl), 353S, 1995.
25. Braun, M.J., Meta, M.D., Schneider, P., and Reiners, Chr., Clinical evaluation of a high-resolution new peripheral quantitative computerized tomography (pQCT) scanner for the bone densitometry at the lower limbs, *Phys. Med. Biol.*, 43, 2279, 1998.
26. Pistoia, W., van Rietbergen, B., Laib, A., and Rüegsegger, P., High-resolution three-dimensional-pQCT images can be an adequate basis for in-vivo microFE analysis of bone, *J. Biomech. Eng.*, 123, 176, 2001.
27. Jones, A.C., Sakellariou, A., Limaye, A., Arns, C.H., Senden, T.J., Sawkins, T., Knachstedt, M.A., Rohner, D., Hutmacher, D.W., Brandwood, A., and Milthorpe, B.K., Investigation of microstructural features in regenerating bone using micro computed tomography, *J. Mater. Sci. Mater. Med.*, 15(4), 529, 2004.
28. Naitoh, M., Katsumata, A., Mitsuya, S., Kamemoto, H., and Ariji, E., Measurement of mandible with microfocus x-ray computerized tomography and compact computerized tomography for dental use, *Int. J. Oral Maxillofac. Implants*, 19(2), 239, 2004.
29. van Oossterwyck, H., Duyck, J., van der Sloten, J., van der Perre, G., Jansen, J., Wevers, M., and Naert, I., Use of microfocus computerized tomography as a new technique for characterizing bone tissue around oral implants, *J. Oral Implantol* 26(1), 5, 2000.
30. Bar, I., Xilberman, Y., Zeira, E., Galun, E., Honigman, A., Turgeman, G., Clemens, T., Gazit, Z., and Gazit, D., Molecular imaging of the skeleton: quantitative real-time bioluminescence monitoring gene expression in bone repair and development, *J. Bone Mineral Res*,, 18(3), 570, 2003.
31. Muche, B., Bollow, M., Francois, R.J., Sieper, J., Hamm, B., and Braun, J., Anatomic structures involved in early- and late-stage sacroiliitis in spondylarthritis: a detailed analysis by contrast-enhanced magnetic resonance imaging, *Arthritis Rheum* 48(5),1374, 2003.
32. Cayi, S.R., Kocak, A., Alkan, A., and Kirimliogclu, H., Is there a clinical correlate to the histological and radiological evidence of inflammation in trans-ligamentous extruded and sequestered lumbar disc herniation? *Br. J. Neurosurg.*, 18(6), 576, 2004.

Section D

Advanced Biomaterials, Technologies, and Sought Applications

12 Mechanical Adaptation of Bone: Bioreactors for Orthopedic Tissue Engineering Applications

Jiro Nagatomi

CONTENTS

12.1 INTRODUCTION

Human bone exists in a very dynamic environment and is constantly exposed to various forms of mechanical force stimuli through weight-bearing, daily activities, and exercise. It has been well documented in the literature that the mechanical force stimuli generated by loading the skeleton are important regulators of bone development and homeostasis. For example, individuals who perform high-impact exercises (e.g., gymnastics) have been shown to exhibit higher bone mineral densities compared with the ones that perform low-impact exercises (e.g. swimming).[1] In contrast, when loading is removed from bones and joints because of immobilization, bone mineral densities decrease.[2] These and other examples strongly suggest that the cells within bone tissue are sensitive to mechanical force stimuli and are capable of adjusting the bone structure to the mechanical demands either by adding or removing tissue. During the last few decades, advancement of tissue and cell culture models has allowed investigators to examine the direct effects of various forms of mechanical force stimuli on bone cell functions. Although the exact mechanism by which the bone cells respond to mechanical loading are yet to be fully understood, a number of *in vitro* studies have demonstrated that osteoblasts (the bone-forming cells), osteocytes (mature osteoblasts), and osteoclasts (bone-resorbing cells) in cultures do respond to applied hydrostatic pressure, stretch, and fluid shear stress in ways that are consistent with *in vivo* observations (i.e., application of mechanical forces lead to enhancement of bone formation and inhibition of bone resorption).[3–13]

The field of bone tissue engineering has met with some success in addressing issues associated with three-dimensional scaffold materials and architecture.[14–18] date, however, very limited *in vitro* bone tissue growth on these polymers has been achieved, even in the presence of osteoinductive molecules such as bone morphogenetic proteins.[14,15,19,20] It has been suggested that the poor growth of new bone tissue observed in static cultures is partially due to inadequate nutrient transport to the cells. At the same time, it is speculated that the limited bone tissue growth *in vitro* results from lack of mechanical stimuli that the bone cells would be routinely subjected to *in vivo*. For these reasons, considerable interest has been generated in the field of bone tissue engineering in developing dynamic tissue culture techniques that can provide convection of nutrient media and mechanical stimuli to the cells on polymer scaffolds.[21–24] These studies using bioreactors in conjunction with three-dimensional cultures of bone (and progenitor) cells are of extreme interest to the scientific community because they meet two purposes; they not only provides various means to facilitate formation of new tissue *in vitro* for bone grafting, but may also offer some insights into the potential cellular and molecular mechanisms involved in the mechanical adaptation of bone.[25]

This chapter briefly discusses the basic science of bone biology, reviews the current literature reports on mechanobiology of bone from the past two decades, and describes the most recent development of bone tissue engineering bioreactors. The final section summarizes and discusses the considerations for future design of bioreactors for orthopedic tissue engineering applications.

12.2 BONE TISSUE DEVELOPMENT, HOMEOSTASIS, AND REPAIR

12.2.1 Skeletal Tissue Development and Maintenance

In humans and animals, the skeleton is formed during the fetal period and maintained throughout the life of the organism. Following the initial formation, the newly synthesized bone tissues constantly change their shapes and sizes to make more mechanically sound structures by processes called growth and modeling. In mature skeletons, a different process called bone remodeling takes place to maintain the systemic calcium homeostasis as well as to remove microdamage that accumulates within bone tissues. In addition to modeling and remodeling, bone is capable of repairing fractures through direct (intramembranous) bone formation at the fracture ends and/or indirect (endochondral) bone formation, which is achieved by formation of callus and replacement with bone.

During growth, modeling, and repair, the amount of bone formation must exceed bone resorption to add new tissue to the ends of the existing bone. In contrast, during bone remodeling, to achieve constant bone mass, a balance must be maintained between bone resorption (to remove the old tissues) and bone formation (to fill the voids with newly synthesized tissues). When these delicately balanced activities of osteoblasts and osteoclasts are shifted in one direction or another, pathological conditions such as osteoporosis (porous, fragile bones) and osteopetrosis (dense, brittle bones) are experienced. The functional and structural integrity of the skeleton is maintained because of the special functions of these cells under many biochemical and mechanical factors.

12.2.2 Skeletal Cells and Their Functions

Osteoblasts are derived from mesenchymal stem cells found in the bone marrow. Once committed, the osteoblast precursor cells proliferate and differentiate into osteoblasts under the control of a transcription factor, core-binding factor–α1 (Cbfa1; also known as Runx2, Osf2).[27] Active osteoblasts synthesize nonmineralized extracellular matrix called osteoid, which is composed of 90% collagenous (mainly type-1 collagen) and 10% noncollagenous proteins. The noncollagenous proteins that are synthesized by osteoblasts include alkaline phosphatase, osteocalcin, osteopontin, osteonectin, bone sialoprotein, and other glycosaminoglycan-containing proteins. Among these proteins, only osteocalcin is bone specific and is often used as a marker of osteoblast maturation. In addition, because of the high abundance within the cells during the early phase of differentiation, alkaline phosphatase is also used as a marker of osteoblast differentiation. Although the exact function of each of these proteins is yet to be fully elucidated, many of them are considered to play roles in binding and carrying of calcium to be incorporated into the osteoid to form mineralized bone tissues. Following the completion of bone formation, osteoblasts that are encased in the newly mineralized tissue cease their synthetic activities and differentiate into osteocytes within the space called lacunae. Osteocytes, the most abundant cells in bone, extend numerous, thin processes that run through canaliculi to form a lacuno-canaliculi network, connected via gap junctions, with the neighboring osteocytes and with the bone-lining cells on the bone surface.

Osteoblast differentiation from their progenitor cells, bone formation (and repair), and subsequent differentiation into osteocytes are influenced by several major growth factors including bone morphogenetic proteins (BMP-2, -3, -4, and -7), fibroblast growth factor (FGF-1, and -2), insulinlike growth factor (IGF-1, and -2), platelet-derived growth factor (PDGF-AA, -AB, and -BB), and transforming growth factor –β (TGF-β-1 and -2) via the serine–threonine receptor kinase and receptor tyrosine kinase pathways.[29] Thus, use of recombinant growth factors such as BMPs and FGFs for induction of osteoblast differentiation from stem cells and for stimulation of bone tissue growth *in vitro* has become a common practice in the field of cell biology and bone tissue engineering.[24,30,31]

Osteoclasts are derived from hematopoietic precursors found in the bone marrow. The multinucleated, bone-resorbing cells are formed by fusion of committed precursors (monocytes) under the control by two main regulatory factors that are secreted by osteoblastic or stromal cells, namely, osteoclast differentiation factor [ODF, also known as receptor mediator of NF-kB ligand (RANKL) or osteoprotegerin ligand, (OPGL)] and osteoclastogenesis inhibitory factor (OCIF, also known as osteoprotegerin, OPG).[33] Besides the main function, that is, the bone resorption capability, osteoclasts differ from macrophages by expression of calcitonin receptors and tartrate-resistant acid phosphatase, both of which are often used as the phenotypic markers of osteoclasts.[32] The bone resorption process begins with osteoclast adhesion and formation of a sealed zone on the bone surface. The tightly adhered osteoclasts then secrete H^+ ions and proteolytic enzymes to demineralize and digest the bone matrix in the sealed zones underneath. Following the cessation of bone resorption, osteoclasts migrate from the bone surface into adjacent marrow space and undergo apoptosis. Activation, bone resorption, and apoptosis of osteoclasts are also regulated by the action of OPG and RANKL along with other cytokines and growth factors such as interleukins (IL-1, IL-6), tumor necrosis factor (TNF- transforming growth factor (TGF-β), and macrophage colony stimulating factor (MCSF).[32,33]

12.2.3 Relationship between Physiological Loading and Skeletal Tissue

The growth, maintenance, and repair of the skeletal tissues that are governed by the functions of osteoblasts and osteoclasts are influenced not only by biochemical growth factors but also by biophysical factors that result from mechanical loading on the skeleton. The initial observations and reports that mechanical loading affects bone structure were made as early as the 1890s.[34] The advent of the space era in the 1960s, however, brought significant attention to the disuse bone loss in microgravity conditions experienced by the astronauts.[35] In long-term space flights, as much as 7% of bone mass is lost, especially in the lower limbs of the astronauts despite the countermeasures such as performing resistance exercises.[36] These observations were dissected further and raised numerous research questions about the effects of different aspects of functional loading on the bone such as the dependence on location in the body (foot, legs, skull, etc.) and types of exercise (jumping, running, playing racquetball, swimming, etc.). However, these physical activities (or lack thereof) are only qualitative, and it is difficult to make one-to-one correlations with measurable physical quantities such as magnitudes of force and deformation with biological events, bone formation, and/or resorption. Moreover, the mechanical stimuli can be defined even more specifically (e.g., hydrostatic pressure, shear stress, tensile stress, etc.) and the cellular and/or molecular events can be deduced to many facets of bone formation and resorption (osteoblast proliferation, bone-related protein synthesis, mineralization, osteoclast formation, etc.). Because of the complexity of the phenomenon, the number of questions has kept on growing. As a result, mechanical adaptation of the skeletal tissues, often referred to as mechanobiology of bone, has become a large field of study and produced a vast literature during the past few decades.

12.3 MECHANOBIOLOGY OF BONE

12.2.1 *In Vivo* Studies of Mechanobiology

To systematically study the effects of mechanical loading on the skeletal tissue, the researchers have used various *in vivo* animal models. The majority of these studies was performed with mammals (mice, rats, rabbits, dogs, sheep), while a few used avian models as well.[37–41] These models were designed to study the effects of either unloading (disuse) or excessive loading on bone remodeling.

In disuse models, unloading of limbs is achieved by various techniques that include resections of local nerves to paralyze the lower limbs, casting of one limb, or suspension by the tail to remove loading on one or both limbs.[40,42] In general, all of these unloading models induce localized bone losses that are site specific, but the rate of bone loss and the time to reach the steady state bone mass varies depending on the species and methods of immobilization. More specifically, it has been reported that disuse (immobilization) leads to more bone loss in the weight-bearing extremities, especially in the distal portions of the limbs compared with the non–weight-bearing extremities; over the 60-week period of immobilization by forelimb casting in adult beagles; the third metacarpal lost up to 50% while the humerus loss was less than 20%.[38] Moreover, the rate of bone loss is higher in the trabecular bone than in the cortical bone, partly as a result of the difference in surface-to-volume ratio of bone tissue adjacent to bone marrow; the loss of trabecular bone occurred mostly in the first 4 weeks following sciatic nerve resection in rats while the cortical bone loss continued to occur in the 8- and 12-week periods.[42] These immobilization-induced bone loss responses are characterized mainly by shifted bone remodeling (acute increase in bone resorption and decrease in new bone formation), which reduces bone mass adjacent to marrow.

Animal models of skeletal loading include both whole-body exercise models (e.g., treadmill running) and isolated limb loading models (e.g., four-point bending of tibia, compression of tail vertebrae), which have advantages and disadvantages.[39,43,44] While the whole-body exercise models are noninvasive, it is almost impossible to relate the local strain level or strain rates with the outcome of increased bone formation and/or decreased bone resorption. In contrast, the isolated limb models allow application of controlled loading to the skeleton, but most of them are either invasive or have results that are difficult to interpret. One of the examples of difficulty in interpretation occurs when the loads are applied through other tissue structures, such as the periosteum, that are highly sensitive to the contact pressure and could trigger responses indirectly related to bone. Despite several disadvantages, these skeletal loading models provided significant amounts of information with regard to mechanical adaptation of the skeleton. These studies demonstrated that bone formation was influenced by various experimental parameters such as the duration of each loading episode, intervals between loading, maximum strain rate, peak strain amplitude, and frequency of cyclic loading. For example, daily loading (36 cycles) of cyclic compression to the rat tail vertebra induced a 30-fold increase in bone formation while a single loading (360 cycles) induced a 4-fold increase. Moreover, when the daily loading episodes were separated by short intervals of rest, the effects on increase in bone formation were enhanced compared with continuous loading episodes.[46]

In addition to identifying the loading parameters that are important for mechanical adaptation of bone, the results obtained from *in vivo* studies have suggested several mechanistic pathways. For example, a single period of loading on the skeleton could induce the periosteal cells and osteocytes to increase enzyme activity of glucose-6-phosphate dehydrogenase within 6 min or osteocytes to increase c-fos and IGF-1 mRNA expression within 6 h, suggesting that these molecules may be mediating the initial osteogenic responses to mechanical loading.[47–49] Furthermore, the results of other *in vivo* studies of mechanobiology have provided evidence that prostaglandins (PGs), cyclooxygenase (COX-2), and nitric oxide (NO) may be mediators of mechanically induced bone formation. Single-dose application of inhibitors to these compounds given to the animals immediately before the exposure to mechanical loading episodes abolished the osteogenic responses that were observed otherwise.[49]

Based on these *in vivo* findings, and because of their locations and abundance within the bone matrix, osteocytes are considered to be the candidate cells that sense and respond to the mechanical loading on the skeleton. The important research questions now are what are the forms of mechanical stimuli osteocytes that are sensitive to and how do osteocytes communicate with osteoblasts and osteoclasts to cause the observed changes in bone remodeling. It is also possible that mechanical force can directly stimulate osteoclasts, osteoblasts, and/or their precursors without the mediation by osteocytes. To date, the exact mechanisms by which these bone cells convert the mechanical signals into biochemical signals are still a topic of debate. In the meantime, the results of *in vivo* studies of mechanobiology and advancement of the cell culture techniques have inspired numerous *in vitro* studies in attempts to elucidate the underlying mechanisms by which the bone cells respond to mechanical force stimuli.

12.3.2 *In Vitro* Studies of Mechanobiology

To simplify the *in vivo* complexity and to investigate the potential mechanisms of mechanical adaptation of bone, researchers have developed various *in vitro* experimental devices to expose cultured bone tissues and cells to different forms of mechanical stimuli. The types of stimuli used in these studies include hydrostatic compression, uniaxial or biaxial stretch of deformable cell culture substrates, and fluid flow.[3–5,7,9,13,50–56] The majority of these studies took advantage of established, osteoblastlike (MC3T3-E1 and osteosarcoma cells) and osteocytelike (MLO-Y4) cell lines while others used primary and low-passaged cultures of rat calvaria osteoblasts and bone marrow cells.[3,4,7,9,50,53,54,56–59]

Hydrostatic compression is one of the mechanical stimuli often studied in mechanobiology of bone. Pressure (both static and dynamic) is usually applied to cultured bone cells using compressed gasses above the supernatant media, and various changes in cellular responses have been observed. For example, exposure of MC3T3-E1 cells to sustained pressure of 2 atm above ambient for 2 days led to increased release of prostaglandins E2 and decreased alkaline phosphatase activity.[58] In a different study, a similar level of sustained hydrostatic pressure (2 atm) inhibited formation of osteoclasts from their precursors and expression of MCSF mRNA, one of the regulators of osteoclast formation and differentiation.[60] In addition, cyclic (dynamic) pressure has been reported to exhibit significant effects on bone cell function. When MC3T3-E1 and ROS 17/2.8 osteoblastlike cells were exposed to dynamic pressure (13 kPa at 0.3 Hz), cell proliferation decreased, but alkaline phosphatase activity increased.[53,61] A more recent study revealed that the effects of dynamic pressure on osteoblasts were dependent on the frequency and duration of the applied stimuli; osteoblasts responded to 1.0 Hz frequency 1-h exposure, but not to either 0.25 Hz frequency or 20-min exposure to similar pressure.[3]

Application of mechanical strain to bone cells *in vivo* is achieved by stretching flexible substrates on which these cells were cultured. Because of the commercial availability of the cell culture stretch devices, the number of studies to examine the effects of strain on bone cell function is continuing to grow. It has been reported that osteoblasts responded to strains of magnitudes ranging from 0.1 to 5%, either applied continuously or cyclically, by increasing cell proliferation but decreasing expression of phenotypic markers such as osteocalcin and alkaline phosphatase.[7,50,54,62,63] Furthermore, it has been shown that exposure to cyclic strain (5% at 0.167 Hz) significantly inhibited osteoclast differentiation from their precursors.[64]

In addition to hydrostatic pressure and mechanical strains, fluid flow–induced shear stress has been shown to elicit cellular responses by osteoblasts, osteoclasts, and osteocytes. *In vitro*, well defined fluid flow–induced shear stress is applied to a monolayer of bone cells using parallel-plate flow chambers.[9,56,65,66,69] It has been reported in the literature that exposure of osteoblasts and/or osteocytes to flow-induced shear stress (up to 24 dyn/cm^2) resulted in increased production of PGE2, COX-2, and NO, all of which are implicated as necessary components for mechanical adaptation of bone.[49,55,56,67]

In some studies, comparisons were made between the types of mechanical stimuli or the types of bone cells. Osteocytes, but not osteoblasts or periosteal fibroblasts, reacted most to application of pulsatile fluid flow with a sustained release of prostaglandin E2.[65] Furthermore, both intermittent hydrostatic compression and substrate deformation are less stimulatory to osteocytes compared with fluid flow as evidenced by lower synthesis of PGE2 and lower expression of osteopontin mRNA by these cells.[65,66] The authors of these studies concluded that osteocytes are the most mechanosensitive cells in bone and that fluid flow is the stimulus involved in the transduction of mechanical loading on the bone into a biological response. To date, however, the definitive conclusions regarding the exact mechanism of bone mechanotransduction are yet to be drawn because the experimental conditions are still far from the *in vivo* environment in which bone cells reside. Nevertheless, many of the mechanical stimuli tested, to different degrees, elicited the bone cell responses pertinent to bone homeostasis and similar to mechanically induced changes observed in *in vivo* studies of mechanobiology. Regardless of the level of current understanding of bone mechanobiology, it is important to note that these studies did inspire the recent technology of bioreactor-based bone tissue engineering.

12.3.3 Traditional and Current Theories of Mechanobiology of Bone

Because there is a great deal of experimental data on mechanobiology of bone, there are theories that arise from previous results and drive further experimental work. It is interesting to note that the paradigms and beliefs of the scientific community concerning the mechanobiology of bone have shifted over time. Since the time of Wolff in the 1890s, the phrase "Wolff's Law" has been used interchangeably with the concept that bone responds to its mechanical environment. While the theoretical details of the initial claim made by Wolff have been criticized and disputed by many researchers in the past century, a number of new hypotheses have arisen. For example, the mechanostat hypothesis proposed by Frost states that there exists a range of effective strains that defines the set point to determine the overload and underload. This and other similar strain-based theories derived from clinical observations or computational studies motivated the experimental work that examined the effects of strains on bone cell function. One fundamental paradox, however, was that tissue-level strains are typically less than 0.2% while the vast range of experimental work demonstrated that the strains must be an order of magnitude higher for cells to respond.[69] For this reason, a new theoretical model was proposed by Weinbaum et al., who hypothesized that osteocytes are excited by interstitial fluid flow through canaliculi and send biochemical signals to osteoblasts to initiate the cascade of events leading to bone remodeling.[70] This popular theory motivated a new set of studies that examined the effects of fluid flow over cultured osteoblasts and osteocytes.[13,55,66,71,72] Based on these *in vitro* results, many investigators believe that the fluid shear stress is the mechanical signal that drives adaptation of bone. At the same time, there is a hypothesis that it is the convection of nutrients to osteocytes due to interstitial flow, and not the mechanical stimulus itself, that mediates the mechanical loading on the skeleton and biological responses.[73] Others hypothesize that loading-induced increase in the bone (intramedullary) pressure or the resulting pressure gradient and interstitial fluid flow through the micropores of the cortical bone are the mechanical stimuli important for mechanical adaptation of bone.[5,74–76] Interestingly, the group that initially proposed the fluid flow–induced shear stress theory has now proposed a new theory stating that the strains amplified in osteocyte processes because of their structure, but not fluid shear stress, are the mechanical signal that stimulates osteocytes to initiate the cascade of events leading to mechanical adaptation.[70,77] These new theories can perhaps motivate a new line of experimental work to generate more data. Thus, careful review and comparison with previous findings are absolutely necessary to fully understand mechanobiology of bone.

12.4 ADVANCES IN BIOREACTORS FOR BONE TISSUE ENGINEERING APPLICATIONS

12.4.1 Motivations and Functional Requirements

Bone tissue engineering approaches that are currently employed typically combine the pertinent type of isolated cells, osteoblasts or mesenchymal stem cells, with resorbable, porous, three-dimensional polymer scaffolds. The central issues with regards to the current techniques are that seeded cells grow only on the peripheral surfaces of the scaffolds, and as a result, there is nonuniform formation of the mineralized extracellular matrix.[14] One of the reasons for this inhomogeneous cell distribution is the lack of nutrient delivery to the interior of tissue engineering constructs. In addition, it is possible that the lack of appropriate mechanical stimuli for osteoblasts and their precursors in the culture impedes adequate bone formation *in vitro*. Currently several bioreactor technologies have been proposed and are under investigation to overcome the nutrient convection problem and to achieve uniform distribution of mineralized tissues on three-dimensional scaffolds for bone tissue engineering applications.

12.4.2 Current Designs of Bioreactors

The current designs of bioreactors for bone tissue engineering include spinner flasks, rotating-wall vessels, and perfusion chambers of various designs. The main goal of all these bioreactors is to provide the nutrients necessary for survival of cells, to remove waste products from the cells, and to consequently deliver mechanical force stimuli to trigger osteogenic differentiation by the progenitors and osteoblastic cells. The simplest bioreactor design is the spinner flask. The cell-seeded scaffolds are suspended by needles embedded in the flask stopper and mixing of culture media is maintained by spinning a magnetic stir bar on the bottom of the spinner flask.[24,78] A study using rat bone marrow stromal cells, seeded on three-dimensional porous 75:25 poly(D,L-lactic-co-glycolic acid) (PLAGA) biodegradable scaffolds demonstrated that compared with static controls, the cells cultured in spinner flasks exhibited an increase in cell proliferation, alkaline phosphatase activity, osteocalcin synthesis, and calcium deposition.[78]

Another popular design of bioreactors for bone tissue engineering is a rotating wall vessel (RWV), originally designed for culturing cells and tissue in a simulated microgravity field under very low shear stress.[79] A typical RWV consists of a stationary inner cylinder that allows gas and nutrient exchange through the permeable membrane and a rotating outer cylinder that generates centrifugal force in the culture medium. Cells seeded on polymer scaffolds or microcarriers are suspended by the force balance between the weight of the cell-seeded constructs (gravitational force) and the slowly moving culture media (centrifugal force) due to the constant rotation of the outer wall. When rat calvarial osteoblasts were seeded on a PLAGA (85:15) hollow microsphere-based three-dimensional, lighter-than-water scaffold in a rotating wall bioreactor, the phenotypic markers, alkaline phosphatase activity and osteoclacin expression, were enhanced at 4 and 7 days compared with a static control.[23]

The final category of bioreactor designs is the perfusion chamber. This type of bioreactor directly pumps culture media through the internal pores of the cell-seeded scaffolds and provides enhanced delivery of the nutrients to and removal of wastes from the cells inside the constructs. Typically, cell-seeded constructs are confined within cylindrical chambers with media inlets and outlets on opposite ends to ensure the flow of medium through the interior, but not exterior, of the constructs; peristaltic pumps are used to circulate the culture media through a closed flow circuit.[21,22,24,80] When rat bone marrow stromal cells were seeded on starch-based, porous three-dimensional scaffolds and cultured in a perfusion chamber under 0.3 mL/min flow for up to 15 days, cell proliferation and alkaline phosphatase activity were both similar to those of the static control, but calcium accretion was significantly enhanced compared with the control.[80] In another study, MC3T3-E1 cells were seeded on devitalized trabecular bone scaffolds and cultured under perfusion at various flow rates (0.01, 0.1, 0.2, and 1.0 mL/min) for 1 week.[22] At the highest flow rate

(1.0 mL/min), substantial cell death was observed throughout the constructs.[22] contrast, at the low flow rate, there was significantly higher cell proliferation compared with the static control.[22]

More recently, a comparison was made between two bioreactor designs while keeping all the other conditions constant; human mesenchymal stem cells seeded on collagen scaffolds were cultured in either a spinner flask (mixing with a magnetic stir bar at 50 rpm) or a perfusion cartridge (perfusion at 0.2 mL/min flow rate) for 5 weeks.[24] Microcomputerized tomography (μCT) of the constructs revealed that mineralized bone rods, 0.5–1.0 mm in length, were present on the peripheral regions of the scaffolds cultured in the spinner flask while the constructs cultured in the perfusion chamber contained fewer and smaller mineralized rods distributed throughout the volume.[24] Generally speaking, the perfusion systems seem be the most logical choice of bioreactor for mitigating the nutrient convection problems in the interiors of the bone tissue engineering scaffolds. The results of these studies so far, however, demonstrated that they were less effective in stimulating expression of osteogenic genes and formation of mineralized matrix by the cells. It should be understood that there are still many technical issues to be addressed in the designs of bioreactors for bone tissue engineering. The advantages and disadvantages of these bioreactor designs are summarized in Table 12.1.

TABLE 12.1

Current Designs of Bone Tissue Engineering Bioreactors

Bioreactor Type	Spinner Flask	Rotating Wall Vessel	Perfusion Chamber
	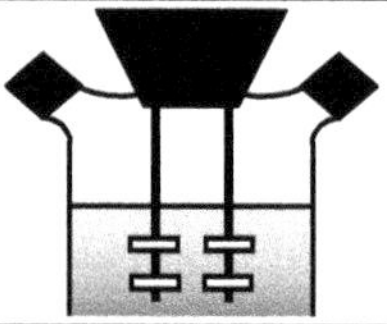	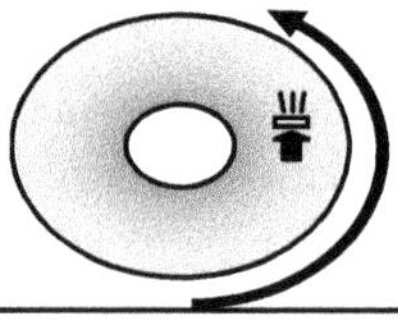	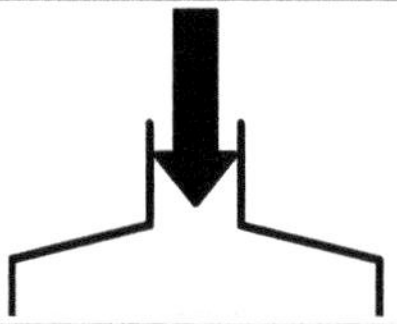
Advantages	• Simple design • Commercially available • Low shear stress on cells	• Commercially available • Low shear stress on cells • Performance well characterized	• Nutrient media delivered to the interior of scaffolds by convection • Mechanical stimuli on cells
Disadvantages	• Media convection only on the peripheral regions of scaffold • Nutrient delivery to the interior by diffusion only	• Media convection only on the peripheral regions of scaffold • Nutrient delivery to the interior by diffusion only • Simulated microgravity may inhibit bone	• Require custom design and fabrication • Potentially high shear on cells

12.4.3 Assessment of Performance of Bioreactors

As routinely performed in most bone tissue engineering studies, the effectiveness of the bioreactors must be assessed on the basis of osteogenic function of the cultured bone cells in comparison with the static control. Cell number and distribution, mRNA and protein expression for osteoblast differentiation markers such as Cbfa-1 (Runx2), alkaline phosphatase, osteocalcin, as well as calcium deposition in the extracellular matrix are commonly quantified using the standard techniques after several days to weeks from the onset of the experiments. Cell proliferation is routinely quantified using various DNA assays and MTT assay, and is also qualitatively determined by fluorescence staining and microscopy.[22–24,80] The markers of osteoblast differentiation are quantified at the message level using real-time PCR with custom primers and probes.[22] Synthesis, release, and activities of proteins are quantified using commercially available enzyme-linked immunosorbent assay and biochemical assays specific for each compound.[22–24,80,81] Mineralization of the extracellular matrix can be examined using microcomputerized tomography[24] as well as quantifying the calcium solubilized in acid using commercially available colorimetric-based calcium assay kits.[22–24,80,81]

In addition to examining the osteogenic markers, the performance of the bioreactors must be routinely assessed for further improvement and development of devices. For example, the culture media within the bioreactors must be periodically monitored for temperature, pH, pO_2, pCO_2 levels as well as for degradation products of polymer scaffolds, glucose levels, and dead cells. Moreover, fluid dynamics and mass transport parameters in each bioreactor system with various scaffold types with different composition, geometry, and pore architecture should be well characterized.[82,83] The delivery of nutrients to and removal of wastes from the cells occur through both convection and diffusion, which are significantly altered by the flow conditions of bioreactors as well as by the scaffold architecture.[83] Furthermore, enhanced degradation of scaffolds and excessive shear stress due to fluid flow can lead to inadvertent and premature removal of the cells from the tissue engineering constructs.[22,24] Both analytical and computational methods are useful in modeling the fluid dynamics and mass transport environments of the interior and exterior of cell-seeded constructs within bone tissue engineering bioreactors.

12.5 CONCLUSION AND PERSPECTIVE ON THE FUTURE

The current advancement of bioreactor technology for bone tissue engineering was motivated by the need to overcome the problems of inadequate nutrient transport to the cells seeded on resorbable polymer scaffolds. Several designs of bioreactors that incorporate dynamic culturing methods have been tested and, with advantages and disadvantages associated with each design, proven to be more effective in induction of osteogenic markers compared with the conventional static culture. From the experimental and theoretical work on mechanobiology of bone, it has become evident that fluid flow over cultured bone cells is one of the mechanical stimuli important for induction of osteogenic function. To date, the exact mechanism by which mechanical loading influences bone homeostasis is still a major topic of debate. While the study of mechanobiology can benefit greatly from the experimental work on bioreactor-based bone tissue engineering, the design of these devices can be advanced and improved by the vast literature reports on the effects of various mechanical force stimuli on bone cell functions. The forms of stimuli and parameters to be controlled in bioreactors are yet to be exhausted; as exemplified by bioreactors for soft tissue engineering applications, other mechanical and/or chemical stimuli in combination with fluid flow may be more beneficial than the fluid flow and mixing alone.[84] creating more realistic, *in vivo*–like three-dimensional culture conditions, the studies of mechanobiology can obtain experimental data that will help us better understand the complex phenomena of mechanical adaptation of bone. The ultimate goals of researchers are to fully understand what combinations of mechanical stimuli regulate bone homeostasis *and* to develop the enabling technology for generating implantable, functional tissues that contain 60% calcium phosphate mineral and 35% organic extracellular matrix (90% of which is type-I collagen) that have highly vascularized structures in the most timely and economical manner.

REFERENCES

1. Courteix, D., Lespessailles, E., Peres, S.L. et al., Effect of physical training on bone mineral density in prepubertal girls: a comparative study between impact-loading and non-impact-loading sports, *Osteoporosis Int.*, 8(2), 152–158, 1998.
2. Leblanc, A.D., Schneider, V.S., Evans, H.J. et al., Bone mineral loss and recovery after 17 weeks of bed rest, *J.Bone Mineral Res.*, 5(8), 843–850, 1990.
3. Nagatomi, J., Arulanandam, B.P., Metzger, D.W. et al., Frequency- and duration-dependent effects of cyclic pressure on select bone cell functions, *Tissue Eng.*, 7, 717–728, 2001.
4. Nagatomi, J., Arulanandam, B.P., Metzger, D.W. et al., Effects of cyclic pressure on bone marrow cell cultures, *J. Biomech. Eng.*, 124(3), 308–314, 2002.
5. Nagatomi, J., Arulanandam, B.P., Metzger, D.W. et al., Cyclic pressure affects osteoblast functions pertinent to osteogenesis, *Ann. Biomed. Eng.*, 31(8), 917–923, 2003.
6. Klein-Nulend, J., Veldhuijzen, J.P., van Strien, M.E. et al., Inhibition of osteoclastic bone resorption by mechanical stimulation *in vitro*, *Arthritis and Rheumatism*, 33(1), 66–72, 1990.
7. Hasegawa, S., Sato, S., Suzuki, Y. et al., Mechanical stretching increases the number of cultured bone cells synthesizing DNA and alters their pattern of protein synthesis, *Calcified Tissue Int.*, 37, 431–436, 1985.
8. Duncan, R.L. and Turner, C.H., Mechanotransduction and the functional response of bone to mechanical strain, *Calcified Tissue Int.*, 57, 344–358, 1995.
9. McAllister, T.N., Du, T., and Frangos, J.A., Fluid shear stress stimulates prostaglandin and nitric oxide release in bone marrow-derived preosteoclast-like cells, *Biochem. Biophys. Res. Comm.*, 270(2), 643–648, 2000.
10. Reich, K.M., Gay, C.V., and Frangos, J.A., Fluid shear stress as a mediator of osteoblast cyclic adenosine monophosphate production, *J. Cell. Physiol.*, 143(1), 100–104, 1990.
11. Batra, N.N., Li, Y.J., Yellowley, C.E. et al., Effects of short-term recovery periods on fluid-induced signaling in osteoblastic cells, *J. Biomech.*, 38(9), 1909–1917, 2005.

12. Donahue, T.L., Haut, T.R., Yellowley, C.E. et al., Mechanosensitivity of bone cells to oscillating fluid flow induced shear stress may be modulated by chemotransport, *J. Biomech.*, 36(9), 1363–71, 2003.
13. Jacobs, C.R., Yellowley, C.E., Davis, B.R. et al., Differential effect of steady versus oscillating flow on bone cells, *J. Biomech.*, 31(11), 969–976, 1998.
14. Ishuag, S.L., Crane, G.M., Miller, M.J. et al., Bone formation by three-dimensional stromal osteoblast culture in biodegradable polymer scaffolds, *J. Biomed. Mater. Res.* 36, 17–28, 1997.
15. Ishuag-Riley, S.L., Crane-Kruger, G.M., Yaszemski, M.J. et al., Three-dimensional culture of rat calvarial osteoblasts in porous biodegradable polymers, *Biomaterials* 19, 1405–1412, 1998.
16. Ma, P.X., Zhang, R., Xiao, G. et al., Engineering new bone tissue in vitro on highly porous poly(alpha-hydroxyl acids)/hydroxyapatite composite scaffolds, *J. Biomed. Mater. Res.*, 54(2), 284–293, 2001.
17. Webster, T.J. and Smith, T.A., Increased osteoblast function on PLGA composites containing nanophase titania, *J. Biomed. Mater. Res. Part A.*, 74(4), 677–686, 2005.
18. Karageorgiou, V. and Kaplan, D., Porosity of 3D biomaterial scaffolds and osteogenesis, *Biomaterials*, 26(27), 5474–5491, 2005.
19. Ren, T., Ren, J., Jia, X. et al., The bone formation in vitro and mandibular defect repair using PLGA porous scaffolds, *J. Biomed. Mater. Res. Part A.*, 74(4), 562–569, 2005.
20. Karageorgiou, V., Meinel, L., Hofmann, S. et al., Bone morphogenetic protein-2 decorated silk fibroin films induce osteogenic differentiation of human bone marrow stromal cells, *J. Biomed. Mater. Res. Part A*, 71(3), 528–537, 2004.
21. Bancroft, G.N., Sikavitsas, V.I., and Mikos, A.G., Design of a flow perfusion bioreactor system for bone tissue-engineering applications, *Tissue Eng.*, 9(3), 549–554, 2003.
22. Cartmell, S.H., Porter, B.D., Garcia, A.J. et al., Effects of medium perfusion rate on cell-seeded three-dimensional bone constructs in vitro, *Tissue Eng.*, 9(6), 1197–1203, 2003.
23. Yu, X., Botchwey, E.A., Levine, E.M. et al., Bioreactor-based bone tissue engineering: the influence of dynamic flow on osteoblast phenotypic expression and matrix mineralization, *Proc. Natl. Acad. Sci. USA*, 101(31), 11203–11208, 2004.
24. Meinel, L., Karageorgiou, V., Fajardo, R. et al., Bone tissue engineering using human mesenchymal stem cells: effects of scaffold material and medium flow, *Ann. Biomed. Eng.*, 32(1), 112–122, 2004.
25. Sorkin, A.M., Dee, K.C., and Knothe Tate M.L., "Culture shock" from the bone cell's perspective: emulating physiological conditions for mechanobiological investigations, *Am. J. Physiol. Cell Physiol.*, 287(6), C1527–C1536, 2004.
26. Manolagas, S.C. and Jilka, R.L., Bone marrow, cytokines, and bone remodeling. emerging insights into the pathophysiology of osteoporosis, *New Engl. J. Med* 332(5), 305–311, 1995.
27. Ducy, P., Zhang, R., Geoffroy, V. et al., Osf2/Cbfa1: a transcriptional activator of osteoblast differentiation, *Cell*, 89(5), 747–754, 1997.
28. Jee, W., Integrated bone tissue physiology, in *Bone Mechanics Handbook*, S. Cowin, Ed., CRC Press, Boca Raton, FL, 2001, pp. 1–34.
29. Barnes, G.L., Kostenuik, P.J., Gerstenfeld, L.C. et al., Growth factor regulation of fracture repair, *J. Bone Miner. Res.*, 14(11), 1805–1815, 1999.
30. Hanada, K., Dennis, J.E., and Caplan, A.I., Stimulatory effects of basic fibroblast growth factor and bone morphogenetic protein-2 on osteogenic differentiation of rat bone marrow-derived mesenchymal stem cells, *J. Bone Miner. Res.*, 12(10), 1606–1614, 1997.

31. Sun, J.S., Wu, S.Y., and Lin, F.H., The role of muscle-derived stem cells in bone tissue engineering, *Biomaterials*, 26(18), 3953–3960, 2005.
32. Suda, T., Takahashi, N., and Martin, T.J., Modulation of osteoclast differentiation, *Endocrine Rev.*, 13(1), 66–80, 1992.
33. Yasuda, H., Shima, N., Nakagawa, N. et al., Osteoclast differentiation factor is a ligand for osteoprotegerin/osteoclastogenesis-inhibitory factor and is identical to TRANCE/RANKL, *Proc. Natl. Acad. Sci. USA*, 95(7), 3597–3602, 1998.
34. Wolff, J., *Das Gesetz der Transfomation der Knochen*. (1892), Maraquet, P. and Furlong, R., Transl., Springer-Verlag, Berlin, 1986.
35. Vogel, J.M. and Whittle, M.W., Bone mineral changes: the second manned Skylab mission, *Aviat Space Environ. Med.*, 47(4), 396–400, 1976.
36. Goodship, A.E. and Cunningham, J.L., Pathophysiology of functional adaptation of bone in remodeling and repair *in vivo*, in *Bone Mechanics Handbook*, Cowin, S.C., ed., CRC Press: Boca Raton, FL, 2001, pp. 1–31.
37. Skerry, T.M. and Lanyon, L.E., Interruption of disuse by short duration walking exercise does not prevent bone loss in the sheep calcaneus, *Bone*, 16(2), 269–274, 1995.
38. Uhthoff, H.K. and Jaworski, Z.F., Bone loss in response to long-term immobilisation, *J. Bone Joint Surg*., Br., 60-B(3), 420–429, 1978.
39. Turner, C.H., Akhter, M.P., Raab, D.M. et al., A non-invasive, *in vivo* model for studying strain adaptive bone modeling, *Bone*, 12(2), 73–79, 1991.
40. Simske, S.J., Luttges, W.M. and Wachtel, H., Age dependent development of osteopenia in the long bones of tail-suspended mice, *Biomed. Sci. Instrum*., 26, 87–94, 1990.
41. Lanyon, L.E. and Rubin, C.T., Static vs dynamic loads as an influence on bone remodeling, *J. Biomech.*, 17(12), 897–905, 1984.
42. Zeng, Q.Q., Jee, W.S., Bigornia, A.E. et al., Time responses of cancellous and cortical bones to sciatic neurectomy in growing female rats, *Bone*, 19(1), 13–21, 1996.
43. Iwamoto, J., Yeh, J.K., and Aloia , J.F., Differential effect of treadmill exercise on three cancellous bone sites in the young growing rat, *Bone*, 24(3), 163–169, 1999.
44. Chambers, T.J., Chow, J.W., Fox, S.W. et al., The role of prostaglandins and nitric oxide in the response of bone to mechanical stimulation, *Adv. Exp. Med. Biol.*, 433, 295–298, 1997.
45. Chambers, T.J., Evans, M., Gardner, T.N. et al., Induction of bone formation in rat tail vertebrae by mechanical loading, *Bone Miner.*, 20(2), 167–178, 1993.
46. Robling, A.G., Hinant, F.M., Burr, D.B. et al., Shorter, more frequent mechanical loading sessions enhance bone mass, *Med. Sci. Sports Exerc*., 34(2), 196–202, 2002.
47. Skerry, T.M., Bitensky, L., Chayen, J. et al., Early strain-related changes in enzyme activity in osteocytes following bone loading *in vivo*, *J. Bone Miner. Res*., 4(5), 783–788, 1989.
48. Lean, J.M., Jagger, C.J. Chambers, T.J. et al., Increased insulin-like growth factor I mRNA expression in rat osteocytes in response to mechanical stimulation, *Am. J. Physiol*., 268(2 Pt 1), E318–E327, 1995.
49. Chambers, T.J., Fox, S., Jagger, C.J. et al., The role of prostaglandins and nitric oxide in the response of bone to mechanical forces, *Osteoarthritis Cartilage*, 7(4), 422–423, 1999.
50. Brighton, C.T., Fisher J.R., Levine, S.E. et al., The biochemical pathway mediating the proliferative response of bone cells to a mechanical stimulus, *J. Bone Joint Surg* (Am.), 78(9), 1337–1347, 1996.
51. Burger, E., Klein-Nulend, J., and Veldhuijzen, J., Modulation of osteogenesis in fetal bone rudiments by mechanical stress *in vitro*, *J. Biomech*., 24(Suppl 1), 101–109, 1991.
52. Klein-Nulend, J., Veldhuijzen, J., van de Stadt, R. et al., Influence of intermittent compressive force on proteoglycan content in calcifying growth plate cartilage *vitro*, *J. Biol. Chem.*, 262(32), 15490–15495, 1987.

53. Kubota, T., Yamauchi, M., Onozaki, J., Sato, S., Suzuki, Y., and Sodek, J., Influence of an intermittent compressive force on matrix protein expression by ROS 17/2.8 cells, with selective stimulation of osteopontin, *Arch. Oral Biol.*, 38(1), 23–30, 1993.
54. Stanford, C., Morcuende, J., and Brand, R., Proliferative and phenotypic responses of bone-like cells to mechanical deformation, *J. Orthopaed. Res.*, 13(5), 664–670, 1995.
55. Klein-Nulend, J., Semeins, C.M., Ajubi, N.E. et al., Pulsating fluid flow increases nitric oxide (NO) synthesis by osteocytes but not periosteal fibroblasts — correlation with prostaglandin upregulation, *Biochem. Biophys. Res. Commun.*, 217(2), 640–648, 1995.
56. Reich, K M. and Frangos, J.A., Effect of flow on prostaglandin E2 and inositol trisphosphate levels in osteoblasts, *Am. J. Physiol.*, 261(3 Pt 1), C428–C432, 1991.
57. Klein-Nulend, J., Roelofsen, J., Semeins, C.M. et al., Mechanical stimulation of osteopontin mRNA expression and synthesis in bone cell cultures, *J. Cell. Physiol.* 170(2), 174–181, 1997.
58. Ozawa, H., Imamura, K., Abe, E. et al., Effect of a continuously applied compressive pressure on mouse osteoblast-like cells (MC3T3-E1) *in vitro*, *J. Cell. Physiol.*, 142, 177–185, 1990.
59. Reilly, G.C., Haut, T.R., Yellowley, C.E. et al., Fluid flow induced PGE2 release by bone cells is reduced by glycocalyx degradation whereas calcium signals are not, *Biorheology*, 40(6), 591–603, 2003.
60. Rubin, J., Biskobing, D., Fan, X. et al., Pressure regulates osteoclast formation and MCSF expression in marrow culture, *J. Cell. Physiol.*, 170(1), 81–87, 1997.
61. Burger, E.H., Gregoire, M., Hagen, J.W. et al., Osteogenic effects of mild mechanical stress on bone cell- and organ cultures, in *The Biochemical Mechanisms of Tooth Movement and Craniofacial Adaptation*, Z. Davidovitch, Ed., Ohio State University College of Dentistry, Columbus, OH, 1992, pp. 187–193.
62. Winter, L.C., Walboomers, X.F., Bumgardner, J.D. et al., Intermittent versus continuous stretching effects on osteoblast-like cells *in vitro*, *J. Biomed. Mater. Res. Part A*, 67(4), 1269–1275, 2003.
63. Stanford, C., Stevens, J., and Brand, R., Cellular deformation reversibly depresses RT-PCR detectable levels of bone-related mRNA, *J. Biomech.*, 28(12), 1419–27, 1995.
64. Rubin, J., Fan, X., Biskobing, D.M. et al., Osteoclastogenesis is repressed by mechanical strain in an *in vitro* mode, *J. Orthopaed. Res.*, 17(5), 639–645, 1999.
65. Klein-Nulend, J., van der Plas, A., Semeins, C. et al., Sensitivity of osteocytes to biomechanical stress *in vitro*, *FASEB J.*, 9(5), 441–445, 1995.
66. You, J., Yellowley, C.E., Donahue, H.J. et al., Substrate deformation levels associated with routine physical activity are less stimulatory to bone cells relative to loading-induced oscillatory fluid flow, *J. Biomech. Eng.*, 122(4), 387–393, 2000.
67. Burger, E.H. and Klein-Nulend, J., Microgravity and bone cell mechanosensitivity, *Bone*, 22(5 Suppl), 127S–130S, 1998.
68. Frost, H.,M., The mechanostat: a proposed pathogenic mechanism of osteoporoses and the bone mass effects of mechanical and nonmechanical agents, *Bone Miner.* 2(2), 73–85,1987.
69. Fritton, S.P. and Rubin, C.T., *In vivo* measurements of bone deformations using strain gauges, in *Bone Mechanics Handbook*, Cowin, S.C., Ed., CRC Press, Boca Raton, FL, 2001, 8.1–8.41.
70. Weinbaum, S., Cowin, S.C., and Zeng, Y., A model for the excitation of osteocytes by mechanical loading-induced bone fluid shear stresses, *J. Biomech.*, 27(3), 339–360, 1994.
71. Cherian, P.P., Cheng, B., Gu, S. et al., Effects of mechanical strain on the function of gap junctions in osteocytes are mediated through the prostaglandin EP2 receptor, *J. Biol. Chem.*, 278(44), 43146–56,2003.

72. Cherian, P.P., Siller-Jackson, A.J., Gu, S. et al., Mechanical strain opens connexin 43 hemichannels in osteocytes: a novel mechanism for the release of prostaglandin, *Mol. Biol. Cell.*, 16(7), 3100–3106, 2005.
73. Knothe Tate, M.L., Knothe, U., and Niederer, P., Experimental elucidation of mechanical load-induced fluid flow and its potential role in bone metabolism and functional adaptation, *Am. J. Med. Sci.*, 316(3), 189–195, 1998.
74. Qin, Y.X., Kaplan, T., Saldanha, A. et al., Fluid pressure gradients, arising from oscillations in intramedullary pressure, is correlated with the formation of bone and inhibition of intracortical porosity, *J. Biomech.*, 36(10), 1427–1437, 2003.
75. Hillsley, M.V. and Frangos, J.A., Bone tissue engineering: the role of interstitial fluid flow, *Biotechnol. Bioeng.*, 43(7), 573–581, 1994.
76. Stevens, H.Y., Meays, D.R., Yeh, J. et al., COX-2 is necessary for venous ligation-mediated bone adaptation in mice, *Bone*, 38(1), 93, 2006.
77. Han, Y., Cowin, S.C., Schaffler, M.B. et al., Mechanotransduction and strain amplification in osteocyte cell processes, *Proc. Natl. Acad. Sci. USA*, 101(47), 16689–16694, 2004.
78. Sikavitsas, V.I., Bancroft, G.N., and Mikos, A.G., Formation of three-dimensional cell/polymer constructs for bone tissue engineering in a spinner flask and a rotating wall vessel bioreactor, *J. Biomed. Mater. Res.*, 62(1), 136–148, 2002.
79. Schwarz, R.P., Goodwin, T.J., and Wolf, D.A., Cell culture for three-dimensional modeling in rotating-wall vessels: an application of simulated microgravity, *J. Tissue Cult. Methods*, 14(2), 51–57, 1992.
80. Gomes, M.E., Sikavitsas, V.I., Behravesh, E. et al., Effect of flow perfusion on the osteogenic differentiation of bone marrow stromal cells cultured on starch-based three-dimensional scaffolds, *J. Biomed. Mater. Res. Part A*, 67(1), 87–95, 2003.
81. Sikavitsas, V.I., Bancroft, G.N., Lemoine, J.J. et al., Flow perfusion enhances the calcified matrix deposition of marrow stromal cells in biodegradable nonwoven fiber mesh scaffolds, *Ann. Biomed. Eng.*, 33(1), 63–70, 2005.
82. Botchwey, E.A., Pollack, S.R., Levine, E.M. et al., Quantitative analysis of three-dimensional fluid flow in rotating bioreactors for tissue engineering, *J. Biomed. Mater. Res. Part A*, 69(2), 205–15, 2004.
83. Botchwey, E.A., Dupree, M.A., Pollack, S.R. et al., Tissue engineered bone: measurement of nutrient transport in three-dimensional matrices, *J. Biomed. Mater. Res. Part A*, 67(1), 357–367, 2003.
84. Altman, G.H., Lu, H.H., Horan, R.L. et al., Advanced bioreactor with controlled application of multi-dimensional strain for tissue engineering, *J. Biomech. Eng* 124(6), 742–749, 2002.

13 Synthetic Scaffolds Used for Orthopedic Tissue Engineering

Mark Borden

CONTENTS

13.1 INTRODUCTION

Over the years, orthopedic implants have been designed to restore the normal physiological function and mechanical stability of diseased or damaged musculoskeletal tissues. Typically, this has been accomplished through the use of high strength metals such as stainless steel, titanium, cobalt chromium alloys, and nonresorbable polymers such as polyethylene. These materials have been used to create a wide array of orthopedic devices designed to replace human joints and stabilize severe fractures. Although these structural implants have functioned adequately in their restorative role, the surgeon's preference would be to minimize or eliminate the use of permanent materials in the body and have the site heal itself.

Historically, surgeons have used biological grafts to supplement or replace permanent implants. In these procedures, the musculoskeletal graft is placed at the surgical site in hope of supporting and stimulating the normal healing process. It is common to use biological grafts consisting of bone, tendon, ligament, or cartilage harvested from the patient's own body (autograft) or from a tissue donor (allograft).[1–14] These types of biological grafts have both advantages and disadvantages. For an autograft taken from the patient's own body, the largest advantage is that it has the highest biocompatibility with no chance of rejection or disease transfer. Additionally, autografts such as bone can be harvested in such a manner that the majority of the cells within the tissue can survive the transplantation process and ultimately contribute to the healing of the graft site.[15,16] For an allograft, on the other hand, the benefit is that it is from a donor site outside the body, so these grafts do not compromise previously healthy tissue and there is greater flexibility in the size and amount of graft available.

Unfortunately, these graft materials are not without their limitations. Patients who undergo autograft harvesting often suffer from complications at the donor site. In particular, patients receiving bone grafts taken from their iliac crest often complain of continued pain at the donor site even though their surgical site has fully healed.[17–22] Although an allograft avoids the donor site problems because of its alternate source, the tissue coming from a cadaver is often unpredictable, with properties that vary from donor to donor. Depending on how the tissue is processed, there can also be a small chance of disease transmission with the donor tissue.

Although biological grafting has become the gold standard in a variety of orthopedic applications, the limitations of these materials have driven the search for synthetic alternatives. These efforts have used tissue engineering principles that combine concepts from biology, materials science, and engineering to create synthetic alternatives to biological tissues. The goal of this work is to develop graft materials that can provide viable substitutes for patient- and donor-derived grafts.

13.2 ORTHOPEDIC TISSUE ENGINEERING

Based on the fundamental understanding of the structure and healing mechanisms of various musculoskeletal tissues, orthopedic tissue engineering research has focused on developing implants to regenerate new tissue and provide mechanical support to the site. In general, tissue healing consists of a cascade of events that are the result of several components working together. The fundamental concepts for tissue engineering were originally established at MIT in the laboratories of Robert Langer. It was through this work that the concepts of using cells, scaffolds, and growth factors together to replace or repair tissue were first introduced.[23]

During tissue regeneration, each of these components plays a unique role in the healing process. The scaffold serves as a trellis for eventual tissue regeneration and provides initial mechanical support while the growth factors stimulate the cells to create new tissue. In this triad of regeneration, the components work together to fully restore the tissue. Although the general concepts of tissue engineering can be applied to orthopedic surgery, the unique structure and properties of bone, ligament, tendon, and cartilage require customized approaches. This can be achieved by developing scaffolds specific to each tissue.

As previously discussed, the scaffold portion of a tissue-engineered graft serves as the substrate for tissue growth and provides mechanical support to the site. During healing, initial cell attachment and regeneration takes place in the porosity of the scaffold. In designing scaffolds for specific applications, the three-dimensional (3D) structure of the pore system must be based on the type of tissue being replaced. Bone, tendon, ligament, and cartilage all have their own unique microarchitecture that gives these tissues distinct properties and functions. In addition to supporting cell growth through its pore system, the scaffold also serves as a means of mechanically stabilizing the site. This makes designing a scaffold a challenging task because of the inverse relationship between mechanical strength and porosity. As the porosity of a scaffold increases to allow for more tissue regeneration, the overall strength of the construct decreases because of the degradation of the scaffold materials. Therefore, it is important to find the balance between porosity, strength, and degradation that will allow the device to support appropriate tissue ingrowth while still providing mechanical stabilization throughout the healing process.

13.2.1 Bone Scaffolds

The gold standard of bone grafting is the use of a cancellous autograft. The effectiveness of this graft is attributed to the optimal structure–property relationship that provides both strength and porosity. A scanning electron micrograph of cancellous bone is shown in Figure 13.1. As seen from the image, uniform pores penetrate throughout the tissue. Composed mainly of collagen and hydroxyapatite mineral, the struts within the cancellous structure provide the mechanical support while the open channels allow for bone ingrowth.

In developing a tissue engineering alternative to cancellous bone, the goal is to mimic the structure and properties as closely as possible. Based on the work of Robert Langer at MIT in the early 1990s, several researchers have developed polymer processing techniques aimed at creating three-dimensional scaffolds for bone repair. These scaffolds have been primarily composed of resorbable poly(hydroxy acids) such as poly(lactic acid) [PLA], poly(glycolic acid) [PGA], and the copolymer poly(lactide-co-glycolide) [PLG]. One method developed by Borden et al. uses polymer microspheres to create a three-dimensional porous structure.[24] In this technique, loose microspheres are added to a mold and heated past the glass transition temperature of the polymer. This causes the contact points between the spheres to fuse without melting the polymer. Because of the random packing of the spheres in 3D space, the voids between the spheres become the porosity of the scaffold.

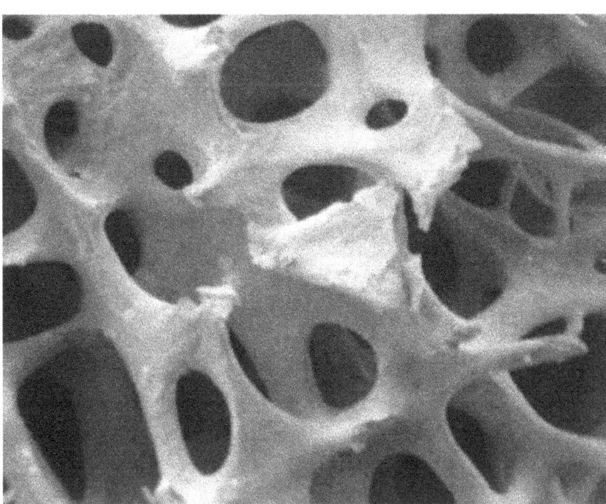

FIGURE 13.1 Electron micrograph of the structure of cancellous bone.

With no dead end channels or fully encapsulated voids, the pore system is 100% interconnected. An example of a microsphere scaffold is shown in Figure 13.2. This scaffold was created by sintering PLG microspheres that had a diameter of 600–700 μm. As seen from the image, the packing of the microspheres has created porosity throughout the structure. Work by Borden et al. has shown that the structure could be modified by changes to sintering temperature and time, and microsphere diameter.[24,25] In addition, biological evaluation of these implants demonstrated that the microsphere structure possessed adequate porosity and mechanical strength for a cancellous bone replacement and was found to support bone growth in an *in vivo* bone defect model.[24–27]

Another technique used to create porous polymer scaffolds involves particulate leaching. In this process, water soluble particles are mixed into a solution of polymer dissolved in an organic solvent. After the mixture is cast into a mold and freeze dried to remove the solvent, the composite is soaked in water to remove the void forming particles. Because of the high particulate content (typically a 9 to 1 particulate to polymer ratio), the dissolution of the void forming particles results in a

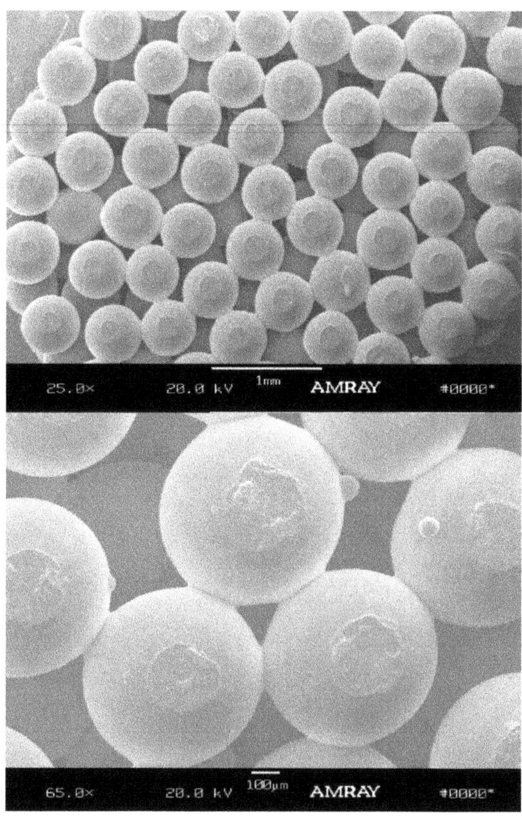

FIGURE 13.2 Images of a porous bone repair scaffold fabricated from a sintered microsphere technique.

highly porous foam. Mikos and coworkers first developed this technique using particles of sodium chloride to create PLG and PLA scaffolds.[28–31] Studies aimed at optimizing the structure showed that it was dependent on NaCl particle size,and concentration. In addition, cell culture results showed that the scaffold was capable of supporting osteoblast attachment and proliferation. In a modification to the salt leaching method, Chen and Ma used paraffin microspheres embedded in a PLA matrix to improve upon the interconnected porosity and give a more uniform 3D structure.[32] Shown in Figure 13.3, the use of paraffin spheres resulted in highly porous foams with spherical shaped pores. Other variations to increase interconnectivity have included using vibration during the casting phase,[33,34] using effervescing salts to create additional porosity,[35] and fusing the salt particles using humidity prior to addition of the polymer solution.[36]

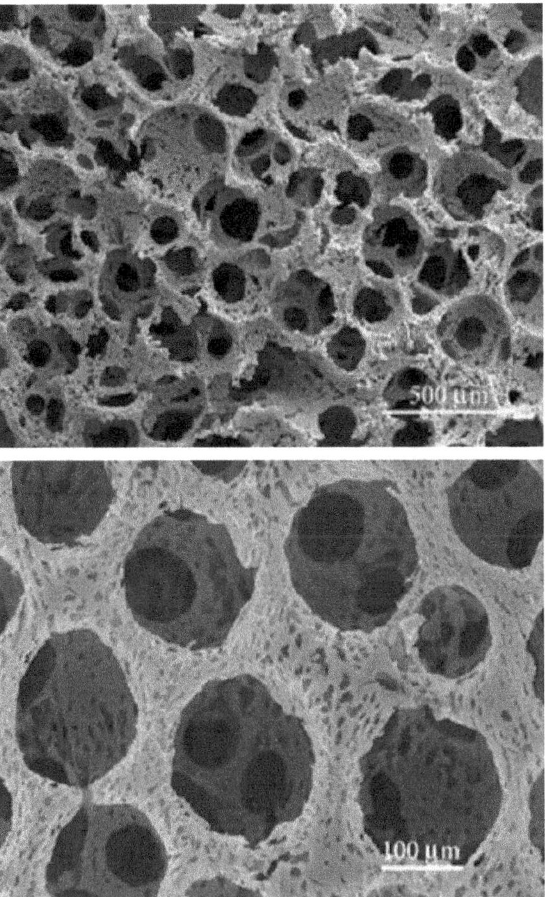

FIGURE 13.3 Images of a porous bone repair scaffold fabricated from a particulate leaching technique.

Another foam technique for creating bone scaffolds is based on the principle of solution phase separation between polymers and their solvents. Coombes and Heckman used various solvents to create PLA and PLG gels that contained separate polymer and solvent phases.[37,38] The gels were then frozen to lock in the 3D orientation of the phases, and then vacuum dried to remove the solvent. This resulted in highly porous foams with interconnected porosity. Ma and coworkers also used the phase separation technique to create PLA composites with hydroxyapatite.[39–41] this method, temperature control and polymer concentration were used to change the morphology of the resulting foams (Figure 13.4). *In vitro* cell culture studies with osteoblasts showed that the scaffold was capable of supporting cell growth and proliferation throughout the porosity of the scaffold.[39] Other composites of PLA and Bioglass[42]; chitosan and hydroxyapatite[43]; and chitosan and tricalcium phosphate have also been created with the phase separation technique.

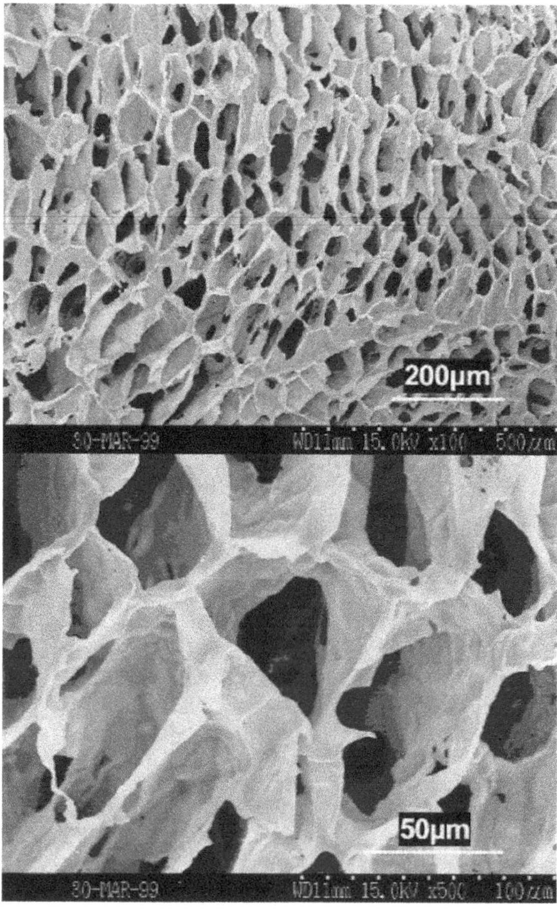

FIGURE 13.4 Images of a porous bone repair scaffold fabricated from a phase separation technique.

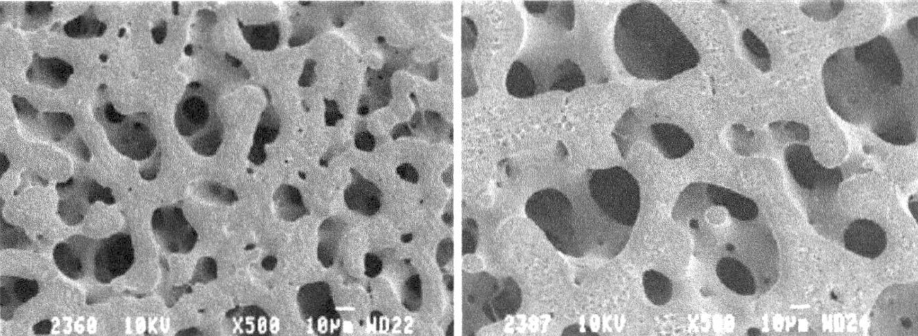

FIGURE 13.5 Images of a porous bone repair scaffold fabricated from a melt blending technique.

In a new approach related to phase separation, Favis and coworkers have utilized a molten polymer blending technique to creating 3D bone scaffolds.[45–47] In this method, two immiscible polymers with different solubilities are blended in a molten state to produce a continuous, two phase composite. Because of the continuous nature of both phases and the differences in polymer solubility, a solvent extraction step is used to dissolve one of the phases to create a 3D interconnected pore system. As seen in Figure 13.5, the scaffold is characterized by a uniform porosity similar in architecture to cancellous bone. With a significant amount of optimization and characterization work, Favis was able to produce polymer scaffolds with compressive strengths and porosities similar to cancellous bone.

As seen from the variety of techniques, there has been a significant effort in developing scaffolds for bone tissue engineering. The examples discussed represent a partial list of the various types of processing that can result in porous polymer scaffolds. Although a variety of 3D structures have been developed, the largest challenge with fabricating these scaffolds has been providing enough strength. Tissue engineering foams for bone repair have been shown to effectively support cell growth and proliferation in cell culture studies, but most do not have the strength to be used during aggressive grafting techniques seen in clinical practice. During graft placement, surgeons often use tamps and other instruments to press the graft in place. If the compressive resistance of the scaffold is too low, it will collapse, thereby eliminating the pore structure and preventing bone ingrowth. This limitation has prevented these scaffolds from transitioning from the laboratory to the orthopedic operating room. However, with further optimization of the structure–property relationship, researchers are close to having the first polymer scaffolds on the market.

13.2.2 Ligament and Tendon Scaffolds

Tendons and ligaments are fibrous tissues that are composed of highly organized type I collagen fibers, fibroblast cells, and extracellular matrix. Figure 13.6 shows the fibrous hierarchy found in a typical tendon. As seen from the illustration, the fibrous structure is the result of the packing of individual collagen fibers into larger

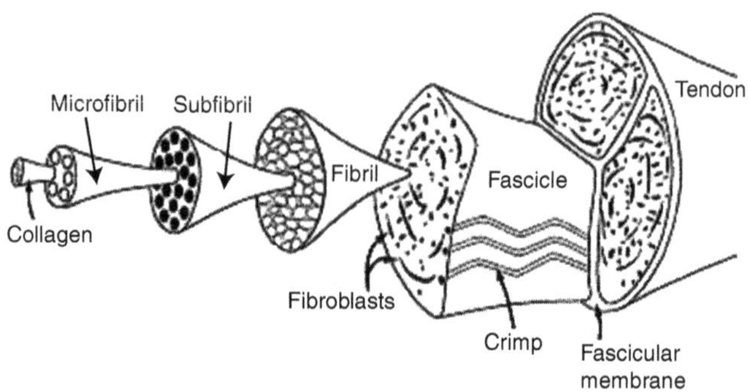

FIGURE 13.6 Illustration of the fibrous hierarchy of tendon. (Kastelic and Baer, Deformation in tendon collagen. In *The Mechanical Properties of Biologic Materials,* Cambridge University Press, Cambridge, U.K., 1980.)

and larger fiber bundles. This cablelike organization of the collagen allows both tendons and ligaments to support very high tensile loads with a minimal amount of elongation.[48] From a healing standpoint, tendons and ligaments have the capacity to heal on their own because of the presence of collagen producing fibroblasts. However, when these injuries result in a large gap between the ends of the damaged tissue, the regenerating fibroblasts cannot span the defect to re-create the collagen fiber structure. Injuries to the Achilles tendon and the anterior cruciate ligament fall into this category and require surgical intervention.

The challenge with engineering a replacement for tendons and ligaments is that the device must maintain its tensile strength for at least 12 months. This is the minimum amount of time it takes for fibrous tissue to regenerate and remodel throughout the device.[49,50] Tendon and ligament prostheses aimed at completely replacing the tissue with synthetic alternatives have, for the most part, resulted in disappointing outcomes. Historically, nonresorbable synthetic fibers such as carbon, Dacron, Teflon, nylon, and silicone have been evaluated as tendon and ligament replacements.[51–57] Although these fibers were shown to possess sufficient mechanical strength and did function as a scaffold by supporting fibrous tissue growth, issues with biocompatibility, fatigue failure, and inflammation have resulted in long term complications that eventually led to device failures.[58–60] It was clear from this work that resorbable, tissue engineered devices were needed.

To avoid the issues with permanent devices, researchers have evaluated resorbable fibers for tendon and ligament repair.[61–63] Based on decades of experience in textile processing, weaving and braiding techniques have been used to create a multitude of 3D structures that can be used for tissue engineering applications. The largest challenge, however, lies in designing a fiber construct that can maintain its strength for the needed 12 months of healing. This requires a resorbable device to immediately support the tensile load of the site in addition to providing a scaffold for eventual tissue regeneration. Since the degradation process of a resorbable polymer is mediated by hydrolysis and is independent of tissue healing, the device will begin to lose its strength as soon as it comes in contact with body fluid. Therefore, it is vital to the success of the implant that the fibroblasts responsible for re-creating the collagen framework can quickly attach to and proliferate within the resorbable fiber scaffold.

Based on these concepts, several resorbable devices have been evaluated for tendon and ligament repair. Table 13.1 shows a listing of the current polymers being

TABLE 13.1
Resorbable Polymer Fibers Used for Ligament and Tendon Tissue Engineering

Type of stuy	Ref.	Polymer	*In Vitro/In Vivo* Results
26-week intro and *in vivo* degradation study	71	Chitin (poly-*N*-acetyl-D-glucoseamine)	Chitin implants were infiltrated with fibrous tissue but degraded too quickly.
		Poly-ε-caprolactone [PCL]	PCL grafts showed good strength retention but fibrous tissue ingrowth was limited.
		PCL/chitin combination 50:50	Combined fiber construct showed good tissue ingrowth and strength retention.
		Poly(lactic acid) [PLA]	PLA implants showed good tissue ingrowth and strength retention.
72-week *in vitro* degradation study	63	Poly(lactic acid) [PLA]	Braided construct showed a complete loss in strength and stiffness at 60–72 weeks.
		Poly(lactide-co-glycolide) [PLG] 90:10	Braided constructs showed a complete loss of strength and stiffness in 24–48 weeks.
10 week *in vitro* degradation, cell attachment studies, and *in vivo* implantation	74	Copolymer of poly(dimethyltrimethyle ne carbonate) [DTMC] and poly (trimethylene carbonate) [TMC] 90:10	Degradation study showed 87% strength retention at 10 weeks; cell studies showed fibroblast attachment and proliferation; animal study showed significant tissue ingrowth at 26 weeks.
Cell culture attachment studies, *in vitro* degradation, and structure-property analysis	72,73	Poly(glycolic acid) [PGA]	PGA implant showed highest time zero mechanical strength but showed poor strength retention properties and the lowest cell attachment numbers.
		Poly(lactic acid) [PLA]	PLA fibers had the best cell attachment and strength retention profile.
		Poly(lactide-co-glyocilde) [PLG] 82:18	PLG fibers showed moderate levels of cell attachment and strength retention.
Cell attachment study	70	Collagen	Fibroblast cell study showed that collagen fibers supported fibroblast attachment and proliferation.
Subcutaneous tissue ingrowth study;	78	Poly(DTE carbonate) [PDTEC]	Degradation study showed 87% strength retention at 30 weeks; *in vivo* study showed 40% strength retention at 8 weeks with tissue ingrowth.
		Poly(lactic acid) [PLA]	Degradation study showed 7% strength retention at 30 weeks; *in vivo* study results showed 7% strength retention at 8 weeks with tissue ingrowth.

evaluated for this application. One of the first materials to be evaluated has been collagen. These devices consist of cross-linked type I collagen fibers that were formed into a multifiber prosthesis, and then embedded in a non–cross-linked collagen substrate. Several studies evaluated the *in vivo* effect of using varying cross-linking methods such as exposure to cyanamide, glutaraldehyde, or carbodiimide, and dehydrothermal cross-linking.[65–70] In general, the results showed that the collagen implants supported the growth of new tendon around and within the device. The devices were functional and able to support tensile loads. The studies agreed that cyanamide or carbodiimide cross-linking resulted in implants that had better tissue incorporation and faster new tissue formation than the glutaraldehyde implants. However, the long term strength of these constructs at 1 year was still below the strength of normal tendon.[67]

With a limit on the ultimate strength of collagen, researchers began looking for fibers with better strength retention profiles. Based on prior success in the suture areas, resorbable polymers such as poly(lactic acid) [PLA], poly(glycolic acid) [PGA], poly(lactide-co-glycolide) [PLG], poly(-caprolactone) [PCL], and poly(carbonates) were evaluated for tendon and ligament repair. In a series of degradation studies, these new fibers were evaluated for their ability to maintain adequate tensile strength through the degradation process. In a study by Sato, fibers composed of PLA, PCL, and chitin were evaluated alone or in combination with one another in a rabbit Achilles tendon model.[71] The 6-month degradation showed that PLA fiber implants and the PCL–chitin fiber composite had the best combination of tissue ingrowth and strength retention. Another study by Dürselen evaluated the *in vitro* degradation of PLA and PLG fibers in 37°C buffer for 72 weeks.[63] The results showed that PLA had a better degradation profile than PGA with strength retention past 1 year. However, the stiffness of the construct remained the same until the very end of degradation and did not result in effective load transfer. It was speculated that a combined fiber construct of slow and fast resorbing fibers would result in optimal load transfer to the regenerating tissue.

Laurencin and coworkers also evaluated PLA and PLG fibers fabricated into a 3D braid.[72,73] Designed for ACL repair, the scaffold shown in Figure 13.7 consisted of a three-phase 3D braid that mimicked the bone–tendon–bone graft commonly used in ACL repair. The denser braids at the end of the construct were designed to support bone growth while the parallel fibers in the central area of the implant were intended for ligament regeneration. The physical characterization of these braided fiber constructs showed that fiber orientation affected tensile properties while porosity remained constant in the range of 54–57%. In addition, an *in vitro* cell culture study showed that a fibronectin coating on the scaffold significantly improved cell attachment.[73]

In addition to poly(hydroxy acid) polymers, fibers from the poly(carbonate) family were also evaluated. Shieh et al. evaluated a new copolymer of dimethyltrimethylene carbonate [DTMC] and trimethylene carbonate [TMC].[74] Although the degradation study only went out 10 weeks, the results showed that the polymer had only lost 15% of its strength. In addition, *in vivo* studies out to 26 weeks showed significant fibrous tissue ingrowth. Choueka et al., Hooper et al., and Kohn and Langer also examined a new amino acid–based poly(carbonate) developed at

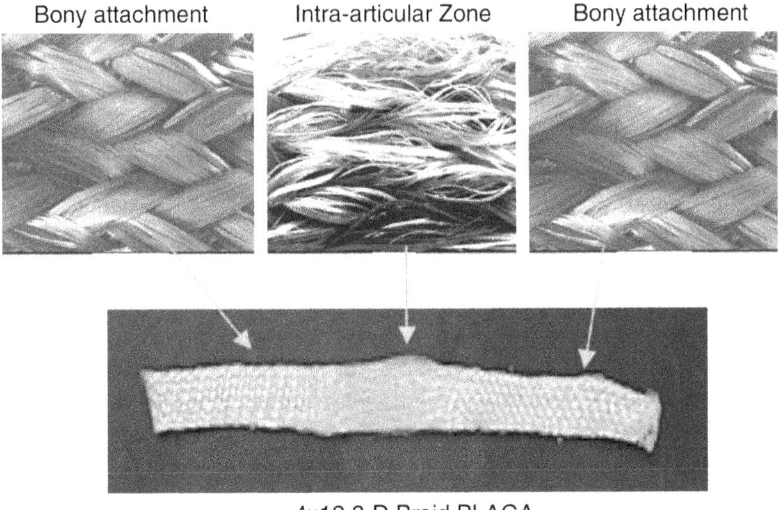

FIGURE 13.7 Images of a braided fiber scaffold for ligament repair.

Rutgers University called poly(DTE carbonate) [PDTEC].[75–77] In comparison studies with PLA, PDTEC showed similar tissue ingrowth capabilities, but showed much higher 8-week *in vivo* strength retention values (40% for PDTEC compared with 7% for PLA).[78]

Although these studies evaluated short term degradation of the fibers, the initial results were very promising. It was shown that the strength retention properties of the fiber constructs were highly dependent on variations in fiber geometry, fiber processing, polymer molecular weight, and 3D architecture. One characteristic linking the studies was the conclusion that slow resorbing polymers were better suited for ligament and tendon replacement than their fast resorbing counterparts. However, it was also concluded that the degradation of the slow fibers must also allow for load transfer to the regenerating tissue. The challenge with developing a tendon and ligament replacement lies in creating a construct that resorbs at a rate that allows for adequate tissue ingrowth but also maintains it strength for the appropriate period.

One feasible approach that may allow for optimization of the strength–tissue ingrowth relationship is the use several fiber types within the scaffold as described by Dürselen et al. and Sato et al.[63,71] In such a hybrid fiber construct, the fast resorbing fibers would add to the immediate tensile properties of the implant but would then quickly make room for newly regenerating fibrous tissue. The slow resorbing fibers would be able to support this immature tissue throughout the healing process until it fully remodeled into a load bearing collagen network. Once the fibroblasts had successfully remodeled into mature, load bearing tissue, the slow resorbing fibers would be completely absorbed by the body leaving no sign of the implant. In this optimal scenario, the device would perform its required function and then be completely replaced by healthy tissue.

13.2.3 Articular Cartilage Scaffolds

Similar to bone, tendon, and ligament, articular cartilage is often surgically repaired because of trauma and pathological degeneration. Found on the surface of joints throughout the body, articular cartilage aids joint motion by functioning as a lubricating surface at the end of bones and also as a shock absorber. Figure 13.8 shows an illustration of the cellular and fibrous organization found in articular cartilage. The combination of water (65–80%), type II collagen (10–20%), proteoglycans (5%), and cells (chondrocytes) in a layered fibrous structure allows cartilage to function as an effective joint surface that resists wear throughout a person's life.[79]

However, cartilage does not have the regenerative abilities to heal itself like other soft tissue. Although it is highly cellular, the local cells are trapped within a thick, fibrous matrix and cannot migrate to the site of the damaged tissue.[80–82] The complete lack of blood vessels within articular cartilage prevents the needed cells, proteins, and extracellular molecules from migrating to the site to aid in regeneration. With limited healing and constant exposure to dynamic motion, any damage caused by trauma or disease can have a debilitating effect on the joint. Once the cartilage is injured or begins to degenerate, the damage at the articular surface accumulates and can result in a complete failure of the joint surface. In these cases, the loss of

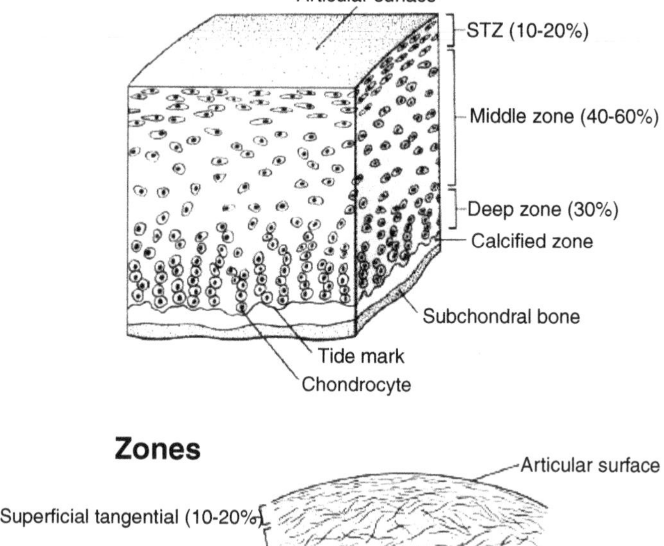

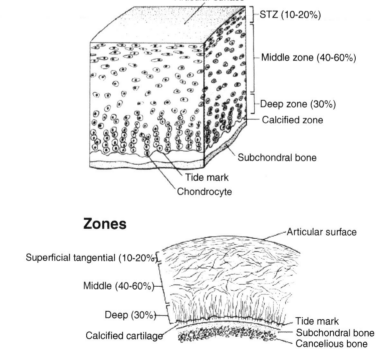

FIGURE 13.8 Illustration of the cellular and fibrous structure of articular cartilage. (Mow, V.C. and Lai, W.M., Some surface characteristics of articular cartilage, *J. Biomechanics* 7(5), 449–456, 1974.)

the articulating surface causes immobility and pain, and often requires replacement of the joint with a prosthetic implant.

From the patient's and surgeon's standpoint, this is clearly not a desired outcome. The alternative would be to provide an artificial construct that has all the components needed for cartilage regeneration. Because of the challenging nature of cartilage healing, a more comprehensive tissue engineering approach must be used. For cartilage repair, it is important that the implant contain both the scaffold and the cells needed for cartilage regeneration. Unlike other musculoskeletal scaffolds that rely on the migration of cells and growth factors from the local blood supply, cartilage scaffolds must contain the appropriate cells prior to implant placement.

To provide a high porosity scaffold to contain the cells and to mimic the fibrous structure of cartilage, resorbable fiber meshes have been evaluated for cartilage repair. These scaffolds consist of resorbable polymer fibers fabricated into 3D constructs that are capable of supporting chondrocyte growth within their porosity. Similar to tendon and ligament scaffolds, synthetic polymers such as poly(lactic acid), poly(glycolic acid), poly(lactide-co-glycolide), and poly(-caprolactone) have been evaluated for cartilage repair.[83–89] In addition, natural materials such as collagen, gelatin, hyaluronic acid, and chitosan have also been evaluated as resorbable fiber constructs.[90–94]

The scaffolds created from these fibers have used woven and nonwoven textile processing techniques to create the 3D architecture. The versatility of these techniques allows for creation of constructs with a range of 3D structures and properties suitable for cartilage repair. In one example, Chen et al. created a woven mesh of PLG fibers and then added an additional collagen web to improve the surface area for chondrocyte attachment.[91,95,96] Shown in Figure 13.9, this structure consists of a

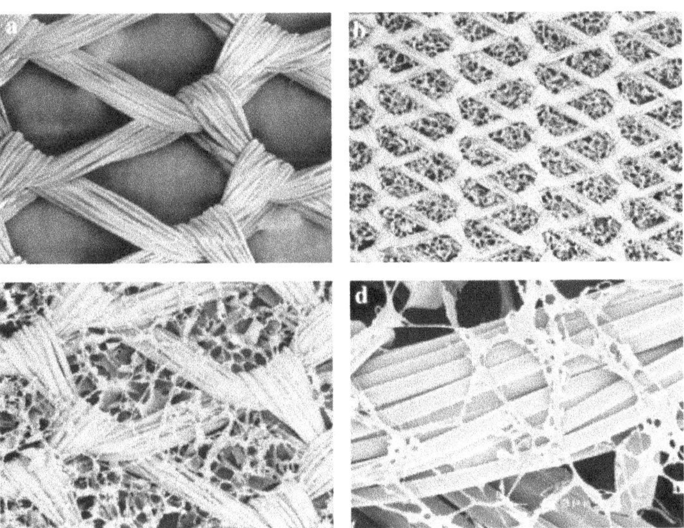

FIGURE 13.9 Images of a woven polymer mesh with embedded collagen fibers for cartilage repair.

polymer–collagen framework designed to provide uniform cell seeding throughout the mesh. *In vitro* analysis showed that the composite mesh seeded with bovine chondrocytes resulted in significant cell attachment and proliferation. These fiber–cell constructs were then implanted to assess *in vivo* cartilage formation. The results showed that the cells survived transplantation and the mesh effectively supported cartilage growth throughout the structure.[91,96]

In addition to woven fiber meshes, nonwoven structures have also been evaluated for cartilage repair.[83–85,92] Composed of PLA, PGA, PLG, and hyaluronic acid, these scaffolds consist of randomly oriented fibers that are typically pressed into mats during a melt spinning process.[84] The fiber diameter in these mats ranged from 10–15 μm with a range in porosity from 90–95%. Although the nonwoven meshes were shown to effectively support cellular attachment and proliferation, a result of the loose arrangement of the polymer fibers, the mechanical properties of the meshes have been low. To compensate for this problem, Langer et al. developed a coated PGA nonwoven mesh that has resulted in greater mechanical properties.[97] In this technique, the PGA mesh is created and dipped in a solution of PLA. After the scaffold is coated, the solvent is evaporated and the result is a bonded nonwoven mesh with a coating of PLA on the surface of PGA fibers. In a study by Moran et al., increasing the thickness of the PLA layer was shown to have a significant effect on the strength and degradation time of the mesh.[86] However, cell culture studies showed less chondrocyte attachment on PLA coated scaffold compared with PGA controls. A compromise may be a coating of collagen or fibronectin on these scaffolds to achieve both good cell attachment and mechanical strength.

In addition to the woven and nonwoven scaffolds, some newer techniques have also been used to create novel structures for cartilage repair. Recent work has shown that tissue engineering scaffolds can be fabricated using rapid prototyping technology.[98–103] One of these techniques, fiber deposition, has shown promising results for cartilage repair.[104] In this method, the polymer is melted and extruded as a fiber through a computer controlled nozzle (Figure 13.10). Following a preprogrammed

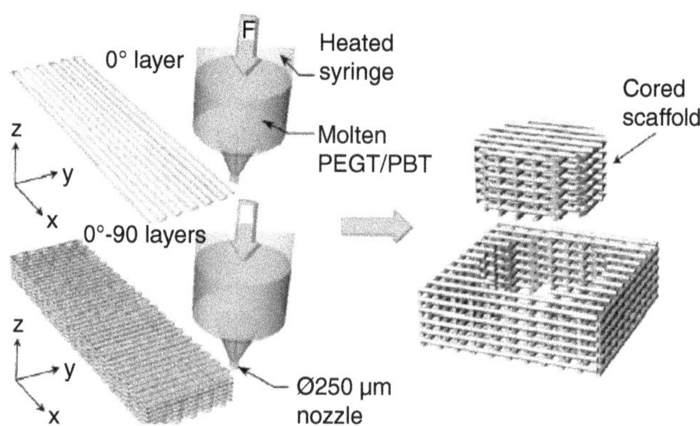

FIGURE 13.10 Illustration of a 3D fiber deposition process used to create scaffold for cartilage repair.

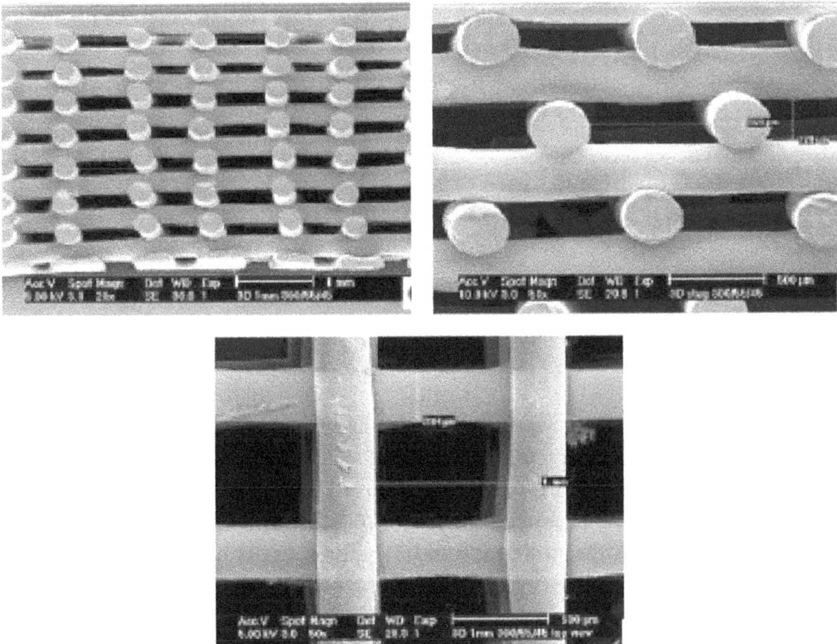

FIGURE 13.11 Images of a porous fiber scaffold for cartilage repair fabricated from a fiber deposition technique.

path, the nozzle deposits the molten fiber into a 3D pattern one layer at a time. In a study by Woodfield, a poly(ethylene glycol) based copolymer was formed into a highly uniform fibrous scaffold.[104] As shown in Figure 13.11, the structures consisted of the uniform arrangements of fibers to create 3D scaffolds. Biological testing of the scaffold showed a homogenous cell distribution throughout the scaffold as well as cartilage tissue formation within the porosity.

In addition to the fiber deposition process, another new technique, electrospinning, has also been evaluated for tissue engineering applications.[105–110] The nanofiber mesh shown in Figure 13.12 is characterized by the random arrangement of small fibers in a 3D orientation. The advantage of a nanofiber based mesh is the significant increase in porosity and available surface compared with standard fiber sizes. Li et al. used the electrospinning technique to create a dispersion of PLG nanofibers.[108] this method, the polymer solution was placed in a syringe that was held in place over a metal collecting tray. The syringe tip and metal tray were connected to an electrical supply, which caused an electrostatic charge to form between the positively charged droplet and the negatively charged tray. As the voltage was slowly increased, small nanofibers were ejected from the droplet and collected on the tray. Because of the small size of the fibers (500–800 nm), the polymer solution rapidly dried as it was sprayed. This resulted in a randomly oriented mesh with an interconnected porosity of 91%. *In vitro* cell studies showed that cells proliferated throughout the structure and showed significant increases in cell number over time.[108]

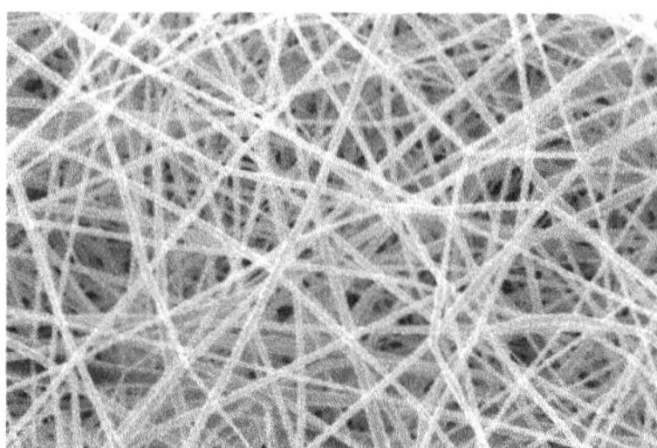
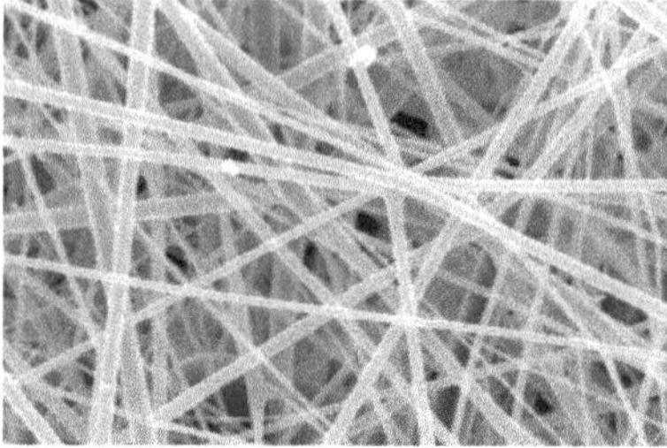

FIGURE 13.12 Image of a nanofiber scaffold for cartilage repair fabricated from an electrospinning technique.

Li et al. also evaluated 3D nanofiber meshes for cartilage repair.[106,107] In this study, the electrospinning technique was used with poly (-caprolactone) to create meshes with an average fiber diameter of 700 nm. Instead of chondrocytes, human bone marrow cells were cultured on the scaffold in the presence of the growth factor TGF-. In this approach, the full spectrum of tissue engineering scaffolds, cells, and growth factors were used. Because bone marrow contains stem cells capable of forming a variety of musculoskeletal tissues, TGF- was used to cause these cells to differentiate into chondrocytes. The results showed that the scaffold was capable of supporting the growth and proliferation of the cells throughout the structure. In addition, the exposure of the marrow derived stem cells to TGF- showed that the cells did show chondrocyte characteristics as seen by the production of cartilage-associated extracellular matrix and gene expression.

Overall, the woven and nonwoven meshes evaluated as cartilage scaffolds demonstrated adequate cell proliferation and matrix synthesis throughout the structures. However, the dependence of these implants on the cellular component has severely limited their use in the operating room. The process of obtaining a patient's own chondrocytes, transferring them to a processing facility for cell culture, seeding the scaffold, and then sending it back to the surgeon for implantation is logistically complicated. This has prevented most companies from getting involved in providing these devices to surgeons.

However, Li's marrow approach may open the door to more surgeon friendly practices.[108] It is entirely feasible for an implant loaded with differentiating growth factors such as TGF- to be opened at the time of surgery and then soaked in a bone marrow aspirate. After a few minutes of cellular attachment, the entire construct could then be placed at the cartilage defect site. This would not only provide the complete spectrum of components needed for cartilage healing but could do so in a surgeon-friendly manner.

13.3 CONCLUSION AND PERSPECTIVE ON THE FUTURE

Through a variety of novel polymer and fiber processing techniques, resorbable polymers have been used to create several tissue engineering scaffolds for bone, tendon, ligament, and cartilage repair. The unique structure of each of these tissues has directed the development of their respective scaffold. The success of tissue engineering devices lies in the interaction between the degrading implant and regenerating tissue. It is important that the relationship between implant and tissue results in adequate tissue function throughout the healing process. Cell culture studies, degradation work, and animal implantations have all paved the way for significant progress in the design and optimization of these scaffolds. The results to date have been very promising with the development of scaffolds capable of supporting significant tissue ingrowth throughout the structure and providing some degree of mechanical stabilization. The last hurdle for creating a clinically feasible device is to ensure that the final resorption of the scaffold results in healthy tissue that has the same histological appearance and mechanical integrity as normal bone, tendon, ligament, or cartilage. Once this has been accomplished, a new generation of musculoskeletal grafts will be available to orthopedic surgeons.

REFERENCES

1. Gadzag, A.R., Lane, J.M., Glaser, D., and Forster RA, Alternative to autogenous bone graft: efficacy and indications, *J. Am. Acad. Ortho. Surg.,* 3(1), 1, 1995.
2. Stevenson, S. and Arnoczky, S.P., Transplantation of musculoskeletal tissue, in *Orthopaedic Basic Science,* American Academy of Orthopaedic Surgeons, Rosemont, IL, 2000, chap. 23.
3. Khan, S.N., Cammisa, F.P., Jr., Sandhu, H.S., Diwan, A.D., Girardi, F.P., and Lane, J.M., The biology of bone grafting, *J. Am. Acad. Orthop. Surg,* 13(1), 77, 2005.
4. Spindler, K.P., Kuhn, J.E., Freedman, K.B., Matthews, C.E., Dittus, R.S., and Harrell, F.E., Jr., Anterior cruciate ligament reconstruction autograft choice: bone-tendon-bone versus hamstring: does it really matter? A systematic review, *Am. J. Sports Med.,* 32(8), 1986, 2004.
5. Barrett, G.R., Noojin, F.K., Hartzog, C.W., and Nash, C.R., Reconstruction of the anterior cruciate ligament in females: a comparison of hamstring versus patellar tendon autograft, *Arthroscopy,* 18(1), 46, 2002.
6. Chang, S.K., Egami, D.K., Shaieb, M.D., Kan, D.M., and Richardson, A.B., Anterior cruciate ligament reconstruction: allograft versus autograft, *Arthroscopy,* 19(5), 453, 2003.
7. Chun, C.H., Han, H.J., Lee, B.C., Kim, D.C., and Yang, J.H., Histologic findings of anterior cruciate ligament reconstruction with Achilles allograft, *Clin. Orthop. Relat. Res.,* (421), 273, 2004.
8. Siebold, R., Buelow, J.U., Bos, L., and Ellermann, A., Primary ACL reconstruction with fresh-frozen patellar versus Achilles tendon allografts, *Arch. Orthop. Trauma Surg.,* 123(4), 180, 2003.
9. Linn, R.M., Fischer, D.A., Smith, J.P., Burstein, D.B., and Quick, D.C., Achilles tendon allograft reconstruction of the anterior cruciate ligament-deficient knee, *Am. J. Sports Med.,* 21(6), 825, 1993.
10. Andres, B.M., Mears, S.C., Somel, D.S., Klug, R., and Wenz, J.F., Treatment of osteoarthritic cartilage lesions with osteochondral autograft transplantation, *Orthopedics,* 26(11), 1121, 2003.
11. Hangody, L., Rathonyi, G.K., Duska, Z., Vasarhelyi, G., Fules, P., and Modis, L., Autologous osteochondral mosaicplasty. Surgical technique, *J. Bone Joint Surg. Am.,* 86-A (Suppl. 1) 65, 2004.

12. Williams, R.J., III, Dreese, J.C., and Chen, C.T., Chondrocyte survival and material properties of hypothermically stored cartilage: an evaluation of tissue used for osteochondral allograft transplantation, *Am. J. Sports Med.,* 32(1), 132, 2004.
13. Kelley, T.F., Sutton, F.M., Wallace, V.P., and Wong, B.J., Chondrocyte repopulation of allograft cartilage: a preliminary investigation and strategy for developing cartilage matrices for reconstruction, *Otolaryngol. Head Neck Surg.,* 127(4), 265, 2002.
14. Tomford, W.W., Mankin, H.J., Friedlaender, G.E., Doppelt, S.H., and Gebhardt, M.C., Methods of banking bone and cartilage for allograft transplantation, *Orthop. Clin. North Am.,* 18(2), 241, 1987.
15. Frolke, J.P., Nulend, J.K., Semeins, C.M., Bakker, F.C., Patka, P., and Haarman, H.J., Viable osteoblastic potential of cortical reamings from intramedullary nailing, *J. Orthop. Res.,* 22(6), 1271, 2004.
16. Tydings, J.D., Martino, L.J., Kircher, M., Alfred, R.H., and Lozman, J., Viability of intramedullary canal bone reamings for continued calcification, *Am. J. Surg.,* 153(3), 306, 1987.
17. Arrington, E.D., Smith, W.J., Chambers, H.G., Bucknell, A.L., and Davino, N.A., Complications of iliac crest bone graft harvesting, *Clin. Orthop.,* (329), 300, 1996.
18. Banwart, J.C., Asher, M.A., and Hassanein, R.S., Iliac crest bone graft harvest donor site morbidity. A statistical evaluation, *Spine,* 20(9), 1055, 1995.
19. Cricchio, G. and Lundgren, S., Donor site morbidity in two different approaches to anterior iliac crest bone harvesting, *Clin. Implant. Dent. Relat. Res.,* 5(3), 161, 2003.
20. Hill, N.M., Horne, J.G., and Devane, P.A., Donor site morbidity in the iliac crest bone graft, *Aust. N.Z. J. Surg.,* 69(10), 726, 1999.
21. Silber, J.S., Anderson, D.G., Daffner, S.D., Brislin, B.T., Leland, J.M., Hilibrand, A.S., Vaccaro, A.R., and Albert, T.J., Donor site morbidity after anterior iliac crest bone harvest for single-level anterior cervical discectomy and fusion, *Spine,* 28(2), 134, 2003.
22. Summers, B.N. and Eisenstein, S.M., Donor site pain from the ilium. A complication of lumbar spine fusion, *J. Bone Joint Surg. [Br],* 71(4), 677, 1989.
23. Langer, R. and Vacanti, J.P., Tissue engineering, *Science,* 260, 920, 1993.
24. Borden, M., Attawia, M., Khan, Y., and Laurencin, C.T., Tissue engineered microsphere-based matrices for bone repair: design and evaluation, *Biomaterials,* 23(2), 551, 2002.
25. Borden, M., El Amin, S.F., Attawia, M., and Laurencin, C.T., Structural and human cellular assessment of a novel microsphere-based tissue engineered scaffold for bone repair, *Biomaterials,* 24(4), 597, 2003.
26. Borden, M., Attawia, M., and Laurencin, C.T., The sintered microsphere matrix for bone tissue engineering: in vitro osteoconductivity studies, *J. Biomed. Mater. Res.,* 61(3), 421, 2002.
27. Borden, M., Attawia, M., Khan, Y., El-Amin, S.F., and Laurencin C.T., Tissue-engineered bone formation in vivo using a novel sintered polymeric microsphere matrix, *J. Bone Joint Surg. Br.,* 86-B(8), 1200, 2004.
28. Ishaug-Riley, S.L., Crane-Kruger, G.M., Yaszemski, M.J., and Mikos, A.G., Three-dimensional culture of rat calvarial osteoblasts in porous biodegradable polymers, *Biomaterials*, 19(15), 1405, 1998.
29. Mikos, A.G., Sarakinos, G., Leite, S.M., Vacanti, J.P., and Langer, R., Laminated three-dimensional biodegradable foams for use in tissue engineering, *Biomaterials* 14(5), 323, 1993.
30. Mikos, A.G., Thorsen, A.J., Czerwonka, L.A., Bao, Y., and Langer, R., Preparation and characterization of poly (*l*-lactic acid) foams, *Polymer,* 35, 1068, 1994.

31. Thomson, R.C., Yaszemski, M.J., Powers, J.M., and Mikos, A.G., Fabrication of biodegradable polymer scaffolds to engineer trabecular bone, *J. Biomater. Sci. Polym. Ed.,* 7(1), 23, 1995.
32. Chen, V.J. and Ma, P.X., Nano-fibrous poly(L-lactic acid) scaffolds with interconnected spherical macropores, *Biomaterials,* 25(11), 2065, 2004.
33. Agrawal, C.M., McKinney, J.S., Huang, D., and Athanasiou, K.A., The use of the vibrating particle technique to fabricate highly permeable biodegradable scaffolds, in *STP:1396 Synthetic Bioabsorbable Polymers for Implants,* American Society for Testing and Materials, Philadelphia, 2000.
34. Chim, H., Ong, J.L., Schantz, J.T., Hutmacher, D.W., and Agrawal, C.M., Efficacy of glow discharge gas plasma treatment as a surface modification process for three-dimensional poly (D,L-lactide) scaffolds, *J. Biomed. Mater. Res. A,* 65(3), 327, 2003.
35. Yoon, J.J. and Park, T.G., Degradation behaviors of biodegradable macroporous scaffolds prepared by gas foaming of effervescent salts, *J. Biomed. Mater. Res.,* 55(3), 401, 2001.
36. Murphy, W.L., Dennis, R.G., Kileny, J.L., and Mooney, D.J., Salt fusion: an approach to improve pore interconnectivity within tissue engineering scaffolds, *Tissue Eng.,* 8(1), 43, 2002.
37. Coombes, A.G. and Heckman, J.D., Gel casting of resorbable polymers. 2. In-vitro degradation of bone graft substitutes, *Biomaterials,* 13(5), 297, 1992.
38. Coombes, A.G. and Heckman, J.D., Gel casting of resorbable polymers. 1. Processing and applications, *Biomaterials,* 13(4), 217, 1992.
39. Ma, P.X., Zhang, R., Xiao, G., and Franceschi, R., Engineering new bone tissue in vitro on highly porous poly(alpha-hydroxyl acids)/hydroxyapatite composite scaffolds, *J. Biomed. Mater. Res.,* 54(2), 284, 2001.
40. Wei, G. and Ma, P.X., Structure and properties of nano-hydroxyapatite/polymer composite scaffolds for bone tissue engineering, *Biomaterials,* 25(19), 4749, 2004.
41. Zhang, R. and Ma, P.X., Porous poly(L-lactic acid)/apatite composites created by biomimetic process, *J. Biomed. Mater. Res.,* 45(4), 285, 1999.
42. Blaker, J.J., Gough, J.E., Maquet, V., Notingher, I., and Boccaccini, A.R., *In vitro* evaluation of novel bioactive composites based on bioglass-filled polylactide foams for bone tissue engineering scaffolds, *J. Biomed. Mater. Res. A,* 67(4), 1401, 2003.
43. Zhang, Y., Ni, M., Zhang, M., and Ratner, B., Calcium phosphate-chitosan composite scaffolds for bone tissue engineering, *Tissue Eng.,* 9(2), 337, 2003.
44. Zhang, Y. and Zhang, M., Synthesis and characterization of macroporous chitosan/calcium phosphate composite scaffolds for tissue engineering, *J. Biomed. Mater. Res.,* 55(3), 304, 2001.
45. Sarazin, P., Roy, X., and Favis, B.D., Controlled preparation and properties of porous poly(L-lactide) obtained from a co-continuous blend of two biodegradable polymers, *Biomaterials,* 25(28), 5965, 2004.
46. Sarazin, P. and Favis, B.D., Morphology control in co-continuous poly(L-lactide)/polystyrene blends: a route towards highly structured and interconnected porosity in poly (L-lactide) materials, *Biomacromolecules,* 4(6), 1669, 2003.
47. Yuan, Z., and Favis B.D., Macroporous poly(L-lactide) of controlled pore size derived from the annealing of co-continuous polystyrene/poly(L-lactide) blends, *Biomaterials,* 25(11), 2161, 2004.
48. Woo, S.L., An, K., Frank, C.B., Livesay, G.A., Ma, C.B., Zeminski, J., Wayne, J.S., and Myers, B.S., Anatomy, biology, and biomechanics of tendon and ligament, in *Orthopaedic Basic Science: Biology and Biomechanics of the Musckuloskeletal System,* American Academy of Orthopaedic Surgeons, Rosemont, IL, 2000, chap. 24.

49. Kasperczyk, W.J., Bosch, U., Oestern, H.J., and Tscherne, H., Staging of patellar tendon autograft healing after posterior cruciate ligament reconstruction. A biomechanical and histological study in a sheep model, *Clin. Orthop. Relat. Res.,* (286), 271, 1993.
50. Bosch, U., Kasperczyk, W.J., Oestern, H.J., and Tscherne, H., The patellar tendon graft for PCL reconstruction. Morphological aspects in a sheep model, *Acta. Orthop. Belg.,* 60 (Suppl. 1) 57, 1994.
51. Mendes, D.G., Iusim, M., Angel, D., Rotem, A., Mordehovich, D., Roffman, M., Lieberson, S., and Boss, J., Ligament and tendon substitution with composite carbon fiber strands, *J. Biomed. Mater. Res.,* 20(6), 699, 1986.
52. Park, J.P., Grana, W.A., and Chitwood, J.S., A high-strength Dacron augmentation for cruciate ligament reconstruction. A two-year canine study, *Clin. Orthop. Relat. Res.,* (196), 175, 1985.
53. Kolarik, J., Vanicek, J., and Migliaresi, C., Preparation and strength of poly(ethylene terephthalate) fiber bundles for model synthetic tendons, *J. Biomed. Mater. Res.,* 18(1), 115, 1984.
54. Hunter, J.M., Singer, D.I., Jaeger, S.H., and Mackin, E.J., Active tendon implants in flexor tendon reconstruction, *J. Hand Surg. [Am.],* 13(6), 849, 1988.
55. Aoki, M., Manske, P.R., Pruitt, D.L., and Larson, B.J., Tendon repair using flexor tendon splints: an experimental study, *J. Hand Surg. [Am.],* 19(6), 984, 1994.
56. Hunter, J.M., Sattel, A.B., Belkin, J., and Masada, K., Collateral ligament reconstruction of the metacarpophalangeal and proximal interphalangeal joints using porous Dacron tendon, *Hand Clin.,* 7(3), 557, 1991.
57. Peterson, W.W., Manske, P.R., Lesker, P.A., Kain, C.C., and Schaefer, R.K., Development of a synthetic replacement for the flexor tendon pulleys — an experimental study, *J. Hand Surg. [Am.],* 11(3), 403, 1986.
58. Koob, T.J., Biomimetic approaches to tendon repair, *Comp. Biochem. Physiol. A Mol. Integr. Physiol.,* 133(4), 1171, 2002.
59. Margevicius. K.J., Claes, L.E., Durselen, L., and Hanselmann, K., Identification and distribution of synthetic ligament wear particles in sheep, *J. Biomed. Mater. Res.,* 31(3), 319, 1996.
60. Rushton, N., Dandy, D.J., and Naylor, C.P., The clinical, arthroscopic and histological findings after replacement of the anterior cruciate ligament with carbon-fibre, *J. Bone Joint Surg. Br.,* 65(3), 308, 1983.
61. Cabaud, H.E., Feagin, J.A., and Rodkey, W.G., Acute anterior cruciate ligament injury and repair reinforced with a biodegradable intraarticular ligament. Experimental studies, *Am. J. Sports Med.,* 10(5), 259, 1982.
62. Laitinen, O., Pohjonen, T., Tormala, P., Saarelainen, K., Vasenius, J., Rokkanen, P., and Vainionpaa, S., Mechanical properties of biodegradable poly-L-lactide ligament augmentation device in experimental anterior cruciate ligament reconstruction, *Arch. Orthop. Trauma Surg.,* 112(6), 270, 1993.
63. Durselen, L., Dauner, M., Hierlemann, H., Planck, H., Claes, L.E., and Ignatius, A., Resorbable polymer fibers for ligament augmentation, *J. Biomed. Mater. Res.,* 58(6), 666, 2001.
64. Ko, F.K., Preform fiber architecture for ceramic-matrix composites, *Am. Ceram. Soc. Bull.,* 68(2), 401, 1989.
65. Dunn, M.G., Avasarala, P.N., and Zawadsky, J.P., Optimization of extruded collagen fibers for ACL reconstruction, *J. Biomed. Mater. Res.,* 27(12), 1545, 1993.
66. Goldstein, J.D., Tria, A.J., Zawadsky, J.P., Kato, Y.P., Christiansen, D., and Silver, F.H., Development of a reconstituted collagen tendon prosthesis. A preliminary implantation study, *J. Bone Joint Surg. Am.,* 71(8), 1183, 1989.

67. Kato, Y.P., Dunn, M.G., Zawadsky, J.P., Tria, A.J., and Silver, F.H., Regeneration of Achilles tendon with a collagen tendon prosthesis. Results of a one-year implantation study, *J. Bone Joint Surg. Am.,* 73(4), 561, 1991.
68. Kato, Y.P., Goldstein, J.D., Christiansen, D., Zawadsky, J.P., Tria, A.J., and Silver, F.H., Short term assessment of reconstituted collagen tendon/ligament prosthesis, *Biomed. Sci. Instrum.,* 24, 87, 1988.
69. Wasserman, A.J., Kato, Y.P., Christiansen, D., Dunn, M.G., and Silver, F.H., Achilles tendon replacement by a collagen fiber prosthesis: morphological evaluation of neo-tendon formation, *Scanning Microsc.,* 3(4), 1183, 1989.
70. Dunn, M.G., Liesch, J.B., Tiku, M.L., and Zawadsky, J.P., Development of fibroblast-seeded ligament analogs for ACL reconstruction, *J. Biomed. Mater. Res.,* 29(11), 1363, 1995.
71. Sato, M., Maeda, M., Kurosawa, H., Inoue, Y., Yamauchi, Y., and Iwase, H., Reconstruction of rabbit Achilles tendon with three bioabsorbable materials: histological and biomechanical studies, *J. Orthop. Sci.,* 5(3), 256, 2000.
72. Cooper, J.A., Lu, H.H., Ko, F.K., Freeman, J.W., and Laurencin, C.T., Fiber-based tissue-engineered scaffold for ligament replacement: design considerations and *vitro* evaluation, *Biomaterials,* 26(13), 1523, 2005.
73. Lu, H.H., Cooper, J.A., Jr., Manuel, S., Freeman, J.W., Attawia. M.A., Ko, F.K., and Laurencin, C.T., Anterior cruciate ligament regeneration using braided biodegradable scaffolds: *in vitro* optimization studies, *Biomaterials,* 26(23), 4805, 2005.
74. Shieh, S.J., Zimmerman, M.C., and Parsons, J.R., Preliminary characterization of bioresorbable and nonresorbable synthetic fibers for the repair of soft tissue injuries, *J. Biomed. Mater. Res.,* 24(7), 789, 1990.
75. Choueka, J., Charvet, J.L., Koval, K.J., Alexander, H., James, K.S., Hooper, K.A., and Kohn, J., Canine bone response to tyrosine-derived polycarbonates and poly(L-lactic acid), *J. Biomed. Mater. Res.,* 31(1), 35, 1996.
76. Hooper, K.A., Macon, N.D., and Kohn, J., Comparative histological evaluation of new tyrosine-derived polymers and poly (L-lactic acid) as a function of polymer degradation,
77. Kohn, J. and Langer R., Poly(iminocarbonates) as potential biomaterials, *Biomaterials,* 3, 176, 1986.
78. Bourke, S.L., Kohn, J., and Dunn, M.G., Preliminary development of a novel resorbable synthetic polymer fiber scaffold for anterior cruciate ligament reconstruction, *Tissue Eng.,* 10(1–2), 43, 2004.
79. Mankin, H.J., Mow, V.C., Buckwalter, J.A., Iannotti, J.P., and Ratcliffec A., Articular cartilage structure, composition, and function, in *Orthopaedic Basic Science,* American Academy of Orthopaedic Surgeons, Rosemont, IL, 2000, chap. 17.
80. Buckwalter, J.A. and Mankin, H.J., Articular cartilage: tissue design and chondrocyte-matrix interactions, *Instr. Course Lect.,* 47, 477, 1998.
81. Mankin, H.J., The reaction of articular cartilage to injury and osteoarthritis (second of two parts), *New Engl. J. Med.,* 291(25), 1335, 1974.
82. Mankin, H.J., The reaction of articular cartilage to injury and osteoarthritis (first of two parts), *New Engl. J. Med.,* 291(24), 1285, 1974.
83. Cohen, S.B., Meirisch, C.M., Wilson, H.A., and Diduch, D.R., The use of absorbable co-polymer pads with alginate and cells for articular cartilage repair in rabbits, *Biomaterials,* 24(15), 2653, 2003.
84. Sittinger, M., Reitzel, D., Dauner, M., Hierlemann, H., Hammer, C., Kastenbauer, E., Planck, H., Burmester, G.R., and Bujia, J., Resorbable polyesters in cartilage engineering: affinity and biocompatibility of polymer fiber structures to chondrocytes, *J Biomed. Mater. Res.,* 33(2), 57, 1996.

85. Freed, L E., Grande, D.A., Lingbin, Z., Emmanual, J., Marquis, J.C., and Langer, R., Joint resurfacing using allograft chondrocytes and synthetic biodegradable polymer scaffolds, *J. Biomed. Mater.,* 28(8), 891, 1994.
86. Moran, J.M., Pazzano, D., and Bonassar, L.J., Characterization of polylactic acid-polyglycolic acid composites for cartilage tissue engineering, *Tissue Eng.,* 9(1), 63, 2003.
87. Lee, S.H., Kim, B.S., Kim, S.H., Kang, S.W., and Kim, Y.H., Thermally produced biodegradable scaffolds for cartilage tissue engineering, *Macromol. Biosci.,* 4(8), 802, 2004.
88. Freed, L.E., Marquis, J.C., Nohria, A., Emmanual, J., Mikos, A.G., and Langer, R., Neocartilage formation in vitro and in vivo using cells cultured on synthetic biodegradable polymers, *J. Biomed. Mater. Res.,* 27(1), 11, 1993.
89. Chu, C.R., Coutts, R.D., Yoshioka, M., Harwood, F.L., Monosov, A.Z., and Amiel, D., Articular cartilage repair using allogeneic perichondrocyte-seeded biodegradable porous polylactic acid (PLA): a tissue-engineering study, *J. Biomed. Mater. Res.,* 29(9), 1147, 1995.
90. Yoo, H.S., Lee, E.A., Yoon, J.J., and Park, T.G., Hyaluronic acid modified biodegradable scaffolds for cartilage tissue engineering, *Biomaterials,* 26(14), 1925, 2005.
91. Chen, G., Sato, T., Ushida, T., Hirochika, R., Shirasaki, Y., Ochiai, N., and Tateishi, T., The use of a novel PLGA fiber/collagen composite web as a scaffold for engineering of articular cartilage tissue with adjustable thickness, *J. Biomed. Mater. Res. A,* 67(4), 1170, 2003.
92. Aigner, J., Tegeler, J., Hutzler, P., Campoccia, D., Pavesio, A., Hammer, C., Kastenbauer, E., and Naumann, A., Cartilage tissue engineering with novel nonwoven structured biomaterial based on hyaluronic acid benzyl ester, *J. Biomed. Mater. Res.,* 42(2), 172, 1998.
93. Xia, W., Liu, W., Cui, L., Liu, Y., Zhong, W., Liu, D., Wu, J., Chua, K., and Cao, Y., Tissue engineering of cartilage with the use of chitosan-gelatin complex scaffolds, *J. Biomed. Mater. Res. B Appl. Biomater.,* 71(2), 373, 2004.
94. Solchaga, L.A., Dennis, J.E., Goldberg, V.M., and Caplan, A.I., Hyaluronic acid-based polymers as cell carriers for tissue-engineered repair of bone and cartilage, *J. Orthop. Res.,* 17(2), 205, 1999.
95. Chen, G., Liu, D., Tadokoro, M., Hirochika, R., Ohgushi, H., Tanaka, J., and Tateishi, T., Chondrogenic differentiation of human mesenchymal stem cells cultured in a cobweb-like biodegradable scaffold, *Biochem. Biophys. Res. Commun.,* 322(1), 50, 2004.
96. Chen, G., Sato, T., Ushida, T., Ochiai, N., and Tateishi, T, Tissue engineering of cartilage using a hybrid scaffold of synthetic polymer and collagen, *Tissue Eng.,* 10(3–4), 323, 2004.
97. Mikos, A.G., Bao, Y., Cima, L.G., Ingber, D.E., Vacanti, J.P., and Langer, R., Preparation of poly(glycolic acid) bonded fiber structures for cell attachment and transplantation, *J. Biomed. Mater. Res.,* 27(2), 183, 1993.
98. Landers, R., Hubner, U., Schmelzeisen, R., and Mulhaupt, R., Rapid prototyping of scaffolds derived from thermoreversible hydrogels and tailored for applications in tissue engineering, *Biomaterials,* 23(23), 4437, 2002.
99. Dhariwala, B., Hunt, E., and Boland, T., Rapid prototyping of tissue-engineering constructs, using photopolymerizable hydrogels and stereolithography, *Tissue Eng.,* 10(9–10), 1316, 2004.
100. Vozzi, G., Flaim, C., Ahluwalia, A., and Bhatia, S., Fabrication of PLGA scaffolds using soft lithography and microsyringe deposition, *Biomaterials,* 24(14), 2533, 2003.

101. Leong, K. F, Cheah, C.M., and Chua, C.K., Solid freeform fabrication of three-dimensional scaffolds for engineering replacement tissues and organs, *Biomaterials,* 24(13), 2363, 2003.
102. Vozzi, G., Previti, A., De Rossi, D., and Ahluwalia, A., Microsyringe-based deposition of two-dimensional and three-dimensional polymer scaffolds with a well-defined geometry for application to tissue engineering, *Tissue Eng.,* 8(6), 1089, 2002.
103. Ciardelli, G., Chiono, V., Cristallini, C., Barbani, N., Ahluwalia, A., Vozzi, G., Previti, A., Tantussi, G., and Giusti, P., Innovative tissue engineering structures through advanced manufacturing technologies, *J. Mater. Sci. Mater. Med.,* 15(4), 305, 2004.
104. Woodfield, T.B., Malda, J., de Wijn, J., Peters, F., Riesle, J., and van Blitterswijk, C.A., Design of porous scaffolds for cartilage tissue engineering using a three-dimensional fiber-deposition technique, *Biomaterials,* 25(18), 4149, 2004.
105. Laurencin, C.T., Ambrosio, A.M., Borden, M.D., and Cooper. J.A., Jr., Tissue engineering: orthopedic applications, *Ann. Rev. Biomed. Eng.,* 1(19), 1999.
106. Li, W.J., Tuli, R., Okafor, C., Derfoul, A., Danielson, K.G., Hall, D.J., and Tuan, R.S., A three-dimensional nanofibrous scaffold for cartilage tissue engineering using human mesenchymal stem cells, *Biomaterials,* 26(6), 599, 2005.
107. Li, W.J., Danielson, K.G., Alexander, P.G., and Tuan, R.S., Biological response of chondrocytes cultured in three-dimensional nanofibrous poly(epsilon-caprolactone) scaffolds, *J. Biomed. Mater. Res. A,* 67(4), 1105, 2003.
108. Li, W.J., Laurencin. C.T., Caterson, E.J., Tuan, R.S., and Ko, F.K., Electrospun nanofibrous structure: a novel scaffold for tissue engineering, *J. Biomed. Mater. Res.,* 60(4), 613, 2002.
109. Bhattarai, N., Edmondson, D., Veiseh, O., Matsen, F.A., and Zhang, M., Electrospun chitosan-based nanofibers and their cellular compatibility, *Biomaterials,* 26(31), 6176, 2005.
110. Bhattarai, S.R., Bhattarai, N., Yi, H.K., Hwang, P.H., Cha, D.I., and Kim, H.Y., Novel biodegradable electrospun membrane: scaffold for tissue engineering, *Biomaterials,* 25(13), 2595, 2004.

14 Polymeric Controlled Release Systems for Management of Bone Infection

Marc Shalaby and Shalaby W. Shalaby

CONTENTS

14.1 INTRODUCTION

Osteomyelitis is a bacterial infection involving bone that is characterized by progressive inflammatory destruction of bone tissue. And while much progress has been made with regards to antibiotic development and the prevention of postsurgical bone infection, osteomyelitis remains a significant cause of morbidity. Osteomyelitis may be the result of hematogenous seeding of bacteria, spread of infection from a contiguous area, surgical inoculation of bacteria into bone, or trauma coincident with contamination.[1] The presence of foreign bodies, such as components of an artificial joint, increases the likelihood of osteomyelitis. Once infection of such devices occurs, removal of these components may be inevitable for complete eradication of the infection.[2] Traditionally, treatment of osteomyelitis is accomplished through prolonged intravenous antibiotic therapy, and often includes surgical debridement of the infected area and any necrotic tissue.

Reviews in the general area of musculoskeletal infections have been the subject of a 2003 book edited by Calhoun and Mader, which focused on (1) the basic science of infection, (2) the management of osteomyelitis, (3) osteomyelitis at different biological sites, (4) antibiotic activities and toxicities, (5) effectiveness of adjunctive therapy, and (6) gene therapy in musculoskeletal repair.[3] Collectively, the book is directed mostly to the biological aspects of musculoskeletal infections and commonly accepted treatments using antibiotics. Accordingly, the present chapter, for the most part, addresses (1) common route causes, clinical diagnosis, and approaches to successful prophylaxis and treatment of osteomyelitis, (2) device-centered infections as they pertain to biomaterial scientists and engineers as well as clinicians, (3) evolution of the localized treatment of bone infection, and (4) advances toward new approaches to the treatment of osteomyelitis and its management.

14.1.1 Common Causes of Different Forms of Osteomyelitis and Their Diagnoses

Normally, bone is very resistant to infection, but in the presence of trauma, foreign bodies, or large inocula, bacteria can adhere to bone, multiply, and cause destruction. In addition, patient comorbidities such as diabetes, rheumatoid arthritis, or vascular disease can limit the body's ability to fight infection. During infection, phagocytes attempt to contain the invading organisms, but in the process, generate proteolytic enzymes and free radicals that contribute to local destruction of bone tissue. As the inflammatory process continues, pus spreads into vascular channels and raises the intraosseous pressure. This rise in pressure ultimately impairs blood flow and results in necrosis of bone. Devascularized fragments, called sequestra, then separate from bone.[4] Established infection may stay contained in the bone, spread to adjacent structures or joints, or develop into an abscess with or without sinus tract formation.

Acute osteomyelitis is a term used to describe a newly recognized bone infection. Often there is pain, redness, and swelling over the infected bone. Acute infection may involve the medullary space, the cortex, or the periosteum. When there are clinical signs of infection lasting 10 or more days, it is considered chronic osteomyelitis and correlates with the development of necrotic bone.[4] Chronic osteomyelitis is a more longstanding process that is characterized by the presence of sequestra, bone sclerosis, and a lower grade of inflammation. Chronic osteomyelitis may smolder for a number of weeks to months. This indolent course sometimes delays proper diagnosis and treatment.

Osteomyelitis after injury is the most prevalent form of osteomyelitis and is usually the result of an open fracture or, less commonly, a complication of reconstructive surgery.[4] This is likely to continue and perhaps become more prevalent given the increasing interest in competitive sports and the increasing survival seen with high-speed automobile accidents. In addition, penetrating trauma such as gunshot wounds or nail punctures may give rise to bone infection. Gram-positive organisms such as *Staphylococcus aureus* or *S. epidermitis*, which normally colonize the skin, are common culprit organisms involved in osteomyelitis after injury.

Arterial vascular insufficiency also contributes to the development of osteomyelitis. This is a well-recognized complication in patients with advanced diabetes mellitus. This type of osteomyelitis is almost exclusively seen in the feet, and lesions often develop insidiously with skin trauma. Infection can then burrow into the deep tissues and ultimately settle in the bones of the foot. Often patients with advanced diabetes and vascular compromise have concomitant neuropathy that impairs their ability to feel pain. This further increases the risk of unrecognized trauma and infection. Infection from foot ulcers tends to be polymicrobial with a combination of Gram-positive, Gram-negative, and anaerobic bacteria. Systemic, broad-spectrum antibiotics and sometimes revascularization procedures are necessary to treat such infections.

Osteomyelitis can also develop *de novo* after episodes of transient bacteremia. This scenario occurs most commonly in prepubertal children and the elderly.[4] children, bacteria can be trapped and proliferate in the metaphyseal sinusoidal veins of long bones such as the tibia or femur.[4,5] Children typically present with fever, localized pain, and swelling in the affected region. Blood cultures are often positive in this situation and are helpful in isolating the offending bacteria. In neonates, the most common organisms are *S. aureus* and streptococci. Later in life, *S. aureus* the predominant organism. And while Gram-positive organisms are still the most common organisms responsible for osteomyelitis in the elderly, Gram negative organisms such as Escherichia coli and pseudomonads play a significant role.

14.1.2 Device-Centered Osteomyelitis

Infection in association with prostheses is also an important clinical scenario. The prevalence of infection after total knee or hip arthroplasty is estimated to be 1–2%. If infection occurs within 3 months of the initial surgery, it is considered an acute infection that is a direct result of bacterial inoculation during surgery. Clinical signs often include fever, pain, erythema, and warmth at the implant site.[5,6] Infection recognized between 3 months and 2 years of surgery is considered a delayed infection and is often the result of colonization and infection with less virulent organisms. Delayed or chronic osteomyelitis associated with prostheses often presents with subtle signs such as mild pain or instability of the affected joint. Patients are often afebrile and have a normal white blood cell count. Complicating matters is that culture of fluid from the prosthetic joint space obtained by percutaneous aspiration has a sensitivity of less than 50%.[7] Furthermore, it is often difficult to distinguish between mechanical loosening of the prosthesis and infectious loosening. A biopsy of the bone, the bone cement, or the artificial joint space is often required to diagnose osteomyelitis.[4] Infections of prostheses after 2 years usually occur as a result of hematogenous spread of bacteria during transient bacteremia. Sudden onset of pain and redness at the site of a previously replaced joint is the usual clinical presentation. Hematogenous seeding of a prosthesis is a risk throughout the life of the implant. As such, prophylactic antibiotics are given for procedures that may induce transient bacteremia such as teeth cleaning or urological procedures.

There are inherent drawbacks to prosthetic devices that make them susceptible to infection. For one, not only are they are devoid of microcirculation (which is crucial for host defenses and delivery of antibiotics), they often lead to reduced blood flow to adjacent tissues, which further lowers the threshold for infection.[5,6] addition, soon after implantation, they are coated by host proteins such as collagen, fibrinogen, and fibronectin. The coated surfaces then become ideal places for free-floating bacteria to adhere and multiply. Once bacterial concentration is high enough, the bacteria form a biofilm layer on the surface of the prosthetic. This biofilm is a polymeric matrix in which bacteria develop into organized, complex communities with structural and functional heterogeneity.[8] The polymer matrix also contains fluid channels to allow for the flow of nutrients and waste.[9] The biofilm serves to protect the bacteria from host defenses and antimicrobial agents, thus making them infinitely more resistant to treatment. In addition, bacteria are further protected in the biofilm because they enter a stationary phase of growth. This renders them less susceptible to antimicrobial agents that rely on cell growth and replication to be effective.[6]

Additionally, studies have shown that the presence of implants impedes the normal immune response to infection. Prosthetic implants have been shown to inhibit superoxide production by phagocytes and may actually induce apoptosis by a mechanism known as "frustrated phagocytosis." This occurs when a phagocyte cell encounters a substrate that is beyond its capacity to phagocytize. The ensuing apoptosis that occurs leads to the release of reactive products of oxygen and lysosomal enzymes. This causes further tissue damage and necrosis and increases the risk of infection.[10] So, in sum, prostheses not only serve as a substrate for bacterial adherence, they limit the body's ability to fight infection.

Several factors further influence the risk of infection with prosthetic devices. Joints that tend to be closer to the skin surface and lack significant soft tissue coverage are more at risk for infection. One such example is the elbow athroplasty, which carries an infection rate as high as 7–9%.[11] Host factors such as underlying diabetes, rheumatoid arthritis, malnourishment, and advanced age may also increase the risk of infection.

The most commonly cultured microorganisms in prosthetic joint infections are coagulase negative staphylococci (in 30–43% of cases), *S. aureus* (in 12–23% of cases), mixed flora (~10%), streptococci (~10%), enteroccocci (3-7%), Gram negative bacilli (3–6%), and anaerobes (2–4%).[6]

14.2 CRITICAL REVIEW OF CURRENT TREATMENT OPTIONS FOR OSTEOMYELITIS

14.2.1 Systemic Treatment

Treatment of osteomyelitis is most commonly accomplished with long courses (4 to 6 weeks) of systemic antibiotics administered intravenously, often followed by several weeks of oral therapy. Most intravenous antibiotic regimes are accomplished through the use of an indwelling catheter. Complications and difficulties with this method are catheter failure, catheter infection, high-cost antibiotics and supplies, poor patient compliance, and frequent dosing schedules. And while long courses of intravenous therapy have moved largely from acute care hospitals to skilled nursing facilities or to home intravenous infusion, significant cost and burden has shifted to these arenas. It has been estimated that the cost of antibiotic treatment ranges from more than $200 per day as an outpatient to as much as $700 per day as an inpatient.[12,13] Multiply this daily cost by 28–42 days, and one can see the enormous direct costs associated with intravenous antibiotic therapy.

Many of the current antibiotics in use today have relatively poor bone penetration. As such, higher systemic doses of antibiotics are required to increase local concentrations in bone to treat established infections. These high systemic antibiotic concentrations may lead to serious toxicities and, as a result, require close monitoring. Important examples of antibiotic-related toxicities are the ototoxicty and nephrotoxicity seen with gentamicin therapy. Furthermore, systemic toxicities limit the spectrum of antibiotics that can be used to treat osteomyelitis.

In addition to intravenous antibiotics, surgical debridement of necrotic bone tissue is often necessary to eradicate infection, especially if there is significant bony destruction. And while a necessity, surgical debridement can lead to gaps in the bone, known as "dead space." To fill this dead space, bone reconstruction procedures are often required after the infection has been eradicated. When foreign materials such as joint prostheses are present, surgical intervention often includes removal of the prosthesis. This may be done in a one stage approach where the infected prosthesis is removed and a new one is placed during the same procedure. More commonly, however, a two stage process is used in which the prosthesis is removed, several weeks of antibiotics are given to eradicate the infection, and a new prosthesis is placed. But even after this aggressive therapy, infection manages to recur in about 14% of cases.[14]

Sometimes, if a prosthetic joint infection is caught early enough (usually within 3 weeks), it may be successfully treated with antibiotics alone or in conjunction with debridement without removal of the prosthetic device. The device can be salvaged as long as the implant is stable within the bone and the surrounding tissue is healthy.[5,6] Antibiotic regimes that include several weeks of intravenous antibiotics followed by several months of oral antibiotics are often employed to suppress and eradicate the infection. If the signs of infection are present for over 3 weeks, salvage of the implant should not be attempted.

14.2.2 Significance of Osteomyelitis and Need for New Approaches to its Management

In the 1960s and early 1970s, osteomyelitis was treated with surgical debridement and 4 to 6 weeks of systematic therapy with penicillinase-resistant penicillins, which are effective against Gram-positive pathogens. For the past 15 years, diversity in pathogens causing osteomyelitis made it necessary to seek additional corrective measures. These measures include the systemic application of potent antibiotics, such as gentamicin, tobramycin, and vancomycin, for combating a broad spectrum of microorganisms. Alternatively, the antibiotics can be incorporated into controlled delivery systems for localized delivery to avoid side effects and toxicities. The localized delivery of antibiotics has gained wide acceptance, particularly in prosthetic joint replacement procedures. One such application is the use of poly(methyl methacrylate) (PMMA) beads impregnated with gentamicin, and/or mixing the drug with PMMA bone cement. Unfortunately, the presence of the drug in bone cement appears to compromise its long-term physical properties. Furthermore, in situations where the PMMA beads outlast their function, a second surgical procedure is required for removal of the beads since they are nonabsorbable.

The aforementioned shortcomings of the present treatments of osteomyelitis has led many contemporary investigators to explore the efficacy of controlled delivery systems based on absorbable polyesters, such as those made of lactide and glycolide. The most common form of these systems are solid microcapsules containing antibiotics such as gentamicin. Unfortunately, in most cases, the method of administration and efficacy of the microcapsules are quite dependent on many variables, including their migration from the administration site, and the accessibility, configuration, and biomechanics of the biological site. Recognized, stringent requirements for the prophylactic or therapeutic treatment of osteomyelitis, growing interest in absorbable delivery systems for localized, controlled drug release, and the development of novel, absorbable carriers led Shalaby and coworkers to explore the use of injectable, gel-forming, absorbable controlled antibiotic-release systems.[15]

14.2.3 Local Drug Delivery

Over the past three decades there has been an interest in carriers for local administration of antibiotics in cases of bone infection. There are obvious advantages to local delivery systems. For one, high local concentrations of antibiotics can be administered directly to the site of infection without the systemic toxicities associated with some antibiotics. This is additionally advantageous because it would avoid systemic exposure to unwanted antibiotics, which should reduce the risk of generating bacterial resistance to antibiotics. Another advantage to such systems is that they allow antibiotics to be delivered to areas where blood supply is limited. Bone is not a very vascular structure to start with, but the ischemia and necrosis that occurs as a result of infection further limit the ability of the body to deliver antibiotics to the infected site via the bloodstream. High local levels of antibiotics facilitate delivery of antibiotics by diffusion to avascular areas of wounds that were previously inaccessible by systemic antibiotics. Furthermore, bacteria that are resistant to many antibiotics at levels achieved with systemic therapy may be susceptible to antibiotics at very high local concentrations.[16]

Choice of antimicrobial agent to be used in local delivery devices is based upon the bactericidal profile of the antibiotic, the antibiotic's ability to be released at concentrations much higher than the minimum inhibitory concentration of bacterial pathogens, the ability of the agent not to provoke any local or systemic side effects, its inability to enter systemic circulation, and its stability at body temperature.[17] addition, with delivery systems based on PMMA, the antibiotic needs to be heat stable to withstand the exothermic reaction that occurs during the polymerization process.

Most antibiotic delivery systems utilize aminoglycosides (gentamicin, tobramycin), beta-lactams, fluoroquinolones, and the glycopeptides vancomycin and teicoplanin. For water soluble agents, such as the beta-lactams, drug release is dependent upon the surface area of the carrier and the initial concentration of drug in the prepared system. For insoluble agents, such as the quinolones, the rate of drug release depends on the porosity of the matrix.[18] There are few data with regard to how high dosing needs to be or should be, how long antibiotics should be delivered, and what are the optimal dosing regimes. In addition, traditional antibiotic sensitivity profiles may not be consistent with *in vivo* killing. This is especially true in cases where bacteria reside in a biofilm. These sessile organisms may have different sensitivities than their free-floating counterparts. Often, much higher local concentrations are necessary to eradicate sessile organisms.[19] New antibiotic sensitivity testing modalities may need to be developed.

Local carrier systems are divided into two categories: nonbiodegradable and bioabsorbable systems. The most actively studied and widely accepted standard for local antibiotic delivery is a nonbiodegradable system based on PMMA.[20] PMMA as an antibiotic delivery system was first studied in 1970 by Buchholz and Englebrecht who fashioned bone cement PMMA beads impregnated with gentamicin. While the system was initially used as prophylaxis against postoperative infection, therapeutic applications for the treatment of osteomyelitis quickly emerged. PMMA can be fashioned into beads to be placed at the site of infection site, or it may be prepared as a cement to anchor prostheses, fill dead space, or preserve joint space during a two-stage prosthetic revision. While there has been some controversy, it is generally accepted that the PMMA bead preparations may remain at the site of infection for up to 4 weeks, but then must be removed surgically to allow for bone regeneration or reconstructive surgery. This need to have a second surgical procedure has been the major drawback to the use of PMMA beads.

Antibiotic-loaded PMMA beads have been used to treat a variety of bone infections. One such application has been in the treatment of infected nonunions. Infected nonunions are an important clinical consequence of open fractures. In fact, failure of therapy and amputations rates for patients with osteomyelitis is highest if a nonunion is present.[23] In a study by Evans and Nelson, gentamicin-impregnated PMMA beads were as effective as systemic therapy with gentamicin in a rabbit model of chronic osteomyelitis.[24] In a human study by Calhoun et al., patients with infected nonunions were treated with either systemic antibiotic therapy or local therapy with gentamicin-impregnated PMMA beads after surgical debridement and perioperative antibiotics. One group of patients received intravenous antibiotics for a total 4 weeks followed by reconstructive surgery. The PMMA group had beads implanted and removed after 2 weeks and prior to reconstruction. Similar rates of healing were noted in both groups.[25]

Although the use of antibiotic-loaded PMMA beads is widely accepted in the treatment of osteomyelitis for management of dead space, such beads are rarely used in the treatment of infected knee or hip arthroplasty. After 4 weeks, these beads become surrounded with dense scar tissue, and it becomes difficult to locate and remove them. Given this drawback, other methods of using PMMA have been developed for use in infected arthoplasties. One method is placement of an antibiotic-impregnated cement "spacer" after removal of the infected prosthetic device. The idea is to have antibiotic release to treat the infection but, at the same time, maintain the length and shape of the effective joint space. After the infection has been eradicated, the spacer may be removed, and another prosthesis may be placed. PMMA blocks are, and will likely continue to be, the standard of care in circumstances where structural requirements, in addition to antibiotic delivery, are necessary.[16]

Another method employed is the use of PMMA as a means of cementing prosthetic joints in place. Antibiotic-impregnated bone cement as surgical prophylaxis during primary arthroplasty has been studied. In one study reviewing 10,905 patients undergoing total hip replacement, survival of the prosthesis was greatly prolonged over the first 2 years of follow-up in patients receiving prophylaxis with systemic antibiotics and gentamicin-loaded bone cement compared with those receiving systemic antibiotics alone.[26] And while this data supports the use of antibiotic impregnated cement in primary arthroplasty, there still exists some controversy.[27] Use of such cements is more widely accepted for use during revision surgery for an infected arthroplasty. In one review, two-stage exchange with antibiotic-loaded PMMA cement was associated with a 93% cure rate compared with a 59% cure rate with two-stage exchange without antibiotic-loaded cement. Interestingly, an 86% cure rate was obtained in patients who underwent direct-exchange with antibiotic-loaded cement.[28] The latter is an attractive finding because direct-exchange requires only one surgical procedure.

In addition to the need for surgical removal of PMMA devices, another drawback is their ability to serve as a substrate for bacterial colonization after antibiotic release has been exhausted. PMMA is surface-friendly to biofilm-forming bacteria, and there are concerns that this may hinder treatment efforts to eradicate infection.[29] In a study by Neut et al.,[27] gentamicin-loaded PMMA beads were retrieved from patients who required the use of the beads in the treatment of prosthetic joint infection. The retrieved beads were subjected to routine and then rigorous culturing techniques. The rigorous techniques were far more sensitive than the current, routine microbiology cultures. In 18 of 20 patients, bacteria were cultured from the PMMA beads using the more rigorous culturing technique. Interestingly, 12 of these 18 patients were considered free of infection by routine hospital culture. What is even more notable is that the three patients considered free of infection by routine culture (but not by the highly sensitive culture) eventually went on to develop infection of their new prosthesis.[27] This suggests not only that routine cultures may not be adequate in assessing when an infection has been eradicated, but it may also imply that antibiotic beads designed to clear an infection may lead to persistent or relapsing infections. Furthermore, PMMA has been shown to have an inhibitory effect on polymorphonuclear cells, thus limiting one aspect of host protection from infection.

There are other disadvantages to PMMA as an antibiotic delivery system. For one, the generation of heat during the polymerization process limits antibiotic choices to those that are heat stable. This temperature rise may also damage surrounding tissues, especially when fabricating spacers *in situ*. PMMA is also very inefficient at delivering antibiotics to local tissues. In fact, one study of antibiotic-loaded PMMA in a rabbit model showed that only the outer 1 mm of PMMA cement released antibiotics, leaving the bulk of the antibiotic trapped in the cement.

In addition, release of antibiotics is only seen for 2 to 4 weeks so intravenous antibiotic therapy is often required to eradicate infection.[32]

Currently, there are five commercially available aminoglycoside-bone cement devices that are approved by the U.S. Food and Drug Administration (FDA). The antibiotic concentrations are low and are appropriate only for prophylaxis of infection rather than for treatment of established infection. Therefore, at the present time, PMMA systems for the treatment of osteomyelitis require hand-mixing of higher doses of antibiotics into the bone cement by the treating physician at the time of surgery as a physician-directed application.

Because of the drawbacks with the current PMMA systems, significant attention has been focused on the use bioabsorbable systems for local antibiotic delivery. These systems have the obvious advantage of being able to deliver high local levels of antibiotics without having to be surgically removed after antibiotic delivery has been completed. Bioabsorbable systems for antibiotic delivery are classified into four broad categories: protein-based materials (natural polymers), bone graft, bone graft substitutes or extenders, and synthetic polymers.[33] Currently there are no FDA-approved bioabsorbable materials available for use in the treatment of established bone infection.[20]

Examples of protein-based materials that have been loaded with antibiotics and tested include sponge collagen, albumin, fibrin, thrombin, and a variety of clotted blood products. None of these systems has gained widespread acceptance in the treatment of osteomyelitis, mostly because of rapid elution rates.[29,34–36] One bioabsorbable system that has promise is one based on alginate. Alginate is a product from marine algae and is a linear copolymer of D-mannuronic acid and L-gulonic acid. These two components combine in random sequence to form a linear polymer that undergoes reversible gelation. Alginate beads have been loaded with vancomycin and coated with poly-L-lysine. *In vitro* studies have shown favorable release profiles and no obvious toxicities.[37]

Bone graft (either autograft or allograft) has been used mostly as a means of dead space management after PMMA bead removal or fracture fixation, or to treat bone defects during revision joint surgery. Bone graft as a means of local antibiotic delivery has been in use for over 20 years. Antibiotics are adsorbed to the bone graft surface and are released by first-order kinetics. The idea is to have a system that can release antibiotics and, at the same time, be incorporated into bone. Eventually the bone graft becomes vascularized, which allows for host defenses to participate in prevention and treatment of infection.[33]

Bone graft substitutes and extenders, like bone grafts, have the advantage of being able to provide local antibiotic delivery while participating in the process of bone regeneration. They have an added advantage over allograft bone grafts in that they avoid the risk of transmitting disease pathogens. Furthermore, there is already a variety of bone graft substitutes that are currently available and approved by the FDA.[16] And while the graft substitutes themselves are FDA-approved, to be used as antibiotic delivery systems, antibiotics have to be added by the treating physician at the time of surgery as a clinician-directed application.

There are many bone graft substitutes that have been studied including calcium sulfates, hydroxyapatites (HAP), apatite-wollastonite glass ceramic blocks, antibiotic-coated demineralized bone, and calcium phosphates.[16,38–40] Commercially prepared calcium sulfate is probably the most used of these materials in treating osteomyelitis.[40] Vancomycin- and tobramycin-loaded calcium sulfate preparations have been studied, and a commercially available tobramycin preparation is available in many countries, but not in the United States.[29]

Plaster of Paris (POP), a calcium sulfate derived from gypsum, is a well studied drug delivery system. POP has been in use since the end of the nineteenth century as a means of filling dead space in bones in the treatment of bone cysts and osteomyelitis. During the twentieth century, further studies found that POP provoked little immune response, did not impede bone regeneration, and could be loaded with a variety of antiseptics and antibiotics. In addition, POP is bioabsorbable and allows bone regeneration to occur within weeks to months after implantation.[38,39] In a study done by Mackey et al., favorable *in vitro* release profiles were obtained for the antibiotics fucidin and gentamicin.[39] Dacquet and coworkers studied the kinetics of a system of POP beads loaded with teicoplanin, an antistaphylococcal agent that is structurally related to the vancomycin–ristocetin group of antibiotics. *In vitro* studies revealed that teicoplanin was released rapidly from the POP beads initially but had sustained antibiotic release for a total of 30 days. Furthermore, levels over the minimum inhibitory concentration (MIC) 90 were seen for up to 9 days.[38]

Hydroxyapatite (HAP) is another bone graft substitute that has been well-studied as a drug delivery system for the treatment of osteomyelitis. Synthetic HAP cement has the same elementary chemical composition as bone and has been successfully loaded with antibiotics. The HAP cement shares some of the advantages of the PMMA cement in that it can provide structural support, fill dead space, and serve as a bonding material between bone and prosthesis. One advantage that HAP has over PMMA is that its chemical composition makes it more biocompatible and allows for its potential use as a bone grafting material. *In vitro* studies of HAP cement loaded with cephalexin or norfloxacin have shown favorable release profiles with drug release observed for up to 10 days.[41] While HAP seems the ideal candidate for drug delivery, its use has been hampered by its brittleness and poor strength.

14.2.4 *Staphylococcus aureus* Osteomyelitis — Special Considerations for Treatment

It has been reported that *S. aureus* is responsible for 80% of human osteomyelitis. It is a capable bone pathogen with adhesion molecules that facilitate its binding to bone matrix and toxin secretion that stimulates bone resorption. It also has the ability to colonize the bone matrix and can be internalized by osteoblasts.[32,43–48] *Staphylococcus aureus* can invade and persist within osteoblasts, which, coupled with the presence of antibiotic-resistant strains, makes the treatment of such bone infections difficult. This prompted the pursuit of a study by Ellington and coworkers to check the null hypothesis that antibiotic sensitivities of *S. aureus* do not change after exposure to the osteoblast intracellular environment.[43] In this study, human and mouse osteoblast cultures were infected, and *S. aureus* cells were allowed to invade. Following times 0, 12, 24, and 48 h (plus or minus the addition of erythromycin, clindamycin, and rifampin at times 0 or 12 h), the osteoblasts were lysed and intracellular bacteria enumerated. Transmission electron microscopy was performed on extracellular and intracellular *S. aureus* cells. In mouse osteoblasts, administration of bacteriostatic antibiotics at time 0 prevented the increase in intracellular *S. aureus* When the antibiotics were delayed 12 h, this did not occur. When rifampin (bactericidal) was introduced at time 0 to human and mouse osteoblasts, there was a significant decrease in number of intracellular *S. aureus* cells within osteoblasts compared with the control. When rifampin was delayed 12 h, this did not occur. Significant time-dependent *S. aureus* structural changes were observed after exposure to the osteoblast intracellular environment. Results of these studies suggested that (1) once *S. aureus* is established intracellularly for 12 h, the bacteria became less sensitive to antibiotics capable of eukaryotic cell penetration and (2) antibiotic sensitivity changes could be due in part to the observed structural changes. These observations led to the rejection of the null hypothesis that the antibiotic sensitivities of *S. aureus* are unaltered by their location.[43] Because of this and other mechanisms of resistance, bone infection due to *S. aureus* often becomes chronic in nature. Chronic osteomyelitis commonly results in abnormal bone remodeling and compromises the blood supply to the infected area and often its cure requires extensive bony and soft tissue reconstruction. Use of controlled delivery systems designed to release therapeutic drug levels of antibiotics into necrotic or osteomyelitic bone was required for long-term treatment to prevent infection recurrence.[32]

14.3 EVOLUTION IN BONE INFECTION MANAGEMENT AND DEVELOPMENT OF NEW CONTROLLED DRUG DELIVERY SYSTEMS

Currently, the most active area of research has been the development of synthetic polymers to serve as antibiotic delivery vehicles. Such materials include polyanhydrides, polylactic acid (PLA), polylactides-co-glycolides (PLGA), polyhydroxyalkanoates, polycaprolactone (PCL), polyhydroxybutyrate-co-hydroxyvalerate (PHBV), and cross-linked polydimethylsiloxane (PDMS).[16] Synthetic polymers have several theoretical advantages over the current systems that employ PMMA. For one, biodegradation and release profiles of the synthetic polymers can be adjusted by making small changes to the polymers during fabrication. This permits a wide range of degradation rates and release profiles within each polymer system. Secondly, these systems may allow for the addition of other bioactive agents that may be helpful in the process of bone growth and regeneration such as growth factors. Additionally, there is no need for surgical removal of the beads after antibiotic exhaustion. Lastly, because bioabsorbable beads can dissolve slowly, there may be a reduced need for bone reconstruction because the bone tissue can slowly fill bony defects.[32]

14.3.1 Controlled Release Systems Using Traditional Absorbable and Water-Soluble Polymers

In one study utilizing a rabbit model for osteomyelitis, an implant composed of a 50:50 copolymer of PLGA loaded with gentamicin was compared with both a gentamicin-loaded PMMA implant and systemic antibiotic therapy with gentamicin.

First, *S. aureus* osteomyelitis was established in rabbit tibias. Next, the rabbits received either an implant (PLGA-gentamicin or PMMA-gentamicin) for 6 weeks or systemic antibiotic therapy for 4 weeks. The investigators found that there was significantly better eradication of the infection in the implant groups compared with the systemic antibiotic group. In the antibiotic-only group, 10 of 16 rabbits eradicated the infection while 8 of 9 and 9 of 9 infections were cleared in the PMMA and PLGA groups, respectively. Furthermore, while a surgical procedure was necessary to remove the PMMA implant, the PLGA implants had essentially been absorbed by 6 weeks.[49] Studies using a 70:30 PLGA implant loaded with vancomycin have also shown promise.[32]

One drawback to some of the synthetic absorbable systems has been the development of an inflammatory reaction *in vivo*. Sometimes, this inflammatory reaction is accompanied by sinus tract formation and sterile drainage. This has been seen with polyglycolic acid (PGA), PLA, and to some extent with PLGA implants.[50–52] In reports from Bostman et al., 8% of patients who underwent PGA and PLGA rod placement for internal fixation of bone fractures experienced a noninfectious inflammatory response severe enough to warrant operative drainage.[51,52] It is thought that perhaps these complications were the result of rapid polymer degradation followed by a brisk local inflammatory reaction.[41,51–53] It is known that the breakdown of most bioabsorbable implants occurs in several steps. Initially, the outer surface of the compound is broken down by hydrolysis. This is followed by a cell-mediated response that fragments the surface of the material. Fragments are then phagocytized and broken down further by lysosomes. It has been postulated that the quicker an absorbable system degrades, the greater the local inflammation.[54] In addition, acidic breakdown products such as lactic acid and glycolic may lead to an increased inflammatory response.

It would follow that a slowly degrading system with neutral breakdown products would significantly limit inflammation. PCL is broken down by acid hydrolysis and free radicals. The final breakdown products of PCL are carbon dioxide and water, making it an ideal system that is unlikely to cause significant toxicities. *In vitro* studies of PCL beads loaded with tobramycin have shown favorable and efficient release profiles that are superior to those seen with PMMA beads.[54] *In vivo* studies have compared tobramycin-loaded PMMA rods to tobramycin-loaded PCL rods surgically implanted into rabbit femurs. The PCL system delivered a significantly higher local peak concentration than did the PMMA system and had a more gradual decrease in local antibiotic levels. Local tobramycin levels were higher in the PCL system for the entire duration of the study (56 days). Only 5 of the 60 rabbits in the study ever had detectable levels of tobramycin in serum assays. In the few rabbits that did have detectable systemic levels of tobramycin, the levels were extremely low and had little chance of causing systemic toxicity.[50] Further studies with PCL utilizing a rabbit osteomyelitis model have shown promising results.[55]

Hydrogel systems have also been investigated as a local therapy for osteomyelitis. In a study by Changez et al., hydrogels based on polyacrylic acid and gelatin were loaded with vancomycin or gentamicin. Using a rabbit osteomyelitis model, *in vivo* antibiotic release was observed for up to 6 weeks and infection was eradicated within that same time. This was true as long as high enough drug concentrations were loaded into the hydrogels (44% w/w antibiotic). The hydrogel implants were well tolerated, fully absorbed and, based on histological studies, produced no significant host reaction. In addition, serum levels of both gentamicin and vancomycin were very low, thus significantly limiting the potential for drug toxicity.[42]

Bioabsorbable polyanhydrides have also been studied *in vivo* in a rat osteomyelitis model. While the bacterial counts in the tissues markedly decreased, eradication of the bacteria was not achieved in the 3 weeks the polymer–antibiotic preparation was implanted.[56] Further studies are needed before these systems become more mainstream.

In recent years, there has been rapid development in the field of injectable materials. Injectable products have several advantages over the previous devices described in this chapter. For one, injection is an easy means of applying the materials for local delivery. In addition, these materials have favorable release profiles and sustain higher local antibiotic concentrations than would ever be possible with systemic therapy. And like other biodegradable materials, a second operation is not needed to remove the spent delivery vehicle. Previous studies have focused on the use of liposomes as drug carriers because of their membranelike composition, but their stability and their tendency to have poor local retention have retarded their clinical use.[57–59] As a result, injectable systems based on synthetic polymers are thought to be more favorable because they are stable, remain localized, and their release profiles can be modified during the fabrication process.[60]

Antibiotic-loaded microspheres based on PLA or PLGA have been where the bulk of study has taken place to date. Ambrose et al. tested several formulations composed of varying amounts of 50:50 PLGA copolymer, poly (ethylene glycol) (PEG), and tobramycin. *In vitro* testing was done to select for the preparation that had the most linear antibiotic release over 4 weeks. The selected formulation was then placed into the quadriceps muscles of mice. High local concentrations were observed, and linear release of antibiotic was seen for as long as 6 weeks. In addition, the microsphere compositions exhibited minimal inflammatory response.[61]

Yenice et al. studied teicoplanin-loaded microspheres made from 75:25 PLGA. *In vitro* studies revealed sustained drug elution for a period of 5 weeks. *In vivo* antibiotic release was observed for 10 days when the antibiotic microspheres were implanted intra-articularly into the lateral femoral condyle of rabbits. In addition, antibiotic concentrations remained above the MIC for *S. aureus* throughout the 2-week study period. And while the observed release profiles were desirable, 86% of the animals developed wound infection complications. Whether this was due to lack of sterile procedure, repeated joint aspiration, or as a result of the microspheres themselves is not clear.[62]

14.3.2 Controlled Release of Antibiotics from Absorbable Gel-Forming Formulations

Studies addressed in this section deal specifically with the *in vivo* release of vancomycin as a potent antibiotic from absorbable gel-formers injected about the periosteum of goat tibia.[15,63,64] The studies were divided into primary and secondary segments to deal with formulations with and without an absorbable cation exchanger. The primary study was designed (1) for a total of 16 goats, as 4-goat sets, (2) to obtain release data in terms of drug level in serum and bone at 1, 2, 3, and 4 weeks in all the goats, and (3) to determine extent of drug removal from soft tissue about the administration site for 13 of the 16 goats at the respective study periods. The secondary study was limited to 4 goats, in 2 sets, administered with active gel-formulation devoid of the cation exchanger. One set of goats was monitored over a 2-week period. The second set was monitored over a 4-week period. Drug concentration was determined in the sera and bones of the 4 animals. Tissue samples from 3 goats were analyzed for vancomycin content. Vancomycin concentrations in serum and bone at different periods of the primary and secondary studies were determined and the results indicated that:

1. At all the examined periods, the vancomycin serum level was well below any expected toxic levels based on accepted human toxicity data.
2. For most of the goats in the primary study group, the highest detectable serum level occurred at day one and no vancomycin could be detected beyond the seventh day.
3. For most of the goats in the secondary study group, the highest detectable level occurred at 4 h, and no vancomycin could be detected at and beyond 7 days
4. The majority of the 4-week goats of the primary study group were shown to contain discernible concentrations of vancomycin in the examined part of their explanted tibia, while none of the examined secondary group animals contained any detectable levels of vancomycin in their analyzed bones.
5. Most of the 1-, 2-, and 3-week animals of the primary group were shown to have discernible concentrations of vancomycin in their tibia.
6. Regardless of the number of animals per set in two study groups, the reproducibility of the results in the primary group exceeded that in the secondary group.

At this point, the serum and bone results were noted to demonstrate (1) the feasibility of using the gel-forming systems for the *in vivo* controlled release of vancomycin, (2) the cation-exchanger containing formulation is the preferred system over the CE-devoid formulation, and (3) a good animal model (apart from associated cost constraints) for more comprehensive future study has been developed, and its viability has been demonstrated.

To develop an understanding of the relative concentration of vancomycin found in the tibia and surrounding soft tissue, we related the drug concentrations in bone and similarly prepared tissue homogenates to the actual weights of the respective explanted samples. In calculating these concentrations and the amount of phosphate buffer used in preparing the homogenates, the original mass of the bone or soft tissue were taken into account. Results of these calculations were as follows:

1. They were in concert with the aforementioned conclusions.
2. They show clearly that during practically the entire 4-week study period, goats of the primary group have had detectable concentrations of vancomycin in the analyzed parts of the tibia and surrounding soft tissue.

3. Residual amounts of vancomycin in soft tissues for both groups generally exceeded those residing in bone at the same study periods.
4. Residual amounts of vancomycin in the soft tissue of the primary group were far greater than those of the secondary group
5. For the secondary group, the vancomycin concentrations in the soft tissue were certainly more discernible than those in bone, which were the practically nonexistent .

The overall test results did show that the gel-formulation with the cation exchanger is indeed a viable candidate for the controlled release of vancomycin. In this regard, it was believed that under the prevailing conditions the formulation provides an active depot of vancomycin for at least 4 weeks, a critical period for the treatment of osteomyelitis because it provides continuous release of drug into the bone where it resides for longer periods than the half-life of vancomycin in serum. This is in concert with lower drug serum concentrations as compared with those measured in bone. As to whether the transient, but continuous, presence of a low dose of vancomycin is efficacious for preventing or treating osteomyelitis, short of conducting the study in infected animals, the following postulate was made: The continuous perfusion of vancomycin increases the efficacy of the drug regimen by about two orders of magnitude compared with those administered systemically. In effect, the detected levels of vancomycin in the goat tibia may very well be sufficient for the management of osteomyelitis in infected goats. This is consistent with earlier discussions by Chein who noted the increasing evidence that suggests that the biological potency of drugs is greatly enhanced by continuous administration via a controlled release mechanism.[65] For instance, effective doses of megestrol acetate in rats, hamsters, and rabbits were substantially reduced by subcutaneous administration via a silicone capsule.[66] Thus, the dose was 13–25 times lower as compared with oral administration, and 7–13 times lower as compared with subcutaneous injections. Therefore, it was postulated that for a localized control delivery system, an efficacious dose of vancomycin can be about 100 times lower than that of IV administered formulations. Having such low localized concentrations will certainly eliminate any toxicity risk in blood associated with traditional vancomycin injections.

14.3.3 Advances toward New Approaches to the Treatment of Osteomyelitis

A drawback associated with the use of biodegradable polymer systems in certain orthopedic applications has been the inability of these systems to provide structural integrity. This has led to efforts to develop composite materials that provide drug delivery, participate in the bone regeneration, and provide structural support during implant incorporation.[16] This can very well be a key aspect in the future treatment of osteomyelitis.

LeRay and coworkers noted that functionalized implants associated with bone substitutes wherein the drug is combined with calcium phosphate powder by absorption, isostatic compression techniques, or dynamic compaction do not allow controlled release and drug activity over a long period.[67] This prompted Billion and coworkers to pursue a study to investigate vancomycin microencapsulation in biodegradable poly(lactide-co-glycolide) microparticles. To optimize encapsulation efficiency by the double emulsion, with and without solvent evaporation–extraction process, they studied two parameters: surfactant (Span® 80) rate and external aqueous phase saturation. *In vitro* dissolution studies, laser granulometry, and scanning electron microscopy were performed to characterize the microparticles. The best results were obtained by stabilizing the first emulsion with 0.5% Span® 80 and saturating the external phase with sodium chloride. Such parameters allowed a 95% drug encapsulation efficiency. This process yielded round microparticles with a mean diameter of ~170 μm and having a smooth, nonporous surface. This formulation was reported to induce a sustained drug release at a constant rate over a period of 10 days. It was also noted that such materials could be associated with biphasic calcium phosphate granules to form an antibiotic-loaded injectable bone substitute providing long-term activity *in situ*.[68]

In addition to the aforementioned studies, there have been a number of new studies which included the following:

Niemela, S.M., Ikaheimo, I., Koskela, M., Veiranto, M., Suokas, E., Tormala, P., Waris, T., and Ashamm, H., Ciprofloxacin-releasing bioabsorbable polymer is superior to titanium in preventing *Staphylococcus epidermidis* attachment and biofilm formation *in vitro*, *J. Biomed. Mater. Res. B Appl. Biomater.*, 76(1), 8, 2006.

Goodger, N.M., Wang, J., Smagalski, G.W., and Hepworth, B., Methylmethacrylate as a space maintainer in mandibular reconstruction, *J. Oral Maxillofac. Surg.*, 63(7), 1048, 2005.

Castro, C., Evora, C., Baro, M., Soriano, I., and Sanchez, E., Two-month ciprofloxacin implants for multibacterial bone infections, *Eur. J. Pharm. Biopharm.*, 60(3), 401, 2005.

Mendel, V., Simanowski, H.J., Scholz, H.C. and Heymann, H., Therapy with gentamicin-PMMA beads, gentamicin-collagen sponge, and cefazolin for experimental osteomyelitis due to *Staphylococcus aureus* in rats, *Arch Orthop. Trauma Surg.*, 125(6), 363, 2005.

Joosten, U., Joist, A., Gosheger, G., Liljenqvist, U., Brandt, B., and von Eiff, C., Effectiveness of hydroxyapatite-vancomycin bone cement in the treatment *Staphylococcus aureus* induced chronic osteomyelitis, *Biomaterials*, 26(25), 5251, 2005.

Lucas-Gerot, A., Verdier, M.C., Tribut, O., Sangleboeuf, J.C., Allain, H., and Oudadesse, H., Gentamicin-loaded calcium carbonate materials: comparison of two drug-loading modes, *J. Biomed. Mater. Res. B Appl. Biomater.*, 73(1), 164, 2005.

Buranapanitkit, B., Srinilta, V., Ingviga, N., Oungbho, K., Geater, A., and Ovatlarnporn, C., The efficacy of a hydroxyapatite composite as a biodegradable antibiotic delivery system, *Clin. Orthop. Relat. Res.*, 424, 244, 2004.

Stallmann, H.P., Faber, C., Bronckers, A.L., Nieuw-Amerongen, A.V., and Wuisman, P.I., Osteomyelitis prevention in rabbits using antimicrobial peptide hLF1-11 or gentamicin-containing calcium phosphate cement, *J. Antimicrob. Chemother.*, 54(2), 472, 2004.

Walenkamp, G.H. and Jacobs, J.A., Antibiotic prophylaxis in cases of closed fractures and prostheses, *Orthopaedics,* 33(4), 424, 2004.

Ersoz, G., Oztuna, B., Coskun, B., Eskandari, M.M., Bayarslan, C., and Kaya, A., Addition of fusidic acid impregnated bone cement to systemic teicoplanin therapy in the treatment or rat osteomyelitis, *J. Chemother.*, 16(1), 51, 2004.

14.4 CONCLUSION AND PERSPECTIVE ON THE FUTURE

Significance of perioperative and device-centered infection, persistent osteomyelitic infection, frequency of infection recurrence, and increasing concerns about drug toxicity and antibiotic resistant bacteria are consistent with the growing interest in using absorbable, controlled release systems capable of local delivery of therapeutic levels of the active agents for prescribed periods with minimum or no transport into the systemic route. This justifies the recommendation to allocate a significant fraction of future research on (1) the use and/or optimization of absorbable controlled delivery systems with precise clinically relevant release profiles, (2) the development of active orthopedic and dental implants for achieving perisurgical prophylaxis, (3) the exploration of combined drug therapy, and (4) the use of absorbable gel-forming liquids as injectable drug formulations for use in prophylaxis as well as treatment of persistent infections. About 80% of bone infection is caused by *S. aureus,* and problems of antibiotic resistant strains warrant the pursuit of new studies on its susceptibility to antibacterial agents and combinations thereof beyond antibiotics. The number and effectiveness of available *in vitro* and *in vivo* models for the evaluation of new drug delivery systems are less than optimal and future investigations need to address this issue.

REFERENCES

1. Waldvogel, F.A., Medoff, G., and Swartz, M.W., Osteomyelitis: a review of clinical features, therapeutic considerations, and unusual aspects, *New Engl. J. Med.*, 282, 198, 1970.
2. Dougherty, S.G., Pathology of infection in prosthetic devices, *Rev. Infect. Dis.*, 10, 1102, 1988.
3. Calhoun, J.H. and Mader, J.T., Eds., *Musculoskeletal Infections*, Marcel Dekker, New York, 2003.
4. Lew, D.P. and Waldvogel, F.A., Osteomyelitis, *New Engl. J. Med.*, 336, 999, 1997.
5. Shirtliff, M.E. and Mader, J.T., Acute septic arthritis, *Clin. Microbiol. Rev.*, 15(4), 527, 2002.
6. Zimmerli, W., Trampuz, A., and Ochsner, P.E., Current concepts: prosthetic-joint infections, *New Engl. J. Med.*, 351(16), 1645, 2004.
7. Darouiche, R.O., Treatment of infections associated with surgical implants, *New Engl. J. Med.*, 350, 1422, 2004
8. Costerton, J. W, Stewart, P.S., and Greenberg, E.P., Bacterial biofilms: a common cause of persistent infections, *Science*, 284, 1318, 1999.

9. Donlan, R.M. and Consterton, J.W., Biofilms: survival mechanisms of clinically relevant microorganisms, *Clin. Microbiol. Rev.*, 15, 167, 2002.
10. Roisman, F.R., Walz, D.T., and Finklestein, A.E., Superoxide radical production by human leukocytes exposed to immune complexes: inhibitory action of gold compounds, *Inflammation*, 7, 355, 1983.
11. Garvin, K. and Feschuk, C., Polylactide-polyglycolide antibiotic implants, *Clin. Orthop.*, 437, 105, 2005.
12. Bernard, L., El-Hajj, M., Pron, B., Lotthe, A., Gleizes, V., Signoret, F., Denormandie, P., Gaillard, J.L., and Perronne, C., Outpatient parenteral antimicrobial therapy (OPAT) for the treatment of osteomyelitis: evaluation of efficacy, tolerance and cost, *J. Clin. Pharm. Ther.*, 26, 445, 2001.
13. Craven, P.C., Treating bone and joint infections with teicoplanin: hospitalization vs. outpatient cost issues, *Hosp, Formul.*, 28(Suppl. 1), 41, 1993.
14. Lai, K.A., Shen, W.J., Yang, C.Y., Lin, R.M., Lin, C.J., and Jou, I.M., Two-stage cementless revision of THR after infection: 5 recurrences in 40 cases followed 2.5-7 years, *Acta Orthopaed. Scand.*, 67, 325, 1996.
15. Corbett, J.T., Jerome, J.E., Allan, J.A., Kelley, W., Kline, J., Farris, H., Fulton, L., and Shalaby, S.W., *In vitro* and *in vivo* release of vancomycin and gentamicin from an injectable absorbable gel-forming matrix for treating osteomyelitis, *Mater. Res. Soc., Meeting Abstracts*, Boston, Massachusetts, Material Research Society, Warrendale, PA, Dec. 1997, p. 351.
16. Hanssen, A.D., Local antibiotic delivery vehicles in the treatment of musculoskeletal infection, *Clin. Orthop.*, 437, 91, 2005.
17. Kanellakopoulou, K. and Giamarellos-Bourboulis, E.J., Carrier systems for the local delivery of antibiotics in bone infections, *Drugs*, 59(6), 1223, 2000.
18. Allababidi, S. and Shah, J.C., Kinetics and mechanism of release from glyceryl monostearate-based implants: evaluation of release in a gel simulating *in vivo* implantation, *J. Pharm. Sci.*, 87(6), 738, 1998.
19. Hanssen, A.D., Osmon, D.R., and Patel, R., Local antibiotic delivery systems: where are we and where are we going? *Clin. Orthop.*, 437, 111, 2005
20. Nelson, C.L., The current status of material used for depot delivery of drugs, *Clin. Orthop.*, 427, 72, 2004.
21. Buchholz, H.W. and Englebrecht, H., Depot effects of various antibiotics mixed with Palacos resins, *Der Chirurg*, 41, 511, 1970.
22. Wahlig, H., Gentamicin-PMMA beads: a drug delivery system in the treatment of chronic bone and soft tissue infections, *J. Antimicrob. Chemother.*, 10, 463, 1982.
23. Cierny, III, G., Classification and treatment of adult osteomyelitis, in *Surgery of the Musculoskeletal System,* Evarts, C.M., Ed., Churchill Livingstone, New York, 1990, p. 4337.
24. Evans, R.P. and Nelson, C.L., Gentamicin-impregnated polymethylmethacrylate beads compared with systemic antibiotic therapy in the treatment of chronic osteomyelitis, *Clin. Orthop.*, 295, 37, 1993.
25. Calhoun, J.H., Henry, S.L., Anger, D.M., and Mader, J.T., The treatment of infected nonunions with gentamicin-polymethylmethacrylate antibiotic beads, *Clin. Orthop* 295, 23, 1993.
26. Espehaug, B., Engesaeter, L.B., Vollset, S.E., Havelin, L.I., and Langeland, N., Antibiotic prophylaxis in total hip arthroplasty. Review of 10,905 primary cemented total hip replacements reported to the Norwegian arthroplasty register, 1987-1995. *J. Bone Joint Surg. Br*, 79(4), 590, 1997.

27. Neut, D., van de Belt, H., Strokroos, I., van Horn, J.R., van der Mei, H.C., and Busscher, H.J., Biomaterial-associated infection of gentamicin-loaded PMMA beads in orthopaedic revision surgery, *J. Antimicrob. Chemother.*, 47, 885, 2001.
28. Langlais, F., Can we improve the results of revision arthroplasty for infected total hip replacement? *J. Bone Joint Surg. Br.*,, 85, 637–640, 2003.
29. McLaren, A.C., Alternative materials to acrylic bone cement for delivery of depot antibiotics in orthopaedic infections, *Clin. Orthop.*, 427, 101, 2004.
30. Horowitz, S.M., Gautsch, T.L., Fondoza, C.G., and Riley, Jr., L., Macrophage exposure to polymethylmethacrylate leads to mediator release and injury, *J. Orthop. Res* 9, 406, 1991.
31. Schurman, D.J., Trindade, C., Hirschman, H.P., Moser, K., Kajiyama, G., and Stevens, P., Antibiotic-acrylic bone cement composites. Studies of gentamicin and Palacos, *J. Bone Joint Surg. Am.*, 60, 978, 1978.
32. Calhoun, J.H. and Mader, J.T., Treatment of osteomyelitis with a biodegradable antibiotic implant, *Clin. Orthop.*, 341, 206, 1997.
33. McLaren, A.C., Alternative materials to acrylic bone cement for delivery of depot antibiotics in orthopaedic infections, *Clin. Orthop.*, 427, 101, 1994.
34. Wachol-Drewek, Z., Pfeiffer, M., and Scholl, E., Comparative investigation of drug delivery of collagen implants saturated in antibiotic solutions and a sponge containing gentamicin, *Biomaterials*, 17(17), 1733, 1996.
35. Greco, F., de Palma, L., Spagnolo, N., Rossi, A., Specchia, N., and Gigante, A., Fibrin-antibiotic mixtures; an *in vitro* study assessing the possibility of using a biologic carrier for local drug delivery, *J. Biomed. Mater. Res.*, 25, 39, 1991.
36. Redl, H., Schlag, G., Stanek, G., Hirschi, A., and Seelcih, T., *In vitro* properties of mixtures of fibrin seal and antibiotics, *Biomaterials*, 4, 29, 1983.
37. Ueng, S.W.N., Lee, S.S., Lin, S.S., Chan, E.C., Hsu, B.R., and Chen, K.T., Biodegradable alginate antibiotic beads, *Clin. Orthop.*, 380, 250, 2000.
38. Dacquet, V., Varlet, A., Tandogan, R.N., Tahon, M.M., Fournier, L., Jehl, F., Monteil, H., and Bascoulergue, G., Antibiotic-impregnated plaster of Paris beads — trials with teicoplanin, *Clin. Orthop.*, 282, 241, 1992.
39. Mackey, D., Varlet, A., and DeBeaumont, D., Antibiotic loaded plaster of Paris pellets, *Clin. Orthop.*, 167, 263, 1982.
40. Mousset, B., Benoit, M.A., Delloye, C., Bouillet, R., and Gillard, J., Biodegradable implants for potential use in bone infection: an *in vitro* study of antibiotic-loaded calcium sulfate, *Int. Orthop.*, 19, 157, 1995
41. Yu, D., Wong, J., Matsuda, Y., Fox, J.L., and Higuchi, W.I., Self-setting hydroxyapatite cement: a novel skeletal drug-delivery system for antibiotics, *J. Pharm. Sci.*, 81(6), 529, 1992.
42. Changez, M,, Koul, V., and Dinda, A.K., Efficacy of antibiotics-loaded interpenetrating network (IPNs) hydrogel based on poly(acrylic acid) and gelatin for the treatment of experimental osteomyelitis: *in vivo* study, *Biomaterials*, 26(14), 2095, 2005.
43. Ellington, K., Harris, M., Hudson, M.C., Vishin, S., Webb, L.X., and Sheretz, R., Intracellular *Staphylococcus aureus* and antibiotic resistance: implications for treatment of staphylococcus osteomyelitis, *J. Orthop. Res.*, 24, 87, 2006.
44 McGavin, M.H., Krajewska-Pietrasik, D., Ryden, C., and Hook, M., Identification of a *Staphylococcus aureus* extracellular matrix-binding protein with broad specificity, *Infect. Immunol.*, 61, 2479, 1993.

45. Arora, M., Shah, N., Meghji, S., Henderson, B., Harris, M., Nair, S., Wilson, M., Gray, C.M., Jones, S.J., and Boyde, A., Effect of *Staphylococcus aureus* extracellular proteinaceus fraction in an isolated osteoclastic resportion assay, *J. Bone Miner. Res* 16, 158, 1998.
46. Nair, S., Song, Y., Meghji, S., Reddi, K., Harris, M., Ross, A., Poole, S., Wilson, M., and Henderson, B., Surface-associated proteins from *Staphylococcus aureus* demonstrate potent bone resorbing activity, *J. Bone Miner. Res.*, 10, 726, 1995.
47. Hudson, M.C., Ramp, W.K., Nicholson, N.C., Williams, A.S., and Nousiainen, M.T., Internalization of *Staphylococcus aureus* by cultured osteoblasts, *Microb. Pathog* 19, 409, 1995.
48. Jevon, M., Guo, C., Ma, B., Mordan, J., Nair, S.P., Harris, M., Henderson, B., Bentley, G., and Meghji, S., Mechanisms of internalization of *Staphylococcus aureus* cultured human osteoblast, *Infect. Immunol.*, 67, 2677, 1999.
49. Garvin, K.L., Miyano, J.A., and Robinson, D., Polylactide/polyglycolide antibiotic implants in the treatment of osteomyelitis: a canine model, *J. Bone Joint Surg., Am* 76, 1500, 1994.
50. Hendricks, K.J., Lane, D., Burd, T.A., Lowry, K.J., Day, D., Phaup, J.G., and Anglen, J.O., Elution characteristics of tobramycin from polycaprolactone in a rabbit model, *Clin. Orthop.*, 392, 418, 2001.
51. Bostman, O.M., Current concepts review. Absorbable implants for the fixation of fractures, *J. Bone Joint Surg.*, 73-A, 148, 1991.
52. Bostman, O., Hirvensalo, E., Makinen, J., and Rokkanen, P., Foreign-body reactions to fracture fixation implants of biodegradable synthetic polymers, *J. Bone Joint Surg* 72-B(4), 592, 1990.
53. Tamada, J. and Langer, R., The development of polyanhydrides for drug delivery applications, *J. Biomater. Sci. Polym. Ed.*, 3, 315, 1992.
54. Burd, T.A., Anglen, J.O., Lowry, K.J., Hendricks, K.J., and Day, D., *In vitro* elution of tobramycin from bioabsorbable polycaprolactone beads, *J. Orthop. Trauma*, 15(6), 424, 2001.
55. Rutledge, B., Huyette, D., Day, D., and Anglen, J., Treatment of osteomyelitis with local antibiotics delivered via bioabsorbable polymer, *Clin. Orthop.*, 411, 280, 2003.
56. Laurencin, C.T., Gerhart, T., Witschger, P., Satcher, R., Domb, A., Rosenberg, A.E., Hanff, P., Edsberg, L., Hayes, W., and Langer R., Bioerodible polyanhydrides for antiobiotic drug delivery: *in vivo* osteomyelitis treatment in a rat model system, *J. Orthop. Res.*, 11, 256, 1993.
57. Hatefi, A. and Amsden, B., Biodegradable injectable in situ forming drug delivery systems, *J. Control Release*, 80, 9, 2002.
58. Couvreur, P., Fattal, E., and Andremont, A., Liposomes and nanoparticles in the treatment of intracellular bacterial infections, *Pharm. Res.*, 8, 1079, 1991.
59. Pinto-Alphandary, H., Andremont, A., and Couvreur, P., Targeted delivery of antibiotics using liposomes and nanaoparticles: research and applications, *Int. J. Antimicrob. Agents*, 13, 155, 2000.
60. Yeh, H.Y. and Huang, Y.Y., Injectable biodegradable polymeric implants for the prevention of postoperative infection: implications for antimicrobial resistance, *Am. J. Drug Deliv.*, 1(3), 149, 2003.
61. Ambrose, C.G., Gogola, G.R., Clyburn, T.A., Raymond, A.K., Peng, A.S., and Mikos, A.G., Antibiotic microspheres: preliminary testing for potential treatment of osteomyelitis, *Clin. Orthop.*, 415, 279, 2003.

62. Yenice, I., Calis, S., Atilla, B., Kas, H.S., Ozlap, M., Ekizoglu, M., Bilgili, H., and Hincal, A.A., *In vitro-in vivo* evaluation of the efficiency of teicoplanin-loaded biodegradable microparticles formulated for implantation to infected bone defects, *J. Microencapsulation*, 20(6), 705, 2003.
63. Corbett, J.T., Kelly, W., Farris, H., Fulton, L., Jerome, J.E., Kline, J.D., Allan, J.M., and Shalaby, S.W., Absorbable gel-forming system for controlled release of vancomycin for treating osteomyelitis, *Trans. Soc. Biomater.*, 21, 341, 1998.
64. Corbett, J.T., Kelly, J.W., Dooley, R.L., Fulton, L.K., and Shalaby, S.W., Development of an animal model for evaluation of antibiotic controlled release systems for the management of osteomyelitis, *Trans. Soc. Biomater.,* 24, 292. 2001.
65. Chein, Y.W. in *Drug Delivery Systems,* Juliano, R.L., Ed., Oxford University Press, New York, 1980, chap. 2.
66. Chang, C.C. and Kinal, F.A., Sustained release hormonal preparations. 3. Biological effectiveness of 6-methyl-17-alpha-acetoxypregna-4,6-diene-3,20-dione, *Steroids* 12, 689, 1968.
67. Le Ray, A.M., Chiffoleau, S., Iooss, P., Grimandi, G., Gouyette, A., Daculsi, G., and Merle, C., Vancomycin encapsulation in biodegradable poly(-caprolactone) microparticles for bone implantation. Influence of the formulation process on size, drug loading, *in vitro* release and cytocompatibility, *Biomaterials*, 24, 443, 2003.
68. Billion, A., Chabaud, L., Gouyette, A., Bouler, J.-M., and Merle, C., Vancomycin biodegradable poly(lactide-co-glycolide) microparticles for bone implantation. Influence of the formulation parameters on the size, morphology, drug loading and *in vitro* release, *J. Microencapsulation*, 22(8), 841, 2005.

Index

A

B

C

D

E

F

G

H

I

J

K

L

M

P

Q

R

S

T

U

V

W

X

Z

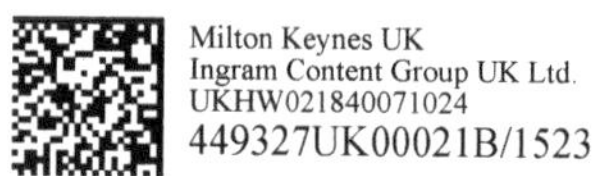
Milton Keynes UK
Ingram Content Group UK Ltd.
UKHW021840071024
449327UK00021B/1523

9 780367 389857